Sjögren's Syndrome

Manuel Ramos-Casals • John H. Stone
Haralampos M. Moutsopoulos

Editors

Sjögren's Syndrome

Diagnosis and Therapeutics

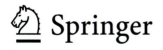 Springer

Editors

Manuel Ramos-Casals, M.D., Ph.D.
Spanish Group of Autoimmune
Diseases (GEAS), Spanish Society
of Internal Medicine (SEMI)
Sjögren Syndrome
Research Group (AGAUR), Laboratory of
Autoimmune Diseases Josep Font
Institut d'Investigacions Biomèdiques
August Pi i Sunyer (IDIBAPS)
Department of Autoimmune Diseases
ICMD Hospital Clínic
Barcelona
Spain

John H. Stone, M.D., M.P.H.
Division of Rheumatology
Allergy and Immunology
Massachusetts General Hospital
Boston, MA
USA

Haralampos M. Moutsopoulos
M.D., F.A.C.P., F.R.C.P.
Department of Pathophysiology
School of Medicine
National University of Athens
Athens
Greece

ISBN 978-0-85729-946-8   e-ISBN 978-0-85729-947-5
DOI 10.1007/978-0-85729-947-5
Springer London Dordrecht Heidelberg New York

British Library Cataloguing in Publication Data
A catalogue record for this book is available from the British Library

Library of Congress Control Number: 2011942749

Springer is part of Springer Science+Business Media (www.springer.com)

To our patients, who have taught us the subtleties and challenges of Sjögren's syndrome, inspired us with their perseverance, and contributed to progress against this condition by participating in research. Along with you, we look forward to a new era of more effective treatments soon

Foreword

We are poised on the verge of major breakthroughs in the understanding and treatment of Sjögren's syndrome (SjS). Though this complex, multi-organ system disorder has been little understood, poorly described, and relatively ignored for decades, successful collaboration on an international scale, careful epidemiologic studies, basic research on the immunological dimensions of this condition, clinical trials, and other investigations have led us to the brink of meaningful advances for patients. As we move forward into an era of individualized medicine for patients with SjS more rational, mechanism-based therapies, it is timely and appropriate to gather collected knowledge from SjS experts around the world on this condition.

This book is divided into four major sections: (I) Scientific Basis; (II) Clinical Manifestations; (III) Diagnosis and Prognosis; and (IV) Therapeutic Aspects. The Scientific Basis chapters address the epidemiology, genetics, proteomics, and immunopathogenesis of SjS. They also discuss the potential roles of viruses in causing SjS, and consider the emerging understanding of the importance of B lymphocytes in the inflammatory symphony of this condition. Within these chapters are themes that promise advances in therapies based upon fundamental understanding of the disease mechanisms of SjS. As the book's editors, we have attempted to carry those themes forward through subsequent sections of the book.

The Clinical Manifestations chapters extend far beyond the sicca symptoms to describe in detail the features of this disorder in virtually every organ system. For example, three separate chapters are devoted to the neurological manifestations of SjS – one each to the central, peripheral, and autonomic nervous system complications of this condition. Similarly, both the vasculitic and non-vasculitic cutaneous features of SjS are given proper attention in separate, well-illustrated chapters. New understandings of pancreatic disease in SjS are elaborated in light of an emerging disease long confused with SjS; namely, autoimmune pancreatitis and IgG4-related disease. Raynaud's phenomenon, the pulmonary complications, and obstetrical/gynecological issues are also given thorough treatments, along with the rest of the organs touched by this protean disorder.

Diagnosis and Prognosis, areas to which the world's SjS have expended much collaborative energy over the past 30 years, are given full consideration with ample reference to consensus documents and evidence-based studies. The lengthy, sometimes contentious, but ultimately fruitful efforts at consensus in the American and

European Classification Criteria are described lucidly. Thorough and practical discussions of the approaches to diagnosis for clinical purposes, an area often confusing for practitioners, are also provided. Aspects of malignancy as they relate to SjS and its prognosis are given appropriate weight in this section, and then considered further in Therapeutic Approaches.

Finally, the growing number of treatment options for SjS are considered in non-overlapping chapters that address the therapy of sicca features; the treatment of B-cell lymphoma; classic immunosuppressive and immunomodulatory drugs for extra-glandular disease; new immunosuppressive and immunomodulatory drugs; B-cell targeted therapies; and experimental treatments.

As co-editors of this book on SjS we would like to thank the 100 contributors who participated as experts in the assembly of this work. You have enabled the creation of a body of knowledge related to SjS not seen on such a scope before. We have learned much from your writing, wisdom, and experience. Our readers will, too.

Finally, two of us – M.R.-C. and J.H.S. – thank the third, H.M.M., for his remarkable contributions to the field of SjS investigation and clinical care that now span more than 30 years. Much of the progress outlined in these pages has stemmed directly from his vision and devotion to fostering new understandings of SjS and to mentoring the next generation of SjS researchers and clinicians. We hope that this book will do the same.

Manel Ramos-Casals
John H. Stone
Haralampos M. Moutsopoulos

Contents

Part III   Diagnosis and Prognosis

Part IV   Therapeutic Aspects

Contributors

Yannis Alamanos, M.D. Department of Public Health, Medical School, University of Patras, Rio, Greece

Graciela S. Alarcón, M.D., M.P.H. Division of Clinical Immunology and Rheumatology, Department of Medicine, School of Medicine, The University of Alabama at Birmingham, Birmingham, AL, USA

María del Carmen Ávila-Casado, M.D., Ph.D. Department of Pathology, Instituto Nacional de Cardiología Ignacio, Chávez, Mexico City, Mexico

Eva Baecklund, M.D., Ph.D. Rheumatology Unit, Department of Medical Sciences, Uppsala University, Uppsala, Sweden

Chiara Baldini, M.D., Ph.D. Rheumatology Unit, Department of Internal Medicine, University of Pisa, Pisa, Italy

Rafael Belenguer, M.D., Ph.D. Rheumatology Unit, Hospital 9 d'Octubre, Valencia, Spain

Jaume Benavent, M.D. Research Group on Primary Care, Institut d'Investigacions Biomèdiques August Pi i Sunyer (IDIBAPS), CAP Les Corts, GesClínic, University of Barcelona, Barcelona, Spain

Stefano Bombardieri, M.D., Ph.D. Rheumatology Unit, Department of Internal Medicine, University of Pisa, Pisa, Italy

Hendrika Bootsma, M.D., Ph.D. Department of Rheumatology and Clinical Immunology, University Medical Center Groningen, University of Groningen, Groningen, The Netherlands

Xavier Bosch, M.D., Ph.D. Department of Internal Medicine, University of Barcelona, ICMiD, Hospital Clínic, Barcelona, Spain

Albert Bové, M.D., Ph.D. Sjögren Syndrome Research Group (AGAUR), Laboratory of Autoimmune Diseases Josep Font, Institut d'Investigacions Biomèdiques August Pi i Sunyer (IDIBAPS), Department of Autoimmune Diseases, Hospital Clínic, Barcelona, Spain

Simon J. Bowman, Ph.D., F.R.C.P Rheumatology Department, University Hospital Birmingham (Selly Oak), Birmingham, UK

Pilar Brito-Zerón, M.D., Ph.D. Sjögren Syndrome Research Group (AGAUR), Laboratory of Autoimmune Diseases Josep Font, Institut d'Investigacions Biomèdiques August Pi i Sunyer (IDIBAPS), Department of Autoimmune Diseases, Hospital Clínic, Barcelona, Spain

Francisco Cárdenas-Velazquez, M.D. Ophthalmology Service, Instituto Nacional de Ciencias Médicas y Nutrición Salvador Zubirán, Mexico City, Mexico

Steven Carsons, M.D. Division of Rheumatology, Allergy and Immunology, Winthrop-University Hospital, Mineola, NY, USA

Department of Medicine, Stony Brook University School of Medicine, Stony Brook, NY, USA

Marinos C. Dalakas, M.D., F.A.A.N. Neuroimmunology Unit, Department of Pathophysiology, Medical School, University of Athens, Athens, Greece

Vikram Deshpande, M.D. Department of Pathology, Massachusetts General Hospital, Boston, MA, USA

Valérie Devauchelle, M.D., Ph.D. EA 2216 "Immunology and Pathology" and IFR 148 ScInBioS, the European University of Brittany and the University of Brest, and the Brest University Medical School Hospital, Brest, France

Cándido Diaz-Lagares, M.D. Sjögren Syndrome Research Group (AGAUR), Laboratory of Autoimmune Diseases Josep Font, Institut d'Investigacions Biomèdiques August Pi i Sunyer (IDIBAPS), Barcelona, Spain

Alexandros A. Drosos, M.D., F.A.C.R. Rheumatology Clinic, Department of Internal Medicine, Medical School, University of Ioannina, Ioannina, Greece

Xavier Forns, M.D., Ph.D. Liver Unit, Ciberehd, IDIBAPS, Hospital Clínic, Barcelona, Spain

Robert I. Fox, M.D., Ph.D. Chief, Rheumatology Clinic, Scripps Memorial Hospital and Research Foundation, La Jolla, CA, USA

Carla M. Fox, R.N. Cheif, Rheumatology Clinic, Scripps Memorial Hospital and Research Foundation, La Jolla, CA, USA

George E. Fragoulis, M.D. Department of Pathophysiology, School of Medicine, National University of Athens, Athens, Greece

Myriam Gandía, M.D. Sjögren Syndrome Research Group (AGAUR), Laboratory of Autoimmune Diseases Josep Font, Institut d'Investigacions Biomèdiques August Pi i Sunyer (IDIBAPS), Department of Autoimmune Diseases, Hospital Clínic, Barcelona, Spain

Rheumatology Department, Hospital Puerta del Mar, Cadiz, Spain

Eleni A. Georgakopoulou, M.D., D.D.S., M.Sc. First Department of Dermatology and Venereology, A. Syggros Hospital, School of Medicine, University of Athens, Athens, Greece

M. Eric Gershwin, M.D. Division of Rheumatology, Allergy and Clinical Immunology, Genome and Biomedical Sciences Facility, University of California at Davis, Davis, CA, USA

Andreas V. Goules, M.D. Department of Pathophysiology, School of Medicine, University of Athens, Athens, Greece

Gabriela Hernández-Molina, M.D., M.S. Immunology and Rheumatology Department, Instituto Nacional de Ciencias Médicas y Nutrición Salvador Zubirán, Mexico City, Mexico

Carmen Hidalgo-Tenorio, M.D., Ph.D. Department of Internal Medicine, Hospital Virgen de las Nieves, Granada, Spain

Sophie Hillion, M.D., Ph.D. EA 2216 "Immunology and Pathology" and IFR 148 ScInBioS, The European University of Brittany and The University of Brest, and The Brest University Medical School Hospital, Brest, France

John A. Ice, Ph.D. Arthritis and Clinical Immunology, Oklahoma Medical Research Foundation, Oklahoma City, OK, USA

David A. Isenberg, M.D., F.R.C.P., F.A.M.S. Department of Rheumatology, University College London Hospital, London, UK

Lennart Jacobsson, M.D., Ph.D. Department of Rheumatology, Skane University Hospital, Malmö, Sweden

Luis J. Jara, M.D. Direction of Education and Research, Hospital de Especialidades, Centro Médico La Raza, IMSS, Universidad Nacional Autónoma de México, Mexico City, DF, Mexico

Cees G.M. Kallenberg, M.D., Ph.D. Department of Rheumatology and Clinical Immunology, University Medical Center Groningen, University of Groningen, Groningen, The Netherlands

Efstathia K. Kapsogeorgou, Ph.D. Department of Pathophysiology, School of Medicine, National University of Athens, Athens, Greece

Stuart S. Kassan, M.D., F.A.C.P. University of Colorado Health Sciences Center, Denver, CO, USA

Munther A. Khamashta, M.D., Ph.D., F.R.C.P. Lupus Research Unit, The Rayne Institute, King's College London School of Medicine at Guy's, King's and St Thomas' Hospitals, St Thomas' Hospital, London, UK

Arezou Khosroshahi, M.D. Division of Rheumatology, Allergy and Immunology, Massachusetts General Hospital, Boston, MA, USA

Eric Kimura-Hayama, M.D. Tomography Department, Instituto Nacional de Cardiología Ignacio, Chávez, Mexico City, Mexico

Christopher J. Lessard, Ph.D. Arthritis and Clinical Immunology, Oklahoma Medical Research Foundation, Oklahoma City, OK, USA

Jacen Maier-Moore, Ph.D. Arthritis and Clinical Immunology, Oklahoma Medical Research Foundation, Oklahoma City, OK, USA

Thomas Mandl, M.D., Ph.D. Department of Rheumatology, Skane University Hospital, Malmö, Sweden

Menelaos N. Manoussakis, M.D. Department of Pathophysiology, School of Medicine, National University of Athens, Athens, Greece

Francis Marchal, M.D., Ph.D. Department of Otolaryngology Head and Neck Surgery, Sialendoscopy Unit, European Sialendoscopy Training Center (ETSC), University Hospital of Geneva, Geneva, Switzerland

Xavier Mariette, M.D., Ph.D. Service de Rhumatologie, Hôpital Bicêtre, Assistance Publique-Hôpitaux de Paris (AP-HP), Université Paris-Sud 11, Le Kremlin Bicêtre, France

Institut Pour la Santé et la Recherche Médicale (INSERM), Paris, France

Clio P. Mavragani, M.D. Department of Pathophysiology, University of Athens Medical School, Laiko University Hospital, Athens, Greece

Department of Experimental Physiology, School of Medicine, University of Athens, Athens, Greece

Gabriela Medina, M.D., Ph.D. Clinical and Epidemiology Research Unit, Hospital de Especialidades Centro Médico La Raza, IMSS, Mexico City, DF, Mexico

Aaron B. Mendelsohn, Ph.D., M.P.H. School of Health Sciences, Walden University, Minneapolis, MN, USA

Courtney G. Montgomery, Ph.D. Arthritis and Clinical Immunology, Oklahoma Medical Research Foundation, Oklahoma City, OK, USA

Katrin E. Morgen, M.D. Department of Psychiatry, Central Institute of Mental Health (CIMH), Mannheim, Germany

Kathy L. Moser, Ph.D. Arthritis and Clinical Immunology, Oklahoma Medical Research Foundation, Oklahoma City, OK, USA

Haralampos M. Moutsopoulos, M.D., F.A.C.P., F.R.C.P., Master ACR Department of Pathophysiology, School of Medicine, National University of Athens, Athens, Greece

Carmen Navarro, M.D., Ph.D. Deputy Director of Clinical Research, Instituto Nacional de Enfermedades Respiratorias, SSA, Mexico City, DF, Mexico

Wan-Fai Ng, M.D., Ph.D. Musculoskeletal Research Group, Institute of Cellular Medicine, Newcastle University, Newcastle Upon Tyne, UK

Roberto Pérez-Alvarez, M.D. Department of Internal Medicine, Hospital Meixoeiro, Vigo, Spain

Marta Pérez-de-Lis, M.D., Ph.D. Department of Internal Medicine, Hospital Meixoeiro, Vigo, Spain

Lucio Pallarés, M.D., Ph.D. Autoimmune Diseases Unit, Hospital Son Espases, Palma de Mallorca, Spain

Pantelis P. Pavlakis, M.D. Neuroimmunology Unit, Department of Pathophysiology, Medical School, University of Athens, Athens, Greece

Jacques-Olivier Pers, M.D., Ph.D. EA 2216 "Immunology and Pathology" and IFR 148 ScInBioS, the European University of Brittany and the University of Brest, and the Brest University Medical School Hospital, Brest, France

James E. Peters, M.D., Ph.D. Department of Rheumatology, University College London Hospital, London, UK

Stephen C. Pflugfelder, M.D. Department of Ophthalmology, Ocular Surface Center, Cullen Eye Institute, Baylor College of Medicine, Houston, TX, USA

Stanley R. Pillemer, M.D. American Biopharma Corporation, Gaithersburg, MD, USA

Guillermo J. Pons-Estel, M.D. Department of Autoimmune Diseases, Institut Clínic de Medicina i Dermatologia, Hospital Clínic, Barcelona, Catalonia, Spain

Division of Clinical Immunology and Rheumatology, Department of Medicine, School of Medicine, The University of Alabama at Birmingham, Birmingham, AL, USA

Bernardo A. Pons-Estel, M.D. Department of Rheumatology, Instituto Cardiovascular de Rosario, Rosario, Argentina

Manuel Ramos-Casals, M.D., Ph.D. Spanish Group of Autoimmune Diseases (GEAS), Spanish Society of Internal Medicine (SEMI), Sjögren Syndrome Research Group (AGAUR), Laboratory of Autoimmune Diseases Josep Font, Institut d'Investigacions Biomèdiques August Pi i Sunyer (IDIBAPS), Department of Autoimmune Diseases, ICMD Hospital Clínic, Barcelona, Spain

Claudia Recillas-Gispert, M.D. Ophthalmology Service, Instituto Nacional de Ciencias Médicas y Nutrición Salvador Zubirán, Mexico City, Mexico

Soledad Retamozo, M.D. Sjögren Syndrome Research Group (AGAUR), Laboratory of Autoimmune Diseases Josep Font, Institut d'Investigacions Biomèdiques August Pi i Sunyer (IDIBAPS), Department of Autoimmune Diseases, Hospital Clínic, Barcelona, Spain

José Rosas, M.D., Ph.D. Department of Rheumatology, Hospital de la Vila-Joiosa, Alicante, Spain

Jorge Sánchez-Guerrero, M.D., M.S. Immunology and Rheumatology Department, Instituto Nacional de Ciencias Médicas y Nutrición Salvador Zubirán, Mexico City, Mexico

Miguel A. Saavedra, M.D., Ph.D. Department of Rheumatology, Hospital de Especialidades Centro Médico La Raza, Universidad Nacional Autónoma de México, Mexico City, DF, Mexico

Alain Saraux, M.D., Ph.D. EA 2216 "Immunology and Pathology" and IFR 148 ScInBioS, The European University of Brittany and The University of Brest, and The Brest University Medical School Hospital, Brest, France

Hal Scofield, M.D. Arthritis and Clinical Immunology, Oklahoma Medical Research Foundation, Oklahoma City, OK, USA

Crispian Scully Division of Maxillofacial Diagnostic, Medical and Surgical Sciences, University College London (UCL) – Eastman Dental Institute, London, UK

Barbara M. Segal, M.D. Division of Rheumatic and Autoimmune Disorders, University of Minnesota Medical School, Minneapolis, MN, USA

Department of Medicine, Hennepin County Medical Center, Minneapolis, MN, USA

Carlo Selmi, M.D., Ph.D. Division of Rheumatology, Allergy and Clinical Immunology, University of California at Davis, Davis, CA, USA

Department of Translational Medicine, IRCCS Istituto Clinico Humanitas, University of Milan, Rozzano (MI), Italy

Karyn Siemasko, M.D. Biological Sciences, Allergan, Inc, Irvine, CA, USA

Antoni Sisó-Almirall, M.D., Ph.D. Research Group on Primary Care, Institut d'Investigacions Biomèdiques August Pi i Sunyer (IDIBAPS), CAP Les Corts, GesClínic, University of Barcelona, Barcelona, Spain

Fotini N. Skopouli, M.D., F.R.C.P. Department of Dietetics and Nutritional Science, Harokopio University of Athens, Athens, Greece

Roser Solans, M.D., Ph.D. Department of Internal Medicine, Hospital Vall d'Hebron, Barcelona, Spain

Richard D. Sontheimer, M.D. Department of Dermatology, University of Utah School of Medicine, Salt Lake City, UT, USA

M. Jose Soto-Cárdenas, M.D., Ph.D. Department of Medicine, University of Cadiz, Department of Internal Medicine, Hospital Puerta del Mar, Cadiz, Spain

Fred K.L. Spijkervet, D.M.D., Ph.D. Department of Oral and Maxillofacial Surgery, University Medical Center Groningen, University of Groningen, Groningen, The Netherlands

Michael E. Stern, M.D., Ph.D. Department of Ophthalmology, Ocular Surface Center, Cullen Eye Institute, Baylor College of Medicine, Houston, TX, USA

John H. Stone, M.D., M.P.H. Division of Rheumatology, Allergy and Immunology, Massachusetts General Hospital, Boston, MA, USA

Peter Szodoray, M.D., Ph.D. Medical and Health Science Center, Clinical Immunology Division, University of Debrecen, Debrecen, Hungary

Rosaria Talarico, M.D. Rheumatology Unit, Department of Internal Medicine, University of Pisa, Pisa, Italy

Elke Theander, M.D., Ph.D. Department of Rheumatology, Skåne University Hospital, Malmö, Sweden

Gabriel Tobón, M.D. EA 2216 "Immunology and Pathology" and IFR 148 ScInBioS, the European University of Brittany and the University of Brest, and the Brest University Medical School Hospital, Brest, France

George E. Tzelepis, M.D. Department of Pathophysiology, School of Medicine, National University of Athens, Athens, Greece

Athanasios G. Tzioufas, M.D. Department of Pathophysiology, School of Medicine, National University of Athens, Athens, Greece

Olga Vera-Lastra, M.D., Ph.D. Department of Internal Medicine, Hospital de Especialidades, Centro Médico Nacional La Raza, IMSS, Universidad Nacional Autónoma de México, Mexico City, DF, Mexico

Arjan Vissink, M.D., Ph.D. Department of Oral and Maxillofacial Surgery, University Medical Center Groningen, University of Groningen, Groningen, The Netherlands

Salvatore deVita, M.D., Ph.D. Rheumatology Clinic, Department of Medical and Biological Sciences, Azienda Ospedaliero-Universitaria, S Maria della Misericordia, Udine, Italy

Claudio Vitali, M.D. Department of Internal Medicine and Section of Rheumatology, 'Villamarina' Hospital, Piombino, Italy

Michael Voulgarelis, M.D., Ph.D. Department of Pathophysiology, School of Medicine, National University of Athens, Athens, Greece

Hobart W. Walling, M.D., Ph.D. Private Practice of Dermatology, Coralville, IA, USA

Rohan R. Walvekar, M.D. Department of Otolaryngology Head and Neck Surgery, LSU Health Sciences Center, Salivary Endoscopy Service and Clinical Research, New Orleans, LA, USA

Fredrick M. Wigley, M.D. Johns Hopkins University, Department of Medicine, Division of Rheumatology, Baltimore, MD, USA

Pierre Youinou, M.D., Ph.D. EA 2216 "Immunology and Pathology" and IFR 148 ScInBioS, the European University of Brittany and the University of Brest, and the Brest University Medical School Hospital, Brest, France

Laboratory of Immunology, Brest University Medical School Hospital, Brest, France

Margit Zeher, M.D., Ph.D. Medical and Health Science Center, Clinical Immunology Division, University of Debrecen, Debrecen, Hungary

Part I
Scientific Basis

Chapter 1
Epidemiology

Yannis Alamanos and Alexandros A. Drosos

Contents

Sjögren's syndrome (SS) is an autoimmune disease characterized by inflammation of exocrine glands, mainly the lacrimal and salivary glands. The disease may occur either independently (primary SS) or in association with other autoimmune diseases such as rheumatoid arthritis, scleroderma, and systemic lupus erythematosus (secondary SS) [1, 2]. The association of SS with other autoimmune rheumatic diseases is discussed in details in Chap. 32. In this chapter we present the epidemiology of primary SS.

1.1 Primary Sjögren's Syndrome

Patients with primary SS may have major complaints, including several systemic features. The impact of these symptoms on disability and quality of life of the subjects affected can be substantial [3, 4]. However, the symptoms of primary SS vary widely and the disease may have an insidious onset, a variable course, and a wide

Y. Alamanos (✉)
Department of Public Health, Medical School, University of Patras,
Rio, Greece

A.A. Drosos
Rheumatology Clinic, Department of Internal Medicine,
Medical School, University of Ioannina, Ioannina, Greece

M. Ramos-Casals et al. (eds.), *Sjögren's Syndrome*,
DOI 10.1007/978-0-85729-947-5_1, © Springer-Verlag London Limited 2012

Table 1.1 Incidence rates (and 95% CIs) of primary SS in studies carried out in adult general populations (cases/100,000)

Study	Population size	Design	Classification criteria	Country	Incidence (95% CI)
Pillemer et al. [15]	~ 100,000 (total population of Olmsted County, Minnesota)	Population-based	Physician diagnosis	USA	3.9 (2.8–4.9)
Plesivcnik et al. [16]	~ 600,000 (total population of Ljubljana region)	Referral center	European (5)	Slovenia	3.9 (1.1–10.2)
Alamanos et al. [14]	~ 500,000 (total population of NW Greece)	Population-based	AECC (12)	Greece	5.3 (4.5–6.1)

spectrum of clinical manifestations. As a consequence, patients with primary SS may be missed or misclassified, or the diagnosis may be delayed. These issues pose several challenges to the study of the epidemiology of primary SS.

1.1.1 Diagnostic Criteria

Diagnostic criteria for primary SS are required in order to provide a rational basis for establishing the diagnosis, assessing prognosis, and guiding therapy. Diagnostic and classification criteria are essential for epidemiologic studies also, because case identification is frequently an important methodological issue in making valid estimations of incidence and prevalence. Several sets of classification criteria for SS have been proposed [5–11], leading to some confusion in the interpretation of some epidemiologic studies. The American–European Consensus criteria (AECC), published in 2002, are the most acceptable for the classification of patients with SS and offer a basis for valid and relatively homogenous epidemiologic studies [12]. The AECC and other sets of classification criteria proposed are reviewed Chap. 29.

The few descriptive epidemiologic studies in primary SS suggest important variations in disease occurrence. These variations may reflect the specific population groups studied, the different classification criteria used, and contrasting methods of case ascertainment [13, 14]. Epidemiologic studies of primary SS in the general population have generally yielded highly heterogeneous results, particularly with regard to disease prevalence. The principal reasons for this stem from differences in diagnostic criteria and study design. As a result, the true prevalence of primary SS in the general population is unclear. In contrast, investigations of the incidence of this condition tend to yield similar results.

1.1.2 Incidence

Table 1.1 summarizes the incidence rates estimated in studies carried out in the general population. The major methodological issues, individual study designs,

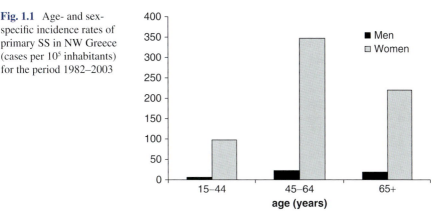

Fig. 1.1 Age- and sex-specific incidence rates of primary SS in NW Greece (cases per 10^5 inhabitants) for the period 1982–2003

and the criteria applied for case identification are also shown. Three incidence studies carried out in Slovenia, Greece, and the USA found an annual incidence of the disease of about 4–5 cases per 100,000 inhabitants. These studies found similar incidence rates even though they used different methods for case ascertainment and case identification. They also found a 10- to 20-fold higher incidence in women than in men, and a peak of age-specific incidence in the age group 50–60.

In a population-based study from Olmsted County, Minnesota, the average annual age- and sex-adjusted incidence of physician-diagnosed Sjögren's syndrome per 100,000 population was estimated to be 3.9 (95% CI=2.8–4.9), with a significantly higher incidence in women (6.9; 95% CI=5.0–8.8) than in men (0.5; 95% CI=0.0–1.2).

In a study carried out in Slovenia the average annual incidence for primary SS in the Ljubljana region was calculated as 3.9 cases per 100,000 inhabitants (95% CI=1.1–10.2). The incidence in women was tenfold higher than in men.

In a study conducted in a defined area of Greece, the age-adjusted mean annual incidence rate for the adult population was 5.3 (95%=CI 4.6–6.3) cases per 10^5 inhabitants (0.5 for men and 10.1 for women).

The mean (SD) age of newly diagnosed cases in the Olmsted County, Minnesota study was 59 (15.8) years, compared with 51.3 (14.5) years (range 19–78) in the Slovenian study and 55.4 (12.5) years (range 18–81) in the Greek study. Figure 1.1 presents the age and sex distribution of incident cases in the Greek study.

The disease is rare in children. Usually only case reports of SS are reported. In a study presenting 13 pediatric patients of primary SS (11 girls and 2 boys) referred during a 15-year period at a rheumatology clinic, the mean (SD) age at disease onset was 9.4 (2.2) years, ranging from 6 to 14 years. In the same period, only two pediatric SS cases associated with juvenile chronic polyarthritis were diagnosed at the same clinic [17].

In a multicenter study of primary SS survey in the pediatric age, a total of 40 cases were identified (35 girls and 5 boys). The age at disease onset ranged from 9.3 to 12.4 years (mean 10.7 years) [18].

Table 1.2 Prevalence estimate rates (and 95% CIs) of primary SS in studies carried out in adult general populations

Study	Population or sample size	Study design	Criteria applied	Country	prevalence (per 100)
Thomas et al. [19]	1,000 (sample)	Sample survey	European (5)	UK	3.3 (2.2–4.4)
Tomsic et al. [20]	889 (sample)	Sample survey	European (5)	Slovenia	0.6 (0.1–2.2)
Dafni et al. [21]	837 (total community population) (female population)	Sample survey	European (5)	Greece	0.6 (0.2–1.4)
Zhang et al. [22]	2,066 (total community population)	Sample survey	San Diego (8) Copenhagen (10)	China	0.34 0.77 (0.44–1.25)
Miyasaka et al. [23]	120,000,000 (Japanese population)	Population-based	Japanese (8)	Japan	0.02 (0.01–0.03)
Alamanos et al. [14]	500,000 (total district population)	Population-based	AECC (12)	Greece	0.09 (0.08–0.10)
Trontzas et al. [24]	8,740 (sample)	Sample survey	AECC (12)	Greece	0.15 (0.09–0.21)
Birlik et al. [25]	2,835 (sample)	Sample survey	European (5)	Turkey	0.35 (0.17–0.65)
Kabasakal et al. [26]	939 (sample of adult women)	Sample survey	AECC (12) European (5)	Turkey	0.6 (0.24–1.39) 1.4 (0.74–2.37)

1.1.3   Prevalence

The prevalence studies of primary SS carried out in general population present wide variations in their prevalence estimates. Table 1.2 summarizes the prevalence estimates for studies conducted in general populations, as well as their major methodological issues, study designs, and criteria for case identification [14, 19–26].

The prevalence estimates vary between 0.2 cases per 1,000 inhabitants (in a study estimating the prevalence of primary SS in the general Japanese population), and 33 cases per 1,000 inhabitants (in a study carried out in a sample of about 1,000 inhabitants in Manchester, UK). These wide variations may partly reflect methodological differences among studies.

Population-based studies using systematic recording of diagnosed cases tend to present lower prevalence estimates than surveys based on the examination of representative samples of general populations. Studies based on systematic recording of diagnosed cases may underestimate the prevalence of an autoimmune rheumatic disease because they miss some cases, mainly the milder cases. On the other hand, sample surveys may overestimate the prevalence of autoimmune rheumatic diseases as they often present relatively low response rates, which may be related to selection bias [27].

Another important methodological issue concerns the different diagnostic criteria applied for case identification. As seen in Table 1.2, even surveys carried out in the same samples gave different prevalence estimates when using different classification criteria.

The results of prevalence studies carried out in different populations suggest a possible role of ethnic differences in the role of the disease. A study carried in the general Japanese population gave a prevalence estimate many fold lower than any other study. On the other hand, a study carried out in a sample of the general population in Manchester, UK, gave a prevalence estimate several fold higher than any other study. These extreme variations are not likely to be due only to methodological differences among studies. The influence of genetic and environmental factors, possibly related to these ethnic differences, remains unclear.

SS in elderly people is relatively common, may be subclinical, and is often associated with a benign clinical course. The disease may also present laboratory and histopathological particularities in this age [28]. In studies analyzing the prevalence estimates by age, the peak of age-specific prevalence was in the age group 66–75 for both sexes. When considering a diagnosis of SS in the elderly, it is important to obtain a thorough drug history. The use of tricyclic antidepressants and antipsychotic agents, which can cause symptoms of dry mouth, is more prevalent in this population. In a population-based study of elderly individuals aged between 65 and 84 years, approximately 27% reported dry eyes or dry mouth [29]. A significant proportion of the population (62%) had sicca symptoms potentially caused by medications, which again emphasizes the importance of the drug history. The prevalence of dry mouth symptoms increases with age and is estimated to be 17% in an elderly population [30]. A minor salivary gland biopsy can be very helpful for diagnosing SS. However, lymphocytic infiltration in minor salivary glands is not specific for SS and has been reported in the healthy elderly, in other autoimmune rheumatic diseases, and occasionally in healthy non-elderly volunteers [31, 32]. In a study performed with 62 elderly volunteers, labial salivary gland biopsy revealed fibrosis and/or fatty infiltration in the majority of individuals examined. This appeared to be related to aging. Three subjects were diagnosed as having primary SS. Four other subjects some histopathological or clinical criteria for SS but could not be classified with certainty as having that condition. All these individuals were asymptomatic, but some of them had anti-Ro (SSA) or anti- La (SSB) autoantibodies [28]. Age-related histological changes of acinar atrophy, fibrosis, and ductal dilatation have been described in the elderly up until the ninth decade [33, 34].

In conclusion, the occurrence of SS likely has important variations among countries and areas of the world. However, the relatively small number of studies for most areas of the world, as well as their methodological differences and the lack of incidence studies for the developing countries, limits our understanding of worldwide SS epidemiology.

References

1. Moutsopoulos HM, Youinou P. New developments in Sjögren's syndrome. Curr Opin Rheumatol. 1991;3:815–22.
2. Moutsopoulos HM. Sjögren's syndrome: autoimmune epithelitis. Clin Immunol Immunopathol. 1994;72:162–5.
3. Strömbeck B, Ekdahl C, Manthorpe R, et al. Health-related quality of life in primary Sjögren's syndrome, rheumatoid arthritis and fibromyalgia compared to normal population data using SF-36. Scand J Rheumatol. 2000;29:20–8.
4. Bowman SJ, Booth DA, Platts RG. UK Sjögren's Interest Group: measurement of fatigue and discomfort in primary Sjogren's syndrome using a new questionnaire tool. Rheumatology (Oxford). 2004;43:758–64.
5. Vitali C, Bombardieri S, Moutsopoulos HM, et al. Preliminary criteria for the classification of Sjögren's syndrome. Results of a prospective concerted action supported by the European Community. Arthritis Rheum. 1993;36:340–7.
6. Vitali C, Moutsopoulos HM, Bombardieri S. The European Community Study Group on diagnostic criteria for Sjögren's syndrome. Sensitivity and specificity of tests for ocular and oral involvement in Sjögren's syndrome. Ann Rheum Dis. 1994;53:637–47.
7. Vitali C, Bombardieri S, Moutsopoulos HM, et al. Assessment of the European classification criteria for Sjögren's syndrome in a series of clinically defined cases: results of a prospective multicentre study. The European Study Group on Diagnostic Criteria for Sjögren's Syndrome. Ann Rheum Dis. 1996;55:116–21.
8. Fox RI, Robinson C, Curd J, et al. First international symposium on Sjögren's syndrome: suggested criteria for classification. Scand J Rheumatol. 1986;61(Suppl):28–30.
9. Homma M, Tojo T, Akizuki M, et al. Criteria for Sjögren's syndrome in Japan. Scand J Rheumatol. 1986;61(Suppl):26–7.
10. Manthorpe R, Oxholm P, Prause JU, et al. The Copenhagen criteria for Sjögren's syndrome. Scand J Rheumatol. 1986;61(Suppl):19–21.
11. Skopouli FN, Drosos AA, Papaioannou T, et al. Preliminary diagnostic criteria for Sjögren's syndrome. Scand J Rheumatol. 1986;61(Suppl):22–5.
12. Vitali C, Bombardieri S, Jonsson R, et al. Classification criteria for Sjögren's syndrome: a revised version of the European criteria proposed by the American-European Consensus Group. Ann Rheum Dis. 2002;61:554–8.
13. Binard A, Devauchelle-Pensec V, Fautrel B, Jousse S, Youinou P, Saraux A. Epidemiology of Sjögren's syndrome: where are we now? Clin Exp Rheumatol. 2007;25:1–4.
14. Alamanos Y, Tsifetaki N, Voulgari PV, et al. Epidemiology of primary Sjögren's syndrome in north-west Greece, 1982–2003. Rheumatology (Oxford). 2006;45:187–91.
15. Pillemer SR, Matteson EL, Jacobsson LT, et al. Incidence of physician-diagnosed primary Sjögren syndrome in residents of Olmsted County, Minnesota. Mayo Clin Proc. 2001;76:593–9.
16. Plesivcnik Novljan M, Rozman B, Hocevar A, et al. Incidence of primary Sjogren's syndrome in Slovenia. Ann Rheum Dis. 2004;63:874–6.
17. Drosos AA, Tsiakou EK, Tsifetaki N, et al. Subgroups of primary Sjögren's syndrome. Sjögren's syndrome in male and paediatric Greek patients. Ann Rheum Dis. 1997;56:333–5.
18. Cimaz R, Casadei A, Rose C, et al. Primary Sjögren syndrome in the paediatric age: a multicentre survey. Eur J Pediatr. 2003;162:661–5.
19. Thomas E, Hay EM, Hajeer A, et al. Sjögren's syndrome: a community-based study of prevalence and impact. Br J Rheumatol. 1998;37:1069–76.
20. Tomsic M, Logar D, Grmek M, et al. Prevalence of Sjögren's syndrome in Slovenia. Rheumatology (Oxford). 1999;38:164–70.
21. Dafni UG, Tzioufas AG, Staikos P, et al. Prevalence of Sjögren's syndrome in a closed rural community. Ann Rheum Dis. 1997;56:521–5.
22. Zhang NZ, Shi CS, Yao QP, et al. Prevalence of primary Sjögren's syndrome in China. J Rheumatol. 1995;22:659–61.

23. Miyasaka N. Epidemiology and pathogenesis of Sjögren's syndrome. Nippon Rinsho. 1995;53:2367–70.
24. Trontzas PI, Andrianakos AA. Sjogren's syndrome: a population based study of prevalence in Greece. The ESORDIG study. Ann Rheum Dis. 2005;64:1240–1.
25. Birlik M, Akar S, Gurler O, et al. Prevalence of primary Sjögren's syndrome in an urban population of Izmir, Turkey. Ann Rheum Dis. 2004;63(Suppl I):502.
26. Kabasakal Y, Kitapcioglu G, Turk T, et al. Prevalence of Sjögren's syndrome in Izmir, Turkey. Ann Rheum Dis. 2004;63(Suppl I):503.
27. Alamanos Y, Voulgari PV, Drosos AA. Epidemiology of rheumatic diseases in Greece. J Rheumatol. 2004;31:1669–70.
28. Drosos AA, Andonopoulos AP, Costopoulos JS, et al. Prevalence of primary Sjögren's syndrome in an elderly population. Br J Rheumatol. 1988;27:123–7.
29. Schein OD, Hochberg MC, Muñoz B, et al. Dry eye and dry mouth in the elderly: a population-based assessment. Arch Intern Med. 1999;159:1359–63.
30. Hochberg MC, Tielsch J, Munoz B, et al. Prevalence of symptoms of dry mouth and their relationship to saliva production in community dwelling elderly: the SEE project. Salisbury Eye Evaluation. J Rheumatol. 1998;25:486–91.
31. Radfar L, Kleiner DE, Fox PC, et al. Prevalence and clinical significance of lymphocytic foci in minor salivary glands of healthy volunteers. Arthritis Rheum. 2002;47(5):520–4.
32. Xu KP, Katagiri S, Takeuchi T, et al. Biopsy of labial salivary glands and lacrimal glands in the diagnosis of Sjögren's syndrome. J Rheumatol. 1996;23:76–82.
33. Pennec YL, Leroy JP, Jouquan J, et al. Comparison of labial and sublingual salivary gland biopsies in the diagnosis of Sjögren's syndrome. Ann Rheum Dis. 1990;49:37–9.
34. Ng KP, Isenberg DA. Sjögren's syndrome: diagnosis and therapeutic challenges in the elderly. Drugs Aging. 2008;25:19–33.

Chapter 2
Genetics, Genomics, and Proteomics of Sjögren's Syndrome

Christopher J. Lessard, John A. Ice, Jacen Maier-Moore, Courtney G. Montgomery, Hal Scofield, and Kathy L. Moser

Contents

2.1 Introduction

Dramatic advances in identifying the genetic basis of many human diseases are transforming our fundamental understanding of etiology and pathogenesis. Over the past decade, large global efforts to characterize sequence variation in the human genome have provided the foundation for this extraordinary progress. Success in mapping disease genes has also been fueled by revolutionary advances in our technical capacity for genotyping and analyzing complex genetic datasets. These advances include the technical capacity for genotyping millions of known variants and have ushered in a new era of powerful, large-scale, and highly successful genome screens for many diseases. Scanning the human genome for association of variants with disease is unbiased and not limited by prior selection of a putative candidate gene for testing. As a result, the genes that are associated with disease can be surprising, oftentimes linking previously unsuspected molecular pathways to

C.J. Lessard • J.A. Ice • J. Maier-Moore • C.G. Montgomery • H. Scofield • K.L. Moser (✉)
Arthritis and Clinical Immunology, Oklahoma Medical Research Foundation,
Oklahoma City, OK, USA

M. Ramos-Casals et al. (eds.), *Sjögren's Syndrome*,
DOI 10.1007/978-0-85729-947-5_2, © Springer-Verlag London Limited 2012

numerous disease phenotypes. In many cases, an association may be located between genes and have no known or obvious functional effect. Thus, a dramatic shift in our knowledge of the genetic architecture of human disease is underway. Still, much remains to be learned.

Pinpointing specific genetic associations with disease and characterizing the effects on gene function offer fundamentally important opportunities for insight into disease etiology and pathogenesis. In Sjögren's syndrome (SS), the etiology remains poorly understood in part due to highly limited knowledge of the underlying genetic architecture. These limitations can largely be attributed to small sample sizes of patient cohorts currently available for study. Similar to most autoimmune diseases, epidemiologic and genetic studies in SS to date strongly support the hypothesis of a complex etiology involving variants in numerous genes with functional consequences across multiple biological pathways. In contrast, the genetics of related autoimmune diseases, such as systemic lupus erythematosus (SLE) and rheumatoid arthritis (RA), are far more advanced and dozens of genetic associations have already been established. A multitude of genes are likely to be involved in SS as well. However, specific genes associated with SS are only beginning to be identified and characterized. In addition, the influences of epigenetic processes and environmental factors on the etiological complexity of SS remain largely undefined.

Gene expression profiling (GEP) and proteomic studies are complementary tools for revealing important disease-associated pathways. Application of these powerful approaches has begun to offer new global views of dysregulated pathways and networks that distinguish patients from controls. Integrating genetic, genomic, and proteomic data can be used for higher level "systems biology" approaches that may prove especially fruitful when combined with detailed clinical data.

In this chapter, we begin by summarizing the evidence for a genetic component to SS, emphasize the underlying concepts and approaches to new gene discovery, and discuss complementary high-throughput RNA and protein-based studies that are providing new and important insight into the underlying molecular pathways leading to this complex disorder. Overall, developing a much more comprehensive understanding of SS is expected in the future as these types of studies progress.

2.2 Genetic Epidemiology of SS

Evidence gathered to date for a genetic etiology in SS is consistent with an important and complex contribution of heritable factors; however, the genetics of SS is substantially understudied. Approximately 40 genetic studies have been reported thus far and are largely focused on candidate genes such as the HLA loci or genes demonstrating association in other autoimmune diseases. In the absence of large-scale genetic studies identifying robust associations, increased concordance rates of disease among monozygotic twins and the frequency of familial aggregation are two measures commonly used as evidence for a genetic component.

A limited number of case reports describing twins with SS have been published, but studies to establish a reliable twin concordance rate are not available [1–4]. For example, Scofield et al. reported adult monozygotic twins with similar serological profiles with respect to high-titer anti-Ro/SSA, severe lymphocytic infiltration of the labial salivary glands, and mild clinical symptoms [4]. Another case of dizygotic twins with SS was reported by Houghton et al., in which one adolescent sister presented with pulmonary symptoms leading to the diagnosis of lymphocytic interstitial pneumonia, while the other sister demonstrated no respiratory symptoms [3]. Interestingly, these dizygotic twins feature both pulmonary involvement and familial aggregation, which are uncommon in juvenile SS. Familial aggregation in SS has also been observed. Several multiplex families with SS have been described, and increased prevalence of other autoimmune diseases in the families of SS patients is quite common (30–35%), including SS (12%), autoimmune thyroid disease (AITD, 14%), RA (14%), and SLE (5–10%) [5].

Clinical and serological features among related autoimmune diseases often demonstrate overlap in which subsets of patients may share similar symptoms (including, but not limited to, arthralgias, myalgias, fatigue, rashes, and visceral involvement from vasculitis) or serological biomarkers such as autoantibody profiles [6]. Many of the clinical features of SS are found in subsets of patients from a variety of other autoimmune disease groups. Direct evidence for associations of common genetic loci shared across related autoimmune disorders has been documented [7]. These studies suggest that sharing of underlying disease mechanisms across related phenotypes may account for overlapping clinical features. Based on phenotypic similarities, increased twin concordance rates in SS could be expected to be between those of RA (15%) and SLE (25%)[8, 9]. Likewise, female sibling or dizygotic twin rates of 2–4% and estimated odds of female sibling concordance (λ_s) between 8 and 30 could be reasonable estimates for SS.

Various human leukocyte antigen (HLA) alleles demonstrate association with many autoimmune diseases, including SS, SLE, RA, and others [10]. A growing list of non-HLA genes have also shown association with multiple autoimmune diseases. For example, associations have been reported for *CTLA4* with AITD, Type 1 Diabetes (T1D), celiac disease, Wegener's granulomatosis, SLE, vitiligo, Addison's disease, and RA [5]. Other associations include *PD-1* with RA, T1D, and SLE, and *PTPN22* with SLE, RA, T1D, Graves's disease, and Hashimoto's thyroiditis [5]. Although most genes associated with SLE, RA, and other autoimmune diseases have not yet been fully evaluated in SS, *IRF5*, *STAT4*, and *BLK* are examples of genes strongly associated with SLE for which there is recent data suggesting association in SS [11]. Thus, although direct evidence overall is limited, the available studies are consistent with a heritable component similar to diseases such as RA and SLE, both of which have well-established genetic associations for dozens of genetic loci.

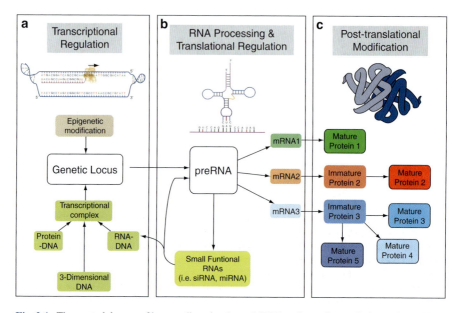

Fig. 2.1 The central dogma of human diversity through RNA and protein regulation and modification. The figure illustrates the stepwise progression of genomic information from DNA to RNA to protein. With 20,000–25,000 genes in the human genome, increased complexity of the human protein repertoires comes from posttranscriptional and posttranslational modification of RNAs and proteins. (**a**) The process of transcribing DNA template into messenger RNA (mRNA) is a tightly controlled process governed by transcription factors, RNA pol II (typically), helicases, and topoisomerases. These molecules coalesce within the proximal promoter region and form the transcription machinery. In order for these molecules to bind the promoter region, the DNA must be open, or "melted." Epigenetic modifications can silence regions of the genome by impeding the melting process. (**b**) Once transcribed, the preRNA can be modified through splicing, addition of the 5′ cap (modified guanine nucleotide), nucleotide editing, and polyadenlyation on the 3' end. Splicing of mRNA can dramatically increase diversity by removing intronic regions and alternatively splicing exons. Some intronic regions form small silencing RNAs (siRNAs) and/or microRNAs (miRNAs). These nonprotein coding RNAs also regulate the transcription and translation process. (**c**) Once mRNA are translated into protein, diversity is further increased by posttranslational modifications such as the addition of functional groups (acetate, phosphate, lipids, and carbohydrates) or structural changes (disulfide bonds)

2.3 Key Concepts in Genetics, Transcriptomics, and Proteomics

The central dogma of information flow from DNA to RNA to protein has grown in complexity over recent years as shown in Fig. 2.1 [12]. The entire human genome contains over 3 billion base pairs, approximately 20,000 genes, and millions of variant sites in the DNA sequence (Fig. 2.2). Genetic associations may occur in DNA coding sequences and alter the structure or function of a protein; however, most associations with complex diseases found to date reside in regions thought to regulate gene expression [12]. Genetic variation may also influence molecular processes

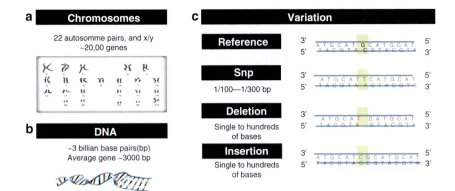

Fig. 2.2 The human genome. The human genome is comprised of 22 autosomal chromosomes and 2 sex chromosomes (*X* and *Y*, panel **a**) consisting of ~3 billion base pairs (panel **b**). The average size of a gene is 3,000 base pairs. (**c**) Every human is ~99.9% identical with the 0.1% of variation leading to benign traits such as eye or hair color, or disease-causing traits such as Sjögren's syndrome. Variation is illustrated in panel c as compared to reference sequence at the top of the panel. The red and blue bases flank the site of variation. Single nucleotide polymorphisms (SNPs) are single base changes and are the most common polymorphisms in the genome (~15 million to date). Deletions and insertions can occur ranging in size from single base units to hundreds of bases

such as splicing and posttranslational modifications that have potential to generate over 100,000 protein isoforms from only 20,000 genetic loci. As the nature and extent of human variation has been revealed over the past decade, it is perhaps not surprising that many complex human diseases now have dozens of variants that are associated with increased risk.

In general, humans are between 99.5% and 99.9% identical, yet there are millions of polymorphic sites scattered throughout the genome that account for individual differences. Many different forms of DNA sequence variation have been discovered in the human genome including: single nucleotide polymorphisms (SNPs, pronounced "snips"), copy number variants (CNVs; variation in which the number of copies of a gene or DNA sequences differ), microsatellites (regions with short tandem repetitive sequences) and insertion/deletion events (indels or DIPs). Any type of variation can influence benign features, such as height, but it can also lead to an increase in the susceptibility of disease development.

SNPs are the most frequent type of polymorphism found in the human genome. Current estimates indicate that one out of every 100–300 base pairs could be a SNP [13]. Estimates of approximately 15,000,000 total SNPs in the human genome continue to increase as additional variants are discovered through ongoing sequencing projects. As such, these common variants are now frequently used to screen the genome when attempting to detect association of specific alleles with disease. Common genetic association study designs are focused on detecting statistically significant differences in allele frequencies for a given SNP between cohorts of cases and controls (Fig. 2.3). Large sample sizes (potentially thousands of subjects) for these types of studies and confirmation in independent cohorts are necessary

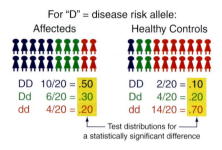

Fig. 2.3 Calculation of association of variants with disease. Every human carries two copies of each chromosome and therefore two copies of every allele, one inherited from their mother and the other from their father. For disease allele D, alleles are counted for both affected individuals and healthy controls. The distribution of alleles between affected individuals and healthy controls is then tested for statistical significance using statistical tests such as Chi-squares (2×2 table) or logistic regression (covariates can be implemented to adjust for confounding)

when the allele frequencies between cases and controls are relatively small, as is the case for many of the associations now established in complex diseases.

When mapping disease loci, not all genetic variation must be genotyped to detect an initial association effect since some variants can serve as markers for causal alleles. Scientists have used the nonrandom, or linked, assortment of loci that occurs during meiotic recombination to map genetic locations on chromosomes. When two loci lie in close proximity on a chromosome, these loci tend to be inherited together more frequently than expected when random crossover events occur. This phenomenon, termed linkage disequilibrium (LD), is measurable by determining correlations between the recombination frequencies of specific alleles at two or more loci. Variable patterns of LD across the genome are defined by the length of the regions in which LD occurs, creating haplotype blocks, and the strength of LD is measured by these correlations [14]. A benefit of understanding these patterns for gene mapping studies lies in the ability to use this knowledge to reduce the genotyping burden while still detecting association of a variant with disease [14]. Essentially, any SNP present on a haplotype block may serve as a tag, or marker, for a causal variant if LD is sufficiently strong. Additional studies can then be used to precisely identify and characterize causal variants (Fig. 2.4).

The dramatic expansion of knowledge regarding human variation has been coupled with revolutionary advances in technologies in order to assay genetic variants. Rapid development of microarrays designed for genotyping have led to the current capacity of assaying up to approximately 2.5 million SNPs in a matter of days and typically capturing information for the majority of variation in Caucasian populations. Thus, it is now possible to efficiently search the entire genome for loci associated with the risk of developing disease in studies referred to as genome-wide association (GWA) scans. Additional genotyping and sequencing can be used to narrow the region of interest further and to identify the disease risk allele (Fig. 2.5).

Many studies of genetically complex diseases have used this approach to identify risk loci with approximately 500 GWA studies reported in the literature and with

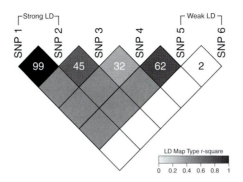

Fig. 2.4 Linkage disequilibrium (LD) between SNPs within the human genome. LD (or correlation) is present between variants within the genome where portions of sequence are inherited nonrandomly as units, and is typically expressed as r^2 values. An example is shown with regions of strong LD and weak LD. Each diamond represents the r^2 values between any 2 *SNPs*. In this example, the r^2 value between SNP1 and SNP2 is $r^2 = 0.99$. The r^2 between SNP5 and SNP6 is 0.20. The shading of each diamond is proportional to the r^2 value. (e.g., black is $r^2 = 1.0$)

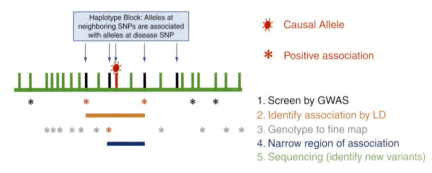

Fig. 2.5 Mapping genetic effects in complex diseases. This figure illustrates the concept of mapping genetic associations within the genome. In the GWA scan phase, markers are selected to take advantage of haplotype block structure and reduce the genotyping burden within a given population. The GWA scan phase will identify SNPs that are in LD with the causal allele and not likely to type it directly. Further genotyping is required to narrow the effect to the region of interest surrounding the causal allele. While LD between SNPs allows researchers to test fewer polymorphisms to capture the majority of variation within an individual genome, it can also pose problems for fine mapping in regions with strong LD. Ultimately, functional assays that test biological effects such as altered transcript levels or changes in coding sequence that modify protein function are usually required to prove causality when multiple markers are in very strong LD with each other

more than 2,400 associations currently identified. Over 30 GWA scans have been reported for autoimmune phenotypes. Collectively, GWA scans have been highly successful in detecting novel associations with disease. For example, associations with over 35 loci have been established with SLE, with the continual confirmation of additional associations [7].

Although GWA studies have proven instrumental in identifying numerous genetic associations, complexities in the underlying architecture of disease can pose significant challenges in the execution of gene mapping studies. The effect size, describing the strength of association between two variables, can be expressed as an odds ratio (OR). Furthermore, GWA scans are neither comprehensive nor very powerful for identifying rare variants (i.e., allele frequency < 1%). The potential for identifying false-positive associations becomes substantial when over a million statistical tests are performed. To compensate for multiple testing, corrections typically place the significance threshold at $p < 5 \times 10^{-8}$. GWA studies to identify low-level risk variants while minimizing false-positive discoveries require large patients cohorts to provide reliable data.

Cohort sizes for genetic association studies published to date in SS have included no greater than a few one-hundred cases (Table 2.1 and Fig. 2.6). In SS, the lack of large patient cohorts available for study has confounded the reliability and reproducibility of genetic associations reported thus far. With such small sample sizes, a seemingly significant association in one study may be nearly impossible to replicate in another given the imprecision in allele frequency estimates or heterogeneity of clinical subjects. This is illustrated in Fig. 2.7, where the power to detect genetic association is influenced not only by the study sample size, but also by the strength of the effect (as quantified by the odds ratio) and the allele frequency. In this context, efforts to build much larger patient cohort resources will be a critical step toward improving statistical power and developing a comprehensive understanding of the contribution of genetics to SS etiology.

2.4   Candidate Genes and SS Pathogenesis

Models of pathogenesis in SS have largely been based on traditional hypothesis-driven studies in which various components of the immune system have been dissected. Genetic studies completed to date have been informative from the perspective that most candidate genes have been chosen for association testing based on these discoveries. Other candidate genes have been evaluated in SS only after associations were identified in other related diseases, such as SLE or RA.

Clearly, the altered function of multiple cell types and molecular pathways is involved in SS, with each possibly having genetic variants that underlie these observations. Evidence to support genetic variants contributing to SS within both the innate and adaptive immune responses has been reported (Fig. 2.6 and Table 2.1). Numerous multifunctional proteins such as cytokines and chemokines have been implicated and are often produced by or act on more than one cell type, adding complexity to disease models. Overall, most of the associations reported to date should be interpreted with caution given that further studies in larger, more statistically powerful sample sets are needed. Additionally, any putative genetic association should also be replicated in independent cohorts. Nevertheless, we can begin to integrate genetic associations into models of disease pathogenesis for variants with significantly differing allele frequencies between cases and controls. We focus the discussion below to include primarily the genes (or loci) with the most

Table 2.1 Summary of non-HLA association studies in Sjögren's syndrome

Locus	Phenotype	Cases	Controls	p-value	OR/RR	Reference
ApoE	Early onset SS	63	64	0.0407	–	Pertovaara et al. Rheumatology (Oxford) 2004;43(12):1484.
BAFF	Anti-Ro/anti-La in SS	123	136	<0.001	–	Nossent et al. Rheumatology (Oxford) 2008;47:1311.
CCR5	SS	39	76	0.043	0.35	Petrek et al. Clin Exp Rheumatol 2002;20(5):701.
CD4A	Anti-Ro or anti-La in SS	391	532	0.00092	0.45	Nordmark et al. Genes Immun 2010:1.
CD40	Anti-Ro or anti-La in SS	391	532	0.00098	0.73	Nordmark et al. Genes Immun 2010:1.
CLTA4	SS	111	156	0.032	1.78	Downie-Doyle et al. Arthritis Rheum 2006;54(8):2432.
EBF1	SS	540	532	0.000099	1.68	Nordmark et al. Genes Immun 2010:1.
	Anti-Ro or anti-La in SS	391	532	0.00051	1.65	Nordmark et al. Genes Immun 2010:1.
FAM167A-BLK	SS	540	532	0.00047	1.37	Nordmark et al. Genes Immun 2010:1.
	Anti-Ro or anti-La in SS	391	532	0.00082	1.40	Nordmark et al. Genes Immun 2010:1.
Fas	Anti-Ro/anti-La negative SS	101	108	0.04	–	Mullighan et al. Ann Rheum Dis 2004;63(1):98.
FCGR3B	SS with <2 copies of FCGR3B	774	409	0.074	2.01	Mamtani et al. Genes Immun 2010;1:155.
	SS with >2 copies of FCGR3B	774	409	0.048	2.26	Mamtani et al. Genes Immun 2010;1:155.
GSTM1	SS	106	143	0.035	1.72	Morinobu et al. Arthritis Rheum 1999;42(12):2612.
HA-1	SS	88	271	0.003	–	Harangi et al. Eur J Immunol 2005;35(1):305.

(continued)

Table 2.1 (continued)

Locus	Phenotype	Cases	Controls	p-value	OR/RR	Reference
IL-1RA	SS	36	100	0.04	2.38	Perrier et al. Clin Immunol Immunopathol 1998;87(3):309.
IL2-IL21	SS	94	368	0.033	0.46	Maiti et al. Arthritis Rheum 2010;62(2):323.
IL-4Rα	SS	45	74	0.035	2.6	Youn et al. Immunogenetics 2000;51(8–9):743.
IL-6	SS	66	400	<0.0001	–	Hulkkonen et al. Rheumatology (Oxford) 2001;40(6):656.
IL-10	s-IgG concentration in SS	28[a]	9[a]	0.012	–	Origuchi et al. Ann Rheum Dis 2003;62:1117.
	SS	129	96	0.036	2.25	Gottenberg et al. Arthritis Rheum 2004;50(2):570.
	Early onset SS	63	150	0.001	–	Font et al. Rheumatology (Oxford) 2002;41(9):1025.
ILT6	SS	149	749	0.0093	2.65	Kabalak et al. Arthritis Rheum 2009;60(10):2923.
Ig KM	Anti-La in SS	6[b]	56[b]	0.016	–	Pertovaara et al. J Rheumatol 2004;31:2175.
	LSG histological severity in SS	35[b]	27[b]	0.004	–	Pertovaara et al. J Rheumatol 2004;31:2175.
	p-IgG3 in SS	35[b]	27[b]	0.002	–	Pertovaara et al. J Rheumatol 2004;31:2175.
	s-β2-m concentration in SS	35[b]	27[b]	0.024	–	Pertovaara et al. J Rheumatol 2004;31:2175.
IRF5	SS	210	154	0.01	1.93	Miceli-Richard et al. Arthritis Rheum 2007;56(12):3989.
	SS	368	711	0.000024	1.49	Nordmark et al. Genes Immun 2009;10:68.
	SS	368	711	0.00032	1.57	Nordmark et al. Genes Immun 2009;10:68.

Table 2.1   (continued)

Locus	Phenotype	Cases	Controls	*p*-value	OR/RR	Reference
IRF-5/ TNPO3	SS	540	532	0.0000055	1.70	Nordmark et al. Genes Immun 2010:1.
	Anti-Ro or anti-La in SS	391	532	0.0000017	1.81	Nordmark et al. Genes Immun 2010:1.
IκBα	SS	98	110	<0.001	16.2	Ou et al. J Clin Immunol 2008;28:440.
	SS	98	110	<0.007	34.14	Ou et al. J Clin Immunol 2008;28:440.
MBL	SS	104	143	0.011	–	Wang et al. Ann Rheum Dis 2001;60(5):483.
	SS	104	143	0.024	1.93	Wang et al. Ann Rheum Dis 2001;60(5):483.
	SS	14	129	0.0479	–	Tsutsumi et al. Genes Immun 2001;2(2):99.
MECP2	SS	460	1828	0.0016	1.33	Cobb et al. Ann Rheum Dis 2010;69:1731.
PTPN22	SS	70	308	0.01	2.42	Gomez et al. Genes Immun 2005;6(7):628.
Ro52	Anti-Ro52 SS vs. healthy controls	38	72	0.00003	–	Nakken et al. Arthritis Rheum 2001;44(3):638.
	Anti-Ro52 (+) vs. anti-Ro (−) in SS	39[c]	23[c]	0.011	2.67	Imanishi et al. Clin Exp Rheumatol 2005;23(4):521.
STAT4	SS	120	1,112	0.01	1.47	Korman et al. Genes Immun 2008;9(3):267.
	SS	368	711	0.0014	1.41	Nordmark et al. Genes Immun 2009;10:68.
	SS	540	532	0.00070	1.40	Nordmark et al. Genes Immun 2010:1.
	Anti-Ro or anti-La in SS	391	532	0.00069	1.44	Nordmark et al. Genes Immun 2010:1.
TAP2	Anti-Ro (+) vs. anti-Ro (−) in SS	51	57	0.001	–	Kumagai et al. Arthritis Rheum 1997;40(9):1685.

(continued)

Table 2.1 (continued)

Locus	Phenotype	Cases	Controls	p-value	OR/RR	Reference
TCRBV	SS	61	121	0.018	3.0	Lawson et al. Ann Rheum Dis 2005;64(3):468.
TGFβ1	SS with anti-La	129	96	0.0006[c]	10.2	Gottenberg et al. Arthritis Rheum 2004;50(2):570.
TNF2	SS	129	96	0.00028[c]	2.86	Gottenberg et al. Arthritis Rheum 2004;50(2):570.
TNFSF4	SS	540	532	0.00074	1.34	Nordmark et al. Genes Immun 2010:1.
	Anti-Ro or anti-La in SS	391	532	0.000076	1.46	Nordmark et al. Genes Immun 2010:1.

[a]This study compares the allele frequencies of codon 54 wild type in subjects with SS by Fisher's exact t-test, and has case and control groups comprised of these patients.
[b]There are more subclinical phenotypes referenced in the paper that exhibit statistical significance than are listed here.
[c]This study used Fisher's exact t-test to compare subjects with primary Sjögren's syndrome producing serum IgG >15g/L with those producing serum IgG <15g/L, and consists of case and control groups of SS subjects producing IgG.

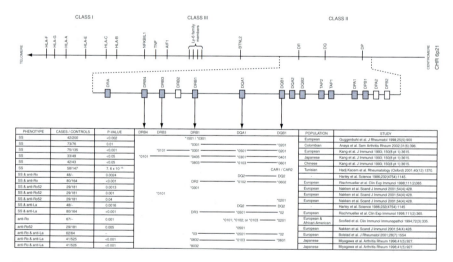

Fig. 2.6 HLA associations with Sjögren's syndrome. This figure summarizes studies that have identified the association of certain alleles and/or haplotypes from the HLA region with Sjögren's syndrome and/or the production of anti-Ro/anti-La autoantibodies. Note the small cohort sizes. Shaded blue boxes denote functional genes. Lines connecting alleles denote haplotype structure. DQ CAR1/CAR2 represents polymorphic CA repeat microsatellites located between the HLA-DQA1 and -DQB1 genes [42]. Note that DR2, DR3, DQ1, and DQ2 are older forms of HLA nomenclature based on serotype groups. These serotype groups are most commonly associated with: DRB1 for DR2 and DR3; DQA1 for DQ1; and DQB1 for DQ2

Fig. 2.7 Power to detect association. This graph illustrates three different scenarios for studies with sample sizes of 100 cases/100 controls (majority of manuscripts published to date), 1,000 case/1,000 controls (current GWA scan), and 5,000 cases/5,000 controls (future GWA scan). Power to detect genetic association is a function of not only sample size, but also the allele frequency and the odds ratio of causal alleles

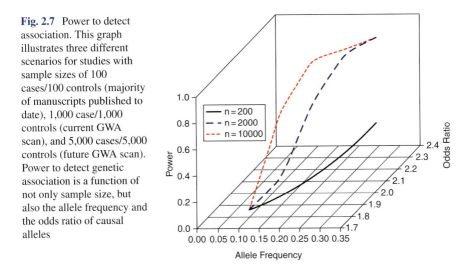

statistically significant evidence ($p < 0.001$) and those which were evaluated in at least 200 cases, including *IRF5, STAT4, TNFSF4, HLA-DR/DQ, FAM167A-BLK*, and *EBF1*. We underscore that unbiased, genome-wide searches for novel genetic associations in SS will undoubtedly provide new details for existing disease paradigms and will most likely reveal new avenues for future study.

Innate immune processes in SS proceed with the activation of interferon (IFN) pathways, followed by cytokine and chemokine production by cells such as monocytes/macrophages and dendritic cells, and then with the presentation of antigen to lymphocytes to generate adaptive responses that ultimately lead to autoantibody production (Table 2.1). Evidence for association with genes involved in IFN pathways has been reported in SS and notably includes interferon regulatory factor 5 (*IRF5*) and signal transducer and activator of transcription 4 locus *STAT4* [11, 15–17]. *IRF5* is a transcription factor that acts downstream of the toll-like receptors and type I interferons to promote the expression of numerous antiviral and pro-inflammatory proteins [18, 19]. Associations with several independent genetic effects within the *IRF5* locus have been documented for SLE and are found in Asian, Caucasian, Hispanic, and African -American populations [20–26]. In SS patients, the GT or TT genotype at an *IRF5* SNP (rs2004640) was found to be more prevalent when compared to controls. The T allele results in the expression of the exon 1B isoform and significant overexpression of IRF5 in cell lines, likely driving increased expression of Type I IFN [27]. Moreover, an association in the "G" risk allele of *TNPO3* at the SNP rs13246321, which is in linkage disequilibrium with rs10488631 within the *IRF5-TNPO3* locus previously demonstrated to have association with SS, was observed in a combined cohort of Norwegian and Swedish SS patients [17].

Genetic association has also been reported in SS with a SNP (rs7574865) found in (*STAT4*) involved in IFN signaling [11]. SNPs in *STAT4* have also been found to show strong association with SLE and RA [27]. *STAT4* encodes a lymphocyte signal transduction molecule that responds to Type 1 IFNs and other cytokines, including interleukin-12 (IL12), IL-13, and interleukin-23 [11]. Upon activation by cytokines, STAT4 translocates to the nucleus and acts as a transcription factor to stimulate expression of IFN-γ, a key inducer of T cell differentiation into type 1 T helper cells. The STAT4 protein is also required to regulate T helper cell responses [28, 29]. In addition to association analyses of SS with single variants, evaluation for more complex genetic models supports additive effects between the major risk alleles in *IRF5* and *STAT4* [16].

Plasmacytoid dendritic cells (pDCs) are a major producer of IFNs and have been observed in salivary gland tissues from SS patients [30]. Infiltrating macrophages secrete cytokines including IL-1, IL-6, macrophage chemotactic factor (MCP-1), and chemokines that can recruit and T and B cells [31]. Lymphocytic salivary gland infiltrates consist of approximately 70% CD4+ T cells and 20% B cells [32]. The CD4+ T cells primarily express the α/β T cell receptor and produce Th1 proinflammatory cytokines (TNF-α, interferon-γ, TGF-β, IL-6, and IL-10), several of which have been implicated, but not yet established, as robust genetic effects (Table 2.1). These cells become activated upon encountering antigens, secreting matrix metalloproteinases and additional chemokines and cytokines. These signaling cascades further exacerbate the immune response, promoting the continued production of Type I interferon and interferon-inducible genes, while driving loss of tolerance and ultimately creating a cycle of autoimmune reactivity [33–38].

Central to the interface between innate and adaptive immunity is antigen presentation. Additional genetic associations of SS with genes involved in this critical process have been identified and include several loci within the Major Histocompatibility Complex (MHC). Historically, studies evaluating alleles in the human leukocyte antigen (HLA) genes for association with SS dominated the literature prior to 1995 (Fig. 2.6). The extended MHC region, located at chromosome 6p21.31, covers approximately 7.6 megabases (Mb) of genomic DNA and encodes for approximately 252 genes and 139 pseudogenes [39]. HLA genes are the subset that encodes cell surface antigen-presenting proteins. Alleles of these genes are well-documented risk factors for the development of autoimmune disorders [40, 41]. The HLA genes found to be associated with SS vary in different ethnic groups and are summarized in Table 2.1 [42]. In general, studies have primarily focused on alleles at the Class II HLA-DR and -DQ loci. The most consistent associations to date have been with DR2 and DR3 alleles at the DRB1 locus in Caucasian populations (Fig. 2.6).

Interestingly, most HLA associations are stronger when evaluated in subsets of patients with anti-Ro/SSA and anti-La/SSB autoantibody responses. Particularly strong associations with these antibody responses were identified in patients heterozygous for DQw1 and DQw2 [43]. Other genes may also be involved in autoantibody production in SS, including the genes Transporter 2, ATP-binding cassette, sub-family B (*TAP2*), and Transforming Growth Factor-β1 (*TGF-β1*) (Table 2.1). The *TAP* genes, which are mapped to the MHC region, are important in peptide loading and cell surface expression of HLA Class I molecules. *TGF-β1*, mapped to chromosome 19q13.1, is a pro-fibrotic, immunosuppressive cytokine expressed by many cell types and is known to be underexpressed in the salivary glands of SS patients [44]. Gottenberg et al. identified an allele at codon 10 of *TGF-β1* with an elevated allele frequency in SS patients who had the HLA-DRB1*3 haplotype and elevated levels of anti-La/SSB autoantibodies [44]. They hypothesized that both the *TGF-β1* polymorphism and the HLA-DRB1*3 haplotype act in combination to promote the production of anti-La/SSB autoantibodies.

Several genes that function in adaptive immune responses, particularly in T and B cells, have been implicated in SS. A genetic association of SS has been recently identified by Nordmark et al. with tumor necrosis factor super family member 4 (*TNFSF4/OX40L*), a gene relevant to T cell functions [17]. *TNFSF4* is expressed on the surface of multiple cell types including pDCs, B cells, NK cells, and vascular endothelial cells. This ligand is involved in signal transduction leading to T cell proliferation and cytokine production. Significantly, binding of this ligand to its receptor, TNFSF4R (Ox40R), inhibits production of regulatory T cells that produce IL-10, plays a critical role in maintenance of peripheral tolerance, and can inhibit the development of autoimmune disease [45]. This interaction drives the Th1 T cell response and production of Type I interferon by pDCs. Candidate gene association studies demonstrated association with *TNFSF4* in Swedish and Norwegian SS patients (Table 2.1) [17].

Several genetic variants with evidence for association with SS could influence B cell function. B cells and plasma cells are important in the mechanisms leading up to glandular dysfunction, as is IgG deposition in the salivary glands and lacrimal ducts targeting receptors important in parasympathetic signaling. Furthermore, autoreactive lymphocytosis and an increase in circulating IgG antibodies have been implicated in the development of extraglandular effects prior to, during, or after glandular disease origination. There is significant autoreactive B cell expansion, hyperreactivity, and antibody formation in the exocrine glands [46]. Salivary infiltrates of some SS patients even demonstrate ectopic germinal centers (GC) with follicular dendritic cell networks lacking follicular zone expansion [47]. The number of anti-Ro/SSA- and anti-La/SSB-producing B cells present in the salivary infiltrate of patients with SS directly correlates with the number of anti-Ro60 producing B cells and the serum titer of circulating anti-Ro/SSA antibody [48].

An interesting example of a genetic association in SS with potential relevance to B cells has recently been identified in the region comprising two genes, *FAM167A* and the B lymphoid tyrosine kinase (*BLK*) locus [17]. *FAM167A* and *BLK* are transcribed in opposite directions, possibly from common promoter elements, and expression levels are inversely correlated. While the function of *FAM167A* remains unknown, *BLK* is expressed in B cells and is involved in cell signaling that results in activation of multiple nuclear transcription factors. Reduced expression of *BLK* is hypothesized to lead to a breakdown in tolerance by allowing autoreactive cells to escape deletion [17].

Early B cell factor 1 (*EBF1*) is a vital transcription factor involved in the enhancement of transcriptional activity during B cell development. EBF1 initiates demethylation of DNA and activates PAX5, driving expression of important B cell activation markers. Immunoglobulin production also requires EBF1. Decreased or altered expression of EBF1 can lead to impaired B cell development. Association was observed with the presence of the "T" risk allele at a SNP (rs3843489) located in the tenth intron and in another SNP (rs869593) located in the sixth intron that appear to be independent genetic effects [17].

Significantly, increased levels of B-cell activating factor (BAFF, BLyS), a member of the tumor necrosis factor family, have been identified in the serum of SS patients compared to healthy controls and directly correlate to the degree of clinical activity and titer of circulating autoantibodies [49–51]. BAFF is essential for B cell maturation [52]. Three receptors have been identified almost exclusively on B cells that bind BAFF, including the BAFF-R (BR3), the cyclophilin ligand activator (TACI), and the B cell maturation antigen (BCMA) [53]. Increased expression of these receptors during B cell development in the presence of BAFF influences the differentiation of mature GC B cells into plasma cells [54]. BAFF levels are increased in the serum of SS patients and gene expression is upregulated in labial salivary gland tissue. Disease susceptibility for anti-Ro/SSA- and anti-La/SSB-positive SS has been associated with the CTAT haplotype of 4 SNPs located in the 5′ regulatory region of the *BAFF* gene, while the TTTT haplotype has been associated with elevated BAFF levels in SS [55].

To facilitate understanding of how genetic variants identified to date can contribute to SS, it is helpful to view them in the context of their effect on relevant pathological pathways. As outlined above, many genetic associations have been observed within pathways important in the immune response, including interferon pathway signaling, antigen processing/presentation, and lymphocyte function. Other pathways with potential genetic associations include intracellular signaling, apoptosis, and inflammatory cytokine/chemokine regulation and cell recruitment. In related diseases such as SLE, multiple genes within a more limited number of common pathways have been observed. Other approaches, including genome-wide gene expression and proteomic studies, have also identified potential genes and pathways for further investigation and are highly complementary to the genetic studies outlined above.

2.5   Gene Expression Studies in SS

Genome-wide gene expression profiling (GEP) studies measure the levels of RNA transcripts for each active genetic locus in a given sample. These studies have identified multiple loci that are differentially expressed in either mRNA isolated from minor salivary glands or peripheral blood of SS patients when compared to healthy controls. This approach utilizes microarrays with oligonucleotides affixed to a glass slide, representing the various transcripts presently annotated in the human genome. When labeled test samples are hybridized to these arrays, the resultant binding yields a florescent signal that can be used to quantitate the mRNA level for a given gene within a given sample. Current generation microarrays can interrogate the levels of ~48,000 transcripts in a single experiment. The analysis of this data often involves comparing transcript levels between groups such as patients and controls, and shows common expression patterns across subsets of presumably co-regulated genes, called signatures. The overexpression or underexpression of sets of genes in patients when compared to controls may point to dysregulation of recognized pathways and provide insight into disease mechanisms.

A review of four genome-wide GEP studies (three from mRNA isolated from labial salivary glands and one from peripheral blood) shows a significant and consistent dysregulation of IFN-inducible genes [30, 56–58]. These genes are overexpressed in SS patients relative to controls and form an "IFN signature" that has been observed in many related autoimmune diseases, such as SLE and RA [59, 60]. Genetic association studies in SS and other autoimmune diseases have found transcription factors, such as IRF5 and STAT4, to be risk factors for disease that may contribute to the overexpression of the genes found within the IFN signature. Of interest, the overexpression of IFITM1 (interferon-induced transmembrane protein 1) was observed in all four studies, and the genetic polymorphisms associated with SS in *IRF5* and *STAT4* correlate with expression levels of IFITM1. Furthermore, the peripheral blood GEP study found positive correlations between anti-Ro/SSA and anti-La/SSB titers and expression levels of the genes comprising the IFN signature in SS.

Other pathways that are dysregulated in SS patients have also been identified through GEP. For example, cytokine and chemokine signaling is important in the recruitment of inflammatory cells into tissues. Hjelmervik et al. and Pérez et al. found that the cytokine interleukin 6 (IL-6) was overexpressed within the labial salivary glands of SS patients when compared to healthy controls [56, 57]. Interestingly, while differences in IL-6 levels in peripheral blood have not been observed, downstream molecules in the IL-6 pathway do appear to be differentially expressed between patients and controls. Genetic association studies have found suggestive evidence that IL-6 is a risk factor for SS. However, additional studies will be required to establish a robust genetic effect and determine whether associated variants contribute to expression differences of IL-6 pathways. Other pathways identified in gene expression studies have been identified and relevance to disease pathogenesis is an active area of ongoing investigation.

2.6 Protein Expression Studies in SS

Although mRNA is an important intermediary molecule between DNA and proteins, not every mRNA molecule is translated into a functional protein. Therefore, the study of differential protein expression within tissues is critical to more clearly understand the functional impact on disease. Proteomics (the study of the structure, function, and modification of proteins) is also rapidly developing in the field of autoimmune disease research. Multiple research tools are available to analyze the complex protein constituents in human tissues. Some of these include 2-dimensional gel electrophoresis, matrix-assisted laser desorption/ionization time-of-flight (MALDI-TOF) mass spectroscopy, and multiple protein microarray chips having the capability to detect and quantify protein constituents in biological samples. Mapping of the SS proteome holds significant promise for revealing valuable biomarkers useful in the diagnosis and classification of the disease. It also stands to aide in drug discovery and monitoring of treatment efficacy with the goal of early treatment to prevent disease progression.

Recent studies aimed at cataloguing the normal human proteome have identified over 1,100 proteins in human saliva [55]. Multiple studies have evaluated the proteomes of whole saliva and minor salivary glands in SS [61–65]. Several hundred proteins have been described that differ in expression between SS patients and controls [61–63, 65]. At least two major trends have been observed in these studies. First, proteins involved in inflammation, including IFN pathways, are present at increased levels in salivary gland tissues and saliva from SS patients. Second, secretory proteins and other typical salivary proteins are decreased in samples from SS patients. The majority of proteins described thus far have not been evaluated as candidate genes in SS. Thus, one goal of future genetic studies will be to determine if specific variants contribute to the differences observed at the protein level, perhaps providing insight into the tissue specificity of autoimmune responses that are characteristic of SS.

2.7   Future Directions

Genetic, genomic, and proteomic studies are rapidly evolving and are expected to continue enhancing our understanding of SS etiology and pathogenesis. The next stage of SS genetics research will be to perform unbiased genome-wide association scans and large-scale replication studies in much larger patient cohorts. Initial efforts are underway. These studies require extensive collaboration and contribution from clinicians and researchers since no single group will be able to independently recruit the large number of well-characterized cases needed. Studies of this scale are expected to elicit many new associated loci and pathways not previously evaluated. Whole genome sequencing is now becoming feasible and the cost will likely be at a sufficiently low level to make this technique feasible on a broad scale in the next 5 or so years. This will be an important phase in SS genetic studies as many rare variants have yet to be explored and GWA scans are typically designed to evaluate more common variants. Transcriptome sequencing and expanded proteomics studies will also provide important insight. Integration of these rich datasets, coupled with detailed clinical information, will undoubtedly be informative in the coming years for dissecting the complex etiology and disease mechanisms in SS.

References

1. Besana C, Salmaggi C, Pellegrino C, et al. Chronic bilateral dacryo-adenitis in identical twins: a possible incomplete form of Sjogren syndrome. *Eur J Pediatr.* 1991;150:652–5.
2. Bolstad AI, Haga HJ, Wassmuth R, et al. Monozygotic twins with primary Sjogren's syndrome. *J Rheumatol.* 2000;27:2264–6.
3. Houghton KM, Cabral DA, Petty RE, et al. Primary Sjogren's syndrome in dizygotic adolescent twins: one case with lymphocytic interstitial pneumonia. *J Rheumatol.* 2005;32:1603–6.
4. Scofield RH, Kurien BT, Reichlin M. Immunologically restricted and inhibitory anti-Ro/SSA in monozygotic twins. *Lupus.* 1997;6:395–8.
5. Cobb BL, Lessard CJ, Harley JB, et al. Genes and Sjogren's syndrome. *Rheum Dis Clin North Am.* 2008;34:847–68. vii.
6. Fox RP. Head and neck findings in systemic lupus erythematosus: Sjogren's syndrome and the eye, ear, and larynx. Philadelphia: Lippencott, Williams, & Wilkins; 2008.
7. Baranzini SE. The genetics of autoimmune diseases: a networked perspective. *Curr Opin Immunol.* 2009;21:596–605.
8. Deapen D, Escalante A, Weinrib L, et al. A revised estimate of twin concordance in systemic lupus erythematosus. *Arthritis Rheum.* 1992;35:311–8.
9. Silman AJ, MacGregor AJ, Thomson W, et al. Twin concordance rates for rheumatoid arthritis: results from a nationwide study. *Br J Rheumatol.* 1993;32:903–7.
10. Graham RR, Ortmann WA, Langefeld CD, et al. Visualizing human leukocyte antigen class II risk haplotypes in human systemic lupus erythematosus. *Am J Hum Genet.* 2002;71:543–53.
11. Korman BD, Alba MI, Le JM, et al. Variant form of STAT4 is associated with primary Sjogren's syndrome. *Genes Immun.* 2008;9:267–70.
12. Feero WG, Guttmacher AE, Collins FS. Genomic medicine – an updated primer. *N Engl J Med.* 2010;362:2001–11.
13. Durbin RM, Abecasis GR, Altshuler DL, et al. A map of human genome variation from population-scale sequencing. *Nature.* 2010;467:1061–73.
14. The International HapMap Consortium. The International HapMap Project. *Nature.* 2003;426:789–96.
15. Miceli-Richard C, Comets E, Loiseau P, et al. Association of an IRF5 gene functional polymorphism with Sjogren's syndrome. *Arthritis Rheum.* 2007;56:3989–94.
16. Nordmark G, Kristjansdottir G, Theander E, et al. Additive effects of the major risk alleles of IRF5 and STAT4 in primary Sjogren's syndrome. *Genes Immun.* 2009;10:68–76.
17. Nordmark G, Kristjansdottir G, Theander E, et al. Association of EBF1, FAM167A(C8orf13)-BLK and TNFSF4 gene variants with primary Sjogren's syndrome. *Genes Immun.* 2011; 12(2):100–9.
18. Takaoka A, Yanai H, Kondo S, et al. Integral role of IRF-5 in the gene induction programme activated by Toll-like receptors. *Nature.* 2005;434:243–9.
19. Taniguchi T, Ogasawara K, Takaoka A, et al. IRF family of transcription factors as regulators of host defense. *Annu Rev Immunol.* 2001;19:623–55.
20. Demirci FY, Manzi S, Ramsey-Goldman R, et al. Association of a common interferon regulatory factor 5 (IRF5) variant with increased risk of systemic lupus erythematosus (SLE). *Ann Hum Genet.* 2007;71:308–11.
21. Graham RR, Kozyrev SV, Baechler EC, et al. A common haplotype of interferon regulatory factor 5 (IRF5) regulates splicing and expression and is associated with increased risk of systemic lupus erythematosus. *Nat Genet.* 2006;38:550–5.
22. Kelly JA, Kelley JM, Kaufman KM, et al. Interferon regulatory factor-5 is genetically associated with systemic lupus erythematosus in African Americans. *Genes Immun.* 2008;9: 187–94.
23. Kozyrev SV, Lewen S, Reddy PM, et al. Structural insertion/deletion variation in IRF5 is associated with a risk haplotype and defines the precise IRF5 isoforms expressed in systemic lupus erythematosus. *Arthritis Rheum.* 2007;56:1234–41.

24. Reddy MV, Velazquez-Cruz R, Baca V, et al. Genetic association of IRF5 with SLE in Mexicans: higher frequency of the risk haplotype and its homozygozity than Europeans. *Hum Genet.* 2007;121:721–7.
25. Shin HD, Sung YK, Choi CB, et al. Replication of the genetic effects of IFN regulatory factor 5 (IRF5) on systemic lupus erythematosus in a Korean population. *Arthritis Res Ther.* 2007;9:R32.
26. Sigurdsson S, Nordmark G, Goring HH, et al. Polymorphisms in the tyrosine kinase 2 and interferon regulatory factor 5 genes are associated with systemic lupus erythematosus. *Am J Hum Genet.* 2005;76:528–37.
27. Remmers EF, Plenge RM, Lee AT, et al. STAT4 and the risk of rheumatoid arthritis and systemic lupus erythematosus. *N Engl J Med.* 2007;357:977–86.
28. Morinobu A, Gadina M, Strober W, et al. STAT4 serine phosphorylation is critical for IL-12-induced IFN-gamma production but not for cell proliferation. *Proc Natl Acad Sci USA.* 2002;99:12281–6.
29. Nishikomori R, Usui T, Wu CY, et al. Activated STAT4 has an essential role in Th1 differentiation and proliferation that is independent of its role in the maintenance of IL-12R beta 2 chain expression and signaling. *J Immunol.* 2002;169:4388–98.
30. Gottenberg JE, Cagnard N, Lucchesi C, et al. Activation of IFN pathways and plasmacytoid dendritic cell recruitment in target organs of primary Sjogren's syndrome. *Proc Natl Acad Sci USA.* 2006;103:2770–5.
31. Lefkowitz DL, Lefkowitz SS. Macrophage-neutrophil interaction: a paradigm for chronic inflammation revisited. *Immunol Cell Biol.* 2001;79:502–6.
32. Fox RI, Carstens SA, Fong S, et al. Use of monoclonal antibodies to analyze peripheral blood and salivary gland lymphocyte subsets in Sjogren's syndrome. *Arthritis Rheum.* 1982;25:419–26.
33. Fox RI, Kang HI, Ando D, et al. Cytokine mRNA expression in salivary gland biopsies of Sjogren's syndrome. *J Immunol.* 1994;152:5532–9.
34. McGeehan GM, Becherer JD, Bast Jr RC, et al. Regulation of tumour necrosis factor-alpha processing by a metalloproteinase inhibitor. *Nature.* 1994;370:558–61.
35. Moutsopoulos HM, Hooks JJ, Chan CC, et al. HLA-DR expression by labial minor salivary gland tissues in Sjogren's syndrome. *Ann Rheum Dis.* 1986;45:677–83.
36. Perez P, Goicovich E, Alliende C, et al. Differential expression of matrix metalloproteinases in labial salivary glands of patients with primary Sjogren's syndrome. *Arthritis Rheum.* 2000;43:2807–17.
37. Wu AJ, Lafrenie RM, Park C, et al. Modulation of MMP-2 (gelatinase A) and MMP-9 (gelatinase B) by interferon-gamma in a human salivary gland cell line. *J Cell Physiol.* 1997;171:117–24.
38. Ogawa N, Dang H, Lazaridis K, et al. Analysis of transforming growth factor beta and other cytokines in autoimmune exocrinopathy (Sjogren's syndrome). *J Interferon Cytokine Res.* 1995;15:759–67.
39. The MHC sequencing consortium. Complete sequence and gene map of a human major histocompatibility complex. *Nature.* 1999;401:921–3.
40. Merriman TR, Todd JA. Genetics of autoimmune disease. *Curr Opin Immunol.* 1995;7:786–92.
41. Nepom GT. MHC and autoimmune diseases. *Immunol Ser.* 1993;59:143–64.
42. Bolstad AI, Jonsson R. Genetic aspects of Sjogren's syndrome. *Arthritis Res.* 2002;4:353–9.
43. Harley JB, Reichlin M, Arnett FC, et al. Gene interaction at HLA-DQ enhances autoantibody production in primary Sjogren's syndrome. *Science.* 1986;232:1145–7.
44. Gottenberg JE, Busson M, Loiseau P, et al. Association of transforming growth factor beta1 and tumor necrosis factor alpha polymorphisms with anti-SSB/La antibody secretion in patients with primary Sjogren's syndrome. *Arthritis Rheum.* 2004;50:570–80.

45. Ito T, Wang YH, Duramad O, et al. OX40 ligand shuts down IL-10-producing regulatory T cells. *Proc Natl Acad Sci USA*. 2006;103:13138–43.
46. Ramos-Casals M, Font J. Primary Sjogren's syndrome: current and emergent aetiopathogenic concepts. *Rheumatology (Oxford)*. 2005;44:1354–67.
47. Larsson A, Bredberg A, Henriksson G, et al. Immunohistochemistry of the B-cell component in lower lip salivary glands of Sjogren's syndrome and healthy subjects. *Scand J Immunol*. 2005;61:98–107.
48. Tengner P, Halse AK, Haga HJ, et al. Detection of anti-Ro/SSA and anti-La/SSB autoantibody-producing cells in salivary glands from patients with Sjogren's syndrome. *Arthritis Rheum*. 1998;41:2238–48.
49. Groom J, Kalled SL, Cutler AH, et al. Association of BAFF/BLyS overexpression and altered B cell differentiation with Sjogren's syndrome. *J Clin Invest*. 2002;109:59–68.
50. Mariette X, Roux S, Zhang J, et al. The level of BLyS (BAFF) correlates with the titre of autoantibodies in human Sjogren's syndrome. *Ann Rheum Dis*. 2003;62:168–71.
51. Pers JO, Daridon C, Devauchelle V, et al. BAFF overexpression is associated with autoantibody production in autoimmune diseases. *Ann N Y Acad Sci*. 2005;1050:34–9.
52. Schneider P, MacKay F, Steiner V, et al. BAFF, a novel ligand of the tumor necrosis factor family, stimulates B cell growth. *J Exp Med*. 1999;189:1747–56.
53. Mackay F, Browning JL. BAFF: a fundamental survival factor for B cells. *Nat Rev Immunol*. 2002;2:465–75.
54. Daridon C, Pers JO, Devauchelle V, et al. Identification of transitional type II B cells in the salivary glands of patients with Sjogren's syndrome. *Arthritis Rheum*. 2006;54:2280–8.
55. Nossent JC, Lester S, Zahra D, et al. Polymorphism in the 5′ regulatory region of the B-lymphocyte activating factor gene is associated with the Ro/La autoantibody response and serum BAFF levels in primary Sjogren's syndrome. *Rheumatology (Oxford)*. 2008;47: 1311–6.
56. Hjelmervik TO, Petersen K, Jonassen I, et al. Gene expression profiling of minor salivary glands clearly distinguishes primary Sjogren's syndrome patients from healthy control subjects. *Arthritis Rheum*. 2005;52:1534–44.
57. Perez P, Anaya JM, Aguilera S, et al. Gene expression and chromosomal location for susceptibility to Sjogren's syndrome. *J Autoimmun*. 2009;33:99–108.
58. Emamian ES, Leon JM, Lessard CJ, et al. Peripheral blood gene expression profiling in Sjogren's syndrome. *Genes Immun*. 2009;10:285–96.
59. Baechler EC, Gregersen PK, Behrens TW. The emerging role of interferon in human systemic lupus erythematosus. *Curr Opin Immunol*. 2004;16:801–7.
60. Sozzani S, Bosisio D, Scarsi M, et al. Type I interferons in systemic autoimmunity. *Autoimmunity*. 2010;43:196–203.
61. Fleissig Y, Deutsch O, Reichenberg E, et al. Different proteomic protein patterns in saliva of Sjogren's syndrome patients. *Oral Dis*. 2009;15:61–8.
62. Hu S, Wang J, Meijer J, et al. Salivary proteomic and genomic biomarkers for primary Sjogren's syndrome. *Arthritis Rheum*. 2007;56:3588–600.
63. Giusti L, Baldini C, Bazzichi L, et al. Proteome analysis of whole saliva: a new tool for rheumatic diseases – the example of Sjogren's syndrome. *Proteomics*. 2007;7:1634–43.
64. Ryu OH, Atkinson JC, Hoehn GT, et al. Identification of parotid salivary biomarkers in Sjogren's syndrome by surface-enhanced laser desorption/ionization time-of-flight mass spectrometry and two-dimensional difference gel electrophoresis. *Rheumatology (Oxford)*. 2006;45:1077–86.
65. Hjelmervik TO, Jonsson R, Bolstad AI. The minor salivary gland proteome in Sjogren's syndrome. *Oral Dis*. 2009;15:342–53.

Chapter 3
Pathogenetic Aspects of Primary Sjögren's Syndrome

Athanasios G. Tzioufas, Efstathia K. Kapsogeorgou,
Menelaos N. Manoussakis, and Haralampos M. Moutsopoulos

Contents

3.1 Introduction

Sjögren's syndrome (SjS) is an ideal model for dissecting the pathogenetic aspects of autoimmune disorders because the affected organs, the labial minor salivary glands, are easily accessible with minimal morbidity to the patient, and patient's sera are rich with autoantibodies directed against organ-specific and non-organ specific antigens. Two major biologic phenomena underlie the autoimmune nature of SjS: (1) the peri-epithelial lymphocytic infiltration of the affected tissues; and (2) B lymphocyte hyperreactivity. Several studies in the past several years have pointed to the central role of the epithelial cell in the pathogenesis of the disease, suggesting

A.G. Tzioufas (✉) • E.K. Kapsogeorgou • M.N. Manoussakis • H.M. Moutsopoulos
Department of Pathophysiology, School of Medicine, National
University of Athens, Athens, Greece

M. Ramos-Casals et al. (eds.), *Sjögren's Syndrome*,
DOI 10.1007/978-0-85729-947-5_3, © Springer-Verlag London Limited 2012

that the condition, in effect, is an "autoimmune epithelitis" [1]. The importance of B cell hyperreactivity is demonstrated by the presence of hypergammaglobulinemia and the large array of autoantibodies associated with SjS.

The extraglandular organ involvement in primary SjS can be categorized into two major groups, peri-epithelial disease and extra-epithelial disease. The peri-epithelial organ involvement, which includes interstitial nephritis, liver involvement, and obstructive bronchiolitis, is the result of lymphocytic invasion into the epithelial tissues of organs beyond the exocrine glands. These clinical features appear early in the disease and usually have a benign course. In contrast, the extra-epithelial manifestations, palpable purpura, glomerulonephritis, and peripheral neuropathy, result from immune complex deposition that is a consequence of ongoing B cell hyperactivity. These disease complications are associated with increased morbidity and risk for lymphoma development.

The etiopathogenic factors that lead to the loss of the immune balance and the massive infiltration of the exocrine glands in SjS are unknown. Incessant activation, defective regulation, or inherent defects of the immune system may all participate. The development of SjS can be conceptualized in three steps. First, autoimmunity is triggered by a given environmental factor or factors acting upon a particular genetic background. Second, the autoimmune response is augmented, becoming chronic through aberrant immune regulatory mechanisms. And third, the lymphoepithelial lesion and eventually tissue damage occur. These are the consequences of the ongoing inflammatory process.

3.2   Characteristics of Autoimmune Lesions

The immunopathology of SjS has been studied extensively in the minor salivary glands. The histopathologic lesions of the exocrine glands consist of lymphocytic infiltrates that tend to develop around ducts and display variable intensity. They extend from mild, focal infiltrates that do not significantly affect the gland organization to diffuse, severe lesions associated with concomitant loss of epithelial structures and tissue architecture [2]. The lymphocytic infiltrates within salivary glands often organize around ectopic structures that resemble germinal centers [3]. T and B lymphocytes comprise the vast majority of infiltrating mononuclear cells in minor salivary gland lesions, whereas macrophages, dendritic cells, and natural killer (NK) cells comprise only a small proportion (approximately 5–10%) [4]. Most of T lymphocytes bear the CD4 phenotype (50–70% of total T cells) [4]. The incidence of T and B cells, macrophages, and interdigitating dendritic cells varies according to the severity of the lesion (Fig. 3.1 and Table 3.1) [4]. T cells predominate in mild lesions (up to 60% of total infiltrating mononuclear cells), whereas B cells predominate in advanced ones (up to 50% of total infiltrating mononuclear cells) [4]. The frequency of macrophages increase, whereas that of interdigitating dendritic cells decrease with lesion severity. The numbers of infiltrating T cells and interdigitating dendritic cells correlate inversely with infiltration severity [4]. In contrast, the numbers of B cells and macrophages correlate directly.

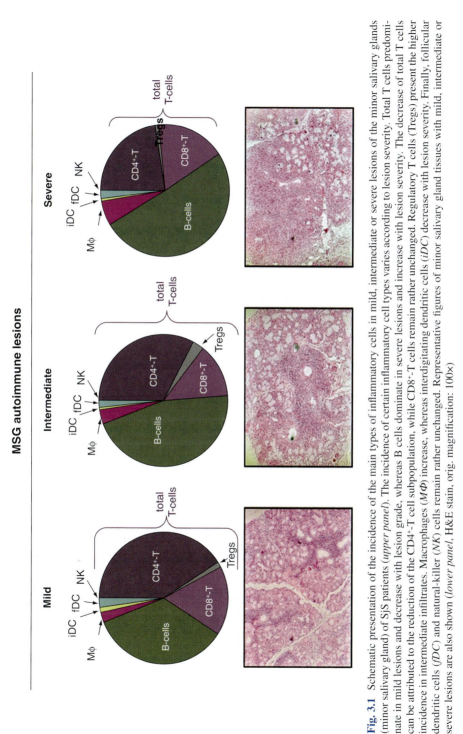

Fig. 3.1 Schematic presentation of the incidence of the main types of inflammatory cells in mild, intermediate or severe lesions of the minor salivary glands (minor salivary gland) of SjS patients (*upper panel*). The incidence of certain inflammatory cell types varies according to lesion severity. Total T cells predominate in mild lesions and decrease with lesion grade, whereas B cells dominate in severe lesions and increase with lesion severity. The decrease of total T cells can be attributed to the reduction of the CD4+-T cell subpopulation, while CD8+-T cells remain rather unchanged. Regulatory T cells (Tregs) present the higher incidence in intermediate infiltrates. Macrophages (*Mϕ*) increase, whereas interdigitating dendritic cells (*iDC*) decrease with lesion severity. Finally, follicular dendritic cells (*fDC*) and natural-killer (*NK*) cells remain rather unchanged. Representative figures of minor salivary gland tissues with mild, intermediate or severe lesions are also shown (*lower panel*, H&E stain, orig. magnification: 100×)

Table 3.1 Frequency of the inflammatory mononuclear cell (MNCs) types (mean values ± SE) in minor salivary gland tissues of SjS patients with variable infiltration grade

Type of infiltrating MNCs	SjS autoimmune infiltrates			
	Total	Mild	Intermediate	Severe
CD3⁺-T cells	48.07 ± 1.81	58.61 ± 2.90	48.12 ± 1.94	40.28 ± 2.43
CD4⁺-T cells	32.94 ± 1.91	41.69 ± 2.38	35.10 ± 2.39	23.49 ± 2.65
CD8⁺-T cells	15.42 ± 0.95	16.37 ± 2.02	13.33 ± 1.84	16.72 ± 0.90
Foxp3⁺ -Tregs	1.86 ± 0.25	1.34 ± 0.43	2.80 ± 0.45	1.42 ± 0.32
CD20⁺-B cells	44.19 ± 1.83	34.69 ± 3.15	45.21 ± 2.18	50.28 ± 2.73
CD3⁺-T/CD20⁺-B cells	1.26 ± 0.12	1.91 ± 0.26	1.12 ± 0.10	0.90 ± 0.14
CD68⁺-MΦ	4.48 ± 0.67	2.40 ± 0.59	3.75 ± 0.82	6.60 ± 1.35
S100⁺-iDC	0.70 ± 0.10	1.32 ± 0.24	0.47 ± 0.11	0.45 ± 0.06
Fascin⁺- fDC	1.89 ± 0.22	2.29 ± 0.49	1.60 ± 0.29	1.85 ± 0.37
CD56⁺-NK cells	0.044 ± 0.003	0.036 ± 0.007	0.040 ± 0.004	0.053 ± 0.005

Table 3.2 Features indicative of the activation of T and B lymphocytes that infiltrate the minor salivary glands of SjS patients

Infiltrating cell types	Features indicative of lymphocytic activation	
T cells	Expression of molecules:	CD45-Ro memory
		HLA-DR
		LFA-1
		IL-2R/CD25
		IL-2 cytokine
	Oligoclonal expansion	
	Detection of Ro(SjSA)-52 kDa reactive T cells	
B cells	Producing:	Rheumatoid factors
		Autoantibodies to Ro(SjS-A) and La(SjSB)
	Predominance of IgG and IgM producing plasma cells	
	Accumulation of memory B cells (CD20⁺/CD27⁺)	
	Oligoclonal or monoclonal expansion	

The decline of T cell population with lesion severity is attributable to a decrease in CD4⁺ T cells because the frequency of infiltrating CD8⁺ T cells remains relatively stable [4]. In addition, regulatory T (Treg) cells, which represent a subpopulation of CD4⁺-T cells with pivotal suppressive role in the regulation of immune responses [5], are differentially distributed in minor salivary gland lesions of distinct severity: a higher incidence of Treg cells is observed in lesions of intermediate severity as opposed to mild or severe infiltrates (Fig. 3.1) [6].

The majority of infiltrating T lymphocytes (77%) in the inflammatory SjS lesions express the CD45-Ro memory helper/inducer marker and are activated, as judged by the expression of HLA class-II molecules, interleukin-2 receptor (IL-2R/CD25), and lymphocyte function-associated antigen-1 (LFA-1), as well as by the production of interleukin-2 (IL-2) (Table 3.2) [7, 8]. The T cell receptor (TCR) repertoire of the infiltrating T lymphocytes is not restricted, but certain TCR variable (V) region genes (Vα2, Vα11.1, Vα17.1, Vβ2 and Vβ13) are predominant in expression, suggesting limited heterogeneity of the infiltrating T cells [8–11]. These findings, along with the detection of clonal expansion of T lymphocytes [9] and the presence within minor salivary gland tissues of Ro(SSA)-52 kDa reactive T cells [12], support an antigen-driven proliferation of T cells at this site of disease.

Clinical and laboratory features including hypergammaglobulinemia, circulating immune complexes apparently seen in some patients as small vessel vasculitis, the plethora of autoantibodies, along with the altered distribution of peripheral B cell subpopulations, the oligoclonal B cell expansion, and the increased risk of B cell lymphomas indicate the occurrence of B cell disturbances in SjS (Table 3.2) [3]. In the minor salivary glands of SjS patients, an accumulation of memory B cells (CD20+/CD27+) has been observed, whereas the infiltrating B lymphocytes are hyperreactive, as indicated by the expression of elevated levels of immunoglobulins (Ig) with autoantibody activity [3, 13, 14]. In fact, the distribution of the plasma cells producing the distinct Ig isotypes is altered within the inflammatory lesions of SjS patients, where the IgG- and IgM-producing plasma cells predominate [15–17]. In normal salivary glands, the main plasma cell isotype bears IgA.

The increased numbers of salivary gland IgG-producing plasma cells correlated with increasing IgG concentrations in the serum [16]. In addition, B lymphocytes producing rheumatoid factors or antibodies reactive against the ribonucleoproteins Ro/SS-A and La/SS-B, the major targets of SjS autoimmune responses, have been identified within the salivary glands of SjS patients [18–21].

Several pieces of data suggest that antigen driven monoclonal or oligoclonal B cell expansion may occur within the salivary glands of patients with SjS and it appears to be associated with the development of B cell lymphomas [3, 22–25]. Among others, the elevated expression of B cell-activating factor (BAFF) by infiltrating mononuclear and epithelial cells in minor salivary gland tissues has been implicated in the expansion of autoreactive B lymphocytes, the altered B cell differentiation and distribution, the formation of ectopic germinal centers, and the lymphoma transformation [26–28].

The association between the local T and B lymphocyte activation in the salivary glands and the production of autoantibodies or the development of lymphoma suggests that the local immune responses are linked to the systemic manifestations of the disorder. This is indicated further by the correlations between certain types of infiltrating immune cells and disease parameters. Thus, the low incidence of Tregs and the high incidence of IL-18 producing macrophages correlate with persistent salivary gland enlargement and C4-hypocomplementemia [6, 29]. As discussed elsewhere in this book, these features are adverse prognostic indicators of a heightened risk of lymphoma development [30–34]. Furthermore, elevated levels of macrophage infiltration have been observed in the minor salivary gland lesions of SjS patients with MALT lymphoma [4], and intense salivary gland inflammation is associated with extraglandular systemic manifestations (such as Raynaud's phenomenon, vasculitis, lymph node/spleen enlargement, and leucopenia) [35].

3.3   Epithelial Cells as Key Regulators of Autoimmune Responses

A plethora of histopathological studies of the inflamed salivary gland tissues of patients have indicated that the ductal and acinar salivary gland epithelial cells display features of in situ activation and immune-competent function, including the aberrant redistribution of the Ro/SSA and La/SSB autoantigens in the cytoplasm [36, 37], the expression of the proto-oncogene c-myc [38], and the expression of a number of other immunoreactive molecules that are implicated in immune-cell homing, activation, differentiation, and proliferation (Table 3.3). Thus, epithelial cells in the salivary glands of SjS patients have been shown to express:

- T-cell-attracting and germinal-center forming chemokines (such as CCL3/MIP-1α, CCL4/MIP-1β, IL-8, CCL5/RANTES, STCP-1/MDC, CXCR3, CXCL-9/Mig, CXCL-10/IP-10, CXCL12/SDF-1, CXCL13/BCA-1, CCL17/TARC, CCL19/ELC, CCL20/LARC, CCL21/SLC/TCA) [21, 39–43]
- Proinflammatory cytokines involved in lymphoid-cell differentiation (including IL-1, IL-6, TNFα, IL-18, adiponectin, B cell-activating factor/BAFF) [26, 29, 44–48]
- MHC class-I and class-II molecules [49–51]
- B7, PD-L1 and CD40 costimulatory molecules [51–54]
- Several adhesion molecules [51, 55, 56]

In addition, elevated epithelial apoptosis and increased expression of apoptosis-related molecules have been detected within minor salivary gland lesions [57], suggesting that this pathway participates in autoantigen release and the expansion of autoimmune responses of SjS (Table 3.3).

These histopathological studies provide indirect evidence for the immunoregulatory role of glandular epithelia in the autoimmune lesions of SjS patients. However, such approaches cannot offer direct support for the functional capacity of epithelia to interact with immune cells, nor can they resolve the pathophysiological basis of the "activated" phenotype of epithelial cells that is observed in the tissues of SjS patients. The activated epithelial cell phenotype, in fact, may owe much to microenvironmental factors such as those occurring from cell-to-cell interactions with infiltrating mononuclear cells or from their products (secreted cytokines and chemokines), or to intrinsic cellular activation processes may operate within epithelial tissues.

The establishment of a reproducible in vitro system for the long-term cultivation of nonneoplastic salivary gland epithelial cell lines enabled the study of the glandular epithelial cells under conditions devoid of the effect of other types of cells and tissue microenvironmental factors [58]. As a means to the study of epithelial cells, the in vitro cultivation of salivary gland epithelial cell provided fruitful insights into the phenotypic and functional properties of these cells. In addition, with this approach, the comparative analyses of cells derived from SjS patients and those from disease controls with nonspecific sialadenitis confirmed a distinctive feature of the former cells, namely, their constitutively activated status, which is highly indicative of an intrinsic activation process. Importantly, for a large number of immuno-active molecules

Table 3.3 Molecules and cellular products expressed by salivary gland epithelial cells (salivary gland epithelial cell) that indicate their potential to regulate local autoimmune responses in SjS patients

Process		Molecules expressed by salivary gland epithelial cell
T cell activation	MHC class-I	HLA-ABC
	MHC class-II	HLA-DR
		HLA-DP, HLA-DQ
	Costimulatory	B7-1 (CD80), B7-2 (CD86)
		PD-L1
		CD40
B cell survival, maturation, and differentiation		B cell activating factor (BAFF)
Immune-cell homing	Adhesion	ICAM-1 (CD54)
		VCAM (CD106)
		E-selectin
Expansion/perpetuation/ organization of infiltrates	Cytokines	IL-1
		IL-6
		TNFα
		IL-18 (pro-active)
		Adiponectin
	T-cell attracting/germinal-center-forming chemokines	CCL3/MIP-1α, CCL4/MIP-1β, IL-8, CCL5/RANTES, CCL20/LARC, STCP-1/ MDC, CXCL-9/Mig, CXCL-10/IP-10, CXCL12/ SDF-1, CXCL13/BCA-1, CXCR3, CCL17/TARC, CCL19/ELC CCL21/SLC/ TCA
Innate immunity-related	Toll-like receptors	TLR-1, TLR-2, TLR-3, TLR-4, TLR-7 and TLR-9
		CD91
Apoptosis-related		Fas
		FasL
Exosomes	Autoantigens	Salivary gland epithelial cell

studied, the comparative analysis of non-neoplastic SGEC lines derived from SS patients and those from disease controls had revealed significantly higher constitutive expression in the former cell lines. Such higher constitutive expression has been found stable after several months of culture (59) and was hitherto shown for MHC class-I, costimulatory molecules (CD80/B7.1 and CD86/B7.2), adhesion molecules (CD54/ ICAM-1), apoptosis-related molecules (CD95/Fas and CD95L/Fas-ligand), CD40, TLR molecules (TLR-1, TLR-2, TLR-3 and TLR-4), and immunoregulatory cytokines (BAFF/BLys and adiponectin) [47, 49, 53, 55, 56, 60, 61, 65]. The elevated expression of plethora of molecules by long-term cultured SGECs derived from SS patients, as well as the expression consistency and independence from culture conditions and time, most likely denotes the intrinsic activation of epithelial cells in SS patients [59, 71]. The nature of factors that contribute in such intrinsic activation remains to be identified.

Nevertheless, it is tempting to speculate that latent viral infections, which are long thought to participate in the development of SS and other autoimmune diseases, may be also causally implicated in the epithelial activation of SS patients.

As in the case of in situ expression, long-term cultured nonneoplastic salivary gland epithelial cells also demonstrate that these cells express various immunoactive molecules, either on a sustained, constitutive basis or inducible by various triggering factors. Such factors include MHC molecules (class I and II), costimulatory molecules (CD80/B7.1, CD86/B7.2, and CD40), adhesion molecules (CD54/ICAM-1), and apoptosis-related molecules (CD95/Fas and CD95L/Fas-ligand) [51, 52, 54, 55, 59–62].

The expression of functional B7 costimulatory proteins [60] deserves particular attention, since these proteins are typically expressed by classical antigen-presenting cells and are critical for the regulation of naive T-cell activation. The B7.2/CD86 molecules that are expressed by salivary gland epithelial cells have been shown to present unique binding properties denoted by the functional interaction with the stimulating CD28-receptor and reduced binding to the negative regulator of immune responses CTLA4 [60]. Furthermore, the expression pattern of the distinct B7.2/CD86 isoforms by salivary gland epithelial cells is similar to that of monocytes [61], one of the major antigen-presenting cells.

The functional expression of such immunoreactive molecules indicates that salivary gland epithelial cells are likely able to mediate the presentation of antigenic peptides and the transmission of activation signals to T-cells. In addition, the constitutive expression of functional Toll-like receptors (TLRs; TLR-1, TLR-2, TLR-3, TLR-4, TLR-7, and TLR-9) and CD91 molecules by cultured salivary gland epithelial cells [63–65] suggests that they are implicated in the induction of local innate immune responses. TLR signaling in salivary gland epithelial cells results in the upregulation of MHC-I, CD54/ICAM-1, CD40, and CD95/Fas proteins expression, thus linking the innate and adaptive immune responses [64]. Cultured salivary gland epithelial cells produce several immunoregulatory cytokines and chemokines, including BAFF [42, 46, 48, 65, 66], implicating salivary gland epithelial cells in the altered B cell differentiation [26] and the formation of ectopic germinal-center-like structures that characterize SjS [67].

Finally, in addition to apoptosis, epithelial cells seem to participate in autoantigen release via an alternative pathway for the presentation of intracellular self-components to the immune system that involves small vesicles (30–100 nm) of endosomal origin, called exosomes [68]. Exosomes, which are distinct from apoptotic bodies, participate in physiological processes such as the exclusion of obsolete proteins and membranes, the exchange of cellular material, and intercellular communication [68]. Exosomes are thought to represent an acellular mechanism for the transfer of antigens to antigen-presenting cells and the stimulation or inactivation of T cells, directly or indirectly by the transfer of antigens to dendritic cells [68].

Analyses of culture supernatants indicate that nonneoplastic salivary gland epithelial cells constitutively release increased amounts of exosomes, which contain the autoantigenic proteins Ro/SS-A, La/SS-B, and Sm, all of which are major targets of immune responses in several autoimmune disorders, particularly SjS and SLE [69]. In this context, exosomal production by epithelial cells may represent a physiologic mechanism for the transport of intracellular constituents to classic antigen-presenting cells and a pathway by which epithelial cells communicate their contents and status to the immune system.

The expression of immune-modulatory molecules outlined above suggests that salivary gland epithelial cell are suitably equipped to mediate the recruitment, activation, amplification, differentiation, and maturation of inflammatory cells. These data strongly implicate these cells in the regulation of local autoimmune responses in salivary glands and justify the term "autoimmune epithelitis" [1] in relationship to SjS.

3.4   Tissue Injury and Repair

3.4.1 Functional Impairment of Glands and Autonomic Nervous System Involvement

Exocrine secretion is controlled by the peripheral autonomic system. Salivary glands are enriched with neuroendocrine-related molecules. Besides the muscarinic and cholinergic receptors, several other molecules including the vasointestinal peptide (VIP) or neuropeptide Y (NPY) are located in the exocrine glands. Unmyelinated afferent nerve fibers provide signals from the lacrimatory and salivatory nuclei of the midbrain to the exocrine glands. These nuclei are under the influence of higher cortical centers, as indicated by the common and reversible side effect of centrally acting medications (e.g., tricyclic antidepressants, clonidine) that cause oral and ocular dryness [70].

In the salivary glands, the neuronal signals from CNS affect the epithelial and stromal tissues via the interaction of the neurotransmitters with their receptors and other neurotransmitters located on the surface of these cells. The main signaling neurotransmitters that have been described so far are acetylcholine and VIP. Cholinergic nerves stimulate mucous saliva secretion through the interaction of the released acetylcholine with muscarinic receptors of the epithelial cells (mainly types M1 and M3) [71]. VIP acts through specific receptors, helping to achieve a maximal degree of secretion [72].

In the peripheral tissue, it is still unknown how the autoimmune lesion and the locally produced inflammatory molecules interact with the neuroendocrine molecules. Although biopsies of salivary and lacrimal glands from patients with SjS have focal lymphocytic infiltrates and partial destruction of glandular secretory units, in some patients, the degree of dryness is higher than that anticipated for the level of glandular destruction. This suggests that additional mechanisms leading to dryness are operating. The impairment of the secretory function in these cases may be explained by either the destruction of neural innervations of the residual glandular elements and the relative density of acetylcholine receptors on the glandular cells, or by the action of cytokines (e.g., TNF-alpha and IL-1), autoantibodies, and other inflammatory mediators (e.g., metalloproteinases) produced locally. These substances may lead to an impaired release of neurotransmitters, a decreased response of the residual glandular cells to available neurotransmitters, or even blockade of their receptors.

Studies of animal models of SjS gave some insights on the complex interaction between innate and adaptive immunity and salivary gland dysfunction. These studies revealed that, as in human disease, inflammation and dysfunction are discordant in some animals. In New Zealand white (NZB/W) F1 mice, incomplete Freund's adjuvant, a nonspecific inflammatory stimulus, accelerates glandular hypofunction by a manner that was not associated with a strong adaptive autoimmune response in the early stages of the disease [73]. Furthermore, Toll-like receptor-3 (TLR3) activation associated with type-1 interferon (IFN) upregulation leads to rapid onset but reversible hyposalivation in the absence of glandular inflammation [74]. The underlying cause of these abnormalities, related to the autonomic nervous system, has not yet been defined, but they may potentially be mediated through the muscarinic receptor signaling, since the major stimulus for saliva production is provided by acetylcholine through muscarinic acetylcholine receptors of which the type-3 receptor (M3R) is responsible for saliva production. The local stimuli for saliva secretion result in the activation of compensatory mechanisms, including the upregulation of the muscarinic receptors on the epithelial cells [75].

The upregulation of specific proteins in inflamed and regenerating tissues has been implicated as a mechanism for autoantigen presentation and autoantibody production [76]. Thus, autoantibodies recognizing the M3 muscarinic receptors have been described in patients with SjS [77]. The description of autoantibodies against the M3R generated much interest and controversy over the last decade. Some groups have found anti-M3R antibodies in up to 90% of SjS patients using peptide ELISAs, whereas others were unable to detect the antibodies by immunological methods. The best evidence for their existence comes from functional studies, in which IgG from SjS patients inhibited acetylcholine-induced bowel or bladder contraction [78]. These autoantibodies, particularly those directed against the third extracellular loop of M3R, have been shown to inhibit the carbachol-evoked increase of intracellular Ca^{2+} directly, suggesting a direct role of antibodies in reducing saliva secretion in patients with SjS [78].

The secretory function of salivary glands is highly dependent upon specific aquaporins (AQP), which are present in five isoforms. These proteins lie on the apical surface of the secretory cell membrane. Of interest, AQP5 is distributed intracellularly rather than on the cell surface in salivary gland epithelial cells of patients with SjS. Acetylcholine treatment of the cells induces the translocation of AQP5 from the cytoplasm to the apical surface of these cells. In addition, AQP5 knockout mice have reduced salivary gland secretion rates even after pilocarpine stimulation compared to the wild type [78].

Cholinergic agonists, particularly pilocarpine and cevimeline, have been widely used for symptom control of xerostomia and dry eyes. Both cholinergic agents respond to the upregulated muscarinic receptors of salivary and lacrimal gland, possibly by antagonizing antimuscarinic receptor antibodies. A more complete description of the interplay between the inflammatory component and the locally expressed neuroendocrine molecules may provide further insights, not only into the pathogenesis of the disease, but also into effective therapeutic approaches to SjS.

3.4.2 Extracellular Matrix and Tissue Damage

Several mechanisms may account for tissue damage and epithelial cell destruction and/or dysfunction in SjS, including the induction of apoptosis, the effect of cytotoxic T cells or autoantibodies, and cell matrix degradation. Several lines of evidence suggest an important role of epithelial cell apoptosis in the pathogenesis of SjS [57, 59, 79]. Elevated levels of epithelial apoptotic cell death have been detected in the minor salivary gland tissues of SjS patients [57]. Several apoptotic mechanisms have been implicated in the apoptosis of the glandular epithelia in SjS. These include the classical Fas/Fas-Ligand (FasL) apoptotic pathway, as well as the cytotoxic effect of proteases, such as perforin and granzymes, and/or cytokines, such as IFNγ, that are produced in SjS autoimmune lesions [57, 59, 79, 80]. Long-term cultured salivary gland epithelial cells obtained from patients with SjS display significantly higher surface constitutive expression of Fas and FasL molecules than those derived from controls [59]. However, salivary gland epithelial cells are resistant to anti-Fas-mediated apoptosis and become sensitive after protein or RNA synthesis inhibition. These facts suggest the importance of anti-apoptotic mechanisms operative within salivary gland epithelial cells. Such mechanisms include the anti-apoptotic proteins cFLIP and Bcl-2, which are expresses constitutively by these cells [59].

Treatment with IFNγ, a cytokine that is abundant within SjS autoimmune lesions, overcomes the resistance of salivary gland epithelial cells and promotes their apoptotic death via the Fas/FasL pathway and anoikia [59], providing thus a mechanism for the elevated epithelial apoptotic cell death observed in the minor salivary glands of SjS patients [57]. In addition, recent data suggest that the overexpression of Ro52 autoantigens in the epithelia may contribute in the reduced epithelial proliferation and increased apoptotic cell death observed in SjS [81].

Cell–matrix interactions are important for cellular functions of the epithelial cell, including response to growth factor signals, proliferation, and ability for cellular regeneration. In lacrimal gland cells grown in vitro, cell–matrix interactions are necessary for secretory responses to muscarinic M3 agonists and are further augmented by novel non-matrix proteins such as BM180 [82, 83]. Proteases such as matrix metalloproteinases and lysosomal cysteine proteinases (cathepsins) play important roles during normal embryonic development of glandular tissue [84]. They mediate cellular migration and differentiation, via the controlled degradation of extracellular matrix (ECM) [84]. Numerous studies have demonstrated a close association of proteases with various diseases, such as rheumatoid arthritis and osteoarthritis [85].

Increased levels of matrix metalloproteinases are also implicated in the progression of SjS [86]. Persisting action of matrix metalloproteinases may lead to destruction and atrophy of exocrine tissues, resulting in sicca symptoms [87]. The epithelial cells express a family of specific receptors including integrins to these matrix proteins, the expression of which is elevated in SjS patients [88]. Moreover, the extracellular matrix in the affected glands may be modified by collagenases and other metalloproteinases [86, 88].

Cytokines such as IL-1, IL-6, IL-8, and TNF-alpha are transcribed in increased amounts by conjunctival epithelial cells of SjS patients [89]. The local production of cytokines by mononuclear cells and also epithelial cells might contribute to the immune-mediated destruction of exocrine glands in primary SjS. Tissue damage appears to start very early during the disease process. Studies of lacrimal glands in the nonobese diabetic (NOD) mice revealed that the initial infiltrating cells at

6 weeks of age, consisting mainly of T-lymphocytes, are responsible for the increased MMP and cathepsin-H expression, initiating the ECM degradation [90].

3.5 Pathogenetic Factors

3.5.1 Genetic Predisposition

The role of genetics in SjS is addressed in detail in Chap. 2. However, a genetic predisposition for the development of SjS is indicated by several clinical and molecular associations. Family members of SjS patients have a higher incidence of SjS and a higher prevalence of serological autoimmune abnormalities than do age- and sex-matched controls. SjS is associated with increased frequencies of HLA-B8, HLA-Dw3, and HLA-DR3 [91, 92]. Molecular immunogenetics have shown that the majority of primary SjS patients carry the DQA1*0501 allele independent of racial and ethnic differences, suggesting that this allele may be a determining factor in the predisposition of certain individuals to primary SjS [93].

The limited number of genome-wide association studies performed in SjS to date have revealed significant genetic associations [94]. Associations of gene polymorphisms outside the HLA-locus with SjS are noteworthy, particularly those that influence the type-I IFN response. In this regard, the genetic association of IRF5 rs2004640 T allele with predisposition to SjS has been confirmed [95]. Another study has found a correlation between IRF5 (CGGGG indel, SNP rs10488631) and STAT4 (SNP rs7582694) polymorphisms and SjS development in a Swedish and Norwegian cohort [96]. The odds ratio in subjects with the risk alleles from both genes was 6.78-fold larger than that found in SLE. These findings indicate that a genetic susceptibility favoring a higher IFN response to different stimuli could be a key event in the onset or perpetuation of the disease.

3.5.2 Environmental Factors

As for many autoimmune diseases, environmental factors and particularly viral infections have been also considered as the main triggering agents for SjS. Viral implication is suggested by three observations. First, the aberrant immune response in SjS cannot be explained solely by activation factors, attributed to the inflammatory microenvironment. Thus, the majority of the infiltrating lymphocytes are CD4+/CD45RO+/Bcl-2+ [7, 57] memory T cells whose antigenic specificity, self or nonself, remains unknown. In addition, in chronic lesions, B cells undergo oligoclonal expansion and organize with T cells and dendritic cells (DCs) to form ectopic follicles. The factor(s) of the ectopic germinal center formation is(are) unknown. Furthermore, epithelial cells produce proinflammatory cytokines in the relative absence of professional antigen-presenting cells implying an activated phenotype that is not directly explained by an autoimmune process against epithelial cell antigens [97].

Table 3.4 List of viruses that have been implicated in SjS pathogenesis

Type of virus	References
Cytomegalovirus (CMV)	Shillitoe et al., Arthritis Rheum. 1982; 25:260
	Venables et al., Ann Rheum Dis. 1985; 2:439
Epstein–Barr (EBV)	Fox et al., J Immunol. 1986; 137:3162
	Saito et al., J Exp Med. 1989; 169:2191
Retroviruses	Talal et al., Arthritis Rheum. 1990; 33:774
	Brookes SM et al., Br J Rheumatol. 1992; 31:735
Human herpes virus type 6 (HHV6)	Saito I et al., Arch Oral Biol. 1991; 36:779
Human T lymphotropic virus type I (HTLV-1)	Shattles et al., Clin Exp Immunol. 1992; 89:46
Human herpes virus type 8 (HHV-8)	Couty JP et al., Clin Exp Rheumatol. 1997; 15:333
Coxsackievirus	Triantafyllopoulou et al., Arthritis Rheum. 2004; 50:2897

Finally, studies with the use of complementary DNA (cDNA) microarray in salivary gland biopsies have shown overexpression of type I IFN-inducible genes, including IFN-stimulated transcription factor 3γ (ISGF3G), and IFN-induced transmembrane proteins such as IFITM1 [98, 99]. Increased production of type I IFNs can be initiated in response to "pathogen-associated molecular patterns" (PAMPs) detected by cell surface or endosomal Toll-like receptors (TLRs). TLRs 3, 4, 8, and 9, as well as the receptor CD91 (involved in antigen presentation to MHC class I and II molecules, via cross priming mechanisms) are functionally expressed in epithelial cells [63–65]. TLR8 and TLR9 sense nucleic acids (single-stranded RNA and prokaryotic unmethylated CpG-DNA, respectively) on endosomal membranes.

The identity of the IFN-inducing nucleic acids in the affected salivary glands remains elusive, and their role in the induction of IFN response genes is still unidentified. Taken all together, it is still unclear whether the syndrome is initiated or perpetuated by an exogenous pathogen such as a persisting single-stranded RNA or DNA virus (activating TLR8 or TLR9 PAMP receptors, respectively) or an endogenous small nuclear or cytoplasmic RNA, associated with the Ro or La autoantigens [100].

Second, certain known viruses, such as the hepatitis C virus (HCV), have often been detected in salivary gland epithelial cells of patients with chronic sialadenitis. This provides evidence that a single-stranded epitheliotropic RNA virus has the capacity of establishing a persistent epithelial cell infection of the salivary glands associated with lymphocytic periductal infiltrates that are often indistinguishable from primary SjS when examining salivary gland biopsies. The difference with primary SjS is mainly clinical, since HCV patients present with different systemic manifestations as well as an increased risk of lymphoma development arising from the salivary glands. These patients do not have circulating anti-Ro/SS-A and anti-La/SS-B autoantibodies.

Third, several studies have shown that certain viruses harbor the salivary glands of SjS patients (Table 3.4). Epstein–Barr virus genes and reactivation antigens, endogenous retroviral particles, and coxsackieviral sequences and capsid proteins have been detected in salivary glands pointing to possible areas of convergence of exogenous pathogen stimulation with the innate and adaptive immune response. The viral effect in the epithelial cell appears to be nonlytic, suggesting that low copy numbers of the candidate viruses harbor cells. Persisting residence of the viral genetic material in a low copy number, within the epithelial cell may alter its biologic properties and initiate an aberrant immune response. The characterization and sequencing of such viral genes need sophisticated techniques, able to detect minute amounts of viral genes, such as the pyrosequencing.

3.5.3 Hormonal

The strong female predominance observed in SjS suggests sex-specific predisposing factors. It appears that a lack of estrogens predisposes to the disease. This is supported by the fact that in the majority of patients the disease is expressed in the perimenopausal period of life of females. Studies have shown that estrogen receptor(ER) and ER mRNA have been detected in salivary tissue and cultured human nonneoplastic salivary gland epithelial cells [101–103]. Studies in normal mice have shown that estrogen suppresses the development of SjS, whereas ovariectomy leads to a condition mimicking SjS [104]. In addition, estrogen can ameliorate T cell recruitment in salivary glands [105] and prevent cell death in the lacrimal glands in murine experimental models [106]. Administration of normal doses of estrogens in MRL/lpr mice, which serve as a model of secondary SjS, prevented the development of sialadenitis. Finally, mice lacking the aromatase gene that encodes the enzyme which catalyzes the production of estrogens develop lymphocytic exocrinopathy resembling SjS [107]. These results indicate that long-term estrogen deficiency may cause autoimmune exocrinopathy, but further studies are needed to obtain a more precise view of human disease.

3.6 Conclusions/Summary

The etiopathogenesis of Sjögren's syndrome (SjS) has not been delineated. However, emerging data suggest that SjS is a multifactorial disorder. Genetic predisposition, hormonal, and environmental factors are all likely to contribute to the development of disease. Tissue destruction is associated with the infiltration by mononuclear inflammatory cells (mainly activated T and B cells). The epithelial cells, which are the targets of SjS autoimmune responses, seem to be key regulators of the local inflammatory procedures. Thus, the epithelial cells of the affected organs (such as minor salivary glands) display a phenotype indicative of intrinsic activation. The etiologic factor of this "intrinsic activation" is not known; however, a persistent viral infection has long been considered to contribute. Most importantly, the "activated" epithelial cells of SjS appear to be suitably equipped to participate in the

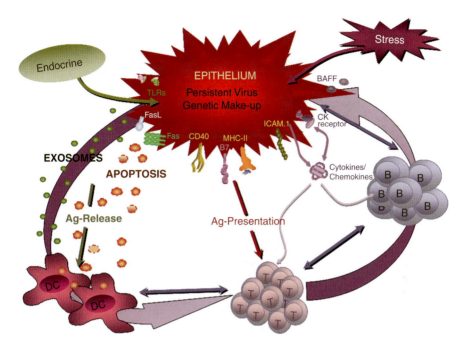

Fig. 3.2 A hypothetical model for SjS pathogenesis. In genetically predisposed individuals, a hormonal or environmental stress results in loss of immune balance and autoimmune responses. The epithelial cells in the target organs become activated, most likely due to intrinsic factors (such as a persistent viral infection) and are capable to recruit, activate, and promote the differentiation of immune cells, which in turn further activate the epithelial cells by the secretion of cytokines/chemokines, establishing thus, a vicious cycle of activation. Furthermore, the activated epithelial cells produce either physiologically (exosomes) or by experiencing apoptotic cell death (apoptotic blebs) vesicles that contain intracellular antigens. These vesicles can be captured by antigen-presenting cells, thus promoting the antigen-specific autoimmune responses. These processes result in the incessant activation of immune system and ultimately lead to the perpetuation of the glandular inflammatory processes and tissue destruction, which characterize the disorder

initiation and perpetuation of the local autoimmune inflammatory responses, including the recruitment, activation and differentiation of inflammatory cells, as well as the release and presentation of autoantigens in the immune system. A schematic model for SjS pathogenesis, emphasizing in the central role of epithelial cells, is presented in Fig. 3.2.

References

1. Moutsopoulos HM. Sjogren's syndrome: autoimmune epithelitis. Clin Immunol Immunopathol. 1994;72:162–5.
2. Tarpley Jr TM, Anderson LG, White CL. Minor salivary gland involvement in Sjogren's syndrome. Oral Surg Oral Med Oral Pathol. 1974;37:64–74.

3. Hansen A, Lipsky PE, Dorner T. B cells in Sjogren's syndrome: indications for disturbed selection and differentiation in ectopic lymphoid tissue. Arthritis Res Ther. 2007;9:218.
4. Christodoulou MI, Kapsogeorgou EK, Moutsopoulos HM. Characteristics of the minor salivary gland infiltrates in Sjogren's syndrome. J Autoimmun. 2010;34:400–7.
5. Bluestone JA, Tang Q. How do CD4+CD25+ regulatory T cells control autoimmunity? Curr Opin Immunol. 2005;17:638–42.
6. Christodoulou MI, Kapsogeorgou EK, Moutsopoulos NM, Moutsopoulos HM. Foxp3+ T-regulatory cells in Sjogren's syndrome: correlation with the grade of the autoimmune lesion and certain adverse prognostic factors. Am J Pathol. 2008;173:1389–96.
7. Skopouli FN, Fox PC, Galanopoulou V, Atkinson JC, Jaffe ES, Moutsopoulos HM. T cell subpopulations in the labial minor salivary gland histopathologic lesion of Sjogren's syndrome. J Rheumatol. 1991;18:210–4.
8. Ohyama Y, Nakamura S, Matsuzaki G, Shinohara M, Hiroki A, Oka M, et al. T-cell receptor V alpha and V beta gene use by infiltrating T cells in labial glands of patients with Sjogren's syndrome. Oral Surg Oral Med Oral Pathol Oral Radiol Endod. 1995;79:730–7.
9. Matsumoto I, Tsubota K, Satake Y, Kita Y, Matsumura R, Murata H, et al. Common T cell receptor clonotype in lacrimal glands and labial salivary glands from patients with Sjogren's syndrome. J Clin Invest. 1996;97:1969–77.
10. Sumida T, Yonaha F, Maeda T, Tanabe E, Koike T, Tomioka H, et al. T cell receptor repertoire of infiltrating T cells in lips of Sjogren's syndrome patients. J Clin Invest. 1992;89:681–5.
11. Sumida T, Kita Y, Yonaha F, Maeda T, Iwamoto I, Yoshida S. T cell receptor V alpha repertoire of infiltrating T cells in labial salivary glands from patients with Sjogren's syndrome. J Rheumatol. 1994;21:1655–61.
12. Namekawa T, Kuroda K, Kato T, Yamamoto K, Murata H, Sakamaki T, et al. Identification of Ro(SjSA) 52 kDa reactive T cells in labial salivary glands from patients with Sjogren's syndrome. J Rheumatol. 1995;22:2092–9.
13. Hansen A, Odendahl M, Reiter K, Jacobi AM, Feist E, Scholze J, et al. Diminished peripheral blood memory B cells and accumulation of memory B cells in the salivary glands of patients with Sjogren's syndrome. Arthritis Rheum. 2002;46:2160–71.
14. Dorner T, Lipsky PE. Abnormalities of B cell phenotype, immunoglobulin gene expression and the emergence of autoimmunity in Sjogren's syndrome. Arthritis Res. 2002;4:360–71.
15. Matthews JB, Deacon EM, Wilson C, Potts AJ, Hamburger J. Plasma cell populations in labial salivary glands from patients with and without Sjogren's syndrome. Histopathology. 1993;23:399–407.
16. Salomonsson S, Rozell BL, Heimburger M, Wahren-Herlenius M. Minor salivary gland immunohistology in the diagnosis of primary Sjogren's syndrome. J Oral Pathol Med. 2009; 38:282–8.
17. Speight PM, Cruchley A, Williams DM. Quantification of plasma cells in labial salivary glands: increased expression of IgM in Sjogren's syndrome. J Oral Pathol Med. 1990;19:126–30.
18. Halse A, Harley JB, Kroneld U, Jonsson R. Ro/SjS-A-reactive B lymphocytes in salivary glands and peripheral blood of patients with Sjogren's syndrome. Clin Exp Immunol. 1999;115:203–7.
19. Deacon EM, Matthews JB, Potts AJ, Hamburger J, Mageed RA, Jefferis R. Expression of rheumatoid factor associated cross-reactive idiotopes by glandular B cells in Sjogren's syndrome. Clin Exp Immunol. 1991;83:280–5.
20. Fox RI, Chen P, Carson DA, Fong S. Expression of a cross-reactive idiotype on rheumatoid factor in patients with Sjogren's syndrome. J Immunol. 1986;136:477–83.
21. Salomonsson S, Jonsson MV, Skarstein K, Brokstad KA, Hjelmstrom P, Wahren-Herlenius M, et al. Cellular basis of ectopic germinal center formation and autoantibody production in the target organ of patients with Sjogren's syndrome. Arthritis Rheum. 2003;48:3187–201.
22. Gellrich S, Rutz S, Borkowski A, Golembowski S, Gromnica-Ihle E, Sterry W, et al. Analysis of V(H)-D-J(H) gene transcripts in B cells infiltrating the salivary glands and lymph node tissues of patients with Sjogren's syndrome. Arthritis Rheum. 1999;42:240–7.
23. Stott DI, Hiepe F, Hummel M, Steinhauser G, Berek C. Antigen-driven clonal proliferation of B cells within the target tissue of an autoimmune disease. The salivary glands of patients with Sjogren's syndrome. J Clin Invest. 1998;102:938–46.

24. Jordan R, Diss TC, Lench NJ, Isaacson PG, Speight PM. Immunoglobulin gene rearrangements in lymphoplasmacytic infiltrates of labial salivary glands in Sjogren's syndrome. A possible predictor of lymphoma development. Oral Surg Oral Med Oral Pathol Oral Radiol Endod. 1995;79:723–9.
25. Schmid U, Helbron D, Lennert K. Development of malignant lymphoma in myoepithelial sialadenitis (Sjogren's syndrome). Virchows Arch A Pathol Anat Histol. 1982;395:11–43.
26. Groom J, Kalled SL, Cutler AH, Olson C, Woodcock SA, Schneider P, et al. Association of BAFF/BLyS overexpression and altered B cell differentiation with Sjogren's syndrome. J Clin Invest. 2002;109:59–68.
27. Daridon C, Guerrier T, Devauchelle V, Saraux A, Pers JO, Youinou P. Polarization of B effector cells in Sjogren's syndrome. Autoimmun Rev. 2007;6:427–31.
28. Jonsson R, Nginamau E, Szyszko E, Brokstad KA. Role of B cells in Sjogren's syndrome – from benign lymphoproliferation to overt malignancy. Front Biosci. 2007;12:2159–70.
29. Manoussakis MN, Boiu S, Korkolopoulou P, Kapsogeorgou EK, Kavantzas N, Ziakas P, et al. Rates of infiltration by macrophages and dendritic cells and expression of interleukin-18 and interleukin-12 in the chronic inflammatory lesions of Sjogren's syndrome: correlation with certain features of immune hyperactivity and factors associated with high risk of lymphoma development. Arthritis Rheum. 2007;56:3977–88.
30. Skopouli FN, Dafni U, Ioannidis JP, Moutsopoulos HM. Clinical evolution, and morbidity and mortality of primary Sjogren's syndrome. Semin Arthritis Rheum. 2000;29:296–304.
31. Ioannidis JP, Vassiliou VA, Moutsopoulos HM. Long-term risk of mortality and lymphoproliferative disease and predictive classification of primary Sjogren's syndrome. Arthritis Rheum. 2002;46:741–7.
32. Ramos-Casals M, Brito-Zeron P, Yague J, Akasbi M, Bautista R, Ruano M, et al. Hypocomplementaemia as an immunological marker of morbidity and mortality in patients with primary Sjogren's syndrome. Rheumatology (Oxford). 2005;44:89–94.
33. Sutcliffe N, Inanc M, Speight P, Isenberg D. Predictors of lymphoma development in primary Sjogren's syndrome. Semin Arthritis Rheum. 1998;28:80–7.
34. Voulgarelis M, Dafni UG, Isenberg DA, Moutsopoulos HM. Malignant lymphoma in primary Sjogren's syndrome: a multicenter, retrospective, clinical study by the European Concerted Action on Sjogren's syndrome. Arthritis Rheum. 1999;42:1765–72.
35. Gerli R, Muscat C, Giansanti M, Danieli MG, Sciuto M, Gabrielli A, et al. Quantitative assessment of salivary gland inflammatory infiltration in primary Sjogren's syndrome: its relationship to different demographic, clinical and serological features of the disorder. Br J Rheumatol. 1997;36:969–75.
36. Ohlsson M, Jonsson R, Brokstad KA. Subcellular redistribution and surface exposure of the Ro52, Ro60 and La48 autoantigens during apoptosis in human ductal epithelial cells: a possible mechanism in the pathogenesis of Sjogren's syndrome. Scand J Immunol. 2002;56: 456–69.
37. Yannopoulos DI, Roncin S, Lamour A, Pennec YL, Moutsopoulos HM, Youinou P. Conjunctival epithelial cells from patients with Sjogren's syndrome inappropriately express major histocompatibility complex molecules, La(SjSB) antigen, and heat-shock proteins. J Clin Immunol. 1992;12:259–65.
38. Skopouli FN, Kousvelari EE, Mertz P, Jaffe ES, Fox PC, Moutsopoulos HM. c-myc mRNA expression in minor salivary glands of patients with Sjogren's syndrome. J Rheumatol. 1992;19:693–9.
39. Amft N, Bowman SJ. Chemokines and cell trafficking in Sjogren's syndrome. Scand J Immunol. 2001;54:62–9.
40. Barone F, Bombardieri M, Rosado MM, Morgan PR, Challacombe SJ, De Vita S, et al. CXCL13, CCL21, and CXCL12 expression in salivary glands of patients with Sjogren's syndrome and MALT lymphoma: association with reactive and malignant areas of lymphoid organization. J Immunol. 2008;180:5130–40.
41. Cuello C, Palladinetti P, Tedla N, Di Girolamo N, Lloyd AR, McCluskey PJ, et al. Chemokine expression and leucocyte infiltration in Sjogren's syndrome. Br J Rheumatol. 1998;37:779–83.

42. Sfriso P, Oliviero F, Calabrese F, Miorin M, Facco M, Contri A, et al. Epithelial CXCR3-B regulates chemokines bioavailability in normal, but not in Sjogren's syndrome, salivary glands. J Immunol. 2006;176:2581–9.

43. Xanthou G, Polihronis M, Tzioufas AG, Paikos S, Sideras P, Moutsopoulos HM. "Lymphoid" chemokine messenger RNA expression by epithelial cells in the chronic inflammatory lesion of the salivary glands of Sjogren's syndrome patients: possible participation in lymphoid structure formation. Arthritis Rheum. 2001;44:408–18.

44. Bombardieri M, Barone F, Pittoni V, Alessandri C, Conigliaro P, Blades MC, et al. Increased circulating levels and salivary gland expression of interleukin-18 in patients with Sjogren's syndrome: relationship with autoantibody production and lymphoid organization of the periductal inflammatory infiltrate. Arthritis Res Ther. 2004;6:R447–56.

45. Boumba D, Skopouli FN, Moutsopoulos HM. Cytokine mRNA expression in the labial salivary gland tissues from patients with primary Sjogren's syndrome. Br J Rheumatol. 1995;34:326–33.

46. Daridon C, Devauchelle V, Hutin P, Le Berre R, Martins-Carvalho C, Bendaoud B, et al. Aberrant expression of BAFF by B lymphocytes infiltrating the salivary glands of patients with primary Sjogren's syndrome. Arthritis Rheum. 2007;56:1134–44.

47. Fox RI, Kang HI, Ando D, Abrams J, Pisa E. Cytokine mRNA expression in salivary gland biopsies of Sjogren's syndrome. J Immunol. 1994;152:5532–9.

48. Katsiougiannis S, Kapsogeorgou EK, Manoussakis MN, Skopouli FN. Salivary gland epithelial cells: a new source of the immunoregulatory hormone adiponectin. Arthritis Rheum. 2006;54:2295–9.

49. Moutsopoulos HM, Hooks JJ, Chan CC, Dalavanga YA, Skopouli FN, Detrick B. HLA-DR expression by labial minor salivary gland tissues in Sjogren's syndrome. Ann Rheum Dis. 1986;45:677–83.

50. Thrane PS, Halstensen TS, Haanaes HR, Brandtzaeg P. Increased epithelial expression of HLA-DQ and HLA-DP molecules in salivary glands from patients with Sjogren's syndrome compared with obstructive sialadenitis. Clin Exp Immunol. 1993;92:256–62.

51. Tsunawaki S, Nakamura S, Ohyama Y, Sasaki M, Ikebe-Hiroki A, Hiraki A, et al. Possible function of salivary gland epithelial cells as nonprofessional antigen-presenting cells in the development of Sjogren's syndrome. J Rheumatol. 2002;29:1884–96.

52. Dimitriou ID, Kapsogeorgou EK, Moutsopoulos HM, Manoussakis MN. CD40 on salivary gland epithelial cells: high constitutive expression by cultured cells from Sjogren's syndrome patients indicating their intrinsic activation. Clin Exp Immunol. 2002;127:386–92.

53. Kobayashi M, Kawano S, Hatachi S, Kurimoto C, Okazaki T, Iwai Y, et al. Enhanced expression of programmed death-1 (PD-1)/PD-L1 in salivary glands of patients with Sjogren's syndrome. J Rheumatol. 2005;32:2156–63.

54. Manoussakis MN, Dimitriou ID, Kapsogeorgou EK, Xanthou G, Paikos S, Polihronis M, et al. Expression of B7 costimulatory molecules by salivary gland epithelial cells in patients with Sjogren's syndrome. Arthritis Rheum. 1999;42:229–39.

55. Kapsogeorgou EK, Dimitriou ID, Abu-Helu RF, Moutsopoulos HM, Manoussakis MN. Activation of epithelial and myoepithelial cells in the salivary glands of patients with Sjogren's syndrome: high expression of intercellular adhesion molecule-1 (ICAM.1) in biopsy specimens and cultured cells. Clin Exp Immunol. 2001;124:126–33.

56. St Clair EW, Angellilo JC, Singer KH. Expression of cell-adhesion molecules in the salivary gland microenvironment of Sjogren's syndrome. Arthritis Rheum. 1992;35:62–6.

57. Polihronis M, Tapinos NI, Theocharis SE, Economou A, Kittas C, Moutsopoulos HM. Modes of epithelial cell death and repair in Sjogren's syndrome (SjS). Clin Exp Immunol. 1998;114:485–90.

58. Dimitriou ID, Kapsogeorgou EK, Abu-Helu RF, Moutsopoulos HM, Manoussakis MN. Establishment of a convenient system for the long-term culture and study of non-neoplastic human salivary gland epithelial cells. Eur J Oral Sci. 2002;110:21–30.

59. Abu-Helu RF, Dimitriou ID, Kapsogeorgou EK, Moutsopoulos HM, Manoussakis MN. Induction of salivary gland epithelial cell injury in Sjogren's syndrome: in vitro assessment of T cell-derived cytokines and Fas protein expression. J Autoimmun. 2001;17:141–53.
60. Kapsogeorgou EK, Moutsopoulos HM, Manoussakis MN. Functional expression of a costimulatory B7.2 (CD86) protein on human salivary gland epithelial cells that interacts with the CD28 receptor, but has reduced binding to CTLA4. J Immunol. 2001;166:3107–13.
61. Kapsogeorgou EK, Moutsopoulos HM, Manoussakis MN. A novel B7-2 (CD86) splice variant with a putative negative regulatory role. J Immunol. 2008;180:3815–23.
62. Ping L, Ogawa N, Sugai S. Novel role of CD40 in Fas-dependent apoptosis of cultured salivary epithelial cells from patients with Sjogren's syndrome. Arthritis Rheum. 2005;52:573–81.
63. Bourazopoulou E, Kapsogeorgou EK, Routsias JG, Manoussakis MN, Moutsopoulos HM, Tzioufas AG. Functional expression of the alpha 2-macroglobulin receptor CD91 in salivary gland epithelial cells. J Autoimmun. 2009;33:141–6.
64. Spachidou MP, Bourazopoulou E, Maratheftis CI, Kapsogeorgou EK, Moutsopoulos HM, Tzioufas AG, et al. Expression of functional Toll-like receptors by salivary gland epithelial cells: increased mRNA expression in cells derived from patients with primary Sjogren's syndrome. Clin Exp Immunol. 2007;147:497–503.
65. Ittah M, Miceli-Richard C, Eric Gottenberg J, Lavie F, Lazure T, Ba N, et al. B cell-activating factor of the tumor necrosis factor family (BAFF) is expressed under stimulation by interferon in salivary gland epithelial cells in primary Sjogren's syndrome. Arthritis Res Ther. 2006;8:R51.
66. Ittah M, Miceli-Richard C, Gottenberg JE, Sellam J, Eid P, Lebon P, et al. Viruses induce high expression of BAFF by salivary gland epithelial cells through TLR- and type-I IFN-dependent and -independent pathways. Eur J Immunol. 2008;38:1058–64.
67. Jonsson MV, Szodoray P, Jellestad S, Jonsson R, Skarstein K. Association between circulating levels of the novel TNF family members APRIL and BAFF and lymphoid organization in primary Sjogren's syndrome. J Clin Immunol. 2005;25:189–201.
68. Thery C, Zitvogel L, Amigorena S. Exosomes: composition, biogenesis and function. Nat Rev Immunol. 2002;2:569–79.
69. Kapsogeorgou EK, Abu-Helu RF, Moutsopoulos HM, Manoussakis MN. Salivary gland epithelial cell exosomes: a source of autoantigenic ribonucleoproteins. Arthritis Rheum. 2005;52:1517–21.
70. Tzioufas AG, Tsonis J, Moutsopoulos HM. Neuroendocrine dysfunction in Sjogren's syndrome. Neuroimmunomodulation. 2008;15:37–45.
71. Zoukhri D, Kublin CL. Impaired neurotransmitter release from lacrimal and salivary gland nerves of a murine model of Sjogren's syndrome. Invest Ophthalmol Vis Sci. 2001;42:925–32.
72. Tornwall J, Uusitalo H, Hukkanen M, Sorsa T, Konttinen YT. Distribution of vasoactive intestinal peptide (VIP) and its binding sites in labial salivary glands in Sjogren's syndrome and in normal controls. Clin Exp Rheumatol. 1994;12:287–92.
73. Deshmukh US, Ohyama Y, Bagavant H, Guo X, Gaskin F, Fu SM. Inflammatory stimuli accelerate Sjogren's syndrome-like disease in (NZB x NZW)F1 mice. Arthritis Rheum. 2008;58:1318–23.
74. Deshmukh US, Nandula SR, Thimmalapura PR, Scindia YM, Bagavant H. Activation of innate immune responses through Toll-like receptor 3 causes a rapid loss of salivary gland function. J Oral Pathol Med. 2009;38:42–7.
75. Beroukas D, Goodfellow R, Hiscock J, Jonsson R, Gordon TP, Waterman SA. Up-regulation of M3-muscarinic receptors in labial salivary gland acini in primary Sjogren's syndrome. Lab Invest. 2002;82:203–10.
76. Casciola-Rosen L, Nagaraju K, Plotz P, Wang K, Levine S, Gabrielson E, et al. Enhanced autoantigen expression in regenerating muscle cells in idiopathic inflammatory myopathy. J Exp Med. 2005;201:591–601.

77. Li J, Ha YM, Ku NY, Choi SY, Lee SJ, Oh SB, et al. Inhibitory effects of autoantibodies on the muscarinic receptors in Sjogren's syndrome. Lab Invest. 2004;84:1430–8.
78. Dawson L, Tobin A, Smith P, Gordon T. Antimuscarinic antibodies in Sjogren's syndrome: where are we, and where are we going? Arthritis Rheum. 2005;52:2984–95.
79. Manoussakis MN, Moutsopoulos HM. Sjogren's syndrome: current concepts. Adv Intern Med. 2001;47:191–217.
80. Bolstad AI, Eiken HG, Rosenlund B, Alarcon-Riquelme ME, Jonsson R. Increased salivary gland tissue expression of Fas, Fas ligand, cytotoxic T lymphocyte-associated antigen 4, and programmed cell death 1 in primary Sjogren's syndrome. Arthritis Rheum. 2003;48:174–85.
81. Espinosa A, Zhou W, Ek M, Hedlund M, Brauner S, Popovic K, et al. The Sjogren's syndrome-associated autoantigen Ro52 is an E3 ligase that regulates proliferation and cell death. J Immunol. 2006;176:6277–85.
82. Stepp MA, Zhu L, Sheppard D, Cranfill RL. Localized distribution of alpha 9 integrin in the cornea and changes in expression during corneal epithelial cell differentiation. J Histochem Cytochem. 1995;43:353–62.
83. Laurie GW, Glass JD, Ogle RA, Stone CM, Sluss JR, Chen L. "BM180": a novel basement membrane protein with a role in stimulus-secretion coupling by lacrimal acinar cells. Am J Physiol. 1996;270:C1743–50.
84. Patel VN, Rebustini IT, Hoffman MP. Salivary gland branching morphogenesis. Differentiation. 2006;74:349–64.
85. Martel-Pelletier J, Welsch DJ, Pelletier JP. Metalloproteases and inhibitors in arthritic diseases. Best Pract Res Clin Rheumatol. 2001;15:805–29.
86. Garcia-Carrasco M, Fuentes-Alexandro S, Escarcega RO, Salgado G, Riebeling C, Cervera R. Pathophysiology of Sjogren's syndrome. Arch Med Res. 2006;37:921–32.
87. Fox RI, Stern M. Sjogren's syndrome: mechanisms of pathogenesis involve interaction of immune and neurosecretory systems. Scand J Rheumatol Suppl. 2002;116:3–13.
88. Konttinen YT, Kangaspunta P, Lindy O, Takagi M, Sorsa T, Segerberg M, et al. Collagenase in Sjogren's syndrome. Ann Rheum Dis. 1994;53:836–9.
89. Jones DT, Monroy D, Ji Z, Atherton SS, Pflugfelder SC. Sjogren's syndrome: cytokine and Epstein-Barr viral gene expression within the conjunctival epithelium. Invest Ophthalmol Vis Sci. 1994;35:3493–504.
90. Schenke-Layland K, Xie J, Magnusson M, Angelis E, Li X, Wu K, et al. Lymphocytic infiltration leads to degradation of lacrimal gland extracellular matrix structures in NOD mice exhibiting a Sjogren's syndrome-like exocrinopathy. Exp Eye Res. 2010;90:223–37.
91. Fye KH, Terasaki PI, Michalski JP, Daniels TE, Opelz G, Talal N. Relationship of HLA-Dw3 and HLA-B8 to Sjogren's syndrome. Arthritis Rheum. 1978;21:337–42.
92. Mann DL, Moutsopoulos HM. HLA DR alloantigens in different subsets of patients with Sjogren's syndrome and in family members. Ann Rheum Dis. 1983;42:533–6.
93. Reveille JD, Macleod MJ, Whittington K, Arnett FC. Specific amino acid residues in the second hypervariable region of HLA-DQA1 and DQB1 chain genes promote the Ro (SjS-A)/La (SjS-B) autoantibody responses. J Immunol. 1991;146:3871–6.
94. Scofield RH. Genetics of systemic lupus erythematosus and Sjogren's syndrome. Curr Opin Rheumatol. 2009;21:448–53.
95. Miceli-Richard C, Comets E, Loiseau P, Puechal X, Hachulla E, Mariette X. Association of an IRF5 gene functional polymorphism with Sjogren's syndrome. Arthritis Rheum. 2007;56:3989–94.
96. Nordmark G, Kristjansdottir G, Theander E, Eriksson P, Brun JG, Wang C, et al. Additive effects of the major risk alleles of IRF5 and STAT4 in primary Sjogren's syndrome. Genes Immun. 2009;10:68–76.
97. Manoussakis MN, Kapsogeorgou EK. The role of epithelial cells in the pathogenesis of Sjogren's syndrome. Clin Rev Allergy Immunol. 2007;32:225–30.
98. Hjelmervik TO, Petersen K, Jonassen I, Jonsson R, Bolstad AI. Gene expression profiling of minor salivary glands clearly distinguishes primary Sjogren's syndrome patients from healthy control subjects. Arthritis Rheum. 2005;52:1534–44.

99. Gottenberg JE, Cagnard N, Lucchesi C, Letourneur F, Mistou S, Lazure T, et al. Activation of IFN pathways and plasmacytoid dendritic cell recruitment in target organs of primary Sjogren's syndrome. Proc Natl Acad Sci USA. 2006;103:2770–5.
100. Bave U, Nordmark G, Lovgren T, Ronnelid J, Cajander S, Eloranta ML, et al. Activation of the type I interferon system in primary Sjogren's syndrome: a possible etiopathogenic mechanism. Arthritis Rheum. 2005;52:1185–95.
101. Leimola-Virtanen R, Salo T, Toikkanen S, Pulkkinen J, Syrjanen S. Expression of estrogen receptor (ER) in oral mucosa and salivary glands. Maturitas. 2000;36:131–7.
102. Tsinti M, Kassi E, Korkolopoulou P, Kapsogeorgou E, Moutsatsou P, Patsouris E, et al. Functional estrogen receptors alpha and beta are expressed in normal human salivary gland epithelium and apparently mediate immunomodulatory effects. Eur J Oral Sci. 2009;117:498–505.
103. Kassi E, Moutsatsou P, Sekeris CE, Moutsopoulos HM, Manoussakis MN. Oestrogen receptors in cultured epithelial cells from salivary glands of Sjogren's syndrome patients. Rheumatology (Oxford). 2003;42:1120–2.
104. Ishimaru N, Arakaki R, Watanabe M, Kobayashi M, Miyazaki K, Hayashi Y. Development of autoimmune exocrinopathy resembling Sjogren's syndrome in estrogen-deficient mice of healthy background. Am J Pathol. 2003;163:1481–90.
105. Carlsten H, Nilsson N, Jonsson R, Backman K, Holmdahl R, Tarkowski A. Estrogen accelerates immune complex glomerulonephritis but ameliorates T cell-mediated vasculitis and sialadenitis in autoimmune MRL lpr/lpr mice. Cell Immunol. 1992;144:190–202.
106. Ishimaru N, Saegusa K, Yanagi K, Haneji N, Saito I, Hayashi Y. Estrogen deficiency accelerates autoimmune exocrinopathy in murine Sjogren's syndrome through fas-mediated apoptosis. Am J Pathol. 1999;155:173–81.
107. Shim GJ, Warner M, Kim HJ, Andersson S, Liu L, Ekman J, et al. Aromatase-deficient mice spontaneously develop a lymphoproliferative autoimmune disease resembling Sjogren's syndrome. Proc Natl Acad Sci U S A. 2004;101:12628–33.

Chapter 4
Primary Sjögren's Syndrome and Viruses

Manuel Ramos-Casals, Albert Bové, Rafael Belenguer, Xavier Forns, and Salvatore deVita

Contents

The etiopathogenesis of primary Sjögren's syndrome (SS) is probably a sequential, multistep process that leads to selective damage of the exocrine glands and consequent target organ dysfunction. Although understanding of the precise mechanisms involved in etiopathogenesis of SS remains incomplete, the autoimmune origin of the disease (autoimmune epithelitis) [1] is the hypothesis postulated most commonly.

The autoimmune etiopathogenic model of primary SS is based on the existence of an altered immune system incapable of discriminating between "foreign" and

M. Ramos-Casals (✉) • A. Bové
Sjögren Syndrome Research Group (AGAUR), Laboratory of Autoimmune Diseases Josep Font, Institut d'Investigacions Biomèdiques August Pi i Sunyer (IDIBAPS), Department of Autoimmune Diseases, Hospital Clínic, Barcelona, Spain

R. Belenguer
Rheumatology Unit, Hospital 9 d'Octubre, Valencia, Spain

X. Forns
Liver Unit, Ciberehd, IDIBAPS,
Hospital Clínic, Barcelona, Spain

S. deVita
Rheumatology Clinic, Department of Medical and Biological Sciences,
Azienda Ospedaliero-Universitaria S Maria della Misericordia, Udine, Italy

M. Ramos-Casals et al. (eds.), *Sjögren's Syndrome*,
DOI 10.1007/978-0-85729-947-5_4, © Springer-Verlag London Limited 2012

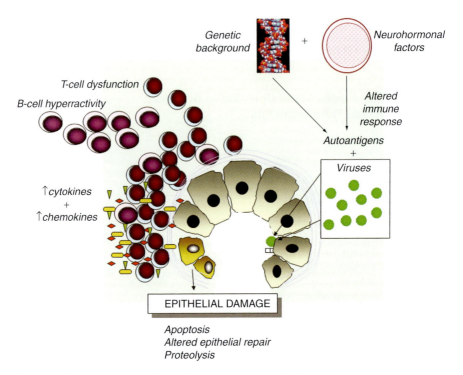

Fig. 4.1 Etiopathogenesis of primary Sjögren syndrome: role of viruses

"self" molecules. This induces an abnormal autoimmune response directed against altered/abnormal self-antigens that are expressed by the epithelium of the exocrine glands. The process is likely to be initiated by a specific combination of intrinsic (e.g., genes) and extrinsic (e.g., infectious agents) factors (Fig. 4.1). The abnormal responses of both T- and B-cells against autoantigens contribute to the histopathological lesion characteristically observed in primary SS, as well as to alterations in the synthesis of numerous intermediate molecules (cytokines and chemokines), thereby helping to perpetuate the autoimmune lesion. The consequent mechanisms of tissue damage leads to chronic exocrine gland inflammation, with fibrosis and loss of physiologic function [2].

Autoimmunity and viral infections are closely related fields. Viruses have been proposed to be the etiologic or triggering agents of a variety of systemic autoimmune diseases. In recent decades, many research groups have focused on the role of viral infection in the etiopathogenesis of SS. Viruses are known to induce the expression of B-cell survival factors such BAFF by salivary gland epithelial cells, through Toll-like receptor (TLR) pathways and mechanisms that are both dependent and independent upon type I interferons (IFN) [3]. Earlier studies suggested that the main candidates are herpesviruses such as Epstein–Barr virus (EBV) and cytomegalovirus (CMV), which have a high seroprevalence (>90%) in the general adult population. However, more recent studies have suggested that other viruses (mainly

Table 4.1 Viruses involved in the etiopathogenesis of Sjögren syndrome

- Hepatitis C virus
- Hepatitis B virus
- Human immunodeficiency virus
- Human T-lymphotropic virus type I
- Endogenous retroviruses
- Coxsackievirus B4
- Epstein–Barr virus
- Herpes simplex virus
- Cytomegalovirus
- Human herpesvirus 6
- Human herpesvirus 8
- Human parvovirus B19

Table 4.2 Extrahepatic sites of hepatitis C virus infection

(a) *Extrahepatic tissues*
  Salivary glands
  Gastric mucous
  Striated muscle
  Peripheral nerve
  Central nervous system
  Myocardium
  Cutaneous lesions
(b) *Circulating blood cells*
  B lymphocytes
  T lymphocytes
  Monocytes
  Neutrophils
  Platelets

hepatitis viruses, retroviruses, and enteroviruses) are also possible etiopathogenic agents in SS (Table 4.1).

4.1 Hepatitis C Virus

The hepatitis C virus (HCV), a linear, single-stranded RNA virus identified in 1989 [4], is recognized as one of the viruses most often associated with autoimmune features. The extrahepatic manifestations common to patients with chronic HCV infection are sometimes sufficient to raise suspicion of an intercurrent autoimmune condition or even to fulfill classification criteria for some idiopathic inflammatory disorders [5, 6]. The specific tropism of HCV for many extrahepatic cell types (Table 4.2) [7–17], especially for circulating blood cells, provides a clear potential link between HCV and autoimmunity.

The true nature of the relationship between HCV and primary SS remains the subject of intense debate. Some believe that the manifestations of HCV infections comprise simply a virus-induced disease that mimics primary SS. Others contend that HCV is the etiopathogenical agent for a subset of patients with primary SS [18]. In 1992, Haddad et al. [19] found histological evidence of SS (Chisholm–Mason classification grade 3 or 4) in 16 of 28 patients with chronic HCV infections. Since then, more than 400 cases of SS-HCV have been reported, making SS one of the systemic autoimmune diseases most closely associated with HCV [20].

According to the HISPAMEC Registry [6], SS accounts for the 47% of the auto-immune conditions associated with HCV reported in the literature. Analysis of these cases has identified considerable overlap between SS classification criteria and extrahepatic features of HCV infection, especially with respect to sicca syndrome (both subjective and objective), histopathological criteria, and immunological markers such as antinuclear antibodies (ANA) and rheumatoid factor (RF). This shows that a clinical diagnosis of SS can be made easily in HCV patients who present with sicca syndrome, a positive ANA, or a positive RF. In contrast, anti-SSA/Ro and anti-SSB/La antibodies are described in only 25% of the SS-HCV patients, a prevalence half that of patients with primary SS. These data suggest that the main differential aspect between primary and HCV-related SS is the immunological pattern; that is, that HCV-related SS tends to have serological markers related to cryoglobulinemia – mixed cryoglobulinemia, RF, and hypocomplementemia – rather than markers traditionally viewed as being more "specific" for primary SS, the anti-SSA/Ro and – SSB/La [6].

Other studies have found a close association between SS and HCV. Sicca syndrome was the second most frequent extraglandular manifestation in the largest series of unselected HCV patients reported [21], with a prevalence of 11%. In another study, SS was diagnosed in 5% of 147 unselected HCV patients, a prevalence fivefold higher than that of the general population [22]. Finally, Caporali et al. [23] recently found that 15% of 501 patients in whom salivary gland biopsy was carried out due to a clinical suspicion of SS were HCV positive.

The lymphotropism of HCV links the virus to the synthesis of cryoglobulins and the development of lymphoma, while its sialotropism may explain the close association with sicca syndrome and SS. Recent experimental studies have found evidence supporting the sialotropism of HCV. Koike et al. [24] described the development of an exocrinopathy resembling SS in the salivary and lacrimal glands of transgenic mice that carry the HCV envelope genes. The findings of that study suggest that the envelope proteins of HCV can recruit lymphocytes into the salivary glands, thereby leading to the formation of lymphocytic infiltrates. De Vita et al. [25] detected HCV in human salivary glands, and two additional studies [7, 8] have demonstrated the capability of HCV to infect and replicate within the salivary gland tissue of HCV patients with sicca syndrome/SS. Arrieta et al. [7] found that HCV infects and replicates in epithelial cells from salivary glands of patients with SS or chronic sialadenitis, a fact also confirmed by Toussirot et al. [8] in 3 SS-HCV patients. The reasons for this predilection of HCV for exocrine gland tissue are unknown.

Chronic HCV infection and primary SS thus appear to have differing etiologies – infectious on the one hand and autoimmune on the other – but share certain etiopathogenic mechanisms. Both entities are characterized by B-cell hyperactivity and are closely associated with B-cell driven processes such as mixed cryoglobulinemia and B-cell lymphoma. The CD5+ B-cell subpopulation, a small group of B-cells involved in the production of natural autoantibodies and RF, may have a possible role in both diseases [26].

These findings have led to HCV infection being considered as an exclusion criterion for the diagnosis of primary SS in the 2002 American-European Criteria [27]. HCV may be considered as an important etiopathogenic agent for SS, with SS-HCV being indistinguishable in most cases from the primary form using the most recent sets of classification criteria. For these patients, we propose the term "SS secondary to HCV" when they fulfill the 2002 Classification Criteria for SS [20]. Chronic HCV infection should be considered an exclusion criterion for the classification of primary SS, not because it mimics primary SS, but because it may be implicated in the etiopathogenesis of SS in a specific subset of patients. However, this etiopathogenic role varies according to the geographical prevalence of HCV infection found in the general population.

4.2   Hepatitis B Virus

Chronic HBV infection is associated with various extrahepatic manifestations including skin rash, arthritis, and glomerular disease [28]. In addition, the association between HBV and some cases of polyarteritis nodosa is well known [29]. Other studies have suggested a possible association between HBV and other systemic autoimmune diseases such as rheumatoid arthritis, polymyalgia rheumatica, antiphospholipid syndrome, and systemic lupus erythematosus [30]. However, there are no data suggestive of a causal role for HBV in these diseases [31], and one study has even suggested a lower frequency of HBV infection in patients with autoimmune diseases [32].

The association between SS and other types of chronic viral hepatitis such as HBV is very infrequent. Only three cases of HBV-related SS have been reported (one associated with HBV vaccination) [33–35], compared with more than 400 cases of HCV-related SS. Similarly, chronic HCV infection also plays an insignificant role in liver disease in SS patients [36]. This predominant etiopathogenic role of HCV is probably due to its specific lymphotropism and sialotropism, which mean it can infect and replicate in both circulating lymphocytes and epithelial cells from the salivary glands.

We have recently reported a prevalence of chronic HBV infection of 0.83% in primary SS [37], very similar to the prevalence in the general population in Spain (0.7%) [38]. In spite of the small number of reported SS-HBV cases, a comparison with primary and HCV-related SS reveals some differences. The clinical expression of SS-HBV is similar with respect to the prevalence of sicca features but shows a higher percentage of patients with joint involvement. With respect to the immunological expression, SS-HBV patients showed a higher frequency of RF but a lower frequency of some immunological features typically described in SS-HCV patients such as hypocomplementemia and cryoglobulinemia [37].

In contrast to the close association between SS and HCV, chronic HBV infection is not associated with SS, with a ratio SS-HBV/SS-HCV cases of 1:10. Although the reasons for the specific predilection of HCV for exocrine tissue are unknown, differences either in the viral structure (HBV is a DNA virus, while HCV is a RNA virus) or in the autoimmune responses they trigger might explain the variation in sialotropism. Thus, Ram et al. have recently suggested a protective role of hepatitis B virus infection against autoimmune disorders given the lower prevalence of hepatitis B core antibody (HBcAb) found in patients with autoimmune diseases (including SS) when compared with healthy controls [39].

4.3   Human Immunodeficiency Virus

In patients with HIV infection, the salivary glands may become infiltrated by lymphocytes in a manner similar to that of HCV infections, leading to a sicca syndrome and a broad spectrum of manifestations. However, salivary gland infiltration is predominantly composed of lymphocytes of the CD8 phenotype (in contrast to primary SS, where CD4+ lymphocytes predominate), and anti-SSA/Ro and anti-SSB/La autoantibodies are usually absent. The HIV-related sicca syndrome is often referred to as "diffuse infiltrative lymphocytosis syndrome" (DILS) [40]. The predominance of CD8 lymphocytes within the salivary glands of HIV patients is not surprising, due to the specific destruction of CD4 cells by the virus.

In 1998, Kordossis et al. described a prevalence of HIV-related sicca syndrome of 8% in Greek patients who were HIV-positive [41]. Kordossis et al. emphasized the clinical similarities between DILS and primary SS. In a similar study conducted in a larger HIV cohort in the USA, a prevalence of 3% was reported [42]. In contrast, data from a labial gland biopsy-based study of 30 unselected, treatment-naive HIV-positive patients in West Africa estimated the prevalence of SS to be 48% [43].

The impact of highly active antiretroviral treatments (HAART) on the incidence and prevalence of DILS is not clear. Panayiotakopoulos et al. [44] described an overall prevalence of HIV-related SS of 1.5% in an unselected HIV-positive population (2 out of 131 patients), substantially lower than the percentage found by the same group in the pre-HAART era (8%), suggesting that SS is rarely found in HIV patients treated with HAART. In contrast, Mastroiani et al. [45] have reported four HIV-positive patients with SS diagnosed 6–48 months after the introduction of HAART. These patients fulfilled objective diagnostic criteria for definite or possible SS, with the most common clinical features being xerostomia, xerophthalmia, fatigue, parotid swelling, and polyarthralgia. Salivary gland biopsy specimens showed diffuse lymphocytic infiltration and patients had abnormal Schirmer's tests, parotid scanning, and ultrasonography. One patient reported a transient, moderate improvement of both xerostomia and xerophthalmia after stopping HAART. All four patients had elevated erythrocyte sedimentation rates, hypergammaglobuline-mia, hypocomplementemia, low HIV viral loads, and absent autoantibodies directed against the SSA/Ro and SSB/La antigens. These authors suggested that HAART plays an important role in the etiology of SS among patients with HIV, and that SS may be a new and important complication of long-term HAART regimens [45].

In summary, HIV-related sicca syndrome has many similarities to SS associated with HCV infection. DILS should be considered a viral-related sicca syndrome rather than a disorder separate from HIV infection [46].

4.4 Human T-lymphotropic Virus Type I

The clinical significance of human T-lymphotropic virus type I (HTLV-I) infection in patients with SS depends on the geographic area. In Japan, where HTLV-I is endemic, a prevalence of nearly 25% [47, 48] was detected in patients with primary SS, suggesting a possible etiopathogenic role for this retrovirus in a subset of cases. Nakamura et al. [49] reported a low prevalence of ectopic germinal center formation in patients with HTLV-I-associated SS.

In contrast, HTLV-I infection is very rare in European countries, although some studies have detected genomic sequences of HTLV-I in patients with primary SS. Mariette et al. [50] detected the HTLV-I *tax* gene within the salivary glands of 15 (30%) of 50 SS patients but also in the 28% of controls. Further investigation of the potential relationship between HTLV-I infection and primary SS is required, but it is possible that this retrovirus has a role in Asian populations that is similar to that of HCV in Mediterranean populations.

4.5 Coxsackieviruses

Recent evidence suggests a role for Coxsackieviruses in the etiopathogenesis of primary SS. Triantafyllopoulou et al. [51] have detected the presence of the Coxsackievirus genome and the main antigenic capsid protein VP1 in 11 of 12 patients with primary SS, 1 of 13 patients with associated SS, and none of 16 controls, suggesting a latent Coxsackievirus infection within the salivary glands of some patients with primary SS. Although the underlying mechanisms of secondary lymphoid structure formation in primary SS are unclear, the authors have proposed an etiopathogenic model which suggests that, in preclinical stages of the disease, lymphocytes transport the virus to its preferential niche (i.e., the epithelial cells of the exocrine glands). During the course of the disease, the virus is cleared from the systemic circulation, but continues to replicate within epithelial cells that become highly specialized antigen-presenting cells. This initiates the recruitment of T and B lymphocytes into exocrine glands and the secretion of chemokines and cytokines.

It is probable that the Coxsackievirus per se induces the formation of secondary lymphoid-like follicles and the exocrine gland pathology, which are the histological hallmarks of primary SS. Coxsackievirus infection and replication in the exocrine glands of patients with primary SS may also contribute to the maintenance of the autoimmune reaction by interaction with host cell proteins.

The same group described a 94 base pair gene with full homology to the P2A gene of the Coxsackievirus B4 [52]. In addition, Coxsackievirus sequences have been detected in cultured epithelial cells eluted from the salivary glands of patients with primary SS, but not in those with associated SS [53], suggesting a chronic infection of the epithelial cells by Coxsackievirus. Stathopolou et al. [52] have reported a cross-reaction between antibodies to the major epitope of Ro60 kD autoantigen and a homologous peptide of Coxsackie virus 2B protein. This cross-reaction might play a role in autoantibody formation and in the perpetuation of the autoimmune response against the SSA/Ro and SSB/La antigens. However, Gottenberg et al. [54] failed to identify Coxsackievirus sequences in the salivary glands of both nine SS patients and nine controls. Further studies are required to define the etiopathogenic role of this enterovirus in larger cohorts of patients with primary SS.

4.6   Herpes Viruses

Herpes viruses, especially Ebstein–Barr virus (EBV), have also been studied in primary SS [55–59]. Dawson et al. [56] detected EBV-DNA in one of six SS patients with lymphoma, and Inoue et al. [57] suggested a possible role for EBV reactivation in increased apoptotic protease activity in SS. Trimeche et al. detected EBV-DNA by PCR in 3/22 (14%) patients with primary SS in comparison with 2/17 (12%) controls [58].

Perrot et al. [55] analysed the prevalence of herpesviruses DNA sequences using degenerated consensus PCR primers in salivary gland biopsies from primary and associated SS. Herpesviruses DNA sequences were isolated from 9/55 (16%) salivary gland specimens (EBV sequences in six cases and herpes simplex virus HSV sequences in the remaining three). With respect to other herpes viruses, Klussman et al. [59] isolated sequences and antigens of HHV-8 in one patient with SS and MALT lymphoma. Due to the high seroprevalence of the herpes viruses in the healthy adult population, a discriminative etiopathogenic role is usually difficult to demonstrate, limiting the significance of isolating sequences of ubiquitous viruses in patients with primary SS.

4.7   Human Parvovirus B19

In 1998, a preliminary study showed that serological evidence of past B19 infection in SS patients was associated with the presence of leukopenia and thrombocytopenia, suggesting a possible relationship between B19 and cytopenia [60]. Two subsequent studies have focused on the etiopathogenic role of B19 in primary SS. De Re et al. [61] analyzed six primary SS patients who had monoclonal lymphoproliferation and detected no B19-DNA within parotid specimens. De Stefano et al. [62] studied salivary gland specimens from ten patients with SS and detected B19-DNA in one (10%), who had a high titer of anti-B19 IgG antibodies but negative IgM assays. Thus, although the presence of B19-DNA in salivary glands of SS patients seems to be infrequent, B19 might persist in some cases.

4.8 Conclusion

In recent decades, many research groups have focused on the role of viral infection in the etiopathogenesis of primary SS, the so-called viral hypothesis. The main earlier candidates were herpesviruses such as EBV and CMV, which have a high seroprevalence in the general population, with more than 90% of adults presenting IgG against these viruses. Recent studies have suggested that other viruses (mainly hepatitis viruses, retroviruses, and enteroviruses) may play a key etiopathogenic role in SS. However, the mechanisms that lead to the aberrant autoimmune responses related to chronic viral infection are not clearly understood.

Because primary infection by these viruses is not always recognized, etiopathogenic studies performed after acute infection are difficult to interpret. Molecular changes induced by first contact with the virus are not susceptible to analysis when the etiopathogenic situation previous to the primary infection is not known. However, the search will be always for the external agent that could trigger the autoimmune response and the development of primary SS. The viral causal agent of SS has not yet been discovered, but many interesting findings on the complex interactions between viruses and SS patients in clinical practice have been made.

References

1. Moutsopoulos HM. Sjögren's syndrome: autoimmune epithelitis. Clin Immunol Immunopathol. 1994;72:162–5.
2. Ramos-Casals M, Font J. Primary Sjögren's syndrome: current and emergent aetiopathogenic concepts. Rheumatology (Oxford). 2005;44(11):1354–67.
3. Ittah M, Miceli-Richard C, Gottenberg JE, et al. Viruses induce high expression of BAFF by salivary gland epithelial cells through TLR- and type-I IFN-dependent and -independent pathways. Eur J Immunol. 2008;38:1058–64.
4. Choo QL, Kuo G, Weiner AJ, et al. Isolation of a cDNA clone derived from a blood-borne non-A, non-B viral hepatitis genome. Science. 1989;244:359–62.
5. Ramos-Casals M, Font J. Extrahepatic manifestations in patients with chronic hepatitis C virus infection. Curr Opin Rheumatol. 2005;17:447–55.
6. Ramos-Casals M, Muñoz S, Medina F, et al. HISPAMEC Study Group. Systemic autoimmune diseases in patients with hepatitis C virus infection: characterization of 1020 cases (The HISPAMEC Registry). J Rheumatol. 2009;36:1442–8.

7. Arrieta JJ, Rodriguez-Inigo E, Ortiz-Movilla N, et al. In situ detection of hepatitis C virus RNA in salivary glands. Am J Pathol. 2001;158:259–64.

8. Toussirot E, Le Huede G, Mougin C, et al. Presence of hepatitis C virus RNA in the salivary glands of patients with Sjögren's syndrome and hepatitis C virus infection. J Rheumatol. 2002;29:2382–5.

9. De Vita S, De Re V, Sansonno D, et al. Gastric mucosa as an additional extrahepatic localization of hepatitis C virus: viral detection in gastric low-grade lymphoma associated with autoimmune disease and in chronic gastritis. Hepatology. 2000;31:182–9.

10. Authier FJ, Bassez G, Payan C, et al. Detection of genomic viral RNA in nerve and muscle of patients with HCV neuropathy. Neurology. 2003;60:808–12.

11. Di Muzio A, Bonetti B, Capasso M, et al. Hepatitis C virus infection and myositis: a virus localization study. Neuromuscul Disord. 2003;13:68–71.

12. Bonetti B, Scardoni M, Monaco S, et al. Hepatitis C virus infection of peripheral nerves in type II cryoglobulinaemia. Virchows Arch. 1999;434:533–5.

13. Radkowski M, Wilkinson J, Nowicki M, et al. Search for hepatitis C virus negative-strand RNA sequences and analysis of viral sequences in the central nervous system: evidence of replication. J Virol. 2002;76:600–8.

14. Okabe M, Fukuda K, Arakawa K, et al. Chronic variant of myocarditis associated with hepatitis C virus infection. Circulation. 1997;96:22–4.

15. Agnello V, Abel G. Localization of hepatitis C virus in cutaneous vasculitic lesions in patients with type II cryoglobulinemia. Arthritis Rheum. 1997;40:2007–15.

16. Crovatto M, Pozzato G, Zorat F, et al. Peripheral blood neutrophils from hepatitis C virus-infected patients are replication sites of the virus. Haematologica. 2000;85:356–61.

17. Ducoulombier D, Roque-Afonso AM, Di Liberto G, et al. Frequent compartmentalization of hepatitis C virus variants in circulating B cells and monocytes. Hepatology. 2004;39: 817–25.

18. Ramos-Casals M, Loustaud-Ratti V, De Vita S, et al. Sjögren syndrome associated with hepatitis C virus: a multicenter analysis of 137 cases. Medicine (Baltimore). 2005;84:81–9.

19. Haddad J, Deny P, Munz-Gotheil C, et al. Lymphocytic sialadenitis of Sjögren's syndrome associated with chronic hepatitis C virus liver disease. Lancet. 1992;339:321–3.

20. Ramos-Casals M, Muñoz S, Zerón PB. Hepatitis C virus and Sjögren's syndrome: trigger or mimic? Rheum Dis Clin North Am. 2008;34:869–84.

21. Cacoub P, Poynard T, Ghillani P, et al. Extrahepatic manifestations of chronic hepatitis C. MULTIVIRC Group. Multidepartment Virus C. Arthritis Rheum. 1999;42:2204–12.

22. Sène D, Ghillani-Dalbin P, Limal N, et al. Anti-cyclic citrullinated peptide antibodies in hepatitis C virus associated rheumatological manifestations and Sjögren's syndrome. Ann Rheum Dis. 2006;65:394–7.

23. Caporali R, Bonacci E, Epis O, Bobbio-Pallavicini F, Morbini P, Montecucco C. Safety and usefulness of minor salivary gland biopsy: retrospective analysis of 502 procedures performed at a single center. Arthritis Rheum. 2008;59:714–20.

24. Koike K, Moriya K, Ishibashi K, et al. Sialadenitis histologically resembling Sjögren syndrome in mice transgenic for hepatitis C virus envelope genes. Proc Natl Acad Sci U S A. 1997;94:233–6.

25. De Vita S, Sansonno D, Dolcetti R, et al. Hepatitis C virus infection within a malignant lymphoma lesion in the course of type II mixed cryoglobulinemia. Blood. 1995;86:1887–92.

26. Ramos-Casals M, García-Carrasco M, Cervera R, et al. Sjögren's syndrome and hepatitis C virus. Clin Rheumatol. 1999;18:93–100.

27. Vitali C, Bombardieri S, Jonsson R, et al. Classification criteria for Sjögren's syndrome: a revised version of the European criteria proposed by the American-European Consensus Group. Ann Rheum Dis. 2002;61:554–8.

28. Han SH. Extrahepatic manifestations of chronic hepatitis B. Clin Liver Dis. 2004;8:403–18.

29. Godeau P, Guillevin L, Bletry O, Wechsler B. Periarteritis nodosa associated with hepatitis B virus. 42 cases. Nouv Presse Med. 1981;10:1289–92.

30. Maya R, Gershwin ME, Shoenfeld Y. Hepatitis B virus (HBV) and autoimmune disease. Clin Rev Allergy Immunol. 2008;34:85–102.
31. Permin H, Aldershvile J, Nielsen JO. Hepatitis B virus infection in patients with rheumatic diseases. Ann Rheum Dis. 1982;41:479–82.
32. Kallenberg CG, Tadema H. Vasculitis and infections: contribution to the issue of autoimmunity reviews devoted to "autoimmunity and infection". Autoimmun Rev. 2008;8:29–32.
33. Toussirot E, Lohse A, Wendling D, Mougin C. Sjögren's syndrome occurring after hepatitis B vaccination. Arthritis Rheum. 2000;43:2139–40.
34. Iakimtchouk K, Myrmel H, Jonsson R. Serological screening for hepatitis B and C and human herpesvirus 6 in Norwegian patients with primary Sjögren's syndrome. J Rheumatol. 1999;26:2065–6.
35. Aprosin ZG, Serov VV, Lopatkina TN. The hepatitis B virus as a probable etiological factor in Sjögren's disease. Ter Arkh. 1993;65:73–8.
36. Font J, Tàssies D, García-Carrasco M, Ramos-Casals M, Cervera R, Reverter JC, et al. Hepatitis G virus infection in primary Sjögren's syndrome: analysis in a series of 100 patients. Ann Rheum Dis. 1998;57(1):42–4.
37. Marcos M, Alvarez F, Brito-Zerón P, et al. Chronic hepatitis B virus infection in Sjögren's syndrome. Prevalence and clinical significance in 603 patients. Autoimmun Rev. 2009;8:616–20.
38. Salleras L, Dominguez A, Bruguera M, Plans P, Costa J, Cardenosa N, et al. Declining prevalence of hepatitis B virus infection in Catalonia (Spain) 12 years after the introduction of universal vaccination. Vaccine. 2007;25:8726–31.
39. Ram M, Anaya JM, Barzilai O, Izhaky D, Porat Katz BS, Blank M, et al. The putative protective role of hepatitis B virus (HBV) infection against autoimmune disorders. Autoimmun Rev. 2008;7:621–5.
40. Itescu S, Winchester R. Diffuse infiltrative lymphocytosis syndrome: a disorder occurring in human immunodeficiency virus-1 infection that may present as a sicca syndrome. Rheum Dis Clin North Am. 1992;18:683–97.
41. Kordossis T, Paikos S, Aroni K, et al. Prevalence of Sjögren's-like syndrome in a cohort of HIV-1-positive patients: descriptive pathology and immunopathology. Br J Rheumatol. 1998;37:691–5.
42. Williams FM, Cohen PR, Jumshyd J, Reveille JD. Prevalence of the diffuse infiltrative lymphocytosis syndrome among human immunodeficiency virus type 1-positive outpatients. Arthritis Rheum. 1998;41:863–8.
43. McArthur CP, Africa CW, Castellani WJ, et al. Salivary gland disease in HIV/AIDS and primary Sjögren's syndrome: analysis of collagen I distribution and histopathology in American and African patients. J Oral Pathol Med. 2003;32:544–51.
44. Panayiotakopoulos GD, Aroni K, Kyriaki D, et al. Paucity of Sjögren-like syndrome in a cohort of HIV-1-positive patients in the HAART era. Part II. Rheumatology (Oxford). 2003;42:1164–7.
45. Mastroianni A. Emergence of Sjögren's syndrome in AIDS patients during highly active antiretroviral therapy. AIDS. 2004;18:1349–52.
46. Ramos-Casals M, Brito-Zerón P, Font J. Lessons from diseases mimicking Sjögren's syndrome. Clin Rev Allergy Immunol. 2007;32:275–83.
47. Hida A, Kawabe Y, Kawakami A, et al. HTLV-I associated Sjögren's syndrome is aetiologically distinct from anti-centromere antibodies positive Sjögren's syndrome. Ann Rheum Dis. 1999;58:320–2.
48. Nakamura H, Kawakami A, Tominaga M, et al. Relationship between Sjögren's syndrome and human T-lymphotropic virus type I infection: follow-up study of 83 patients. J Lab Clin Med. 2000;135:139–44.
49. Nakamura H, Kawakami A, Hayashi T, et al. Low prevalence of ectopic germinal centre formation in patients with HTLV-I-associated Sjögren's syndrome. Rheumatology (Oxford). 2009;48:854–5.

50. Mariette X, Agbalika F, Zucker-Franklin D, et al. Detection of the tax gene of HTLV-I in labial salivary glands from patients with Sjögren's syndrome and other diseases of the oral cavity. Clin Exp Rheumatol. 2000;18:341–7.

51. Triantafyllopoulou A, Tapinos N, Moutsopoulos HM. Evidence for coxsackievirus infection in primary Sjögren's syndrome. Arthritis Rheum. 2004;50:2897–902.

52. Stathopoulou EA, Routsias JG, Stea EA, Moutsopoulos HM, Tzioufas AG. Cross-reaction between antibodies to the major epitope of Ro60 kD autoantigen and a homologous peptide of Coxsackie virus 2B protein. Clin Exp Immunol. 2005;141:148–54.

53. Youinou P, Pers JO, Saraux A, Pennec YL. Viruses contribute to the development of Sjögren's syndrome. Clin Exp Immunol. 2005;141:19–20.

54. Gottenberg JE, Pallier C, Ittah M, et al. Failure to confirm coxsackievirus infection in primary Sjögren's syndrome. Arthritis Rheum. 2006;54:2026–8.

55. Perrot S, Calvez V, Escande JP, Dupin N, Marcelin AG. Prevalences of herpesviruses DNA sequences in salivary gland biopsies from primary and secondary Sjögren's syndrome using degenerated consensus PCR primers. J Clin Virol. 2003;28:165–8.

56. Dawson TM, Starkebaum G, Wood BL, Willkens RF, Gown AM. Epstein-Barr virus, methotrexate, and lymphoma in patients with rheumatoid arthritis and primary Sjögren's syndrome: case series. J Rheumatol. 2001;28:47–53.

57. Inoue H, Tsubota K, Ono M, et al. Possible involvement of EBV-mediated alpha-fodrin cleavage for organ-specific autoantigen in Sjögren's syndrome. J Immunol. 2001;166:5801–9.

58. Trimeche M, Ziadi S, Amara K, Khelifa M, Bahri F, Mestiri S, et al. Prevalence of Epstein-Barr virus in Sjögren's syndrome in Tunisia. Rev Med Interne. 2006;27:519–23.

59. Klussmann JP, Wagner M, Guntinas-Lichius O, Muller A. Detection of HHV-8 sequences and antigens in a MALT lymphoma associated with Sjögren's syndrome. J Oral Pathol Med. 2003;32:243–5.

60. Ramos-Casals M, Cervera R, Garcia-Carrasco M, et al. Cytopenia and past human parvovirus B19 infection in patients with primary Sjögren's syndrome. Semin Arthritis Rheum. 2000;29:373–8.

61. De Re V, De Vita S, Battistella V, et al. Absence of human parvovirus B19 DNA in myoepithelial sialadenitis of primary Sjögren's syndrome. Ann Rheum Dis. 2002;61:855–6.

62. De Stefano R, Manganelli S, Frati E, et al. No association between human parvovirus B19 infection and Sjögren's syndrome. Ann Rheum Dis. 2003;62:86–7.

Chapter 5
Etiopathogenic Role of B Cells in Primary Sjögren's Syndrome

Jacques-Olivier Pers, Sophie Hillion, Gabriel Tobón, Valérie Devauchelle, Alain Saraux, and Pierre Youinou

Contents

Sjögren's syndrome (SjS) is an autoimmune epithelitis [1], the hallmarks of which are a disruption of epithelial cells and the infiltration by lymphocytes of lacrimal and salivary glands. The epithelitis and salivary gland infiltration typically lead to profound salivary gland dysfunction. SjS can develop as a primary disorder or against a background of other readily identified connective tissue disorders [2]. Among the permissive autoimmune settings are rheumatoid arthritis (RA), systemic sclerosis

J.-O. Pers • S. Hillion • G. Tobón • V. Devauchelle • A. Saraux
EA 2216 "Immunology and Pathology" and IFR 148 ScInBioS,
the European University of Brittany and the University of Brest,
and the Brest University Medical School Hospital, Brest, France

P. Youinou (✉)
EA 2216 "Immunology and Pathology" and IFR 148 ScInBioS,
the European University of Brittany and the University of Brest,
and the Brest University Medical School Hospital, Brest, France

Laboratory of Immunology, Brest University Medical School Hospital, Brest, France

M. Ramos-Casals et al. (eds.), *Sjögren's Syndrome*,
DOI 10.1007/978-0-85729-947-5_5, © Springer-Verlag London Limited 2012

Table 5.1 Arguments for Sjögren's syndrome as a "T-cell disease"	• Predominance of T cells in salivary gland infiltrates • Limited heterogeneity of the T-cell antigen receptors • Impaired proliferative potential of circulating T cells • Requirement of T cells for antibody class switching • Importance of T cells in the formation of germinal centers • T helper 1 profile of cytokines in the exocrine glands

(SSc), and systemic lupus erythematosus (SLE). Popular theories regarding the pathogenesis of SjS are that the condition is triggered by viruses [3] and modulated by sex hormones [4]. Its etiologic pathways appear to include a combination of environmental agents and genetic factors [5].

Lymphocytes are central to the pathogenesis of SjS. The epithelial structures of inflamed tissues in SjS are wrapped within a sheath of lymphocytes. However, controversy persists over which lymphocyte subtype initiates the process. Studies beginning in the 1980s focused upon disturbances in the T-cell compartment. SjS patients demonstrate a number of features that imply a greater role for T cells than B cells in the disease (Table 5.1). For example, T-cell infiltrates predominate within the salivary glands of SjS patients [6], have a restricted antigen repertoire, and display impaired proliferative capacity. Regulatory T cells (Treg cells) have been detected in salivary glands from SjS patients more recently [7]. Their presence correlates positively with lesion severity and negatively with their number in the blood [8]. However, the function of circulating Treg cells is believed to be normal in SjS [9]. In summary, one school of thought with regard to SjS pathogenesis holds that the influence of T cells is predominant, and the role of B lymphocytes is confined to antibody production.

Nonetheless, clinical and experimental evidence has sparked substantial interest in the possibility that B cells play critical roles in the pathogenesis of SjS. This greater appreciation of the importance of B cells does not necessarily imply that T cells are not also instrumental in SjS. Major breakthroughs in the understanding of B lymphocytes in health and disease are:

- The widespread availability of targeted recombinations in knock-out mice
- The dissection of B cell developmental stages [10]
- The profiling of B-cell-related gene expression using microarray technology [11]
- The dissection of candidate biomarkers by applying proteomic technologies [12]
- The discovery of two representatives of the tumor-necrosis factor (TNF) ligand family in the late 1990s [13]: A Proliferation-Inducing Ligand (APRIL), and the B-cell-Activating Factor (BAFF) of the TNF Family.

The clinical benefits obtained from the use of anti-B cell monoclonal antibodies have been ascribed to the purging of autoreactive B lymphocytes. It is conceivable that such autoreactive cells are the prime effectors in SjS, as it is known that T cells predominate in mild lesions but B cells become dominant in severe lesions [14].

	T1	T2	T3
IgM	+++	+++	++
IgD	–	–	–
CD21	–	++	++
CD23	–	++	++

Table 5.2 Phenotype of transitional B cells from type-1 (T1) through type-3 (T3)

5.1 The Role of T Cells in SjS

Three observations have weakened the dogma that T cells are central to SjS:

1. The process may occur when interferon (IFN) induces an excessive production of BAFF [15] by dendritic cells (DCs).
2. Antibody responses may develop outside the germinal centers [16].
3. Germinal centers can develop in the total absence of T cells [7]. By the same token, T lymphocytes do not appear to be mandatory for Ig class-switching to occur in SjS.

Germinal center evolution is initiated by immature [17] or mature transitional [18] B lymphocytes that have just migrated from the bone marrow to the peripheral blood. Once in the periphery, transitional B cells are engaged by their B-cell antigen receptor (BCRs) and promoted by follicular T helper (Th) cells and interdigitating dendritic cells upstream from the germinal centers [19] (Table 5.2). The requirement for T cells in this process that once seemed indisputable is now challenged by recent findings. For example, TNF deficiency fails to protect predisposed mice against SjS [20]. This experimental discovery is reminiscent of the clinical observation that a proportion of SjS patients develop ectopic germinal centers independent of T-cell-mediated inflammation [21].

T lymphocytes might also be advantageous for differentiation of naïve B lymphocytes into cytokine-producing B lymphocytes. According to the CD4+ T lymphocyte paradigm, Th1 cells secrete a specific array of cytokines, such as IFN-γ and interleukin (IL)-2. Both of these cytokines favor the T-cell-mediated arm of the response, and Th-2 cells secrete a different array of cytokines, such as IL-4 and IL-6, which prefer its B-cell-mediated arm. The production of IFN-γ and IL-2 by B effector (Be)-1 cells on one side and the elaboration of IL-4 and IL-6 by Be-2 cells on the other are regulated by Th-1 and Th-2 cells, respectively [22]. The beauty of such a model is that Be-1 and Be-2 polarize naïve CD4+ T cells toward Th-1 and Th-2 responses, respectively (Fig. 5.1). The Be-1 cells of the salivary glands of patients with SjS [23] may hence have been imprinted by Th-1 cells, but inversely this latter phenotype, which predominates over the Th2 at that site [24], might have been promoted by Be-1 cells [25].

It has been proposed that the Th-1/Th-2 balance changes with the progress of the immunopathological lesions in primary SjS and, concomitantly, with the cytotoxic T cell and antibody-producing B-cell involvement [26].

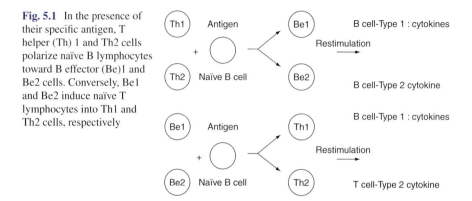

Fig. 5.1 In the presence of their specific antigen, T helper (Th) 1 and Th2 cells polarize naïve B lymphocytes toward B effector (Be)1 and Be2 cells. Conversely, Be1 and Be2 induce naïve T lymphocytes into Th1 and Th2 cells, respectively

5.2 The Role of B Cells in SjS

5.2.1 The Impact of B Cell Cytokines

Acting in synergy with one another, BAFF and APRIL behave as conclusive determinants of the development of autoimmune disorders (reviewed in [27]). These two B cell-specific cytokines have two receptors in common: TACI ("*t*ransmembrane-*a*ctivator, *c*alcium modulator and cytophilin ligand *i*nteractor"), and BCMA ("the *B*-*c*ell *m*aturation *a*ntigen"). In addition, BAFF (but not APRIL) binds to BR3, whereas APRIL (but not BAFF) binds to membrane heparin sulfate proteoglycans. Several reviews have touched on this topic (see for example [28]). When overexpressed in transgenic (Tg) mice, BAFF induces autoimmune disorders, with the emergence of an SLE [29] and the subsequent development of a SjS-like pattern [30].

BAFF are elevated in sera [31], saliva [32], and salivary glands [33] of patients with primary SjS. However, a number of conflicting results have cast doubt on the reliability of the enzyme-linked immunosorbent assays (ELISA) presently in use for its quantification. There is also the intriguing issue of why the serum concentrations of BAFF remain within, or below, normal range in a proportion of patients with SLE [34], RA [35], primary SjS [36], or SSc [37].

In addition, estimates of BAFF fluctuate with changes in inflammatory activity, extent of the damages, and classification criteria chosen by the investigators for the diseases. Furthermore, the disease activity correlates better with leukocyte BAFF messenger RNA amounts than with plasma BAFF protein titers [38]. Awareness of so many flaws prompted us to set up our own ELISA for the measurement of BAFF [39]. This in-house test appeared to be satisfactory, based on the finding that the majority of SjS patients display high serum levels of BAFF. We therefore considered the antibodies raised against synthetic peptides and used in certain ELISAs as capture or revealing agents. We reasoned that, the ELISA polyclonal antibodies or monoclonal antibodies recognize the nonglycosylated form of BAFF but not its glycosylated form, a bias might derive from excessive nonglycosylated BAFF, at the expense of its

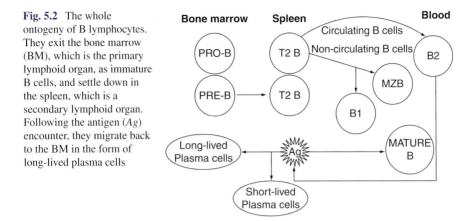

Fig. 5.2 The whole ontogeny of B lymphocytes. They exit the bone marrow (BM), which is the primary lymphoid organ, as immature B cells, and settle down in the spleen, which is a secondary lymphoid organ. Following the antigen (*Ag*) encounter, they migrate back to the BM in the form of long-lived plasma cells

glycosylated form, or from the presence of intergenic splice variants, such as Δ3 [40] and Δ4 BAFF (our unpublished results), or from the predominance of heterotrimers of BAFF and APRIL over homotrimers of BAFF [41] or even from the presence of enormous virus-like structures that contain 60 monomers of BAFF [42].

At first glance, the fact that the Th-17 lymphocyte subpopulation have recently been recognized as dominant within inflammatory tissues [43] does not fit with the B-cell dominance? One may suggest that the Th-17-centric cytokine IL-17 acts in synergy with BAFF to influence B-cell biology in various autoimmune settings. Supporting this hypothesis [44] is the intriguing observation that IL-17 and IL-17 receptor blocker exert opposite effects in mice with SjS.

B lymphocytes are thus stimulated, as reflected by the generation of a vast array of autoantibody-producing cells, including those nicely detected within plasma cells (PCs) in the salivary glands by the Jonsson's group [45]. Furthermore, IgA class rheumatoid factor (RF), IgA-containing immune-complexes [46], monoclonal Ig [47], and their particular presentation as mixed cryoglobulins [48], are not uncommon in these patients. Moreover, they document the existence of a continuum from benign to malignant lymphomas [49]. In this respect, Southern blot methods may detect B cell clonal expansions in the salivary glands of patients with SjS, without circulating monoclonal Ig [50].

5.2.2   *Ontogeny of B Lymphocytes*

A prolific approach to unraveling the function of the different B cell subsets has been to analyze their ontogeny. Figure 5.2 depicts the whole ontogeny from the bone marrow (BM), which is the primary lymphoid organ, to the spleen, which is a secondary lymphoid organ (SLO), and, following the antigen encounter, back to the BM in the form of long-lived PCs. On their arrival to the spleen, immature B cells give rise to type-1 (BT1), type-2 (BT2), and possibly type-3 [51] transitional

B cells. Only a minor fraction of immature B cells survive the shift from immature to the mature naïve stage, so that the transitional B-cell compartment is widely believed to represent a negative selection checkpoint for autoreactive B cells [52].

BAFF facilitates the maintenance of B cells through this checkpoint, to such an extent that crosstalk between BCR and BR3 emerges as a fundamental mechanism to regulate transitional B-cell survival [53]. The consequence of a local excess of BAFF is that self-reactive B cells are unduly rescued from deletion, and thereby offered the possibility to enter forbidden FO and marginal zone (MZ) niches [54]. Such upregulation of BAFF overcomes the reduced competitiveness of autoantigen-engaged B lymphocytes, due to their increased dependence on BAFF [55]. B lymphocytes differentiate into marginal-zone MZ or into FO B cells [56], depending on the affinity of the BCRs to their antigens [57]. Once entered the FO, the BT2 cells initiate the development of novel germinal centers, or colonize preexisting germinal centers [58].

In the salivary glands of patients with primary SjS, these structures have long been acknowledged as similar to those in SLOs. In reality, numerous MZ-like structures arise as aggregates in the tissue, locate distally to the genuine germinal centers, and position away from the epithelium [59]. Even worse, these aggregates and genuine ectopic germinal centers do not exclude autoreactive B cells as established in primary SjS [21], and SLE [60], through the binding of a 9 G4 monoclonal antibody that recognizes the anti-V4.34-encoded autoantibodies. We have compared the B cells of aggregates with those of ectopic genuine germinal centers. Of interesting note in terms of pathophysiology, the activation-induced cytidine deaminase (AID), required for Ig switch as well as somatic hypermutations [61], was detected [62]. This enzyme was expressed within the DC networks and interfollicular large B cells. The presence of AID suggests that these cell aggregates are functional.

5.2.3   Subpopulations of B Cells

Subsequent variations in the expression level of IgD and CD38 have led to a model for Bm homeostasis across the germinal centers. An inference from this proposal is that, once activated, naïve Bm1 lymphocytes become Bm2 cells, and develop into germinal center founder Bm2' cells. They differentiate further into centroblastic Bm3 cells, and centrocytic Bm4 cells, ending with early memory Bm5 and memory Bm5 or PCs. Throughout this process, cells representing each subset are released into the peripheral blood [63]. Patients with primary SjS exhibit disturbances in their distribution, mainly involving intrinsic B cell lymphoma (Bcl)-6 and increase in circulating Bm2/Bm2' cells [64], and a reciprocal decrease in early Bm5 and Bm5 cells [65]. Thus, not only are the B cells hyperactive in patients with SjS, but their distribution in their peripheral blood is disturbed. In these patients, there is a high ratio of increased percentages of circulating Bm2-plus-Bm2' cells to decreased percentages of early Bm5-plus-Bm5 cells that differentiates them (Fig. 5.3) from patients with RA or SLE [66], which is a case for B cells in the pathogenesis of primary SjS. Furthermore, this unique distribution of B cell subsets is a signature for primary SjS, relative to miscellaneous diseases, which might even constitute a diagnostic tool (Fig. 5.3).

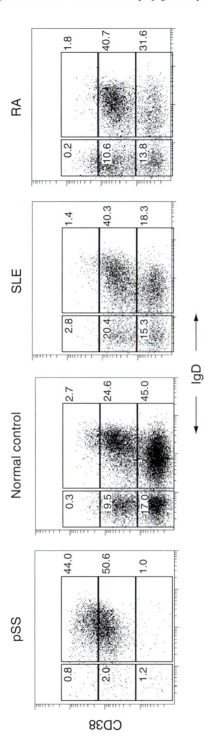
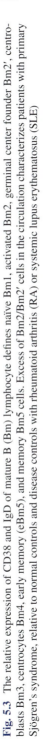

Fig. 5.3 The relative expression of CD38 and IgD of mature B (Bm) lymphocyte defines naïve Bm1, activated Bm2, germinal center founder Bm2′, centroblasts Bm3, centrocytes Bm4, early memory (eBm5), and memory Bm5 cells. Excess of Bm2/Bm2′ cells in the circulation characterizes patients with primary Sjögren's syndrome, relative to normal controls and disease controls with rheumatoid arthritis (RA) or systemic lupus erythematosus (SLE)

5.2.4 B Cell Monoclonal Expansion

Virtually all patients meeting the classification criteria for SjS [67] present with an association between salivary gland lymphocytes foci and ductal epithelial cell proliferation designated as lymphoproliferative sialadenitis. Straightaway, the question arises as to the relevance of such B cell aggregates to the pathophysiology of the syndrome. There are phenotypic findings to support that the salivary gland clusters of B cells are benign [68]. The issue turns as to why lymphoma develops at high frequency on the background of polyclonal proliferation of B cells in patients with SjS [49]. This issue was first addressed by Bunim and Talal who noticed that malignant lymphoma occurred in a patient with primary SjS [69]. Then, Talal and Bunim reported on the association of these two B-cell aberrations [70], and showed that the whole sequence from benign to malignant B proliferations was represented in the patients with primary SjS, but not in those with secondary SjS [71].

This seminal observation changes the view of lymphoma from an all-or-none phenomenon to one of a continuous spectrum of disease [72]. Ensuing studies revealed that widespread deregulation of lymphoid tissue complicates SjS. The clinical course and the evolution of patients with primary SjS and non-Hodgkin's lymphoma (NHL) has underlined the frequency of MZ [73] lymphoma, and extranodal manifestations [74]. Intriguingly, extra-salivary lymphoma may supersede the original autoimmune setting. The long duration of sicca symptoms and the appearance of benign salivary gland lesions indicate that SjS is the first to develop. Such findings highlight the importance to delineate the order of events leading to uncontrollable B-cell transformation. The presence of palpable purpura and low C4 levels at the first visit distinguishes the patients at risk of developing NHL from those with uncomplicated disease [75]. Neutropenia and cryoglobulinemia are also associated with an increased incidence of NHL [76], and RF-producing B lymphocytes are frequently involved in such proliferation [77]. Whatever it is, B cells have come under suspicion as the lymphocyte population that initiates the entire pathological process.

5.3 B Cells Are Not Dispensable

5.3.1 B Cell Chemokines and Antibody Production

Three pieces of evidence deserve now to be discussed to highlight the role of B lymphocytes. The first is the constitutively expressed but functionally impaired chemokine receptor CXCR3 for T cells on epithelial cells [78], coupled with the aberrantly expressed B-cell-attracting chemokine CXCL13 on epithelial cells [79], and lymphoid infiltrates [80] recruit SjS-related B cells expressing CXCR5 into the salivary glands [81]. Organ-specific inflammation might develop through the aberrant expression, of a single chemokine within a given tissue. This process seems, however, to be regulated by the accumulation of a certain mass of cells and the subsequent

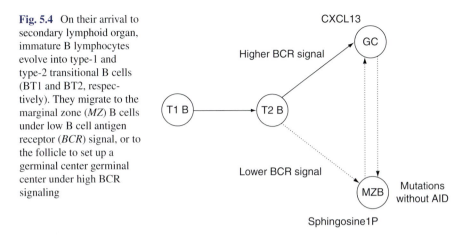

Fig. 5.4 On their arrival to secondary lymphoid organ, immature B lymphocytes evolve into type-1 and type-2 transitional B cells (BT1 and BT2, respectively). They migrate to the marginal zone (*MZ*) B cells under low B cell antigen receptor (*BCR*) signal, or to the follicle to set up a germinal center germinal center under high BCR signaling

production of lymphotoxins (LT). A particularly important function of B cells may be the effect they have on lymphoid neogenesis through the production of LT.

The second evidence for B cells is that certain autoantibodies encountered in this disease are pathogenic. An appealing example is the antimuscarinic receptor antibody that inhibits the mechanism of fluid secretion by human submandibular salivary acinar cells [82], and further alters the stimulated secretion of saliva when infused into nonobese diabetic Ig μ^{null} mice [83]. Similar pathogenic agents are, probably, anticarbonic anhydrase II [84], and, possibly anti-α-fodrin autoantibodies [85].

The third evidence is that treatment of primary SjS with a monoclonal antibody directed against CD20 has proved effective in depleting B cells from the blood [86] and the salivary glands [87] of these patients, and in relieving their complaints (reviewed in [88]).

5.3.2 Peculiarities of B Cell Products: Cytokines and IgA Autoantibodies

Three additional observations support aberrant B-cell function in SjS. Discovery of BAFF was not a tangential development, because BAFF is sufficient to induce a SjS-like disease with an expansion of BT2 and MZ B cells in the salivary glands of the mice [30]. Interestingly, we found similar features in B cells eluted from human salivary glands [21, 59]. Due to sphingosine 1-phosphate (see Fig. 5.4) inserted into its receptor, these MZ B cells might resist the CXCL13-mediated attraction toward the germinal centers [89]. The presence of this receptor on the surface of inflammatory mononuclear cells [90] facilitates the infiltration of these MZ B cells, where the receptor occupancy prevents their migration under the effect of CXCL13 [91]. IL-7 has also been suspected to favor the survival of lymphoid tissue B cells [92]. These findings do not prove that MZ B lymphocytes are pathogenic in SjS, but open up this possibly.

It is also relevant to the dysfunction of B lymphocytes that serum IgA are heavily glycosylated in primary SjS [93], owing to an excessive activity of α2-3- and α2-6-sialyl-transferases in B lymphocytes [94]. As a result, IgA with overexpression of sialic acid in both their Fab and Fc regions are not recognized by asialoglycoprotein receptors, and thereby accumulate in the serum [95]. The most important function of sialic acid is probably its ability to act as a biological mask, via steric hindrance and electrostatic repulsion. One may also speculate that such changes make the Ig pathogenic by influencing their conformation.

In addition, revision of the Ig genes coding for the BCR rescues autoreactive B cells in the periphery, aided by the recombination-activating genes (RAG)1- and RAG2-encoded enzymes [96]. Triple-nested reverse-transcriptase polymerase-chain reactions in single-sorted lymphocytes eluted from the salivary glands of SjS patients detected mRNAs for RAG1 and RAG2 in single B cells, but not in neighboring T cells [97], and their protein products were also identified in the salivary glands. Thus, ongoing B-cell stimulation may overwhelm the capacity of revision to prevent autoimmunity.

5.3.3 Intrinsic Abnormalities of B Cells in Primary SjS

The last three arguments against B cells as the main lymphocyte population in SjS are abnormalities detected in their molecular mechanisms. Pre-switch Ig transcripts are aberrantly retained in circulating post-switch memory B lymphocytes, although an ongoing switch is unlikely in the absence of transcripts for Bcl-6 [98] and AID [21]. Coexistence of transcripts for the two isotypes may perhaps be ascribed to a B cell intrinsic defect.

B cells are also peculiar in that their BCR partition, along with other proteins involved in cell signaling, partition into cholesterol and ganglioside M1-enriched microdomains of the cell membrane [99], termed lipid rafts (LRs). Interestingly, the association of the BCRs with the LRs persists, prolonging the signal transduction [33]. Finally, the single-cell analysis technology has proved that mRNA for BAFF exists in B cells from salivary glands. For this to occur, the downstream negative regulator of BAFF-mediated B-cell survival has to be inhibited [100].

Equally important in distinguishing the role of B cells in the pathogenesis of SjS is that BAFF potentiates the B cell selection with the BCR complex [101], and synergizes with IL-21 at that site [102]. Growing evidence suggests that the signaling mechanisms that maintain B-cell fitness during selection at transitional stages, and survival after maturation rely on cross-talk between BCR and one of the receptors for BAFF (recently highlighted in [103]). Of important note in this regard, there is an inverse correlation between the preexisting levels of BAFF and the number of months B cells take to repopulate the blood of rituximab-treated patients with primary SjS [104]. Supporting this concept are that some patients resist rituximab due to the local overexpression of BAFF in their salivary glands [105], and that human CD20-Tg autoimmune-prone mice with elevated levels of BAFF are resistant to rituximab, a monoclonal antibody directed against CD20 [106]. Thus, B cell infiltration would be modulated by BAFF in salivary glands [107], but not in lupus nephritis [108].

5.4   Conclusion

No doubt, there is a striking revival of interest in B lymphocytes as contributors to the cause of SjS. There are also significant unmet needs in the current approaches to patient management. Management of primary SjS is still palliative, aimed at diminishing symptoms, but new insights into B cell behavior have unveiled new approaches [109]. Treatments that target B lymphocytes for depletion are indeed gaining in popularity [110]. These findings afford a rationale behind the therapeutic use of monoclonal antibodies specific for B lymphocytes. Interestingly, the efficacy of B cell depletion is dissociated from changes in levels of autoantibodies, due to ongoing activity of long-lived PCs. There is a reduction in the level of RF, which derived from short-lived PCs. In the absence of B cells upstream these PCs are not produced anymore. It is all the more convincing that previous monoclonal antibodies aimed at killing the T cells have proved disappointing (reviewed in [111]). On the other hand, the therapeutic use of antagonists of BAFF [112] has thus far been disappointing [113].

Acknowledgments   We are grateful to Geneviève Michel and Simone Forest for cheerful and expert secretarial assistance.

References

1. Moutsopoulos HM. Sjögren's syndrome: autoimmune epithelitis. Clin Immunol Immunopathol. 1994;72:162–5.
2. Delaleu N, Jonsson R, Koller MM. Sjögren's syndrome. Eur J Oral Sci. 2005;113:101–13.
3. Youinou P, Pers JO, Saraux A, Pennec YL. Viruses contribute to the development of Sjögren's syndrome. Clin Exp Immunol. 2005;141:19–20.
4. Forsblad-d'Elia H, Carlsten H, Labrie F, Konttinen YT, Ohlsson C. Low serum levels of steroids are associated with disease characteristics in primary Sjögren's syndrome. Supplementation with DHA restores the concentrations. J Clin Endocrinol Metab. 2009;94:2044–51.
5. Anaya JM, Delgado-Vega AM, Castiblanco J. Genetic basis of Sjögren's syndrome. How strong is the evidence? Clin Dev Immunol. 2006;13:209–22.
6. Adamson 3rd TC, Fox RI, Frisman DM, Howell FV. Immunohistologic analysis of lymphoid infiltrates in primary Sjögren's syndrome using monoclonal antibodies. J Immunol. 1983;130:203–8.
7. Lentz VM, Manser T. Cutting edge: germinal centers can be induced in the absence of T cells. J Immunol. 2001;167:15–20.
8. Christodoulou MI, Kapsogeorgou EK, Moutsopoulos NM, Moutsopoulos HM. Foxp3+ T-regulatory cells in Sjögren's syndrome: correlation with the grade of the autoimmune lesion and certain adverse prognostic factors. Am J Pathol. 2008;173:1389–96.
9. Gottenberg JE, Lavie F, Abbed K, Gasnault J, Le Nevot E, Delfraissy JF, et al. CD4 CD25 high regulatory T cells are not impaired in patients with primary Sjögren's syndrome. J Autoimmun. 2005;24:235–42.
10. Schmidlin H, Diehl SA, Blom B. New insights into the regulation of human B-cell differentiation. Trends Immunol. 2009;30:277–85.
11. Hoheisel JD. Microarray technology: beyond transcript profiling and genotype analysis. Nat Rev Genet. 2006;7:200–10.

12. Baldini C, Giusti L, Bazzichi L, Lucacchini A, Bombardieri S. Proteomic analysis of the saliva: a clue for understanding primary from secondary Sjögren's syndrome? Autoimmun Rev. 2008;7:185–91.
13. Mackay F, Schneider P, Rennert P, Browning J. BAFF and APRIL: a tutorial on B cell survival. Annu Rev Immunol. 2003;21:231–64.
14. Christodoulou MI, Kapsogeorgou EK, Moutsopoulos HM. Characteristics of the minor salivary gland infiltrates in Sjögren's syndrome. J Autoimmun. 2009;34(4):400–7 [Epub ahead of print].
15. Litinskiy MB, Nardelli B, Hilbert DM, He B, Schaffer A, Casali P, et al. DCs induce CD40-independent Ig class switching through BLyS and APRIL. Nat Immunol. 2002;3:822–9.
16. William J, Euler C, Christensen S, Shlomchik MJ. Evolution of autoantibody responses *via* somatic hypermutation outside of germinal centers. Science. 2002;297:2066–70.
17. Lee J, Kuchen S, Fischer R, Chang S, Lipsky PE. Identification and characterization of a human CD5+ pre-naive B cell population. J Immunol. 2009;182:4116–26.
18. Sims GP, Ettinger R, Shirota Y, Yarboro CH, Illei GG, Lipsky PE. Identification and characterization of circulating human transitional B cells. Blood. 2005;105:4390–8.
19. Paus D, Phan TG, Chan TD, Gardam S, Basten A, Brink R. Antigen recognition strength regulates the choice extrafollicular plasma cell and germinal center B cell differentiation. J Exp Med. 2006;203:1081–91.
20. Batten M, Fletcher C, Ng LG, Groom J, Wheway J, Laâbi Y, et al. TNF deficiency fails to protect BAFF transgenic mice against autoimmunity and reveals a predisposition to B cell lymphoma. J Immunol. 2004;172:812–22.
21. Le Pottier L, Devauchelle V, Fautrel A, Daridon C, Saraux A, Youinou P, et al. Ectopic germinal centers are rare in Sjögren's syndrome salivary glands and do not exclude autoreactive B cells. J Immunol. 2009;182:3540–7.
22. Harris DP, Haynes L, Sayles PC, Duso DK, Eaton SM, Lepak NM, et al. Reciprocal regulation of polarized cytokine production by B and T cells. Nat Immunol. 2000;1:475–82.
23. Daridon C, Guerrier T, Devauchelle V, Saraux A, Pers JO, Youinou P. Polarization of B effector cells in Sjögren's syndrome. Autoimmun Rev. 2007;6:427–31.
24. Kolkowski EC, Reth P, Pelusa F, Bosch J, Pujol-Borrell R, Coll J, et al. Th1 predominance and perforin expression in minor salivary glands from patients with primary Sjögren's syndrome. J Autoimmun. 1999;13:155–62.
25. Harris DP, Goodrich S, Gerth AJ, Peng SL, Lund FE. Regulation of IFN-gamma production by B effector 1 cells: essential roles for T-bet and the IFN-gamma receptor. J Immunol. 2005;174:6781–90.
26. Mitsias DI, Tzioufas AG, Veiopoulou C, Zintzaras E, Tassios IK, Kogopoulou O, et al. The Th1/Th2 cytokine balance changes with the progress of the immunopathological lesion of Sjögren's syndrome. Clin Exp Immunol. 2002;128:562–8.
27. Mackay F, Silveira PA, Brink R. B cells and the BAFF/APRIL axis: fast-forward on autoimmunity and signaling. Curr Opin Immunol. 2007;19:327–36.
28. Mackay F, Schneider P. Cracking the BAFF code. Nat Rev Immunol. 2009;9:491–502.
29. Mackay F, Woodcock SA, Lawton P, Ambrose C, Baetscher M, Schneider P, et al. Mice transgenic for BAFF develop lymphocytic disorders along with autoimmune manifestations. J Exp Med. 1999;190:1697–710.
30. Groom J, Kalled SL, Cutler AH, Olson C, Woodcock SA, Schneider P, et al. Association of BAFF/BLyS overexpression and altered B cell differentiation with Sjögren's syndrome. J Clin Invest. 2002;109:59–68.
31. Mariette X, Roux S, Zhang J, Bengoufa D, Lavie F, Zhou T, et al. The level of BLyS (BAFF) correlates with the titre of autoantibodies in human Sjögren's syndrome. Ann Rheum Dis. 2003;62:168–71.
32. Pers JO, Arbonneau F, Devauchelle-Pensec V, Saraux A, Pennec YL, Youinou P. Is periodontal disease mediated by salivary BAFF in Sjögren's syndrome? Arthritis Rheum. 2005;52:2411–4.
33. d'Arbonneau F, Pers JO, Devauchelle V, Pennec Y, Saraux A, Youinou P. BAFF-induced changes in B cell antigen receptor-containing lipid rafts in Sjögren's syndrome. Arthritis Rheum. 2006;54:115–26.

34. Zhang J, Roschke V, Baker KP, Wang Z, Alarcón GS, Fessler BJ, et al. Cutting edge: a role for B lymphocyte stimulator in systemic lupus erythematosus. J Immunol. 2001;166:6–10.
35. Cheema GS, Roschke V, Hilbert DM, Stohl W. Elevated serum B lymphocyte stimulator levels in patients with systemic immune-based rheumatic diseases. Arthritis Rheum. 2001;44: 1313–9.
36. Pers JO, Daridon C, Devauchelle V, Jousse S, Saraux A, Jamin C, et al. BAFF overexpression is associated with autoantibody production in autoimmune diseases. Ann N Y Acad Sci. 2005;1050:34–9.
37. Matsushita T, Hasegawa M, Yanaba K, Kodera M, Takehara K, Sato S. Elevated serum BAFF levels in patients with systemic sclerosis: enhanced BAFF signaling in systemic sclerosis B lymphocytes. Arthritis Rheum. 2006;54:192–201.
38. Collins CE, Gavin AL, Migone TS, Hilbert DM, Nemazee D, Stohl W. B lymphocyte stimulator (BLyS) isoforms in systemic lupus erythematosus: disease activity correlates better with blood leukocyte BLyS mRNA levels than with plasma BlyS protein levels. Arthritis Res Ther. 2006;8:R6.
39. Le Pottier L, Bendaoud B, Renaudineau Y, Youinou P, Pers JO, Daridon C. New ELISA for B cell-activating factor. Clin Chem. 2009;55:1843–51.
40. Gavin AL, Aït-Azzouzene D, Ware CF, Nemazee D. DeltaBAFF, an alternate splice isoform that regulates receptor binding and biopresentation of the B cell survival cytokine, BAFF. J Biol Chem. 2003;278:38220–8.
41. Roschke V, Sosnovtseva S, Ward CD, Hong JS, Smith R, Albert V, et al. BLyS and APRIL form biologically active heterotrimers that are expressed in patients with systemic immune-based rheumatic diseases. J Immunol. 2002;169:4314–21.
42. Liu Y, Xu L, Opalka N, Kappler J, Shu HB, Zhang G. Crystal structure of sTALL-1 reveals a virus-like assembly of TNF family ligands. Cell. 2002;108:383–94.
43. Katsifis GE, Rekka S, Moutsopoulos NM, Pillemer S, Wahl SM. Systemic and local IL-17 and linked cytokines associated with Sjögren's syndrome immunopathogenesis. Am J Pathol. 2009;175:1167–77.
44. Doreau A, Belot A, Bastid J, Riche B, Trescol-Biemont MC, Ranchin B, et al. IL-17 acts in synergy with B cell-activating factor to influence B cell biology and the pathophysiology of systemic lupus erythematosus. Nat Immunol. 2009;10:778–85.
45. Tengnér P, Halse AK, Haga HJ, Jonsson R, Wahren-Herlenius M. Detection of anti-Ro/SjSA and anti-La/SjSB autoantibody-producing cells in salivary glands from patients with Sjögren's syndrome. Arthritis Rheum. 1998;41:2238–48.
46. Bendaoud B, Pennec YL, Lelong A, Le Noac'h JF, Magadur G, Jouquan J, et al. IgA-containing immune complexes in the circulation of patients with primary Sjögren's syndrome. J Autoimmun. 1991;4:177–84.
47. Sugai S, Konda S, Shoraski Y, Murayama T, Nishikawa T. Non-IgM monoclonal gammopathy in patients with Sjögren's syndrome. Am J Med. 1980;68:861–6.
48. Tzioufas AG, Manoussakis MN, Costello R, Silis M, Papadopoulos NM, Moutsopoulos HM. Cryoglobulinemia in autoimmune rheumatic diseases. Evidence of circulating monoclonal cryoglobulins in patients with primary Sjögren's syndrome. Arthritis Rheum. 1986;29:1098–104.
49. Masaki Y, Sugai S. Lymphoproliferative disorders in Sjögren's syndrome. Autoimmun Rev. 2004;3:175–82.
50. Fishleder A, Tubbs R, Hesse B, Levine H. Uniform detection of immunoglobulin-gene rearrangement in benign lymphoepithelial lesions. N Engl J Med. 1987;316:1118–21.
51. Palanichamy A, Barnard J, Zheng B, Owen T, Quach T, Wei C, et al. Novel human transitional B cell populations revealed by B cell depletion therapy. J Immunol. 2009;182:5982–93.
52. Carsetti R, Rosado MM, Wardmann H. Peripheral development of B cells in mouse and man. Immunol Rev. 2004;197:179–91.
53. Smith SH, Cancro MP. Cutting edge: B cell receptor signals regulate BLyS receptor levels in mature B cells and their immediate progenitors. J Immunol. 2003;170:5820–3.
54. Thien M, Phan TG, Gardam S, Amesbury M, Basten A, Mackay F, et al. Excess BAFF rescues self-reactive B cells from peripheral deletion and allows them to enter forbidden follicular and marginal zone niches. Immunity. 2004;20:785–98.

55. Lesley R, Xu Y, Kalled SL, Hess DM, Schwab SR, Shu HB, et al. Reduced competitiveness of autoantigen-engaged B cells due to increased dependence on BAFF. Immunity. 2004;20: 441–53.
56. Weill JC, Weller S, Reynaud CA. Human marginal zone B cells. Annu Rev Immunol. 2009; 27:267–85.
57. Kouskoff V, Famiglietti S, Lacaud G, Lang P, Rider JE, Kay BK, et al. Antigens varying in affinity for the BCR induce differential B lymphocyte responses. J Exp Med. 1998;188: 1453–64.
58. Schwickert TA, Alabyev B, Manser T, Nussenzweig MC. Germinal center reutilization by newly activated B cells. J Exp Med. 2009;206:2907–14.
59. Daridon C, Pers JO, Devauchelle V, Martins-Carvalho C, Hutin P, Pennec YL, et al. Identification of transitional type II B cells in the salivary glands of patients with Sjögren's syndrome. Arthritis Rheum. 2006;54:2280–8.
60. Cappione 3rd A, Anolik JH, Pugh-Bernard A, Barnard J, Dutcher P, Silverman G, et al. Germinal center exclusion of autoreactive B cells is defective in human systemic lupus erythematosus. J Clin Invest. 2005;115:3205–16.
61. Honjo T, Muramatsu M, Fagarasan S. AID: how does it aid antibody diversity? Immunity. 2004;20:659–68.
62. Bombardieri M, Barone F, Humby F, Kelly S, McGurk M, Morgan P, et al. AID expression in follicular dendritic cell networks and interfollicular large B cells supports functionality of ectopic lymphoid neogenesis in autoimmune sialoadenitis and MALT lymphoma in Sjögren's syndrome. J Immunol. 2007;179:4929–38.
63. Pascual V, Liu YJ, Magalski A, de Bouteiller O, Banchereau J, Capra JD. Analysis of somatic mutation in five B cell subsets of human tonsil. J Exp Med. 1994;180:329–39.
64. Bohnhorst JØ, Bjørgan MB, Thoen JE, Natvig JB, Thompson KM. Bm1-Bm5 classification of peripheral blood B cells reveals circulating germinal center founder cells in healthy individuals and disturbance in the B cell subpopulations in patients with primary Sjögren's syndrome. J Immunol. 2001;167:3610–8.
65. Hansen A, Gosemann M, Pruss A, Reiter K, Ruzickova S, Lipsky PE, et al. Abnormalities in peripheral B cell memory of patients with primary Sjögren's syndrome. Arthritis Rheum. 2004;50:1897–908.
66. Binard A, Le Pottier L, Devauchelle-Pensec V, Saraux A, Youinou P, Pers JO. Is the blood B-cell subset profile diagnostic for Sjögren syndrome? Ann Rheum Dis. 2009;68: 1447–52.
67. Vitali C, Bombardieri S, Jonsson R, Moutsopoulos HM, Alexander EL, Carsons SE, et al. Classification criteria for Sjögren's syndrome: a revised version of the European criteria by the American-European Consensus Group. Ann Rheum Dis. 2002;61:554–8.
68. Brandtzaeg P, Johansen FE. Mucosal B cells: phenotypic characteristics, transcriptional regulation, and homing properties. Immunol Rev. 2005;206:32–63.
69. Bunim JJ, Talal N. The association of malignant lymphoma with Sjögren's syndrome. Trans Assoc Am Physicians. 1963;76:45–56.
70. Talal N, Bunim JJ. The development of malignant lymphoma in the course of Sjögren's syndrome. Am J Med. 1964;36:529–40.
71. Anderson LG, Talal N. The spectrum of benign to malignant lymphoproliferation in Sjögren's syndrome. Clin Exp Immunol. 1972;10:199–221.
72. Jonsson R, Kroneld U, Bäckman K, Magnusson B, Tarkowski A. Progression of sialadenitis in Sjögren's syndrome. Br J Rheumatol. 1993;32:578–81.
73. Royer B, Cazals-Hatem D, Sibilia J, Agbalika F, Cayuela JM, Soussi T, et al. Lymphomas in patients with Sjogren's syndrome are marginal zone B-cell neoplasms, arise in diverse extranodal and nodal sites, and are not associated with viruses. Blood. 1997;90:766–75.
74. Voulgarelis M, Dafni UG, Isenberg DA, Moutsopoulos HM. Malignant lymphoma in primary Sjögren's syndrome: a multicenter, retrospective, clinical study by the European Concerted Action on Sjögren's Syndrome. Arthritis Rheum. 1999;42:1765–72.
75. Ioannidis JP, Vassiliou VA, Moutsopoulos HM. Long-term risk of mortality and lymphoproliferative disease and predictive classification of primary Sjögren's syndrome. Arthritis Rheum. 2002;46:741–7.

76. Baimpa E, Dahabreh IJ, Voulgarelis M, Moutsopoulos HM. Hematologic manifestations and predictors of lymphoma development in primary Sjögren syndrome: clinical and pathophysiologic aspects. Medicine (Baltimore). 2009;88:284–93.
77. Martin T, Weber JC, Levallois H, Labouret N, Soley A, Koenig S, et al. Salivary gland lymphomas in patients with Sjögren's syndrome may frequently develop from rheumatoid factor B cells. Arthritis Rheum. 2000;43:908–16.
78. Sfriso P, Oliviero F, Calabrese F, Miorin M, Facco M, Contri A, et al. Epithelial CXCR3-B regulates chemokines bioavailability in normal, but not in Sjögren's syndrome, salivary glands. J Immunol. 2006;176:2581–9.
79. Amft N, Curnow SJ, Scheel-Toellner D, Devadas A, Oates J, Crocker J, et al. Ectopic expression of the B cell-attracting chemokine BCA-1 (CXCL13) on endothelial cells and within lymphoid follicles contributes to the establishment of germinal center-like structures in Sjögren's syndrome. Arthritis Rheum. 2001;44:2633–41.
80. Barone F, Bombardieri M, Manzo A, Blades MC, Morgan PR, Challacombe SJ, et al. Association of CXCL13 and CCL21 expression with the progressive organization of lymphoid-like structures in Sjögren's syndrome. Arthritis Rheum. 2005;52:1773–84.
81. Hansen A, Reiter K, Ziprian T, Jacobi A, Hoffmann A, Gosemann M, et al. Dysregulation of chemokine receptor expression and function by B cells of patients with primary Sjögren's syndrome. Arthritis Rheum. 2005;52:2109–19.
82. Dawson LJ, Stanbury J, Venn N, Hasdimir B, Rogers SN, Smith PM. Antimuscarinic antibodies in primary Sjögren's syndrome reversibly inhibit the mechanism of fluid secretion by human submandibular salivary acinar cells. Arthritis Rheum. 2006;54:1165–73.
83. Robinson CP, Brayer J, Yamachika S, Esch TR, Peck AB, Stewart CA, et al. Transfer of human serum IgG to nonobese diabetic Igmu null mice reveals a role for autoantibodies in the loss of secretory function of exocrine tissues in Sjögren's syndrome. Proc Natl Acad Sci U S A. 1998;95:7538–43.
84. Takemoto F, Katori H, Sawa N, Hoshino J, Suwabe T, Sogawa Y, et al. Induction of anti-carbonic-anhydrase-II antibody causes renal tubular acidosis in a mouse model of Sjogren's syndrome. Nephron Physiol. 2007;106:63–8.
85. Haneji N, Nakamura T, Takio K, Yanagi K, Higashiyama H, Saito I, et al. Identification of alpha-fodrin as a candidate autoantigen in primary Sjögren's syndrome. Science. 1997;276:604–7.
86. Pijpe J, van Imhoff GW, Spijkervet FK, Roodenburg JL, Wolbink GJ, Mansour K, et al. Rituximab treatment in patients with primary Sjögren's syndrome: an open-label phase II study. Arthritis Rheum. 2005;52:2740–50.
87. Devauchelle-Pensec V, Pennec Y, Morvan J, Pers JO, Daridon C, Jousse-Joulin S, et al. Improvement of Sjögren's syndrome after two infusions of rituximab. Arthritis Rheum. 2007;57:310–7.
88. Saraux A. The point on the ongoing B-cell depleting trials currently in progress over the world in primary Sjögren's syndrome. Autoimmun Rev. 2010;9(9):609–14.
89. Cinamon G, Matloubian M, Lesneski MJ, Xu Y, Low C, Lu T, et al. Sphingosine 1-phosphate receptor 1 promotes B cell localization in the splenic marginal zone. Nat Immunol. 2004;5:713–20.
90. Sekiguchi M, Iwasaki T, Kitano M, Kuno H, Hashimoto N, Kawahito Y, et al. Role of sphingosine 1-phosphate in the pathogenesis of Sjögren's syndrome. J Immunol. 2008;180:1921–8.
91. Cinamon G, Zachariah MA, Lam OM, Foss Jr FW, Cyster JG. Follicular shuttling of marginal zone B cells facilitates antigen transport. Nat Immunol. 2008;9:54–62.
92. Meier D, Bornmann C, Chappaz S, Schmutz S, Otten LA, Ceredig R, et al. Ectopic lymphoid-organ development occurs through interleukin 7-mediated enhanced survival of lymphoid-tissue-inducer cells. Immunity. 2007;26:643–54.
93. Basset C, Durand V, Jamin C, Clément J, Pennec Y, Youinou P, et al. Increased N-linked glycosylation leading to oversialylation of monomeric immunoglobulin A1 from patients with Sjögren's syndrome. Scand J Immunol. 2000;51:300–6.
94. Basset C, Durand V, Mimassi N, Pennec YL, Youinou P, Dueymes M. Enhanced sialyltransferase activity in B lymphocytes from patients with primary Sjögren's syndrome. Scand J Immunol. 2000;51:307–11.
95. Basset C, Devauchelle V, Durand V, Jamin C, Pennec YL, Youinou P, et al. Glycosylation of immunoglobulin A influences its receptor binding. Scand J Immunol. 1999;50:572–9.

96. Nemazee D, Weigert M. Revising B cell receptors. J Exp Med. 2000;191:1813–7.
97. Daridon C, Devauchelle V, Hutin P, Le Berre R, Martins-Carvalho C, Bendaoud B, et al. Aberrant expression of BAFF by B lymphocytes infiltrating the salivary glands of patients with primary Sjögren's syndrome. Arthritis Rheum. 2007;56:1134–44.
98. Kusam S, Dent A. Common mechanisms for the regulation of B cell differentiation and transformation by the transcriptional repressor protein Bcl-6. Immunol Res. 2007;37:177–86.
99. Pierce SK. Lipid rafts and B-cell activation. Nat Rev Immunol. 2002;2:96–105.
100. Qian Y, Qin J, Cui G, Naramura M, Snow EC, Ware CF, et al. Act1, a negative regulator in CD40- and BAFF-mediated B cell survival. Immunity. 2004;21:575–87.
101. Hase H, Kanno Y, Kojima M, Hasegawa K, Sakurai D, Kojima H, et al. BAFF/BLyS can potentiate B-cell selection with the B-cell coreceptor complex. Blood. 2004;103:2257–65.
102. Ettinger R, Sims GP, Robbins R, Withers D, Fischer RT, Grammer AC, et al. IL-21 and BAFF/BLyS synergize in stimulating plasma cell differentiation from a unique population of human splenic memory B cells. J Immunol. 2007;178:2872–82.
103. Khan WN. B cell receptor and BAFF receptor signaling regulation of B cell homeostasis. J Immunol. 2009;183:3561–7.
104. Pers JO, Devauchelle V, Daridon C, Bendaoud B, Le Berre R, Bordron A, et al. BAFF-modulated repopulation of B lymphocytes in the blood and salivary glands of rituximab-treated patients with Sjögren's syndrome. Arthritis Rheum. 2007;56:1464–77.
105. Quartuccio L, Fabris M, Moretti M, Barone F, Bombardieri M, Rupolo M, et al. Resistance to rituximab therapy and local BAFF overexpression in Sjögren's syndrome-related myoepithelial sialadenitis and low-grade parotid B-cell lymphoma. Open Rheumatol J. 2008; 2:38–43.
106. Ahuja A, Shupe J, Dunn R, Kashgarian M, Kehry MR, Shlomchik MJ. Depletion of B cells in murine lupus: efficacy and resistance. J Immunol. 2007;179:3351–61.
107. Jonsson MV, Szodoray P, Jellestad S, Jonsson R, Skarstein K. Association between circulating levels of the novel TNF family members APRIL and BAFF and lymphoid organization in primary Sjögren's syndrome. J Clin Immunol. 2005;25:189–201.
108. Fletcher CA, Sutherland AP, Groom JR, Batten ML, Ng LG, Gommerman J, et al. Development of nephritis but not sialadenitis in autoimmune-prone BAFF transgenic mice lacking marginal zone B cells. Eur J Immunol. 2006;36:2504–14.
109. Edwards JC, Cambridge G. B-cell targeting in rheumatoid arthritis and other autoimmune diseases. Nat Rev Immunol. 2006;6:394–403.
110. Blank M, Shoenfeld Y. B cell-targeted therapy in autoimmunity. J Autoimmun. 2007;28:62–8.
111. Ramos-Casals M, Brito-Zerón P. Emerging biological therapies in primary Sjögren's syndrome. Rheumatology (Oxford). 2007;46:1389–96.
112. Kalled SL. BAFF: a novel therapeutic target for autoimmunity. Curr Opin Investig Drugs. 2002;3:1005–10.
113. Dall'Era M, Chakravarty E, Wallace D, Genovese M, Weisman M, Kavanaugh A, et al. Reduced B lymphocyte and immunoglobulin levels after atacicept treatment in patients with SLE: results of a multicenter, phase Ib, double-blind, placebo-controlled, dose-escalating trial. Arthritis Rheum. 2007;56:4142–50.

Part II
Clinical Manifestations

Chapter 6
Oral Involvement

Crispian Scully and Eleni A. Georgakopoulou

Contents

C. Scully (✉)
Division of Maxillofacial Diagnostic, Medical and Surgical Sciences,
University College London (UCL) – Eastman Dental Institute, London, UK

E.A. Georgakopoulou
First Department of Dermatology and Venereology, A. Syggros Hospital,
School of Medicine, University of Athens, Athens, Greece

M. Ramos-Casals et al. (eds.), *Sjögren's Syndrome*,
DOI 10.1007/978-0-85729-947-5_6, © Springer-Verlag London Limited 2012

Table 6.1 Whole saliva flow rates (mL/min)

	Normal	Hyposalivation
Unstimulated (resting)	0.3–0.4 mL/min	<0.1 mL/min
Stimulated	1–2 mL/min	<0.5 mL/min

Whole saliva = total output from the major and minor salivary glands

6.1   Introduction

This chapter summarizes the orofacial involvement in Sjögren syndrome (SS). Oral manifestations of SS are mainly xerostomia and hyposalivation, autoimmune sialadenitis causing salivary gland swelling, and secondary manifestations such as dental caries, oral candidiasis, bacterial sialadenitis, oral malodour, and oral ulcers. These secondary manifestations are the first features of the disease to become evident in approximately half of the patients with primary SS, and their identification is important for early diagnosis. Furthermore, as most SS patients consider oral complications a major factor of quality of life deterioration [1], their treatment should be a priority.

6.2   Definitions

Xerostomia, the subjective complaint of oral dryness, is the most common salivary complaint among patients with SS, but this symptom is not specific for SS. The symptom of xerostomia may or may not reflect decreased salivation (hyposalivation). Hyposalivation is usually defined as an unstimulated whole salivary flow rate <0.1 mL/min.

6.3   Objective Determination of Salivary Flow

The normal salivary flow rate varies widely from person to person. Thus, unless baseline salivary flow rates for individual patients are known, it is rarely possible to determine if there has been a reduction in salivary flow.

Unstimulated salivary flow rate (USFR) measurement of whole saliva uses a simple draining test for 5 min at rest. If the saliva produced during this test is less or equal to 0.1 mL/min, the patient has hyposalivation. Normal and reference values are shown in Table 6.1 [2, 3].

The Saxon test is a simple, reproducible, and low-cost test for xerostomia, which involves chewing on a folded sterile sponge for 2 min. Saliva production is quantified by weighing the sponge before and after chewing. Normal control subjects produce ≥2.75 g of saliva in 2 min [4].

Because salivary flow rates vary over time for each individual, the salivary tests used as a diagnostic aid for SS diagnosis should be performed on several occasions [5].

6.4   Etiology of Xerostomia

Many patients complain of a dry mouth but yet lack objective evidence of hyposalivation (hyposialia). The feeling of oral dryness is associated with a lack of saliva, yet many patients with hyposalivation do not complain of dry mouth. Because oral dryness is a subjective complaint, it is not surprising that there is a huge variation in the patient's threshold of discomfort or other symptoms. Xerostomia is also impacted by tolerance and adaptation over time.

Older patients in particular often complain of a dry mouth; indeed, in the older age groups, up to 25% of patients have this complaint. Medications are usually responsible for this symptom in such cases [6, 7], but 10% of healthy young adults also complain of persistent xerostomia and note that it influences their overall quality of life [8].

A 15-year longitudinal study of xerostomia in people between 50 and 65 years of age showed an almost linear increase with age in the prevalence of xerostomia [9]. Dry mouth is also a common peri- and postmenopausal symptom [10].

In general, however, in HEALTHY men and women, there are NO age-associated differences in parotid and submandibular salivary flow rates, either at rest and with 2% citrate stimulation [11].

Xerostomia can stem from many causes other than SS (Table 6.2). The cause of xerostomia is sometimes simple such as smoking or mouth-breathing [12]. Smokers often complain of daytime xerostomia [9]. Medications are the most common cause. Medications with anticholinergic or sympathomimetic activity are the most frequent offenders. Irradiation of the major salivary glands as part of cancer therapy and bone marrow transplants often lead to xerostomia.

The main other causes of hyposalivation to be considered in the proper circumstances are dehydration, HIV disease, hepatitis C virus infection, and sarcoidosis (Algorithm 6.1).

6.5   Orofacial Manifestations in SS

Diminished salivary gland function and parotid gland enlargement are among the most prevalent manifestations in SS [13] but there are others, as shown in Table 6.3.

SS may affect not only the salivary glands but may also result in neurological manifestations.

6.5.1   Salivary Involvement

Hyposalivation has been recognized as a prominent feature of SS since the first descriptions of the syndrome. Because saliva is essential to oral health, patients who have hyposalivation have difficulty with functions such as swallowing and speech, and may develop oral or salivary gland infections. Some complain of a burning sensation within the mouth [14].

Table 6.2 Causes of xerostomia

- Interference with neural rransmission:
  - Medications/drugs
    Anticholinergic drugs: e.g., atropine, scopolamine
    Sympathomimetic drugs; e.g., ephedrine
    Anti-neoplastic agents that directly damage salivary glands
    Antireflux agents, e.g., proton-pump inhibitors
    Antidepressants
       Selective serotonin reuptake inhibitors
       Tricyclic antidepressants
    Other psychoactive drugs
       Antihistamines
       Benzodiazepines
       Nicotine
       Opioids
       Phenothiazines
    Antihypertensives
       Alpha-1 antagonists (e.g., terazosin and prazosin)
       Alpha-2 agonists (e.g., clonidine)
       Beta blockers (e.g., atenolol, propanolol)
       Drugs that deplete fluid: diuretics
- Autonomic dysfunction
  - Cholinergic dysautonomia
  - Dysautonomia
  - Endocrine (diabetes, hypothyroidism)
  - Ganglionic neuropathy
- Central nervous system conditions
  - Alzheimer disease
  - Anxiety or stress
  - Bulimia nervosa
  - Hypochondriasis
  - Psychogenic disorders
- Dehydration
  - Diabetes mellitus
  - Diabetes insipidus
  - Diarrhea and vomiting
  - Hypercalcemia
  - Renal disease
  - Severe hemorrhage
- Starvation
- Cancer therapy
  - Chemotherapy
  - Chemoradiotherapy
  - Hematopoietic stem cell transplantation/bone marrow transplantation/chronic graft-versus-host disease
  - Irradiation (radiotherapy or radioactive iodine)

Table 6.2 (continued)

• Systemic conditions affecting salivary glands
– Hereditary
Aplasia of salivary glands
Cystic fibrosis
Ectodermal dysplasia
– Inflammatory conditions
Lupus sialadenitis *[How does this differ from Sjögren syndrome occurring in the setting of SLE?]*
Sarcoidosis
Sjögren syndrome
– Infections
Human immunodeficiency virus
Hepatitis C virus
Epstein–Barr virus
Cytomegalovirus
HTLV-1
Others
– Deposits
Amyloidosis
Hemochromatosis
Hyperlipidemia
Others
– IgG4-related systemic disease (see also Mikulicz disease)
Fibromyalgia

Salivary gland swelling may also be seen in SS [15], usually due to autoimmune or myoepithelial sialadenitis. It can occasionally be the presenting feature of SS [16, 17]. If parotid gland enlargement persists or if the glands are hard on palpation and associated with enlarged lymph nodes, the physician should consider the possibility that the benign lymphoproliferation of SS has evolved into a lymphoid malignancy.

6.5.2 Neurological Involvement

Orofacial pain, trigeminal neuropathy and other cranial nerve palsies may also occasionally occur [18].

6.6 Sialochemical Changes in SS

Salivary gland swelling, early dental loss, sialochemistry alterations, and even sialorrhoea have been observed before the onset of typical signs and symptoms of SS [17]. Unstimulated whole saliva (UWS) flow is the measure generally used to

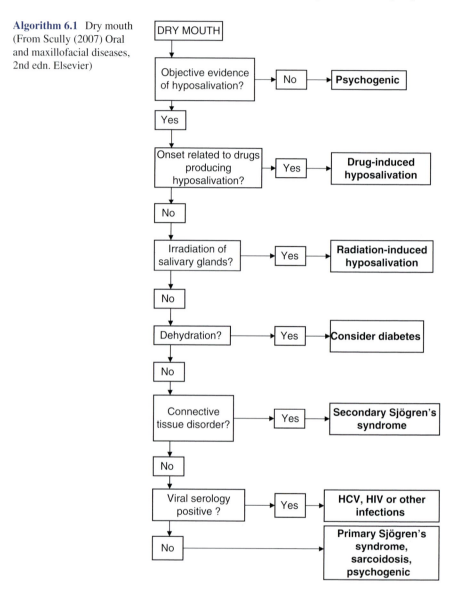

assess the severity of hyposalivation and also proves to be an independent predictor of deteriorated exocrine gland function [19]. Xerostomia is generally associated with reduced quantities rather than altered qualitative properties of saliva. Lower levels of sulfated oligosaccharides within mucinous acini may contribute to xerostomia [20]. The amounts of prostaglandin PGE-2 in saliva and in sera from persons with primary SS are significantly higher than in pre- or post-menopausal women [21]. Saliva from patients with SS has elevated levels of sodium, chloride,

Table 6.3 Orofacial manifestations in Sjögren syndrome

Tissue affected	Consequences	Clinical features
Salivary gland	Hyposalivation	Discomfort, disturbed swallowing and speech, infections (caries, candidiasis, bacterial sialadenitis), taste disturbances, burning sensation
	Sialadenitis	Salivary gland swelling from autoimmune or bacterial sialadenitis, or lymphoma
Neurological		Pain, facial palsy, trigeminal sensory changes, other cranial neuropathies

lactoferrin, beta-2-microglobulin, immunoglobulin A, lysozyme C, and cystatin C, and decreased salivary amylase and carbonic anhydrase [22, 23], but these findings are not specific enough for diagnostic purposes. Antibodies against exocrine gland cholinoreceptors correlate with dry mouth in persons with primary syndromes.

Heat shock proteins, mucins, carbonic anhydrases, enolase, vimentin, and cyclophilin B are among the proteins identified in minor salivary glands. The differences in the proteomes of minor salivary glands from primary SS patients and non-SS controls are mainly related to ribosomal proteins, immunity and stress. Alpha-defensin-1 and calmodulin are among six proteins exclusively identified in primary SS patients [24].

Fibronectin peptides in saliva from SS have recently been suggested as a method of monitoring repetition disease activity in primary SS [25].

6.7 Hyposalivation: Clinical Features and Complications

6.7.1 Clinical Features

Oral complaints (often the presenting feature) can include:

- Xerostomia: often the most frequent and obvious clinical component, although not all patients complain of dry mouth
- Soreness or burning sensation.
- Difficulty eating dry foods (the "cracker sign").
- Difficulties in controlling dentures.
- Difficulties in speech: Difficulty speaking for long periods of time or the development of hoarseness there may be a clicking quality of the speech as the tongue tends to stick to the palate.
- Difficulties in swallowing.
- Complications such as unpleasant taste or loss of sense of taste; oral malodour; caries; candidiasis; sialadenitis.
- Putting a glass of water on the bedside table to drink at night (and sometimes, resulting nocturia).
- Salivary gland enlargement (see below).

A positive response to the following questions is significantly associated with reduced salivary output [26]:

Question	Response
Do you have difficulties swallowing any foods?	Yes/No
Does your mouth feel dry while eating a meal?	Yes/No
Do you sip liquids to aid in swallowing dry foods?	Yes/No
Does the amount of saliva in your mouth seems to be too little, too much, or you don't notice it?	

6.7.2 Examination

The patient should be examined by

- Inspection
- For facial symmetry
- For evidence of enlarged glands
- Of the salivary ducts for pus
- Of the salivary pool under the tongue
- Of the mucosa for erythema, mucositis, angular cheilitis, dryness, or lingual depapillation
- Palpation of the salivary glands
- Parotids
- Submandibular glands

By bimanual palpation of the glands with fingers both inside and outside the mouth.

6.7.3 Clinical Signs of Hyposalivation

Reduced salivation may result in a dry mucosa that becomes sticky. The lips may adhere to each other. There may be lack of salivary pooling in the floor of the mouth and saliva flows poorly, if at all, from the ducts of the major glands upon stimulation or palpation.

Physical findings may include a tendency of the mucosa to stick to a dental mirror or tongue spatula; food residues within the oral cavity; frothiness of saliva, particularly in the lower sulcular reflection; and the absence of frank salivation from major gland duct orifices (Fig. 6.1, 6.2). The tongue may develop a characteristic appearance: a lobulated, red surface with partial or complete depapillation. Salivary gland enlargement, particularly of the parotid glands, is also characteristic of SS (see below). However, not all patients with SS have salivary gland enlargement. Isolated enlargement of the submandibular glands is not typical of SS, but rather is more suggestive of IgG4-related systemic disease.

Fig. 6.1 Dry mouth; food
residues

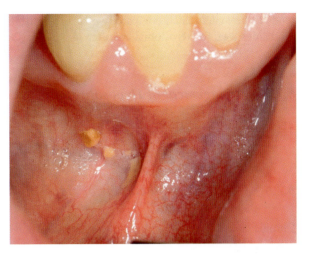

Fig. 6.2 Lobulated tongue

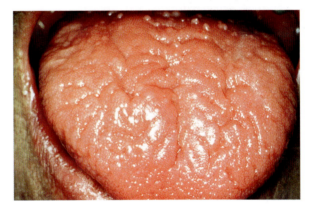

6.7.4 *Effect of Hyposalivation on Quality of Life*

SS has a large impact on health-related quality of life (HR-QOL), employment, and
disability of patients [27]. Furthermore, in SS patients, both the oral health-related
and generic quality of life (QOL) are poor. The salivary flow rate correlates with
both Disease Damage Index and Oral Health Impact Profile (OHIP-14) ratings. The
number of autoimmune symptoms correlates with both oral and generic QOL; and
oral health accounts for a significant percentage of variance in SF-36 domains of
general health and social function [28].

Among patients with rheumatic disorders, xerostomia is common and the prevalence increases with age [29]. Women are more susceptible to rheumatic diseases
than men and more likely to be affected by xerostomia and xerophthalmia. There is
a significant correlation between xerostomia and xerophthalmia, but xerostomia

tends to be undertreated compared with xerophthalmia, partly because treatment modalities used for xerostomia are often ineffective [29].

6.7.5 Management of Hyposalivation

This is discussed in Chap. 36.

6.7.6 Chronic Complications of Hyposalivation

Chronic complications of hyposalivation are shown in Box 6.1:

> **Box 6.1: Chronic Complications of Hyposalivation**
> - Tooth demineralization and caries.
> - Gingival changes
> - Difficulty with chewing.
> - Impairment of denture use.
> - Swallowing difficulties.
> - Oral malodour.
> - Altered taste.
> - Mucosal dryness and sensitivity.
> - Oral infections (candidiasis and bacterial sialadenitis).

6.7.6.1 Dental Caries

SS is often suspected because of a particular predisposition to dental caries [30, 31]. Box 6.2 illustrates the optimal approach to the prevention of dental caries. Dietary control of sucrose intake, the daily use of fluoride toothpastes, other fluoride applications, and frequent visits to the dentist are essential.

Calcium and phosphate are essential components of enamel and dentine. They form highly insoluble complexes, but in the presence of casein phosphopeptide – a group of peptides known as "CPP" – calcium and phosphate remain soluble and biologically available as amorphous calcium phosphate (ACP). A therapeutic CPP-ACP complex can be applied to teeth by means of chewing-gum, toothpaste, lozenges, mouth rinses, or sprays, providing bioavailable calcium and phosphate ions that aid remineralization of white spot lesions in an effect similar to self-applied fluorides. CPP-ACP also reduces the appearance of new caries in patients with xerostomia [32].

Another therapeutic approach to the management of sequelae of xerostomia is the use of a supersaturated calcium phosphate rinse in conjunction with 1.1% NaF for daily use [33].

Box 6.2: Strategies for Reducing Dental Caries in Patients with Sjögren's
Syndrome
- Frequent dental visits for early detection of caries
- Prevention of demineralization and encouragement of remineralization
  through the use of:
  - Sodium fluoride:
    1.1% neutral gel
    Lozenges
    0.05% rinse
    5% varnish
    Difluorosilane 1% varnish
  - Calcium/phosphate:
    Recaldent containing chewing gum
    Caphosol

6.7.6.2   Periodontal Health

Gingival capillary alterations have been described in SS [34], but predilections to
gingivitis and periodontitis are not documented as well as the risk of varies [35–37].
The true relationship between SS and periodontitis, if any, remains unclear.

6.7.6.3   Oral Functional Impairments

Chewing may be impaired but patients with reduced or increased salivary flow do
not show objective alterations in masticatory efficiency [38].

Denture use and function are impaired, but few studies describe the effects of
hyposalivation on denture retention [39].

6.7.6.4   Oral Infections

The risk of oral infections such as candidiasis and bacterial sialadenitis is increased
in SS. Despite effective oral hygiene, more SS subjects than controls have detectable levels of oral yeasts [40]. The load of *Candida* in patients with SS is relevant to
the level of salivary flow rates [41].

Frank candidiasis may be seen, particularly if there are other predisposing factors
(Box 6.3). However, denture-related stomatitis with or without angular stomatitis
(cheilitis) is more common. These are also complications of *Candida* infection.

Box 6.3: Factors Predisposing to Oral Candidiasis
- Disturbed local oral ecology or marked changes in the oral microbial flora
  by antibiotics, corticosteroids, xerostomia, dental appliances [42, 43]
- Heavy smoking

- Systemic conditions
  - Immune defects
    Malnutrition and dietary factors
    HIV/AIDS
    Extreme old age
    Diabetes mellitus
    Malignant and chronic diseases
    Blood dyscrasias
  - Cancer therapy
    Radiation to the head and neck
    Chemotherapy

6.7.6.5 Denture-Induced Stomatitis

Denture-induced stomatitis (denture sore mouth; chronic atrophic candidiasis) consists of mild inflammation of the mucosa beneath a denture – usually a complete upper denture [43]. This is a disease mainly of the middle-aged or older people, more prevalent in women than men. Predisposing factors are xerostomia and the wearing of dentures throughout the night. Dentures can produce a number of ecological changes; they often lower the pH between the maxillary denture and oral mucosa, alter the oral flora, and allow plaque to collect between the mucosal surface of the denture and the palate. The accumulation of microbial plaque (bacteria or yeasts) on dentures and within the fitting surface between the denture and the underlying mucosa produces an inflammatory reaction. When candida is involved, the more common terms "*Candida*-associated denture stomatitis", "denture-induced candidiasis", or "chronic atrophic candidiasis" are used.

The characteristic presenting features of denture-induced stomatitis are chronic erythema and edema of the mucosa that contacts the fitting surface of the denture. Complete upper dentures are the type of dental appliance most often associated with this complication. The erythema is restricted to the denture-bearing area and is usually asymptomatic. Complications are uncommon, but include angular stomatitis.

The denture plaque and fitting surface is infested, usually with *Candida albicans*.

Therefore, to prevent recurrence of denture-induced stomatitis, dentures should be left out of the mouth at night and stored in an antiseptic. Denture cleansing and disinfection that includes removal of *Candida* is a necessary and important factor. Cleansers can be divided into groups according to their main components: alkaline peroxides, alkaline hypochlorites, acids, disinfectants, yeast lytic enzymes, and proteolytic enzymes. The latter are found to be the most effective against *Candida*. Denture soak solution containing benzoic acid is absorbed into the acrylic resin and eradicates *Candida albicans* from the denture surface as well as the internal surface of the prosthesis. An oral rinse containing chlorhexidine gluconate results in complete elimination of *C. albicans* on the acrylic resin surface of the denture, and in reduction of palatal inflammation. A protease-containing denture soak (Alcalase protease) is also an effective way of removing denture plaque, especially when combined with brushing.

The mucosal infection is eradicated by brushing the palate and using miconazole gel, nystatin pastilles amphotericin or fluconazole, administered concurrently with an oral antiseptic such as chlorhexidine which has antifungal activity.

6.7.6.6 Angular Stomatitis

Patients are predisposed to angular stomatitis (perleche, angular cheilitis) by the wearing of dentures. Other risk factors are iron deficiency, hypovitaminosis B, malabsorption states (e.g. Crohn's disease), orofacial granulomatosis, Down's syndrome, HIV infection, diabetes, and other disorders associated with immunodeficiency. Most patients with angular cheilitis also have denture-induced stomatitis. Infective agents can be isolated in up to 54% of lesions, usually *Candida albicans*, but *Staphylococcus aureus* or streptococci may also be cultured from lesions.

Clinical features include soreness, erythema, and symmetrical fissuring at the angles of the mouth. In the treatment of angular cheilitis, it is important to apply an topical antifungal agent such as miconazole gel and to encourage smoking cessation. Lesions that respond poorly to these lesions may require topical fucidin or systemic fluconazole.

6.7.6.7 Candidiasis

Candidiasis may cause soreness or burning and thus should be treated with antifungals until there is neither erythema nor symptoms (Box 6.4).

Box 6.4: Drug Treatment to Manage and Prevent Hyposalivation-Induced Candidiasis
- Clinicians should be aware that some antifungal agents contain sugar products. These contribute to the overgrowth of *Candida*. In contrast, nystatin vaginal tablets do not contain sugar. These can be administered orally two or three times daily to treat oral candidiasis.
- Sips of water should be given as necessary to dissolve the tablets
- Topical antifungal cream should be applied to the denture surface

Topical antifungals in liquid form such as amphotericin suspension are acceptable because the mouth is dry. Other preparations such as miconazole or fluconazole are also effective. However, the sucrose content of the product must be considered due to the impact of sucrose on dental caries, the risk of which is already raised in patients with dry mouth. Nystatin suspension has a high sucrose content (and a small level of alcohol). Fluconazole suspension also has a high sucrose content. Chlorexidine mouth wash has been proved effective in reducing *Candida* carriage in patients with xerostomia and is reported also to increase salivary flow rate [44]. Prosthesis surfaces are frequently infected and so dentures and other removable appliances should be left out of the mouth at night and disinfected by storage in sodium hypochlorite solution, chlorhexidine, or benzalkonium chloride. An antifungal preparation such as miconazole gel or amphotericin or nystatin ointment should be spread on the prosthesis before reinsertion.

6.7.6.8 Bacterial Sialadenitis

Bacterial sialadenitis is most commonly associated with *Streptococcus viridans* and *Staphylococcus aureus* (often penicillin-resistant). The parotid glands are most commonly affected, and it may be seen:

- In SS
- After radiotherapy to the head and neck
- Following gastrointestinal surgery, because of dehydration and xerostomia
- Rarely in otherwise apparently healthy patients, when it is usually due to salivary abnormalities such as calculi, mucus plugs, and duct strictures.

Acute parotitis typically presents with painful and tender enlargement of one parotid gland, reddening of the overlying skin, pus exuding from the parotid duct orifice, and trismus (Fig. 6.3). The diagnosis is a clinical one, but pus milked from Stenson's duct should be sent for culture and sensitivity testing. Sialadenitis is treated most effectively with a penicillinase-resistant antibiotic such as flucloxacillin. Hydration is important and surgical drainage is needed if fluctuance is present.

Sialadenitis can be prevented by the stimulation of salivation and by mouth-wetting agents such as lactoperoxidase gel, which reduce both periodontal-associated pathogens and *Candida* species [45]. Antibacterial agents such as 0.12% or 0.2% chlorhexidine gluconate mouth rinse and xylitol (in sugar-free gums and mints) may also help.

6.7.6.9 Oral Ulceration

Oral ulcers are not uncommon in patients with SS. The management of this complication depends on the underlying cause [46]. Prolonged xerostomia can result in thinner mucosa that is susceptible to tearing after mild trauma. Oral

Fig. 6.3 Sialadenitis

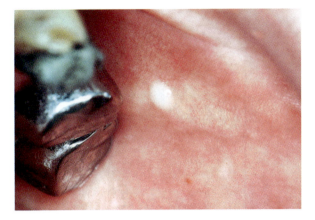

lichen planus has been reported in up to 18% of patients with SS. In addition, lichenoid reactions to drugs used to treat other existing co-morbidities (e.g., non-steroidal anti-inflammatory drugs or hydroxychloroquine) can occur. Other causes of drug-induced oral ulcers in patients with SS are methotrexate and bisphosphonates. Finally, acute erythematous candidiasis can also present as painful oral erosions.

6.8   Salivary Gland Enlargement

There is a wide range of causes of salivary gland enlargement (Table 6.4) (Algorithm 6.2).

Acute salivary gland swellings in adults are mostly unilateral and caused by salivary duct obstruction, but SS or ascending bacterial sialadenitis may be the cause (see below). Ascending bacterial sialadenitis produces symptoms and signs similar to mumps but the pain is generally more intense and pus may be expressed from the duct of the affected gland. Dehydration and atropine use can precipitate this complication in susceptible individuals.

Recurrent salivary gland swelling suggests salivary duct obstruction, particularly that which can be caused by sialolithiasis see also : stone.

Persistent swellings of an entire salivary gland or glands that is painless and associated with a smooth glandular surface can be seen in SS, HIV/AIDS, sialosis (sialadenosis), chronic sclerosing sialadenitis [47] (see also Mikulicz disease) and sarcoidosis. Such swellings may also be caused by certain drugs (e.g., protease inhibitors) or by neoplasms. Persistent swelling of a salivary gland can also be caused by a neoplasm, either benign or malignant. Salivary gland tumors commonly affect the parotid and may encroach upon the pharynx, producing pain or facial palsy (Fig. 6.4).

The non-SS causes of salivary gland enlargement are shown in Box 6.5.

Table 6.4 Main causes of persistent salivary gland swelling

	Sjögren syndrome	Sarcoidosis	HIV-related sialadenitis	HCV-related sialadenitis	Sclerosing sialadenitis (IgG4 related plasmacytic disease)	Sialosis/sialadenosis
Mean age	40–50	25–35 and 45–65	All ages	30–50	50–60	20–60
Sex ratio	F>>>M	F=M	M>F	M=F	M>F	M=F
Sicca symptoms	Present	Present	Present	Present	None to mild	May be present
Response to steroids	Variable	Variable	Non-reported	Non-reported	Very good	Non-reported
SSA	Positive or negative	Negative	Negative	Negative	Negative	Negative
SSB	Positive or negative	Negative	Negative	Negative	Negative	Negative
Salivary gland biopsy (histopathology, immunostaining)	Lymphocytic focal aggregates mainly CD4+ Normal acini replaced by lymphocytes	Non-caseating granulomas	Perivascular, periacinar, periductal lymphocytic infiltrates CD8+, Multicystic lymphoepithelial lesions	SS similar, less inflammation, CD20+ lymphocytes	Infiltration with IgG4 secreting plasmacytes	Acinar cell hypertrophy/also, acinar atrophy and fatty infiltration
Diagnostic work up	American-European consensus criteria	CXR, SACE	Positive HIV serology	Anti-HCV serology	Serum IgG4/IgG high ratio	Investigations for diabetes, alcoholism, endocrinopathy, bulimia, anorexia hyperlipedimia malnutrition, cirrhosis
	Lesional biopsies		Salivary gland biopsy	HCV RNA PCR	Salivary gland biopsy	Salivary gland biopsy

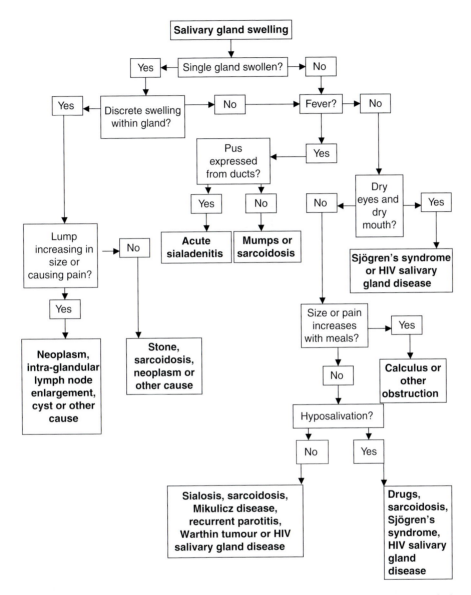

Algorithm 6.2 Salivary gland swelling (From Scully (2007) Oral and maxillofacial diseases, 2nd edn. Elsevier)

Fig. 6.4 Salivary gland enlargement

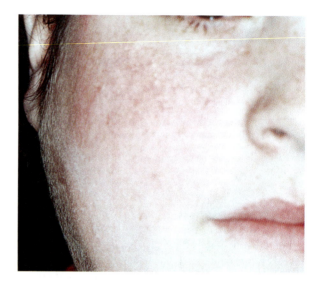

6.9   Salivary Swelling in SS

Salivary swelling does not occur in all patients with SS. The parotid glands are the ones most likely to be swollen in SS. Isolated submandibular gland swelling is highly uncharacteristic of SS and its presence suggests another disorder, e.g., IgG4-related sialadenitis [48–50].

Parotid swelling, which occurs in 25–66% of patients with primary SS but rarely in secondary SS, commonly takes one of several forms [51]:

- Mild, chronic, bilateral, and painless
- Recurrent, bilateral, and painless
- Recurrent, bilateral but asymmetric, and painless
- Unilateral and painful. This presentation usually results from acute bacterial sialadenitis, a complication of SS but not a direct manifestation of the disease itself.
- Massive and bilateral, associated with adenopathy. Such a presentation is often associated with the development of lymphoma.

The most common cause of chronic salivary gland swelling in SS is autoimmune sialadenitis, also termed myoepithelial sialadenitis (MESA) for benign lymphoepithelial lesion. MESA is characterized by persistent, painless, firm swelling of the major salivary glands that can be either unilateral or bilateral. The histopathology reveals lymphocytic and plasmacytic infiltrates, with "islands" of epithelium called "epimyothelial islands" composed of ductal and myoepithelial cells.

The risk of developing a lymphoma for a patient with primary SS is on the order of 4–10%. This has been estimated to be 44 times higher than that of the general population. Among patients with primary SS, the incidence of non-Hodgkin's lymphoma has been estimated to be 320 cases per 100,000 patient-years of follow-up [52]. Most lymphomas occur in the major salivary glands as extranodal marginal zone B-cell non-Hodgkin lymphomas and 80% are MALT lymphomas [53, 54]. The parotid gland is by far the most likely site of such malignancies [55]. Other issues related to the development of lymphoma in patients with SS are discussed elsewhere in this book.

References

1. Fox PC, Bowman SJ, Segal B, Vivino FB, Murukutla N, Choueiri K, et al. Oral involvement in primary Sjögren syndrome. J Am Dent Assoc. 2008;139:1592–601.
2. Ghezzi EM, Lange LA, Ship JA. Determination of variation of stimulated salivary flow rates. J Dent Res. 2000;79:1874M.
3. Navazesh M, Christensen C, Brightman V. Clinical criteria for the diagnosis of salivary gland hypofunction. J Dent Res. 1992;71:1363.
4. Kohler PF, Winter ME. A quantitative test for xerostomia. The saxon test, an oral equivalent of the schirmer test. Arthritis Rheum. 2005;28:1128–32.
5. Jorkjend L, Johansson A, Johansson AK, Bergenholtz A. Resting and stimulated whole salivary flow rates in Sjögren's syndrome patients over time: a diagnostic aid for subsidized dental care? Acta Odontol Scand. 2004;62(5):264–8.
6. Moore PA, Guggenheimer J. Medication-induced hyposalivation: etiology, diagnosis, and treatment. Compend Contin Educ Dent. 2008;29(1):50–5.
7. Turner MD, Ship JA. Dry mouth and its effects on the oral health of elderly people. J Am Dent Assoc. 2007;138(Suppl):15S–20.
8. Thomson WM, Lawrence HP, Broadbent JM, Poulton R. The impact of xerostomia on oral-health-related quality of life among younger adults. Health Qual Life Outcomes. 2006;4:86.

9. Johansson AK, Johansson A, Unell L, Ekbäck G, Ordell S, Carlsson GE. A 15-yr longitudinal study of xerostomia in a Swedish population of 50-yr-old subjects. Eur J Oral Sci. 2009; 117(1):13–9.
10. Meurman JH, Tarkkila L, Tiitinen A. The menopause and oral health. Maturitas. 2009;63(1): 56–62. Epub 2009 Mar 25.
11. Baum BJ, Ship JA, Wu AJ. Salivary gland function and aging: a model for studying the interaction of aging and systemic disease. Crit Rev Oral Biol Med. 1992;4(1):53–64.
12. Yamamoto K, Nagashima H, Yamachika S, Hoshiba D, Yamaguchi K, Yamada H, et al. The application of a night guard for sleep-related xerostomia. Oral Surg Oral Med Oral Pathol Oral Radiol Endod. 2008;106(3):e11–4. Epub 2008 Jul 7.
13. Kassan SS, Moutsopoulos HM. Clinical manifestations and early diagnosis of Sjögren syndrome. Arch Intern Med. 2004;164(12):1275–84.
14. Cho MA, Ko JY, Kim YK, Kho HS. Salivary flow rate and clinical characteristics of patients with xerostomia according to its aetiology. J Oral Rehabil. 2010;37(3):185–93.
15. Longman LP, Higham SM, Bucknall R, Kaye SB, Edgar WM, Field EA. Signs and symptoms in patients with salivary gland hypofunction. Postgrad Med J. 1997;73(856):93–7.
16. Flaitz CM. Parotitis as the initial sign of juvenile Sjögren's syndrome. Pediatr Dent. 2001; 23(2):140–2.
17. Mignogna MD, Fedele S, Lo Russo L, Lo Muzio L, Wolff A. Sjögren's syndrome: the diagnostic potential of early oral manifestations preceding hyposalivation/xerostomia. J Oral Pathol Med. 2005;34(1):1–6.
18. Mellgren SI, Göransson LG, Omdal R. Primary Sjögren's syndrome associated neuropathy. Can J Neurol Sci. 2007;34(3):280–7.
19. Haldorsen K, Moen K, Jacobsen H, Jonsson R, Brun JG. Exocrine function in primary Sjögren syndrome: natural course and prognostic factors. Ann Rheum Dis. 2008;67(7):949–54. Epub Oct 25, 2007.
20. Alliende C, Kwon YJ, Brito M, Molina C, Aguilera S, Pérez P, et al. Reduced sulfation of muc5b is linked to xerostomia in patients with Sjögren syndrome. Ann Rheum Dis. 2008;67(10):1480–7. Epub 2007 Nov 12.
21. Reina S, Orman B, Anaya JM, Sterin-Borda L, Borda E. Cholinoreceptor autoantibodies in Sjögren syndrome. J Dent Res. 2007;86(9):832–6.
22. Mathews SA, Kurien BT, Scofield RH. Oral manifestations of Sjögren's syndrome. J Dent Res. 2008;87(4):308–18.
23. Helenius LM, Meurman JH, Helenius I, Kari K, Hietanen J, Suuronen R, et al. Oral and salivary parameters in patients with rheumatic diseases. Acta Odontol Scand. 2005;63(5): 284–93.
24. Hjelmervik TO, Jonsson R, Bolstad AI. The minor salivary gland proteome in Sjögren's syndrome. Oral Dis. 2009;15(5):342–53. Epub Apr 2, 2009.
25. Silvestre FJ, Puente A, Bagán JV, Castell JV. Presence of fibronectin peptides in saliva of patients with Sjögren's syndrome: a potential indicator of salivary gland destruction. Med Oral Patol Oral Cir Bucal. 2009;14(8):e365–70.
26. Navazesh M. How can oral health care providers determine if patients have dry mouth? J Am Dent Assoc. 2003;134(5):613–8.
27. Meijer JM, Meiners PM, Huddleston Slater JJ, Spijkervet FK, Kallenberg CG, Vissink A, et al. Health-related quality of life, employment and disability in patients with Sjogren's syndrome. Rheumatology (Oxford). 2009;48(9):1077–82. Epub Jun 24, 2009.
28. Stewart CM, Berg KM, Cha S, Reeves WH. Salivary dysfunction and quality of life in Sjögren syndrome: a critical oral-systemic connection. J Am Dent Assoc. 2008;139(3):291–9; quiz 358–9.
29. Guobis Z, Baseviciene N, Paipaliene P, Niedzelskiene I, Janusevičiūte G. Aspects of xerostomia prevalence and treatment among rheumatic inpatients. Medicina (Kaunas). 2008;44(12):960–8.
30. Seo DG, Kim J, Lee CY, Park SH. Diagnosis of Sjögren's syndrome from a xerostomia case accompanied by multiple dental caries. Oper Dent. 2009;34(3):359–64.

31. Llena C, Forner L, Baca P. Anticariogenicity of casein phosphopeptide-amorphous calcium phosphate: a review of the literature. J Contemp Dent Pract. 2009;10(3):1–9.
32. Singh ML, Papas AS. Long-term clinical observation of dental caries in salivary hypofunction patients using a supersaturated calcium-phosphate remineralizing rinse. J Clin Dent. 2009; 20(3):87–92.
33. Scardina GA, Ruggieri A, Messina P. Periodontal disease and Sjögren syndrome: a possible correlation? Angiology. 2010;61(3):289–93.
34. Mutlu S, Porter SR, Richards A, Scully C, Maddison P. Gingival and periodontal health in Sjogren's syndrome and other connective tissue disorders. Clin Exp Rheumatol. 1993;11:95–6.
35. Antoniazzi RP, Miranda LA, Zanatta FB, Islabão AG, Gustafsson A, Chiapinotto GA, et al. Periodontal conditions of individuals with Sjögren's syndrome. J Periodontol. 2009;80(3):429–35.
36. Boutsi EA, Paikos S, Dafni UG, Moutsopoulos HM, Skopouli FN. Dental and periodontal status of Sjögren's syndrome. J Clin Periodontol. 2000;27:231–5.
37. Schiødt M, Christensen LB, Petersen PE, Thorn JJ. Periodontal disease in primary Sjögren's syndrome. Oral Dis. 2001;7(2):106–8.
38. Gomes SG, Custódio W, Cury AA, Garcia RC. Effect of salivary flow rate on masticatory efficiency. Int J Prosthodont. 2009;22(2):168–72.
39. Turner M, Jahangiri L, Ship JA. Hyposalivation, xerostomia and the complete denture: a systematic review. J Am Dent Assoc. 2008;139(2):146–50.
40. Leung KC, McMillan AS, Cheung BP, Leung WK. Sjögren's syndrome sufferers have increased oral yeast levels despite regular dental care. Oral Dis. 2008;14(2):163–73.
41. Radfar L, Shea Y, Fischer SH, Sankar V, Leakan RA, Baum BJ, et al. Fungal load and candidiasis in Sjögren's syndrome. Oral Surg Oral Med Oral Pathol Oral Radiol Endod. 2003;96(3):283–7.
42. Akpan A, Morgan R. Oral candidiasis. Postgrad Med J. 2002;78:455–9.
43. Scully C, El-Kabir M, Samaranayake LP. Candida and oral candidosis. Crit Rev Oral Biol Med. 1994;5:124–58.
44. Torres SR, Peixoto CB, Caldas DM, Akiti T, Barreiros MG, de Uzeda M, et al. A prospective randomized trial to reduce oral *Candida* spp. colonization in patients with hyposalivation. Braz Oral Res. 2007;21(2):182–7.
45. Nagy K, Urban E, et al. Controlled study of lactoperoxidase gel on oral flora and saliva in irradiated patients with oral cancer. J Craniofac Surg. 2007;18:1157.
46. Lundström IM, Lindström FD. Subjective and clinical oral symptoms in patients with primary Sjögren's syndrome. Clin Exp Rheumatol. 1995;13(6):725–31.
47. Bartunková J, Sedivá A, Vencovsky J, Tesar V. Primary Sjögren's syndrome in children and adolescents: proposal for diagnostic criteria. Clin Exp Rheumatol. 1999;17:381–6.
48. Khosroshahi A, Stone JH. IgG4-related systemic disease: overview of the clinical features. Curr Opin Rheumatol. 2011;23:57–66.
49. Yamamoto M, Harada S, Ohara M, Suzuki C, Naishiro Y, Yamamoto H, et al. Clinical and pathological differences between Mikulicz's disease and Sjogren's syndrome. Rheumatology. 2005;44:227–34.
50. Yamamoto M, Harada S, Ohara M, Suzuki C, Naishiro Y, Yamamoto H, et al. A new conceptualization for Mikulicz's disease as an IgG4-related plasmacytic disease. Mod Rheumatol. 2006;16:335–40.
51. Manoussakis MN. Sjogren's Syndrome Orphanet encyclopedia. November 2001 http://www.orpha.net/data/patho/GB/uk-sjogren.pdf.
52. Zintzaras E, Voulgarelis M, Moutsopoulos HM. The risk of lymphoma development in autoimmune diseases: a meta-analysis. Arch Intern Med. 2005;165(20):2337–44.
53. Roh LJ, Huh J, Suh C. Primary non-Hodgkin's lymphomas of the major salivary glands. J Surg Oncol. 2008;97:35–9.
54. Voulgarelis M, Dafni UG, Isenberg DA, Moutsopoulos HM, The Members of the European Concerted Action on Sjögren's Syndrome. Malignant lymphoma in primary Sjögren's syndrome: a multicenter, retrospective, clinical study by the European concerted action on Sjögren's syndrome. Arthritis Rheum. 1999;42:1765–72.

55. Smedby KE et al. Autoimmune disorders and risk of non-Hodgkin lymphoma subtypes: a pooled analysis within the InterLymph Consortium. Blood. 2008;111(8):4029–38.

Key Websites (Accessed Dec 19, 2009)

- http://www.drymouth.info/practitioner/sources.asp
- Miller AV, Ranatunga SKM, Francis ML. Sjögren syndrome: differential diagnoses & workup. http://emedicine.medscape.com/article/332125-diagnosis
- Miller AV, Ranatunga SKM, Francis ML. Sjögren syndrome: treatment & medication. http://emedicine.medscape.com/article/332125-treatment

Chapter 7
Ocular Involvement

Stephen C. Pflugfelder, Karyn Siemasko, and Michael E. Stern

Contents

7.1 Sjögren's Syndrome: A Disease of the Lacrimal Functional Unit

Sjögren's syndrome (SS) is a systemic autoimmune disease characterized by diminished production and secretion of tears by the lacrimal glands and saliva by the salivary glands resulting in keratoconjunctivitis sicca and stomatitis sicca, respectively. The estimated prevalence of primary SS (pSS) in the USA is 1.3 million individuals

S.C. Pflugfelder (✉) • M.E. Stern
Department of Ophthalmology, Ocular Surface Center, Cullen Eye Institute,
Baylor College of Medicine, Houston, TX, USA

K. Siemasko
Biological Sciences, Allergan, Inc, Irvine, CA, USA

M. Ramos-Casals et al. (eds.), *Sjögren's Syndrome*,
DOI 10.1007/978-0-85729-947-5_7, © Springer-Verlag London Limited 2012

and the prevalence is 10–20 greater in women [1–4]. Primary SS is an autoimmune inflammation to self-antigens in the lacrimal and salivary glands in the absence of a defined systemic autoimmune disease. Multiple factors, including defective immunoregulation, genetic background, and environmental insults (e.g., desiccating stress and viral infection) have been proposed in the pathogenesis of glandular and mucosal autoimmunity in pSS [5–7]. In secondary SS, salivary and lacrimal gland inflammation develops in the presence of an existing autoimmune disease, such as rheumatoid arthritis, systemic lupus erythematosus, or scleroderma [8, 9].

The main and accessory lacrimal glands, along with the conjunctiva, cornea, meibomian glands, and their interconnecting neural network comprise the lacrimal functional unit (LFU) [10]. SS causes profound dysfunction of multiple components of the LFU, resulting in severe chronic dry eye [11].

7.2   Components of the Lacrimal Functional Unit

The LFU is essential in maintaining a homeostasis on the ocular surface by maintaining a stable tear film of normal composition. Factors in healthy tears support and protect the conjunctiva and cornea. The tear fluid contains numerous proteins, including enzymes, growth factors (e.g., epidermal growth factors) and antimicrobial factors such as secretory IgA, cystatins, and defensins. The tear film is currently considered to be a hydrated mucin gel [12]. It is composed of three major components, including mucins secreted by the stratified ocular surface epithelial and conjunctival goblet cells, aqueous produced by the lacrimal glands, and lipids secreted by the meibomian glands [13].The conjunctiva and corneal epithelia express membrane-tethered mucins 1, 2, and 16 that make up the glycocalyx that lubricates the ocular surface and binds the tear mucin layer to the hydrophobic epithelial cell surface [14].

MUC5AC is a soluble mucin secreted by conjunctival goblet cells, and the lacrimal glands contribute MUC-7 to the tear film [15–17]. Mucins are thought to clear pathogens, provide ocular surface lubrication, and serve as a barrier function to microbial invasion and inflammatory cellular infiltration of the ocular surface [18, 19]. The aqueous component secreted by the lacrimal glands contains trophic and protective factors including growth factors, immunoglobulin A, lactoferrin, lysozyme, defensins, interleukin-1 receptor antagonist, and electrolytes [13]. Finally, the meibomian glands secrete the lipid layer that functions to decrease tear film evaporation. A stable tear film keeps the cornea surface smooth, continuously lubricates the ocular surface, protects it from microbial infections and environmental insults, and delivers factors to maintain well-being of the epithelial surface. As the primary refracting surface of the eye, a healthy and stable tear film is essential for high quality vision. Tear film instability and the corneal epithelial disease that develops in dry eye can decrease functional vision and contrast sensitivity [20–22]. Consequently, many SS patients experience blurred and fluctuating vision, visual fatigue, and severe photophobia [22, 23]. Even small alterations in tear composition resulting from disease of the LFU in SS can produce deleterious consequences for the ocular surface.

7.3 Lacrimal Gland

The lacrimal gland secretes tears produced by acinar and ductal epithelia on demand. The main lacrimal gland, consisting of the palpebral and orbital lobes, is located in the superior temporal orbit. The accessory lacrimal glands consist of the glands of Krause that are located in the upper fornix and glands of Wolfring in the superior conjunctiva just above the upper edge of the tarsus. The majority of tear secretion by the lacrimal glands is reflexive, in response to neural stimulation [24]. Innervating parasympathetic cholinergic nerves release acetylcholine that binds to the muscarinic 3 acetylcholine receptor (M3R) located on the basolateral cell membranes of lacrimal gland secretory epithelia [25, 26]. In addition, the cholinergic neurotransmitter VIP interacts with the type I and type II VIP receptors on these cells [27]. Binding of acetylcholine and VIP to their respective receptors activates signaling pathways, leading to the fusion of secretory granules with the apical membrane, membrane ion transporter activation, and ion pump insertion to coordinate electrolyte secretion and regulate tear osmolarity. Sympathetic nerves also innervate the lacrimal gland. The binding of norepinephrine to $\alpha 1$- and β-adrenergic receptors increases Ca^+ flux into the cytosol [28]. Finally, the neurotransmitters substance P and calcitonin gene-related peptide (CGRP) are released by sensory nerves in the lacrimal glands [25].

Proteins secreted by the lacrimal gland are synthesized and mannosylated in the endoplasmic reticulum. As the proteins move through the Golgi complex, the carbohydrate groups are modified. While in the trans-Golgi apparatus, proteins are assembled into transport vesicles and packaged into secretory vesicles. The lacrimal gland contains T and B lymphoid follicles and IgA-producing plasma cells that surround the acini. These lymphocytes make up what has been referred to as the mucosal-associated lymphoid tissue (MALT).

7.4 Conjunctiva

The conjunctiva covers the majority of the ocular surface and functions as the major support system for the cornea by producing tear components and supplying immune and inflammatory cells [29]. The conjunctiva has three topographic zones: bulbar, palpebral, and forniceal. The conjunctiva forms a continuous mucosal surface over these three zones. The bulbar conjunctiva covers the anterior surface of the globe, the palpebral conjunctiva lines the inner surface of the eyelids, and the forniceal conjunctiva connects the palpebral and bulbar conjunctiva. The conjunctiva consists of two components, the stratified nonkeratinized secretory epithelium and the underlying stroma. Goblet cells comprise approximately 5–20% of conjunctival epithelial cells. These specialized cells secrete MUC5AC mucin and TGF-β2 into the tears [30]. The conjunctiva is also a source of the sIgA found in tears [31]. The lamina propria of the conjunctiva is vascularized and contains numerous bone marrow-derived cells, including macrophages, mast cells, lymphocytes, plasma cells, and dendritic cells [31].

The adaptive arm of the ocular surface immune response is located in the conjunctiva and is called the conjunctival-associated lymphoid tissue (CALT). The CALT is found mainly in the palpebral conjunctiva and consists of intraepithelial lymphocytes, lymphoid follicles located just below the epithelium and lymphatics, and blood vessels [32]. The CALT initiates and regulates immune responses by sampling and processing antigens on the ocular surface. The CALT is now accepted as a component of the overall mucosa-associated lymphoid tissue (MALT) [31]. Knop and Knop have proposed that the lacrimal drainage-associated lymphoid tissue, lymphocytes in the lacrimal glands, and the CALT all serve as a defensive unit for the ocular surface called the eye-associated lymphoid tissue (EALT) [31].

7.5   Cornea

The cornea is endowed with the highest density of sensory nerve endings of any tissue in the body [33]. The cornea is a unique clear tissue that is the most powerful lens in the eye. Its clarity is due to the surface tear layer, specialized non-keratinizing epithelium with tight junctions, keratocytes, organized collagen lamella, and endothelial cells that pump fluid out of the cornea. The sensory nerve endings that terminate in the corneal epithelium constantly monitor the environment and signal the central nervous system to regulate tear secretion by the lacrimal functional unit in response to environmental challenge. In the healthy state, proteases in the tear film regulate turnover of the differentiated apical cornea epithelial cells. Increased tear protease activity in SS accelerates epithelial turnover and disrupts the protective epithelial barrier [34]. The cornea contains resident MHC class II-negative dendritic cells. These dendritic cells are capable of expressing MHC class II and traveling to the draining lymph nodes to initiate immune reactions in response to proinflammatory stimuli such as increased tear cytokines in SS [35–38].

7.6   Meibomian Glands and Eyelids

The meibomian glands secrete lipids that retard tear film evaporation and stabilize the tear film. Meibomian glands are located in the tarsal plates of the upper and lower eyelids. Lipid is released into the tears from the meibomian gland ducts that are located on the lid margins. Over 100 different lipids are secreted by the meibomian gland that include polar lipids, wax esters, free fatty acids, and cholesterol [39].

7.7   Neural Innervation

An integrated neural network connects the lacrimal glands, cornea, conjunctiva, and the meibomian glands [10]. The primary role of the LFU is to maintain homeostasis on ocular surface. The LFU is regulated by sensory, sympathetic, and parasympathetic nerves. Afferent signals from the ocular surface are transmitted via the ophthalmic division of the trigeminal nerve to the central nervous system where they synapse with autonomic efferent nerves. In response to afferent stimulation, neurotransmitters are released by the efferent nerves innervating the secretory tissues [10, 40]. In addition to stimulating tear secretion, VIP released by efferent parasympathetic nerves can inhibit proinflammatory cytokine and chemokine production and enhance secretion of the anti-inflammatory cytokines TGF-β and IL-10 [41].

7.8   Mechanisms of Dysfunction

SS causes a profound reduction in tear production by components of the LFU, particularly the lacrimal glands and ocular surface epithelium. This results in an unstable tear film of altered composition that inadequately supports the ocular surface and causes symptoms of eye irritation and blurred vision.

7.8.1   Lacrimal Gland

Secretory dysfunction of the lacrimal gland in SS is identified clinically by symptoms of ocular irritation such as dryness and a foreign body sensation that typically worsen with prolonged visual effort or exposure to dry or drafty environments. Patients may complain of inability to produce tears reflexively in response to cold, wind, or emotional stimuli. Lacrimal gland secretory dysfunction in SS occurs by a variety of mechanisms, some reversible, others permanent.

Circulating acetylcholine M3R autoantibodies can inhibit tear secretion by competitively binding to acetylcholine receptors on lacrimal acinar cells [42]. Chronic aqueous tear deficiency may also cause degeneration of the corneal nociceptors, resulting in reduced sensory stimulation of lacrimal secretion [43, 44].

Inflammation can also promote dysfunction or death of lacrimal gland secretory epithelia. Inflammatory cytokines such as IL-1 have been reported to inhibit cholinergic-induced secretion of lacrimal acinar cells [45]. TNF-α and the T-helper 1 (Th1) cytokine IFN-gamma can promote apoptosis of lacrimal acinar cells [46–48].Progressive lymphocytic infiltration may eventually replace most or all of the lacrimal acini.

7.8.2   Ocular Surface

Ocular surface disease in SS results from reduced secretion and altered composition of tears. With loss of the ability to produce tears reflexively, the LFU can no longer respond adequately to stressful environmental conditions on the ocular surface. Tear composition changes in SS include increased osmolarity, decreased concentration of lacrimal secreted factors (lactoferrin and EGF), and increased concentrations of inflammatory mediators [49]. In addition, inflammation on the ocular surface in SS may alter differentiation of the conjunctival epithelium, pushing it toward squamous metaplasia [50, 51]. This changes the normally lubricated conjunctival mucosa to a poorly wettable skin-like phenotype with increased production of cornified envelope precursor proteins by the stratified epithelium and reduced numbers of mucin-filled goblet cells. Evidence suggests these changes are driven by exposure to hyperosmolar tears and to the Th1 cytokine IFN-gamma [50, 52].

Accelerated loss of apical corneal epithelial cells results from proteolytic dissolution of tight junction proteins by activated proteases, such as matrix metalloproteinase 9 (MMP-9) [34]. Similar to the conjunctiva, there may be increased production of cornified envelope precursor proteins and accelerated corneal epithelial cell apoptosis. These changes lead to an irregular and poorly lubricated corneal surface and exposure of sensory nerve endings in the corneal epithelium to noxious environmental stimuli [53].

7.9 Diagnosis of Ocular Involvement in Sjögren's Syndrome

The US-EEC consensus criteria for diagnosis of Sjögren's syndrome require presence of eye irritation symptoms and objective evidence of dry eye (generally rapid tear breakup time, low Schirmer 1 test, or the presence of ocular surface dye staining) [54].

Fluorescein tear breakup time is assessed by staining the tears with fluorescein dye and measuring the time in seconds for discontinuities to develop in the precorneal tear film. The optimal method of performing this test is with a fluorescein-impregnated strip that is wetted with preservative-free saline and touched to the inferior bulbar conjunctiva. Fluorescein TBUT has previously been reported to be rapid in different types of dry eye, including aqueous tear deficiency (both non-SS and SS), mucin deficiency (e.g., Stevens–Johnson syndrome, and meibomian gland disease with lipid deficiency) [55–59].Noninvasive methods to evaluate tear stability, such as videokeratoscopic surface regularity indices, appear to be more sensitive in detecting altered corneal tear layer in eyes with aqueous tear deficiency [60]. The Klyce surface regularity index has been found to correlate with the severity of corneal epithelial disease and therefore it has value in trying to identify eyes with ocular surface disease from SS.

The Schirmer test, originally described in 1903 [61], remains the most commonly used technique for assessing tear secretion. It is performed without (Schirmer 1) or with topical anesthesia (basic secretion test) by placing a folded Schirmer test strip over the lid margin at the junction of the medial and lateral thirds. Aqueous tear production is measured by the millimeters wetted during a 5 min test period [62]. The Schirmer 1 test has the advantage of assessing the ability of the eyes to tear reflexively in response to sensory stimulation, an ability that is lost early in the course of SS [63]. A Schirmer 1 score of ≤5.5 mm in 5 min has been suggested as diagnostic for aqueous tear deficiency [64].

Ocular surface disease in SS is detected by staining the ocular surface with diagnostic dyes. Fluorescein dye is commonly used to detect evidence of corneal epithelial disease. Diffuse punctate staining, including the central cornea, is typically observed

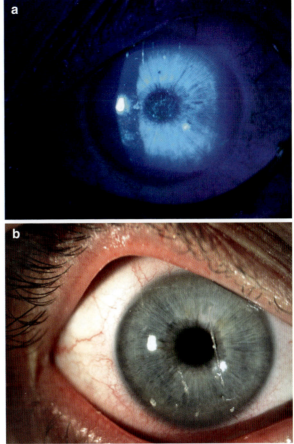

in SS (Fig. 7.1a). More advanced staining is often accompanied by adherent mucus
and epithelial filaments on the cornea (Fig. 7.1b).

Lissamine green and rose bengal dyes have greater sensitivity to detect diseased
conjunctival epithelium in SS. Both dyes characteristically stain in an exposure
zone pattern, but lissamine green is generally better tolerated by patients (Fig. 7.2).
Impression cytology of the conjunctiva can directly show loss of mucin-filled goblet
cells and squamous metaplasia in the conjunctiva that are characteristic findings in
the keratoconjunctivitis of SS [51, 65].

7.10   Treatment of LFU Dysfunction

Consensus and evidence-based algorithms for the treatment of ocular surface disease
associated with dry eyes have been proposed by the Delphi panel and the International
Dry Eye Workshop (DEWS) [66, 67]. Both guidelines recommend therapies based

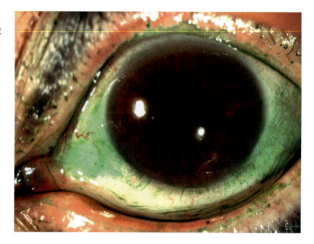

Fig. 7.2 Diffuse exposure zone lissamine green staining of conjunctiva in patient with primary Sjögren's syndrome

on disease severity. Four levels of severity were proposed for each guideline, ranging from mild (level 1) to severe (level 4) disease. Criteria used to grade levels of clinical severity are provided in Table 7.1. Most patients with SS would have level 2 or worse disease and easily fulfill the US-EEC consensus criteria.

Treatment recommendations for each level of clinical severity are provided in Table 7.2. Artificial tears provide transient symptomatic relief for patients who experience intermittent eye irritation when reading or when exposed to dry or drafty environments. Preservative-free preparations are recommended for level 2 and worse disease to prevent surface toxicity from preservatives, particularly benzylkonium chloride. As the disease worsens and patients experience frequent or constant irritation, artificial tears are often inadequate to treat symptoms and ocular surface disease and additional therapies are required.

If moderate-to-severe ocular surface dye staining is present, punctal occlusion is beneficial in increasing tear volume and reducing symptoms, particularly in patients who have lost the ability to tear reflexively and cannot respond to adverse environmental conditions. Punctal occlusion can be accomplished by punctal plugs or thermal cautery. Thermal cautery is permanent but does not carry the risk of microtrauma to the nasal conjunctiva that may occur from silicone punctal plugs.

Patients with central corneal epithelial disease, blurred vision symptoms, or reduced visual acuity from dry eyes require more aggressive therapy that typically includes pulse topical corticosteroid steroid therapy (e.g., loteprednol, etabonate 0.5% four times a day for 2 weeks followed by twice daily for 2 weeks), cyclosporine A 0.05% emulsion two to four times per day, oral doxycycline 40 mg per day (given in one or two doses), and topical autologous serum or plasma. Oral secretogouges have been reported to improve symptoms and dye staining [67, 68]. The Boston Ocular Surface prosthesis has been reported to be an effective therapeutic device for patients with reduced vision and/or moderate to severe irritation or photophobia despite these medical treatments (Fig. 7.3) [69, 70].In the most severe cases with corneal epithelial defects or stromal ulceration, surgical therapies, such as amniotic membrane transplantation or tarsorrhaphy, may need to be considered.

Table 7.1 Dry eye severity grading scheme[a]

Dry eye severity level	1	2	3	4
Discomfort, severity, and frequency	Mild and/or episodic, occurs under environ stress	Moderate or chronic, stress or no stress	Severe, frequent, or constant without stress	Severe and/or disabling and constant
Visual symptoms	None or episodic mild fatigue	Annoying and/or activity limiting, episodic	Annoying, chronic, and/or constant limiting activity	Constant and/or possibly disabling
Conjunctival injection	Mild to none	Mild to none	±	+/++
Conjunctival staining	Mild to none	Variable	Moderate to marked	Marked
Corneal staining (severity/location)	Mild to none	Variable	Marked and central	Severe diffuse
Corneal/tear signs	Mild to none	Mild debris, ↓ meniscus	Filaments, mucus clumping, ↑ tear debris	Filaments, mucus clumping, ↑ tear debris, ulceration
Lid/meibomian glands	MGD variably present	MGD variably present	Frequent	Trichiasis, keratinization, symblepharon
TBUT (s)	Variable	≤ 10	≥ 5	Immediate
Schirmer score (mm/5 min)	Variable	≤ 10	≤ 5	≤ 2

[a]From Dry Eye Workshop Management and Therapy committee report [67]

Environ environmental, *MGD* meibomian gland disease

Table 7.2 Management recommendations for dry eye[a]

Level	Therapy
1	Environmental/dietary modification; eliminate systemic medications with anticholinergic side effects; artificial tears (preservative-free if used >QID); gels and ointments; eyelid therapy for blepharitis
2	If level 1 treatments are inadequate, add: preservative-free artificial tears; anti-inflammatory therapy (cyclosporine A, corticosteroid), oral tetracyclines for posterior blepharitis, punctal plugs if aqueous tear deficiency, oral secretogogues, moisture chamber spectacles
3	If level 2 treatments are inadequate, add: autologous serum/plasma, therapeutic contact lenses (Boston ocular surface prosthesis); permanent punctal occlusion
4	If level 3 treatments are inadequate, add: systemic anti-inflammatory agents, surgery (lid surgery, tarsorrhaphy; mucus membrane, salivary gland, amniotic membrane transplantation)

[a]Treatment recommendations of Dry Eye Workshop Management and Therapy committee [67]

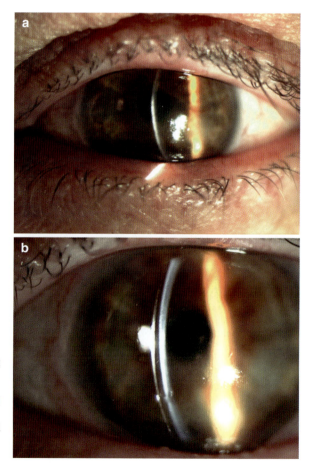

Fig. 7.3 Appearance of cornea with severe epitheliopathy, central stromal haze, and surface irregularity in patient with primary Sjögren's syndrome before (**a**) and after (**b**) fitting with the Boston Ocular Surface Prosthesis. This specially designed fluid-filled scleral contact lens improved corneal surface regularity and visual acuity from 20/100 to 20/30

References

1. Helmick CG, Felson DT, Lawrence RC, Gabriel S, Hirsch R, Kwoh CK, et al. Estimates of the prevalence of arthritis and other rheumatic conditions in the United States. Part I. Arthritis Rheum. 2008;58:15–25.
2. Sullivan DA. Sex hormones and Sjogren's syndrome. J Rheumatol Suppl. 1997;50:17–32.
3. Sullivan DA. Androgen deficiency & dry eye syndromes. Arch Soc Esp Oftalmol. 2004;79:49–50.
4. Toda I, Sullivan BD, Wickham LA, Sullivan DA. Gender- and androgen-related influence on the expression of proto-oncogene and apoptotic factor mRNAs in lacrimal glands of autoimmune and non-autoimmune mice. J Steroid Biochem Mol Biol. 1999;71:49–61.
5. Fox RI. Impact of systemic immune disease on the lacrimal functional unit. In: Pflugfelder SC, Stern ME, Beuerman R, editors. Dry eye and the ocular surface. New York: Marcel Dekker; 2004. p. 269–308.
6. Pflugfelder SC, Crouse CA, Monroy D, Yen M, Rowe M, Atherton S. Epstein-Barr virus and the lacrimal gland pathology of Sjogren's syndrome. Am J Pathol. 1993;143:49–64.
7. Pflugfelder SC, Stern ME, Symposium Participants. Immunoregulation on the ocular surface: 2nd Cullen Symposium. Ocul Surf. 2009;7:67–77.
8. Fox RI, Michelson P. Approaches to the treatment of Sjogren's syndrome. J Rheumatol Suppl. 2000;61:15–21.
9. Fox RI, Maruyama T. Pathogenesis and treatment of Sjogren's syndrome. Curr Opin Rheumatol. 1997;9:393–9.
10. Stern ME, Beuerman RW, Fox RI, Gao J, Mircheff AK, Pflugfelder SC. The pathology of dry eye: the interaction between the ocular surface and lacrimal glands. Cornea. 1998;17:584–9.
11. Pflugfelder SC, Stern ME, Beuerman R. Dysfunction of the integrated functional unit – impact on tear film stability and composition. In: Pflugfelder SC, Stern ME, Beuerman R, editors. Dry eye and the ocular surface. New York: Marcel Dekker; 2004. p. 63–88.
12. Pflugfelder SC, Liu Z, Monroy D, Jones DT, Carvajal ME, Price-Schiavi S, et al. Detection of sialomucin complex (MUC4) in human ocular surface epithelium and tear fluid. Invest Ophthalmol Vis Sci. 2000;41:1316–26.
13. Stern ME, Beuerman R, Pflugfelder SC. The normal tear film and ocular surface. In: Pflugfelder SC, Stern ME, Beuerman R, editors. Dry eye and the ocular surface. New York: Marcel Dekker; 2004. p. 41–62.
14. Govindarajan B, Gipson IK. Membrane-tethered mucins have multiple functions on the ocular surface. Exp Eye Res. 2010;90:655–63.
15. Inatomi T, Spurr-Michaud SJ, Tisdale AS, Zhan Q, Feldman ST, Gipson IK. Expression of secretory mucin genes by human conjunctival epithelia. Invest Ophthalmol Vis Sci. 1996;37:1684–92.
16. Jumblatt MM, McKenzie RW, Steele PS, Emberts CG, Jumblatt JE. MUC7 expression in the human lacrimal gland and conjunctiva. Cornea. 2003;22:41–5.
17. Watanabe H. Significance of mucin on the ocular surface. Cornea. 2002;21:S17–22.
18. Komatsu M, Tatum L, Altman NH, Carothers Carraway CA, Carraway KL. Potentiation of metastasis by cell surface sialomucin complex (rat MUC4), a multifunctional anti-adhesive glycoprotein. Int J Cancer. 2000;87:480–6.
19. Guzman-Aranguez A, Argueso P. Structure and biological roles of mucin-type O-glycans at the ocular surface. Ocul Surf. 2010;8:8–17.
20. Rieger G. The importance of the precorneal tear film for the quality of optical imaging. Br J Ophthalmol. 1992;76:157–8.
21. Rolando M, Iester M, Macri A, Calabria G. Low spatial-contrast sensitivity in dry eyes. Cornea. 1998;17:376–9.
22. Chotikavanich S, de Paiva CS, de Li Q, Chen JJ, Bian F, Farley WJ, et al. Production and activity of matrix metalloproteinase-9 on the ocular surface increase in dysfunctional tear syndrome. Invest Ophthalmol Vis Sci. 2009;50:3203–9.

23. Goto T, Zheng Z, Okamoto S, Ohashi Y. Tear film stability analysis system: introducing a new application for videokeratography. Cornea. 2004;23:65–70.
24. Jordan A, Baum J. Basic tear flow. Does it exist? Ophthalmology. 1980;87:920–30.
25. Dartt DA. Regulation of tear secretion. Adv Exp Med Biol. 1994;350:1–9.
26. Nakamura M, Tada Y, Akaishi T, Nakata K. M3 muscarinic receptor mediates regulation of protein secretion in rabbit lacrimal gland. Curr Eye Res. 1997;16:614–9.
27. Hodges RR, Zoukhri D, Sergheraert C, Zieske JD, Dartt DA. Identification of vasoactive intestinal peptide receptor subtypes in the lacrimal gland and their signal-transducing components. Invest Ophthalmol Vis Sci. 1997;38:610–9.
28. Hodges RR, Dicker DM, Rose PE, Dartt DA. Alpha 1-adrenergic and cholinergic agonists use separate signal transduction pathways in lacrimal gland. Am J Physiol. 1992;262:G1087–96.
29. Knop E, Knop N. A functional unit for ocular surface immune defense formed by the lacrimal gland, conjunctiva and lacrimal drainage system. Adv Exp Med Biol. 2002;506:835–44.
30. Pflugfelder SC, De Paiva CS, Villarreal AL, Stern ME. Effects of sequential artificial tear and cyclosporine emulsion therapy on conjunctival goblet cell density and transforming growth factor-beta 2 production. Cornea. 2008;27:64–9.
31. Knop E, Knop N. Influence of the eye-associated lymphoid tissue (EALT) on inflammatory ocular surface disease. Ocul Surf. 2005;3(4 Suppl):S180–6.
32. Steven P, Gebert A. Conjunctiva-associated lymphoid tissue – current knowledge, animal models and experimental prospects. Ophthalmic Res. 2009;42:2–8.
33. Rosenthal P, Baran I, Jacobs DS. Corneal pain without stain. Is it real? Ocul Surf. 2009;7:28–40.
34. Pflugfelder SC, Farley W, Luo L, Zhuo Chen L, de Paiva CS, Olmos LC, et al. Matrix metalloproteinase-9 (MMP-9) knockout confers resistance to corneal epithelial barrier disruption in experimental dry eye. Am J Pathol. 2005;166:61–71.
35. Hamrah P, Liu Y, Zhang Q, Dana MR. The corneal stroma is endowed with a significant number of resident dendritic cells. Invest Ophthalmol Vis Sci. 2003;44:581–9.
36. Hamrah P, Zhang Q, Liu Y, Dana MR. Novel characterization of MHC class II-negative population of resident corneal Langerhans cell-type dendritic cells. Invest Ophthalmol Vis Sci. 2002;43:639–46.
37. Hamrah P, Huq SO, Liu Y, Zhang Q, Dana MR. Corneal immunity is mediated by heterogeneous population of antigen-presenting cells. J Leukoc Biol. 2003;74:172–8.
38. Hamrah P, Liu Y, Zhang Q, Dana MR. Alterations in corneal stromal dendritic cell phenotype and distribution in inflammation. Arch Ophthalmol. 2003;121:1132–40.
39. McCulley JP, Shine WE. The lipid layer of tears: dependent on meibomian gland function. Exp Eye Res. 2004;78:361–5.
40. Beuerman R, Stern ME, Mircheff A, Pflugfelder SC. The lacrimal functional unit. In: Pflugfelder SC, Stern ME, Beuerman R, editors. Dry eye and the ocular surface. New York: Marcel Dekker; 2004. p. 11–40.
41. Szliter EA, Lighvani S, Barrett RP, Hazlett LD. Vasoactive intestinal peptide balances pro- and anti-inflammatory cytokines in the Pseudomonas aeruginosa-infected cornea and protects against corneal perforation. J Immunol. 2007;178:1105–14.
42. Robinson CP, Brayer J, Yamachika S, Esch TR, Peck AB, Stewart CA, et al. Transfer of human serum IgG to nonobese diabetic Igmu null mice reveals a role for autoantibodies in the loss of secretory function of exocrine tissues in Sjögren's syndrome. Proc Natl Acad Sci USA. 1998;95:7538–43.
43. Benítez-Del-Castillo JM, Acosta MC, Wassfi MA, Díaz-Valle D, Gegúndez JA, Fernandez C, et al. Relationship between corneal innervation with confocal microscopy and corneal sensitivity with non-contact esthesiometry in patients with dry eye. Invest Ophthalmol Vis Sci. 2007;48(1):173–81.
44. Tuominen IS, Konttinen YT, Vesaluoma MH, Moilanen JA, Helintö M, Tervo TM. Corneal morphology and innervation in primary Sjögren's syndrome. Invest Ophthalmol Vis Sci. 2003;44:2545–9.

45. Zoukhri D, Hodges RR, Byon D, Kublin CL. Role of proinflammatory cytokines in the impaired lacrimation associated with autoimmune xerophthalmia. Invest Ophthalmol Vis Sci. 2002;43:1429–36.
46. Kong L, Robinson CP, Peck AB, Vela-Roch N, Sakata KM, Dang H, et al. Inappropriate apoptosis of salivary and lacrimal gland epithelium of immunodeficient NOD-scid mice. Clin Exp Rheumatol. 1998;16:675–81.
47. Cha S, Brayer J, Gao J, Brown V, Killedar S, Yasunari U, et al. A dual role for interferon-gamma in the pathogenesis of Sjogrens syndrome-like autoimmune exocrinopathy in the non-obese diabetic mouse. Scand J Immunol. 2004;60:552–6.
48. Kimura-Shimmyo A, Kashiwamura S, Ueda H, Ikeda T, Kanno S, Akira S, et al. Cytokine-induced injury of the lacrimal and salivary glands. J Immunother. 2002;25 Suppl 1:S42–51.
49. Lam H, Bleiden L, de Paiva CS, Farley W, Stern ME, Pflugfelder SC. Tear cytokine profiles in dysfunctional tear syndrome. Am J Ophthalmol. 2009;147:198–205.
50. De Paiva CS, Villarreal AL, Corrales RM, Rahman HT, Chang VY, Farley WJ, et al. Dry eye-induced conjunctival epithelial squamous metaplasia is modulated by interferon-gamma. Invest Ophthalmol Vis Sci. 2007;48:2553–60.
51. Pflugfelder SC, Tseng SCG, Yoshino K, Monroy D, Felix C, Reis B. Correlation of goblet cell density and mucosal epithelial mucin expression with rose bengal staining in patients with ocular irritation. Ophthalmology. 1997;104:223–35.
52. Chen Z, Tong L, Li Z, Yoon KC, Qi H, Farley W, et al. Hyperosmolarity-induced cornification of human corneal epithelial cells is regulated by JNK MAPK. Invest Ophthalmol Vis Sci. 2008;49:539–49.
53. De Paiva CS, Pflugfelder SC. Corneal epitheliopathy of dry eye induces hyperesthesia to mechanical air jet stimulation. Am J Ophthalmol. 2003;2004(137):109–15.
54. Vitali C, Bombardieri S, Moutsopoulos HM, Balestrieri G, Bencivelli W, Bernstein RM, et al. Preliminary criteria for the classification of Sjögren's syndrome. Results of a prospective concerted action supported by the European Community. Arthritis Rheum. 1993;36:340–7.
55. Pflugfelder SC, Tseng SC, Sanabria O, Kell H, Garcia CG, Felix C, et al. Evaluation of subjective assessments and objective diagnostic tests for diagnosing tear-film disorders known to cause ocular irritation. Cornea. 1998;17:38–56.
56. Nemeth J, Erdelyi B, Csakany B, Gaspar P, Soumelidis A, Kahlesz F, et al. High-speed videotopographic measurement of tear film build-up time. Invest Ophthalmol Vis Sci. 2002;43:1783–90.
57. Lemp MA, Dohlman CH, Kuwabara T, Holly FJ, Carroll JM. Dry eye secondary to mucus deficiency. Trans Am Acad Ophthalmol Otolaryngol. 1971;75:1223–7.
58. McCulley JOP, Sciallis GF. Meibomian keratoconjunctivitis. Am J Ophthalmol. 1877;84:788–93.
59. Zengin N, Tol H, Gunduz K, Okudan S, Balevi S, Endogru H. Meibomian gland dysfunction and tear film abnormalities in rosacea. Cornea. 1995;14:144–6.
60. de Paiva CS, Lindsey JL, Pflugfelder SC. Assessing the severity of keratitis sicca with videokeratoscopic indices. Ophthalmology. 2003;110:1102–9.
61. Schirmer O. Studien zur Physiologie und Pathologie der Tranenabsonderung and Tranenabfuhr. Graefes Arch Clin Exp Ophthalmol. 1903;56:197.
62. Farris RL, Gilbard JP, Stuchell RN, Mandel ID. Diagnostic tests in keratoconjunctivitis sicca. CLAO J. 1983;9:23–8.
63. Tsubota K. The importance of the Schirmer test with nasal stimulation. Am J Ophthalmol. 1991;111:106.
64. van Bijsterveld OP. Diagnostic tests in sicca syndrome. Arch Ophthalmol. 1969;82:10–4.
65. Nelson JD. Diagnosis of keratoconjunctivitis sicca. Int Ophthalmol Clin. 1994;34:37–56.
66. Behrens A, Doyle JJ, Stern L, Chuck RS, McDonnell PJ, Azar DT, et al. Dysfunctional tear syndrome: a Delphi approach to treatment recommendations. Cornea. 2006;25:900–7.
67. Pflugfelder S. Management and therapy of dry eye disease: report of the Management and Therapy Subcommittee of the International Dry Eye WorkShop. Ocul Surf. 2007;5:163–78.

68. Petrone D, Condemi JJ, Fife R, Gluck O, Cohen S, Dalgin P. Double-blind randomized placebo-controlled study of cevimeline in Sjögren's syndrome patients with xerostomia and keratoconjunctivitis sicca. Arthritis Rheum. 2002;46:748–54.
69. Stason WB, Razavi M, Jacobs DS, Shepard DS, Suaya JA, Johns L, et al. Clinical benefits of the Boston Ocular Surface Prosthesis. Am J Ophthalmol. 2010;149:54–61.
70. Rosenthal P, Croteau A. Fluid-ventilated, gas-permeable scleral contact lens is an effective option for managing severe ocular surface disease and many corneal disorders that would otherwise require penetrating keratoplasty. Eye Contact Lens. 2005;31:130–4.

Chapter 8
Ear, Nose, and Throat Manifestations of Sjögren's Syndrome

Rohan R. Walvekar and Francis Marchal

Contents

8.1 Introduction

Sjögren's syndrome (SjS) is an autoimmune disease that primarily affects the secretory function of lacrimal and salivary glands [1]. Dry mouth (xerostomia) is the most common presenting complaint [2], but SjS can affect multiple organs including the kidneys, lungs, liver, blood vessels, and lymph nodes, resulting in a myriad of clinical manifestations [3]. This chapter provides an overview of the key manifestations of SjS associated with the ear, nose, and throat region. We review the otologic, sinus and nasal, laryngopharyngeal, and tracheal manifestations of this disease.

8.2 Otologic Manifestations

The otologic manifestations associated with SjS have not been extensively reported but are generally mild [4]. Most otologic complaints consist of hearing loss (25%), which is often a mild to moderate sensorineural hearing loss in the high frequencies

R.R. Walvekar
Department of Otolaryngology Head and Neck Surgery, LSU Health Sciences
Center, Salivary Endoscopy Service and Clinical Research, New Orleans, LA, USA

F. Marchal (✉)
Department of Otolaryngology Head and Neck Surgery, Sialendoscopy Unit, European
Sialendoscopy Training Center (ETSC), University Hospital of Geneva, Geneva, Switzerland

M. Ramos-Casals et al. (eds.), *Sjögren's Syndrome*,
DOI 10.1007/978-0-85729-947-5_8, © Springer-Verlag London Limited 2012

[3–5]. Although the pathophysiology of this hearing loss is not well understood, it is postulated to be due to the deposition of immune complexes in the inner ear stria vascularis and subsequent ischemia of the inner ear arterial microvasculature. Autoantibodies to cardiolipin and M_3 muscarinic receptors in patient sera are suspected to play a role in the pathogenesis of this hearing loss [3]. Other proposed theories include autoantibodies to ciliar epitopes in patients with increased genetic susceptibility or increased production of gamma interferon and inflammatory cytokines by inner ear cells [3, 6–8].

The deposition of the immune complexes occurs at the basal turn of the cochlea, which represents hearing in the high frequencies [4]. Consequently, patients with SjS have high frequency sensorineural hearing loss that can be either unilateral or bilateral [4]. Studies evaluating otologic symptoms in patients with SjS suggest that the prevalence of hearing loss is lower in patients with primary SjS (4.5–27%) as compared to those with secondary SjS (19.4–46%) [1, 4]. This is consistent with the notion that sensorineural hearing loss is associated with systemic autoimmune disease rather than SjS per se. Current evidence is still insufficient to confirm this hypothesis. Mild to severe sensorineural hearing loss may also be an early manifestation of SjS [3] and consequently could be included in the workup of patients with sicca complex.

Patients with SjS can also present with complaints related to dryness of the external auditory canal skin, otalgia or ear pain, tinnitus, vertigo, and recurrent ear infections. Hearing loss, otalgia, and tinnitus have been reported to occur in 25% of patients presenting with otologic symptoms. These symptoms are proposed to be due to crust or lymphoid masses obstructing the eustachian tube orifice [9].

Doig et al. [1] were the first to report audiological findings in SjS. The study evaluated 22 patients with primary SjS, 31 with secondary SjS (rheumatoid arthritis and SjS), and 21 with RA. Evaluations included a comprehensive otologic history with examination of the ears and audiometry. Audiometric evaluation were graded 1 (normal hearing), 2 (maximum limit of hearing loss acceptable as normal), and 3 (impaired hearing both conductive and sensorineural). The authors reported otalgia and tinnitus in 4.5% (1 of 22) and dryness of the external auditory canal, dry wax, or/and abnormal/perforated ear drum in 9.1% (2 of 22) patients with primary SjS. A low incidence of otologic symptoms was recorded for patients with secondary SjS, as well. However, Campbell et al. [9] reported that dryness of the external canal is more frequent than abnormalities of the tympanic membrane.

Doig et al. also suggested that patients with SjS are at risk for otitis media with effusion. However, in a more recent study, Freeman et al. evaluated 196 patients with SjS including 60 patients with unclassified sicca syndrome (according to the revised 2002 international classification criteria [10]) and did not report an increased prevalence of middle ear pathology or risk for otitis media with effusion [4].

Although the otologic manifestations of SjS are not frequent, they can cause significant quality-of-life impairment. It would be ideal to include a comprehensive otologic workup including a microscopic ear examination, review of otologic symptoms, and objective hearing evaluation (speech audiometry, auditory brainstem-evoked responses, and impedance audiometry) to evaluate external, middle, and inner ear pathology as well as rule out retrocochlear and brainstem lesion that can be associated with sensorineural hearing loss.

Fig. 8.1 Radioactive (^{99m}Tc) scans of salivary glands in Sjögren's syndrome (*below*) and in a normal subject (*above*). The diminished uptake over nasal cavity (*C*) in the patients with Sjögren's syndrome is seen as compared to the normal patient. *C* Nasal cavity, *D* Oral cavity, *A* Parotid glands, *B* Submandibular glands

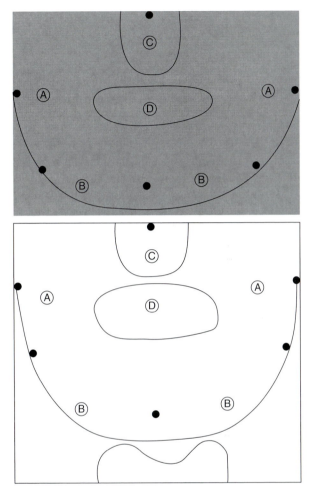

8.3 Sinus and Nasal Manifestations

Nasal function can be altered in patients suffering from SjS as a consequence of the exocrine gland dysfunction in that condition. Nasal mucociliary clearance studies in patients with SjS demonstrate a dissociation of flow between the solid and gel layers of nasal mucus [11]. In addition, hypofunctioning of the nasal glands can be visualized by scanning the nasal cavity using a Technetium 99m scan (^{99m}Tc). Patients with SjS show reduced uptake in the nose, oral cavity, and major salivary glands compared to normal controls (Fig. 8.1) [1]. Much investigation remains to be performed, however, to facilitate a full understanding of the extent of nasal disease in SjS.

Most studies describing the prevalence of nasal symptoms are observational in nature and have reported variable results. Nasal complaints most commonly consist of nasal dryness, crusting, congestion, hyposmia, and epistaxis. Freeman et al. [4] reported nasal symptoms in up to 50% of patients in their study. However, nasal examination with anterior rhinoscopy revealed abnormal findings in only 20% [4]. Nasal dryness has been reported from 18% to 73% in various studies [1, 9, 12, 13], and crusting in 18.5% [1], 44% [12], and up to 50% [9] in different studies. Hyposmia or a decreased sense of smell is present in 30–45% of patients and is often associated with hypoguesia [1, 5, 9, 14]. Chronic sinusitis has also been reported in patients with SjS [5].

Epistaxis is commonly reported in patients with SjS. Doig et al. reported epistaxis in 31% of patients with primary SjS [1]. However, Freeman and colleagues reported a divergent experience [4]. In fact, while Doig et al. and other studies have reported objective findings of nasal crusting, nasal atrophy, and nasal dryness in up to 54% of patients, Freeman and colleagues found abnormal nasal examinations in only 20% of their study population [1, 4]. These differences in presenting symptoms and clinical findings can be explained by individual patient variability, small sample sizes, and geographical variability in study populations.

Although, nasal symptoms are prevalent in patients with SjS, they are often not dominant presenting symptoms. Consequently, it is incumbent on the physician to question patients regarding these symptoms and to perform an evaluation of nasal symptoms and a complete nasal examination, including anterior rhinoscopy and nasal endoscopic evaluation of the nasal cavity and nasopharynx. Smell disturbances can be further quantified utilizing test such as the UPSIT (University of Pennsylvania Smell Identification Test) test (Sensonics Inc, Haddon Heights, NJ). The UPSIT test is a standardized microcapsulated odorant test that can be applied over 15–20 min on an outpatient basis. Scores range from 19 to 40, categorizing patients from severe microsmia to normal smell appreciation [15, 16].

8.4   Laryngopharyngeal and Tracheal Manifestations

The symptom of dry mouth and physical findings consistent with xerostomia are hallmarks of SjS and have been reported in up to 100% and 94% of patients, respectively [1, 9, 17–21]. The oral manifestations of SjS are comprehensively described in Chap. 6. However, it is important to reiterate that dry mouth and xerostomia are intimately related to and often contribute to symptoms and manifestations within the larynx, pharynx, and trachea. Laryngopharyngeal symptoms generally occur with or after the onset of xerostomia [14].

Pharyngeal involvement usually is related to absence of saliva and dryness of the pharyngeal mucosa [9]. Thick, tenacious secretions can also contribute to these symptoms. Most patients complain of food sticking to the mouth, difficulty swallowing food, the need to drink water to wash food down the esophagus, and avoidance of dry foods [9]. Patients may also complain of dry cough and a foreign body or globus sensation in the throat.

Freeman et al. [4] reported that abnormal findings in the throat and larynx were detected in only 24% of patients, despite the fact that approximately 80% of the

Fig. 8.2 Bamboo node: middle third right vocal cord lesion (*black arrow* points to nodule)

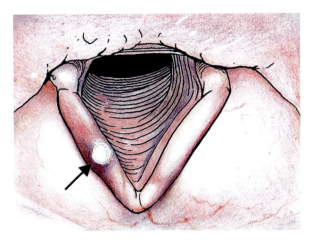

patients in their study had laryngopharyngeal complaints. Previous studies have shown that laryngopharyngeal symptoms are often associated with significant esophageal dysmotility (10%) [22, 23], the presence of esophageal webs, and post-cricoid narrowing [9]. Consequently, throat and laryngeal complaints must be taken seriously and investigated appropriately. A detailed review of esophageal manifestations of SjS is presented in Chap. 16.

Hoarseness and dsyphonia are late manifestations of SjS. Bloch et al. reported hoarseness in 20 (32%) of their 62 patients with primary SjS [24]. Hoarseness is usually related to chronic mucosal dryness or tenacious mucus that coats the vocal cords. Other causes in include cricoarytenoid joint arthritis, laryngitis, granulomatous or nongranulomatous nodules, laryngeal mucosal thickening, or recurrent laryngeal nerve paresis or palsy [25]. Movement of the vocal cords is usually normal on examination, suggesting that cricoarytenoid joint involvement as seen in RA is uncommon in SjS [1]. However, a vocal fold lesion can be the presenting symptom of SjS [5]. In addition, a vocal cord lesion unique to autoimmune diseases known as the "bamboo node" has been described in SjS. The lesion is a white or yellow transverse submucosal lesion typically located in the middle third of the vocal fold (Fig. 8.2) [26]. Murano et al. reported two cases of bamboo nodes in patients with SjS [27].

Granulomatous and nongranulomatous nodules have also been described in SjS. Granulomatous nodules have no site predilection. In contrast, nongranulomatous nodules are symmetrical and characteristically involve the anterior third of the true cords. They are similar in appearance and histology to vocal nodules secondary to vocal abuse [5, 25]. Patients may not have visible laryngeal lesions but can present with hoarseness. Clinical and experimental data suggest that this could be explained by submucosal deposition of immune complexes that may be present for long durations of time prior to development of visible lesions. Gilliam and Cheatum examined the basement membrane of a patient with skin and laryngeal lesion with systemic lupus erythematosus and demonstrated immune complexes that confirmed similar postulations by Cooke in 1972 [25, 28, 29].

Other vocal cord lesions described in association with SjS include a patient with bilateral vocal nodules with different gross appearance: one side presenting with a granuloma and the other with a polypoidal and edematous lesion [25]. Grundy et al. [30] reported a patient with SjS who presented with a rapidly enlarging mass on the left vocal cord that required a temporary tracheostomy and lateral laryngotomy for tumor excision. Pathology could not distinguish between a sarcomatous transformation versus a pseudolymphoma. Another variation includes a patient reported to have presented with progressive hoarseness and dyspnea that was associated with diffuse thickening and narrowing of the glottic and supraglottic structures [31].

Tracheal involvement in SjS includes dryness and thick adherent mucus with erythrema of the mucosa seen in 25% of patients [9]. Crusting is often present and consequently hemoptysis may occur. However, it must be borne in mind that SjS can be associated with actual lymphocytic infiltration and also with pseudolymphoma of the larynx [9, 25, 30]. Consequently, concerning symptoms such as persistent hoarseness, associated dysphagia, laryngeal lesions, and hemoptysis need further evaluation, histopathological confirmation of benign disease, and exclusion of coexistent malignancy of the aerodigestive tract.

Most laryngopharyngeal and tracheal evaluations reported in the literature have been performed by indirect laryngoscopy. In current practice, high-definition tools with recording capabilities have significantly improved quality of head and neck assessments. Flexible laryngoscopy, high-definition imaging, and stroboscopy to delineate vocal fold motion, and transnasal in-office esophagoscopy and bronchoscopy are tools available to the otolaryngologist today.

The diagnosis and treatment of SjS can be challenging. A collaborative effort involving the otolaryngologist, ophthalmologist, internist, rheumatologist, radiologist, pathologist, and dental services to appropriately diagnose, classify, and treat patients effectively and in a comprehensive fashion is needed [2]. There remain many gaps in our understanding of the ear, nose, and throat manifestations of this disorder.

Acknowledgments The authors would like to acknowledge the Louisiana State University (LSU) Department of Otolaryngology Head & Neck Surgery, New Orleans, Louisiana, USA for its support. In particularly, we wish to thank Virginia Plauche (LSU School of Medicine) and Neelima Tammareddi (PGY-2 Otolaryngology Resident), Esther Phelps and Dane Blanchard (academic staff) with LSU Department of Otolaryngology Head Neck Surgery.

The authors would like to thank Eugene New for his help with the illustrations contained in this chapter (medart4u@yahoo.com).

References

1. Doig JA et al. Otolaryngological aspects of Sjogren's syndrome. Br Med J. 1971;4(5785): 460–3.
2. Carsons S. Sjogren's syndrome. In: Firestein G, Budd RC, Harris ED, McInnes IB, Ruddy S, Sergent JS, editors. Firestein: Kelley's textbook of rheumatology. 8th ed. Philadelphia: W.B. Saunders Company; 2008. p. 1148–69.
3. Tucci M, Quatraro C, Silvestris F. Sjogren's syndrome: an autoimmune disorder with otolaryngological involvement. Acta Otorhinolaryngol Ital. 2005;25(3):139–44.

4. Freeman SR et al. Ear, nose, and throat manifestations of Sjogren's syndrome: retrospective review of a multidisciplinary clinic. J Otolaryngol. 2005;34(1):20–4.
5. Mahoney EJ, Spiegel JH. Sjogren's disease. Otolaryngol Clin North Am. 2003;36(4): 733–45.
6. Trune DR. Cochlear immunoglobulin in the C3H/lpr mouse model for autoimmune hearing loss. Otolaryngol Head Neck Surg. 1997;117(5):504–8.
7. Nariuchi H et al. Mechanisms of hearing disturbance in an autoimmune model mouse NZB/kl. Acta Otolaryngol Suppl. 1994;514:127–31.
8. Moysan JF et al. Is the target of anti-cardiolipin antibodies the same in Gougerot-Sjogren syndrome and lupus erythematosus disseminatus? Rev Med Interne. 1987;8(2): 163–8.
9. Campbell SM, Montanaro A, Bardana EJ. Head and neck manifestations of autoimmune disease. Am J Otolaryngol. 1983;4(3):187–216.
10. Vitali C et al. Classification criteria for Sjogren's syndrome: a revised version of the European criteria proposed by the American-European Consensus Group. Ann Rheum Dis. 2002;61(6): 554–8.
11. Takeuchi K et al. Nasal mucociliary clearance in Sjogren's syndrome. Dissociation in flow between sol and gel layers. Acta Otolaryngol. 1989;108(1–2):126–9.
12. Rasmussen N, Brofeldt S, Manthorpe R. Smell and nasal findings in patients with primary Sjogren's syndrome. Scand J Rheumatol Suppl. 1986;61:142–5.
13. Jacobsen H, Johannessen AC, et al. Sjogren's syndrome in Bergen during a two-year period. ENT symptoms in Sjogren's syndrome. In: Transactions of the XXV Congress of the Scandinavian Oto-Laryngological Society. Bergen. 1993.
14. Henkin RI et al. Abnormalities of taste and smell in Sjogren's syndrome. Ann Intern Med. 1972;76(3):375–83.
15. Doty RL, Shaman P, Dann M. Development of the University of Pennsylvania Smell Identification Test: a standardized microencapsulated test of olfactory function. Physiol Behav. 1984;32(3):489–502.
16. Doty RL et al. University of Pennsylvania Smell Identification Test: a rapid quantitative olfactory function test for the clinic. Laryngoscope. 1984;94(2 Pt 1):176–8.
17. Lin DF et al. Clinical and prognostic characteristics of 573 cases of primary Sjogren's syndrome. Chin Med J (Engl). 2010;123(22):3252–7.
18. Garcia-Carrasco M et al. Primary Sjogren syndrome: clinical and immunologic disease patterns in a cohort of 400 patients. Medicine (Baltimore). 2002;81(4):270–80.
19. Skopouli FN et al. Clinical evolution, and morbidity and mortality of primary Sjogren's syndrome. Semin Arthritis Rheum. 2000;29(5):296–304.
20. Davidson BK, Kelly CA, Griffiths ID. Primary Sjogren's syndrome in the North East of England: a long-term follow-up study. Rheumatology (Oxford). 1999;38(3):245–53.
21. Alamanos Y et al. Epidemiology of primary Sjogren's syndrome in north-west Greece, 1982–2003. Rheumatology (Oxford). 2006;45(2):187–91.
22. Kjellen G et al. Esophageal function, radiography, and dysphagia in Sjogren's syndrome. Dig Dis Sci. 1986;31(3):225–9.
23. Anselmino M et al. Esophageal motor function in primary Sjogren's syndrome: correlation with dysphagia and xerostomia. Dig Dis Sci. 1997;42(1):113–8.
24. Bloch KB, Buchanan WW, Wohl MJ, et al. Sjogren's syndrome: a clinical, pathological, and serological study of 62 cases. Medicine. 1965;44:187–231.
25. Prytz S. Vocal nodules in Sjogren's syndrome. J Laryngol Otol. 1980;94(2):197–203.
26. Valter HR, Pillon J, Kosugi EM, Fujita R, Pontes P. Laryngeal assessment in reumatic disease patients. Rev Bras Otorrinolaringol. 2005;71(4):499–503.
27. Murano E et al. Bamboo node: primary vocal fold lesion as evidence of autoimmune disease. J Voice. 2001;15(3):441–50.
28. Cooke TD et al. The pathogenesis of chronic inflammation in experimental antigen-induced arthritis. II. Preferential localization of antigen-antibody complexes to collagenous tissues. J Exp Med. 1972;135(2):323–38.

29. Gilliam JN, Cheatum DE. Immunoglobulins in the larynx in systemic lupus erythematosus. Arch Dermatol. 1973;108(5):696–7.
30. Grundy DJ. Sjogren's disease with widespread lymphoid deposits. Proc R Soc Med. 1972;65(2):167–8.
31. Barrs DM, McDonald TJ, Duffy J. Sjogren's syndrome involving the larynx: report of a case. J Laryngol Otol. 1979;93(9):933–6.

Chapter 9
Fatigue in Primary Sjögren's Syndrome

Barbara M. Segal

Contents

9.1   Epidemiology of Fatigue

Recognition of a syndrome characterized by fatigue in patients without an obvious cardiopulmonary illness dates back to the late nineteenth century [1–3]. Early descriptions of patients with "neurasthenia" focused on the substantial weakness and lassitude accompanying the syndrome, which was particularly prominent among women. Following the conclusion of the First World War, physicians were challenged by the large numbers of battle-scarred veterans afflicted by chronic fatigue [4]. The lack of a generally accepted tool for measuring fatigue impeded progress in understanding that symptom.

Barbara M. Segal
Division of Rheumatic and Autoimmune Disorders,
University of Minnesota Medical School, Minneapolis, MN, USA

Department of Medicine, Hennepin County Medical Center,
Minneapolis, MN, USA

M. Ramos-Casals et al. (eds.), *Sjögren's Syndrome*,
DOI 10.1007/978-0-85729-947-5_9, © Springer-Verlag London Limited 2012

Over the past two decades, reliable instruments for fatigue measurement have been developed that can be used both in day-to-day clinical practice and in clinical trials. Persistent fatigue is a common symptom reported by 15–22% of persons in the general population [5, 6]. Abnormal fatigue, defined as a sense of exhaustion that is not relieved by rest, is also a ubiquitous concomitant of chronic illness. Among patients with autoimmune disease, fatigue is a particularly prevalent and debilitating symptom. It has a profoundly negative impact on quality of life [7].

9.2   Assessing Fatigue

Tools used to measure fatigue include a simple 10 cm visual analog scale (VAS) that provides a global rating, and brief questionnaires in which patients are asked to respond to a series of questions [8–10]. Among the "uni-dimensional" questionnaires that have been used in primary Sjögren's syndrome (SS) studies (Table 9.1), the Functional Assessment of Chronic Illness Therapy (FACIT) Fatigue Scale and the Fatigue Severity Scale (FSS) have acceptable psychometric properties, [9, 39]. Each of these instruments provides a composite fatigue score comparable to the global fatigue rating provided by a VAS [8, 9, 42]. The different questionnaires address slightly different aspects of fatigue, but comparisons between scales demonstrate convergent validity [15, 22] (Table 9.1). The reliability and validity of the FACIT-Fatigue instrument (FACIT-F) and the FSS have been established in a variety of chronic rheumatic and nonrheumatic illnesses [9, 43]. The smallest difference in fatigue score that patients perceive as beneficial (minimal clinically important difference or MCID) has been evaluated with the FSS in RA and in SLE [44, 45]. The MCID of the FACIT-F was assessed in a sample of RA patients [9]. A minimally important difference for a fatigue visual analog scale of about 10% has been suggested for use in RA clinical trials and for interpretation of the fatigue VAS in day-to-day clinical practice [33]. There is need for agreement on a standardized version of a fatigue VAS and additional research to establish the sensitivity to change for the fatigue questionnaires in SS.

Fatigue influences the physical, emotional, cognitive, and even social aspects of life. Moreover, it frequently coexists with factors such as stress, mood disturbance, and sleep disorder that complicate the measurement of fatigue. Instruments with more complex structure such as the Multidimensional Fatigue Inventory and Profile of Fatigue provide a means to investigate relationships between different aspects (domains) of fatigue and physiologic or psychosocial variables [11, 46]. The Profile of Fatigue and Discomfort (PROFAD-SSI) provides specific profile of symptoms based upon descriptors used by patients with primary SS. Examples include fatigue, joint and muscle pain, and cold hands. Important domains are the physical (needing to rest, low stamina, weak muscles) and the mental experience of fatigue (difficulty concentrating and poor memory). The individual domains of physical and mental fatigue obtained with the Profile of Fatigue can vary independently of each other.

Table 9.1 Questionnaires used to measure fatigue in primary Sjögren's syndrome

Instrument(ref)	Comments	Internal consistency (Cronbach's alpha)	Construct validity in primary SS studies	Number of primary SS studies	Citations
MFI [11]	Multidimensional: 20-items that generate 5 dimensions of 4 items each (general, physical, reduced activity, reduced motivation, mental fatigue)	$\alpha=.8$	Moderate to strong correlation with the equivalent facets of the profile fatigue and with a VAS	9	[12] [13] [14] [15] [16] [16] [18] [17] [18]
FSS [9, 10]	9 items scored on a 1–7 scale which address fatigue impact on specific types of functioning during the past week	$\alpha=.93$	Moderate correlations with VAS and somatic domain of the Profile of Fatigue	2	[19, 20] [21, 22]
FACIT-F fatigue scale [8]	13 items (range 0–52). Normative data available on patients with cancer and from the general population	$\alpha=.87$	Strong correlation with the vitality subscale of the SF-36	2	[23, 24] [24]
Dutch fatigue scale [10]	9-item scored on 1–4 point scale	$\alpha=.91$	Validated in normal and medical populations	1	[25]
SF-36 [26]	4-item measure of vitality (energy level and fatigue)			11	[27] [28] [11] [29] [30] [28] [32]

(continued)

Table 9.1 (continued)

Instrument(ref)	Comments	Internal consistency (Cronbach's alpha)	Construct validity in primary SS studies	Number of primary SS studies	Citations
Profile of fatigue [29]	Multidimensional: four somatic and two mental facets comprised of 16 items providing mean score (range 0–7) for 2 domains: somatic and physical	$\alpha = .97$–99	Strong correlation with the VAS and SF36; somatic domain correlates with FSS	9	[34] [30] [31] [37] [15] [21] [38] [127] [11]
Chalder fatigue scale [32]	14 items: measures severity of fatigue in 2 dimensions (mental, physical) with 4 response alternatives (range 0–56)	$\alpha = .89$	CFS failed to discriminate between primary SS patients and controls [40]	2	[33] [34]

The FSS is simple to administer and has been widely used by investigators interested in the impact of fatigue among patients with multiple sclerosis and SLE, as well as primary SS, primary biliary cirrhosis (PBC), and chronic hepatitis C [47–50]. The nine item FSS index emphasizes the behavioral aspects of fatigue and assesses an individual's perception of the degree to which fatigue limits his or her ability to function on a 7-point scale [8]. A score of ≥4 indicates abnormal fatigue that limits physical activity [51]. Interestingly, nearly identical mean FSS scores of between 4.6 and 4.8 have been reported in primary SS, SLE, RA, multiple sclerosis, and primary biliary cirrhosis, disorders with heterogeneous organ manifestations and quite different demographics. The severity of fatigue experienced by persons with chronic inflammatory illness is similar despite differences in gender, age, and disease-specific organ manifestations [21, 39, 45, 47, 48].

Multiple studies have, in fact, demonstrated that psychosocial variables are significant predictors of fatigue in patients with rheumatic disease [27, 52, 53]. In a large cohort of primary SS patients, the predominant factors associated with fatigue as measured by the FSS were pain, depression, and helplessness [22]. Those same three variables predicted 71% of the variance in physical fatigue. Helplessness, a concept defined as the perception that patients have very little control over their symptoms, has been identified as a significant risk factor for fatigue in SLE and in multiple sclerosis as well as in primary SS. The relationship between fatigue and helplessness is consistent with cognitive theory that suggests that persons who see themselves as unable to influence or control their condition are more susceptible to fatigue and depression [54, 55].

In contrast to the associations detected between fatigue and behavioral variables, correlations between fatigue and laboratory variables such as the Westergren erythrocyte sedimentation rate and autoantibody titers are weak or inconsistent [25, 47, 52, 56, 57]. In SLE, variables associated with fatigue include older age, helplessness, abnormal illness behavior, and any previous neurologic disease manifestation, but not laboratory measures or disease activity [58]. Similarly, multiple disease-related variables, including sicca symptom severity, salivary gland function, immunoglobulin titer, hemoglobin concentration, and absolute lymphocyte count were not associated with physical or "mental" fatigue in primary SS [22].

9.3 Prevalence of Fatigue and Impact of Fatigue on Health-Related Quality of Life in Primary SS

In persons with primary SS, the prevalence of abnormal fatigue is about 70% [11, 20, 22, 31]. Seropositive and seronegative patients are equally likely to report clinically significant fatigue [22]. The prevalence of chronic fatigue was reported to be 22% among healthy working adults in a population-based study [59]. Fatigue, pain, and cognitive symptoms comprise a commonly experienced set of overlapping symptoms. The mechanisms underlying such symptom clusters are largely unknown (Table 9.2).

Table 9.2 Hypothesized individual risk factors for symptom clusters associated with primary Sjögren's syndrome

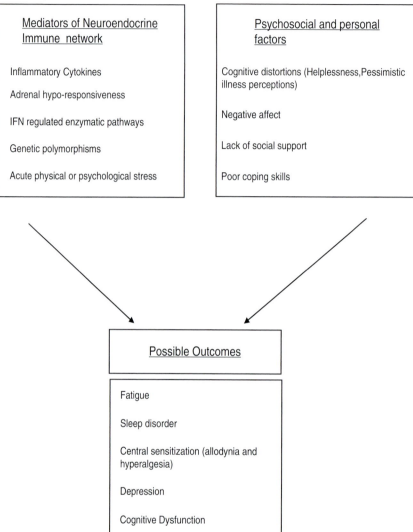

Patients with similar fatigue intensity can have widely divergent levels of disability [26]. Stratification of subjects according to the level of disability is therefore important in assessing fatigue. The SF-36 is a widely used measure of health-related quality of life designed for use in population surveys [60]. Each of the eight SF-36 subscales has a range of 0–100, with 100 indicating very good health status. Any score below 50 is considered below the population average. Population norms are available for demographic subsets categorized by age and gender. SF-36 scale scores provide a means to measure the effects of illness on each of eight domains of health status: physical activity, usual role functioning, pain, general health, vitality, social activity, role functioning difficulties caused by emotional problems, and mental health. The domain scores can be used to derive two summary measures of health status: physical (PCS) and mental (MCS) summary measures. The SF-36 has been applied in multiple rheumatic conditions for the purposes of assessing relative health status, the effectiveness of interventions, and the validity of new disease-specific questionnaires [61, 62].

Substantial reduction in all domains of health-related quality of life has been demonstrated in primary SS comparable to the reduction in quality of life in patients with RA and fibromyalgia.[31] Irrespective of the instrument used to assess fatigue, diminished quality of life is strikingly linked to fatigue in multiple autoimmune disorders including primary SS [31, 49, 57]. In a recent large community survey of primary SS subjects, Physical functioning (mean = 35.0), Energy/fatigue (mean = 38.9), and General Health (mean = 45.5) were the domains that were ranked lowest by primary SS patients [23]. General health among primary SS patients was uniquely predicted by somatic fatigue (pain, mental fatigue, depression, age, and sicca severity were not significant predictors in the model), whereas emotional well-being was predicted by depression and pain severity.

Oral sicca severity as measured by the PROFAD-SSI was also associated with reduced general health, social functioning, and lower energy levels and greater fatigue levels [63]. Patients with the most severe sicca symptoms report the greatest impact on all activities of daily life: physical activity, daily activities, social interactions, mental alertness, sexual relations, career productivity, and choice of occupation. Interestingly, in a large survey of patients with RA, noninflammatory rheumatic disorders, and fibromyalgia, the prevalence of sicca symptoms was increased in all three patient groups. The likelihood of self-reported sicca symptoms was related to illness severity, therapy, and psychological distress [64].

9.4 Relationship of Fatigue to Cognitive Symptoms and to Depression

Affective disorder is associated with fatigue in essentially all studies. In a recent survey of persons with primary SS in the United States, the prevalence of depressive symptoms was 37% [22]. This figure is similar to the prevalence of self-reported depression in SLE (32%) [65]. Fatigue and depression have a dual interaction in that depressed patients typically report the most severe fatigue and patients with fatigue are more likely to be depressed. However, clinicians should be cautious in attributing pain and fatigue to depression in primary SS, because the nature of the relationship between fatigue and depression has not been elucidated. Further, the majority of primary SS patients with fatigue are not depressed [22]. Depression could contribute to fatigue through psychological effects: for example, the patient's reaction to having a chronic illness. It is also possible that parallel but independent biological mechanisms such as dysregulated cytokine networks contribute to the underlying pathophysiology of both fatigue and depression [19].

Patients with primary SS and SLE often refer to a symptom colloquially referred to as "brain fog." Although subjective memory loss and concentration difficulties are frequently reported by primary SS patients, the contribution of cognitive dysfunction to quality of life and to fatigue is less clear. Cognitive symptoms do not contribute to disability independently of depression [23]. Attention and memory are cognitive domains that are very sensitive to depression. Cognitive function measured objectively, particularly performance on verbal memory and attention tests, correlates with perceived problems in memory and attention in primary SS, but larger studies are needed to assess the contribution of depression to mild cognitive dysfunction [66].

The neuroanatomic substrate of cognitive difficulties in primary SS has been explored recently. In unselected primary SS patients, conventional magnetic resonance imaging of the brain did not demonstrate clinically relevant abnormalities [21]. However, two recent pilot studies that combined detailed neuropsychometric assessment with sensitive brain imaging modalities suggest a different picture of neuropathology in primary SS. Cerebral perfusion abnormalities in brain single photon emission computerized tomography (SPECT) imaging in primary SS patients correlated with deficits on psychometric tests of executive function and attention [67]. In addition, a high-resolution quantitative diffusion tensor imaging (MR-DTI) study suggested a very localized pattern of white matter injury in primary SS subjects who complained of subtle cognitive impairment. MR-DTI demonstrated abnormalities localized to the inferior frontal white matter in primary SS patients with mild difficulties in verbal memory and attention [68]. The inferior frontal region is involved in memory processing and regulation of the impact of negative emotion on memory [69–71]. Observation of abnormality localized to inferior frontal white matter in primary SS is especially intriguing in light of recent data that link fatigue in primary SS with elevated levels of inflammatory cytokines within the cerebrospinal fluid [72].

Brain imaging studies have also demonstrated interesting correlations between fatigue and imaging parameters in both multiple sclerosis (MS) and SLE [73, 74]. Functional MRI demonstrated different brain activation patterns in fatigued versus nonfatigued MS patients [75]. Moreover, abnormal recruitment of frontal-thalamic circuitry was associated with interferon-induced fatigue [75]. Another functional MRI study demonstrated that cognitive fatigue in MS, operationally defined by slowed performance on a specific mental task, relates to impaired interactions between functionally related cortical and subcortical areas [76]. Evidence of correlation between decreased perfusion of the thalamus and increased fatigue provides further structural support to theories relating fatigue to impaired connectivity between cortical and subcortical regions [77]. In MS patients studied with proton magnetic resonance spectroscopy, fatigue (FSS) was associated with diffuse axonal injury. This association was independent of T2 lesion volume, age, disease duration, and disability score. These findings suggest that increased recruitment of cortical areas is responsible for the patients' sense that the effort required to perform actions is disproportionately high [78]. In primary SS, a pilot brain diffusion tensor imaging study demonstrated correlation of white matter injury in the caudal anterior cingulate gyrus with physical fatigue (FSS) and with pain severity [79]. Although additional work is needed to confirm the DTI data, quantitative computer-assisted brain imaging has the potential to provide a window into brain microstructure and to provide clues to the origin of the subtle cognitive dysfunction in primary SS.

9.5   Fatigue Viewed From the Physiological Perspective: Relationships Between Fatigue, Sleep Quality, and Neuroendocrine Function

Since the 1920s, attempts to evaluate fatigue from a physiologic perspective have been viewed skeptically. Although fatigue is a subjective experience that can be measured only by asking patients to describe how they feel, the experience of fatigue assessed through the use of fatigue questionnaires has been shown to correlate with physiologic variables. Several studies have addressed cardiopulmonary exercise performance [41, 51, 80]. There are limited data on sleep quality in primary SS and SLE, yet poor sleep quality is reported by as many as 62% of patients with SLE and 75% of patients with primary SS [81–83]. In primary SS and in SLE, fatigue is associated with both reduction in aerobic capacity and with poor sleep quality [41, 73, 84].

Sleep quality is amenable to measurement with validated self-report questionnaires such as the Pittsburg Sleep Quality Index (PSQI) [85] and by objective assessments such as polysomnography and actigraphy. Polysomnography, the classic "sleep study," represents the gold standard for evaluation of sleep quality. However, because of its high cost and intrusive nature, relatively few data are available regarding the effect of sleep quality on daytime fatigue in patients with autoimmune disease. Actigraphy involves the analysis of data obtained with a laser wrist band worn by the subject during the night. The subject records the time he or she goes to bed and the time of awakening in a sleep diary. The propulsive movements of the upper extremity are recorded on a computer chip. Actigraphy, which provides a reliable record of sleep duration and sleep fragmentation, correlates well with polysomnography studies conducted in a sleep laboratory [86]. Recently the relationship between daytime fatigue and objectively measured sleep quality was reported in primary SS and RA subjects [35]. For individuals with both conditions, a night of worse discomfort and poor sleep was followed by more severe fatigue compared with the individual's average.

Disturbed neuroendocrine function has been suggested as a cause of both fatigue and sleep disorder [87]. Adrenal axis hypofunction has been reported in primary SS [88], but the precise nature of the relationship between neuroendocrine function and fatigue in primary SS has been difficult to define. The role of the autonomic nervous system in mediating some aspects of fatigue also remains speculative. There is evidence of both parasympathetic and sympathetic nervous system dysfunction in primary SS compared to controls. Cardiovascular reflexes (tilt test, heart rate variability) are generally reduced in primary SS patients, but the clinical relevance of these findings is unclear [89–91]. High levels of fatigue correlated with hypotension in one study [92]. However, data on autonomic nervous system function must be interpreted cautiously because the correlation between the results of autonomic reflex tests and autonomic nervous system symptoms is poor. Symptoms of autonomic dysfunction, but not the results of reflex tests, are significantly associated with fatigue, anxiety, and depression [36].

In animal models, the behavioral response to infection or injury is a stereotypical behavioral alteration termed sickness behavior [93]. Behavioral aspects of sickness include depression, lethargy, the need to sleep, failure to feed, reduced social behavior, and increased sensitivity to pain [94]. These behavioral manifestations are presumed to be mediated by the effects of inflammatory cytokines acting upon the hypothalamic-pituitary stress response system. Cytokine release provides a signal that triggers the set of metabolic and behavioral changes that are collectively called "sickness" [93]. For example, IL-1 can induce slow wave sleep, loss of appetite, and enhanced production of corticotrophin releasing hormone [88, 95]. The modulation of sleep by inflammatory cytokines is one example of altered homeostasis by centrally acting cytokines which has been well studied in human models of illness [96].

Increased levels of IL-1Ra in cerebral spinal fluid are associated with increasing fatigue in primary SS patients, indicating that the activated IL-1 system is a possible biological factor associated with fatigue [20]. Additional evidence for a link between inflammatory cytokines and fatigue is suggested by the finding that soluble IL6R had a strong inverse correlation with fatigue in one study of primary SS [14]. IL-6 stimulates the HPA axis via IL-6 receptors to produce stress hormones counteracting fatigue. Disruption in neuroendocrine function regulated by IL-6 could play a role in mediating fatigue. However, few studies have explored the link between circulating inflammatory cytokines and fatigue, and the data in primary SS are inconsistent [16]. The IL-6 system is thought to regulate dehydroepiandrosterone sulfate (DHEA-S). While DHEA levels are decreased in primary SS patients [87, 88], DHEA treatment had no effect on fatigue in primary SS in two studies [13, 89]. Although improvement in fatigue did not occur with DHEA, even at supraphysiologic doses, there is evidence consistent with the hypothesis that defective processing of DHEA could contribute to fatigue in primary SS [90].

9.6   Relationship Between Fibromyalgia and SS

Features of fibromyalgia (FM) include fatigue, generalized pain, and the presence of multiple tender points on examination. Patients with chronic widespread pain and 11/18 tender points fulfill the ACR classification criteria for FM [101]. The reported prevalence of FM in the general population is about 2.0% [102]. Controversy continues as to whether FM is a distinct clinical disease entity or a universal human response to illness and stress. Irritable bowel syndrome, irritable bladder, and chronic fatigue syndrome overlap with FM, and clear differentiation between these disorders is often difficult. It has been suggested that FM is not a specific disease entity but rather a condition in which the symptoms reflect difficulties in coping with various types of environmental stresses [103]. However, FM patients are not uniform, and the severity of psychological distress and behavioral disorders vary among patients meeting criteria for FM [104, 105]. Although no specific etiologic factors have been identified as causative of FM, a variety of stressors including trauma, history of abuse, and viral infection have been linked to the onset of the illness.

In patient surveys, as many as 22.1% of patients with SLE and 17.0% of patients with arthritis appear to have clinical features consistent with the diagnosis of FM [106]. Patients recognized as meeting ACR criteria for FM typically present with high levels of polysymptomatic distress including fatigue, cognitive symptoms, sleep disturbance, and decreased pain threshold [107]. The prevalence of FM among patients with definite primary SS is between 12% and 22% [108, 109]. The reason for the increased frequency of FM in persons with rheumatic disease compared to the general population is not well understood. A population-based cohort study demonstrated that high levels of cortisol after dexamethasone and high levels of cortisol in evening saliva were associated with a moderately increased risk of developing chronic widespread pain [110]. Thus, a reasonable hypothesis is that adrenal axis hypofunction predisposes some individuals with systemic autoimmune disease to the development of FM.

FM patients exhibit physiologic disturbances in central pain processing including decreased pain threshold (allodynia) and increased sensitivity to subthreshold pain stimuli (hyperalgesia.) A decreased threshold to multiple types of noxious stimuli including heat and noise has also been demonstrated in FM and is characteristic of central sensitization. Dysregulation of the stress response system could be a final common pathway resulting in diffuse widespread pain and chronic fatigue which are then maintained by central sensitization mechanisms [111, 112]. A unifying hypothesis of FM and related disorders such as irritable bowel syndrome suggests that the somatic components represent biological amplification of sensory input, a paradigm that is supported by the results of functional imaging brain MRI studies in FM [113]. The cause of the abnormalities in central pain processing and the reason that disordered sensory processing at a central level is maintained in FM patients is not known.

The evaluation of pain mechanisms in primary SS patients is complex, because pain of nociceptive and neuropathic origin often coexist. Symptoms suggestive of neuropathic pain (burning, pins and needles sensation, numbness) are very frequently reported by patients with primary SS, but are also frequently reported by patients with FM in whom central sensitization is presumed to be the mechanism. Pain severity and pain interference with activities as measured by the Brief Pain Inventory were substantially greater in primary SS patients with positive sensory symptoms (paresthesia and burning discomfort.) Both positive and negative sensory symptoms (numbness) were more common in patients compared to controls in a recent large survey of primary SS [114]. These differences in sensory symptoms persisted between patients and controls when adjusted for depression and a history of FM, suggesting that nerve damage in the primary SS patients was the more likely explanation.

Table 9.3 Comparison of nociceptive and neuropathic pain

Pain classification	Pain mechanism	Clinical exam	Descriptors/stimulus
I. Neuropathic	Primary lesion (or dysfunction) in the nervous system	Positive and negative sensory signs including stimulus-evoked hypersensitivities often with focal autonomic abnormalities	
A. Spontaneous	Central hyperexcitability possibly due to loss of inhibition due to destruction of peripheral nociceptors	Sensory deficits often marked in the area of pain	Burning, throbbing shooting, stabbing, or electric-like Pins and needles
B. Stimulus-evoked	Maintained by continuing activity from damaged primary afferent nociceptors	Allodynia (pain response to a normally nonpainful stimulus) and mechanical and pressure hyperalgesia	Abnormal sensation produced by pressure, cold or heat, pin, brush,
II. Nociceptive	Activation of peripheral nociceptors	Mechanical or inflammatory tissue damage	Dull aching

Distinguishing FM from primary SS with painful sensory neuropathy is especially challenging because the clinical neurological deficits in patients with primary SS and small-fiber neuropathy can be modest. In some patients with small-fiber neuropathy, the clinical examination is completely normal and ancillary tests (e.g., skin biopsy with evaluation of epidermal nerve fiber density) are required for diagnosis. Both neuropathic pain and nociceptive pain can lead to central sensitization, particularly in individuals with high anxiety and emotional distress [115].

Distinguishing FM from primary SS can also be problematic because of the overlap in clinical presentation. Fatigue is the presenting complaint in as many as 27% of primary SS patients; muscle pain is the presenting symptom in an additional 25% [63, 116]. Similarly, chronic fatigue, atypical Raynaud's phenomenon, depression, and anxiety are highly prevalent in FM. Eighty to 90% of patients with either primary SS or FM are women, and routine laboratory testing, and results of radiologic studies are typically normal in both conditions [117]. Complaints of xerostomia may be present in as many as 70% of FM subjects [118]. The precise cause of the sicca symptoms in FM patients is not known, although it has been suggested that neurologic mechanisms could account for the sicca symptoms in the absence of gland inflammation.

Detailed bedside neurologic evaluation is especially helpful in those with complaints of neuropathic pain (Table 9.3). Evidence of small-fiber neuropathy (manifest by painful distal paresthesia and loss of distal sensation to pinprick) was found in 45% of outpatients with a definite diagnosis of primary SS [119]. The mechanism of sensory neuropathy is not known. Increased amounts of substance P and vasoactive intestinal peptide, in mast cells, plasma cells, and lymphocytes in primary SS, suggest that neuropeptides upregulated by inflammation may play a role in peripheral nerve damage [120]. Abnormalities on sensory testing are often subtle, and electrophysiologic studies are normal in patients with painful, predominantly, small-fiber neuropathy. Epidermal nerve fiber biopsy (EFNB), which is used to demonstrate loss of small unmyelinated nerve fibers, is an elegant technique available in only a few centers and can be useful to confirm an impression of small-fiber neuropathy.

9.7   Management of Pain and Fatigue

Diagnosis and optimal management of SS frequently requires a multidisciplinary approach including objective evaluation of sicca complaints to document the severity and response to topical management. Investigation of neuropathic complaints to detect subtle forms of neuropathy, and evaluation for sleep disorders and depression can be important in the management of chronic fatigue and pain. Pharmacologic therapy of pain, sleep disorder, and affective disorders should be carefully tailored to minimize anticholinergic effects of medications which have the potential to increase sicca complications. Reduction of pain is optimized when all pain sources are addressed. Both central and peripheral pain mechanisms often coexist in patients with primary SS and subclinical neuropathy may be common. Gabapentin and tricyclics are effective for small-fiber neuropathy in diabetics and may have efficacy in primary SS.

The pharmacologic treatment of FM is particularly difficult. NSAIDs and opioids are not effective for central pain [121]. A trial of tricyclics, serotonin–norepinephrine reuptake inhibitors, and/or alpha-2 delta ligands may be modestly helpful in a minority of patients, although promising results obtained in pilot studies of FM have not been duplicated thus far with only about 30% pain reduction in one half of the patients [122]. Fatigue has not been a primary outcome in most primary SS clinical trials; however, recently published randomized controlled trials of rituximab have shown a significant benefit in systemic manifestations such as cryoglobulinemic vasculitis, renal and pulmonary involvement as well as improvement in fatigue [12, 123, 124].

Psychological evaluation as part of the assessment of patients with fatigue and widespread pain is appropriate. Behavioral and psychological variables such as helplessness and poor coping predispose patients with chronic illness to increased pain and fatigue and increase the risk of affective disorder. Educational intervention targeting cognitive appraisal of illness to improve coping abilities is helpful in SLE [125]. The contribution of psychological factors to fatigue was underlined by a clinical trial of DHEA in primary SS which showed that subjects in the placebo arm experienced improvement equal to the effect on subjects in the treatment arm, demonstrating that the expectation of benefit was sufficient to improve fatigue [13]. Nonpharmacologic therapy which may be beneficial includes recommendations regarding exercise and stress management in some patients. Low-impact aerobic exercise gradually increasing in intensity, duration, and frequency may be an effective strategy in reducing fatigue in autoimmune conditions including primary SS [122, 126].

9.8 Summary

Primary SS is a common systemic autoimmune disorder in which diagnosis is frequently delayed. Extraglandular manifestations of primary SS include persistent abnormal fatigue which is present in 70% and can be the presenting symptom. A cluster of symptoms: fatigue, pain, and emotional distress are often the principle reason that patients seek care. Nonspecific constitutional symptoms accompany the sicca manifestations in the majority of primary SS patients and are the predominant predictors of poor quality of life. The clinical presentation may overlap substantially with that of FM. Evaluation of and treatment for neuropathic and nociceptive sources of pain, emotional distress, and sleep quality are required for the optimal management of fatigue and improvement in the overall health status of patients with primary SS.

References

1. Beard GM. Neurosthenia, or nervous exhaustion. Boston Med Surg J. 1869;3:217–20.
2. Shorter E. Chronic fatigue in historical perspective. Ciba Found Symp. 1993;173:6–16.
3. Wessely S. Old wine in new bottles: neurasthenia and "M.E.". Psychol Med. 1990;20:427–36.
4. Muscio B. Is a fatigue test possible? Br J Psychol. 1921;12:31–46.
5. Chen MK. The epidemiology of self-perceived fatigue among adults. Prev Med. 1986;15:74–81.
6. Loge JH, Ekeberg O, Kaasa S. Fatigue in the general Norwegian population: normative data and associations. J Psychosom Res. 1998;45:53–65.
7. Wolfe F, Michaud K, Li T, Katz RS. EQ-5D and SF-36 quality of life measures in systemic lupus erythematosus: comparisons with rheumatoid arthritis, noninflammatory rheumatic disorders, and fibromyalgia. J Rheumatol. 2010;37:296–304.
8. Krupp LB, LaRocca NG, Muir-Nash J, Steinberg AD. The fatigue severity scale: application to patients with multiple sclerosis and systemic lupus erythematosus. Arch Neurol. 1989;46:1121–3.
9. Cella D, Yount S, Sorensen M, Chartash E, Sengupta N, Grober J. Validation of the functional assessment of chronic illness therapy fatigue scale relative to other instrumentation in patients with rheumatoid arthritis. J Rheumatol. 2005;32:811–9.
10. Tiesinga LJ, Dassen TW, Halfens RJ. DUFS and DEFS: development, reliability and validity of the Dutch fatigue scale and the Dutch exertion fatigue scale. Int J Nurs Stud. 1998;35:115–23.
11. Bowman SJ, Booth DA, Platts RG, UK Sjogren's Interest Group. Measurement of fatigue and discomfort in primary Sjogren's syndrome using a new questionnaire tool. Rheumatology. 2004;43:758–64.
12. Meijer JM, Meiners PM, Vissink A, et al. Effective rituximab treatment in primary Sjogren's syndrome: a randomised, double-blind, placebo-controlled trial. Arthritis Rheum. 2010. doi:10.1002/art.27314.
13. Virkki LM, Porola P, Forsblad-d'Elia H, Valtysdottir S, Solovieva SA, Konttinen YT. Dehydroepiandrosterone (DHEA) substitution treatment for severe fatigue in DHEA-deficient patients with primary Sjögren's syndrome. Arthritis Care Res. 2010;62:118–24.
14. d'Elia HF, Bjurman C, Rehnberg E, Kvist G, Konttinen YT. Interleukin 6 and its soluble receptor in a central role at the neuroimmunoendocrine interface in Sjogren syndrome: an explanatory interventional study. Ann Rheum Dis. 2009;68:285–6.

15. Goodchild CE, Treharne GJ, Booth DA, Kitas GD, Bowman SJ. Measuring fatigue among women with Sjogren's syndrome or rheumatoid arthritis: a comparison of the Profile of Fatigue (ProF) and the Multidimensional Fatigue Inventory (MFI). Musculoskeletal Care. 2008;6:31–48.
16. Vriezekolk JE, Geenen R, Hartkamp A, et al. Psychological and somatic predictors of perceived and measured ocular dryness of patients with primary Sjogren's syndrome. J Rheumatol. 2005;32:2351–5.
17. Hartkamp A, Geenen R, Bijl M, Kruize AA, Godaert GL, Derksen RH. Serum cytokine levels related to multiple dimensions of fatigue in patients with primary Sjogren's syndrome. Ann Rheum Dis. 2004;63:1335–7.
18. Zandbelt MM, de Wilde P, van Damme P, et al. Etancercept in the treatment of patients with primary Sjogren's syndrome: a pilot study. J Rheumatol. 2004;31:96–101.
19. Godaert GL, Hartkamp A, Geenen R, et al. Fatigue in daily life in patients with primary Sjogren's syndrome and systemic lupus erythematosus. Ann N Y Acad Sci. 2002;966:320–6.
20. Barendregt PJ, Visser MR, Smets EM, et al. Fatigue in primary Sjogren's syndrome. Ann Rheum Dis. 1998;57:291–5.
21. Harboe E, Beyer MK, Greve OJ, et al. Cerebral white matter hyperintensities are not increased in patients with primary Sjogren's syndrome. Eur J Neurol. 2009;16:576–81.
22. Segal B, Thomas W, Rogers T, et al. Prevalence, severity, and predictors of fatigue in subjects with primary Sjogren's syndrome. Arthritis Rheum. 2008;59:1780–7.
23. Segal B, Bowman SJ, Fox PC, et al. Primary Sjogren's syndrome: health experiences and predictors of health quality among patients in the United States. Health Qual Life Outcomes. 2009;7:46.
24. Walker J, Gordon T, Lester S, et al. Increased severity of lower urinary tract symptoms and daytime somnolence in primary Sjogren's syndrome. J Rheumatol. 2003;30:2406–12.
25. Bax HI, Vriesendorp TM, Kallenberg CGM, Kalk WWI. Fatigue and immune activity in Sjögren's syndrome. Ann Rheum Dis. 2002;61:284.
26. Reeves WC, Lloyd A, Vernon SD, et al. Identification of ambiguities in the 1994 chronic fatigue syndrome research case definition and recommendations for resolution. BMC Health Serv Res. 2003;3:25.
27. Champey J, Corruble E, Gottenberg JE, et al. Quality of life and psychological status in patients with primary Sjögren's syndrome and sicca symptoms without autoimmune features. Arthritis Rheum. 2006;55:451–7.
28. Belanguer R, Ramos-Casals M, Brito-Zeron P, et al. Influence of clinical and immunological parameters on the health-related quality of life of patients with primary Sjögren's syndrome. Clin Exp Rheumatol. 2005;23:351–6.
29. Rostron J, Rogers S, Longman L, et al. Health-related quality of life in patients with primary Sjogren's syndrome and xerostomia: a comparative study. Gerondontology. 2002;10:53–9.
30. Tensing EK, Solovieva SA, Tervahartiala T, et al. Fatigue and health profile in sicca syndrome of Sjogren's and non-Sjogren's syndrome origin. Clin Exp Rheumatol. 2001;19:313–6.
31. Strombeck B, Ekdahl C, Manthorpe R, Wikstrom I, Jacobsson L. Health-related quality of life in primary Sjogren's syndrome, rheumatoid arthritis and fibromyalgia compared to normal population data using SF-36. Scand J Rheumatol. 2000;29:283–8.
32. Thomas E, Hay EM, Hajeer A, et al. Sjogren's syndrome: a community-based study of prevalence and impact. Br J Rheumatol. 1998;37:1069–76.
33. Khanna D, Pope JE, Khanna PP, et al. The minimally important difference for the fatigue visual analog scale in patients with rheumatoid arthritis followed in an academic clinical practice. J Rheumatol. 2008;35:2339–43.
34. Theander L, Strombeck B, Mandl T, et al. Sleepiness or fatigue? Can we detect treatable causes of tiredness in primary Sjogren's syndrome? Rheumatology (Oxford). 2010;49:1177–83.
35. Goodchild CE, Treharne GJ, Booth DA, Bowman SJ. Daytime patterning of fatigue and its associations with the previous night's discomfort and poor sleep among women with primary Sjögren's syndrome or rheumatoid arthritis. Musculoskeletal Care. 2010;8(2):107–17. PMID: 20229610.

36. Mandl T, Hammar O, Theander E, Wollmer P, Ohlsson B. Autonomic nervous dysfunction development in patients with primary Sjogren's syndrome: a follow-up study. Rheumatology (Oxford). 2010;49(6):1101–6.
37. Bowman SJ, Hamburger J, Richards A, et al. Patient-reported outcomes in primary Sjogren's syndrome: comparison of the long and short versions of the profile of fatigue and discomfort–sicca symptoms inventory. Rheumatology (Oxford). 2009;48:140–3.
38. Bowman SJ, Sutcliffe N, Isenberg DA, et al. Sjögren's Systemic Clinical Activity Index (SCAI)--a systemic disease activity measure for use in clinical trials in primary Sjögren's syndrome. Rheumatology (Oxford). 2007;461:845–51.
39. Valko PO, Bassetti CL, Bloch KE, Held U, Baumann CR. Validity of the fatigue severity scale in a Swiss cohort. Sleep. 2008;31:1601–7.
40. Lwin CT, Bishay M, Platts RG, Booth DA, Bowman SJ. The assessment of fatigue in primary Sjögren's syndrome. Scand J Rheumatol. 2003;32:33–7.
41. Strombeck B, Ekdahl C, Manthorpe R, Jacobsson LT. Physical capacity in women with primary Sjogren's syndrome: a controlled study. Arthritis Rheum. 2003;49:681–8.
42. Chalder T, Berelowitz G, Pawlikowska T, et al. Development of a fatigue scale. J Psychosom Res. 1993;37:147–53.
43. Ad Hoc Committee on Systemic Lupus Erythematosus Response Criteria for Fatigue. Measurement of fatigue in systemic lupus erythematosus: a systematic review. Arthritis Rheum. 2007;57:1348–57.
44. Goligher EC, Pouchot J, Brant R, et al. Minimal clinically important difference for 7 measures of fatigue in patients with systemic lupus erythematosus. J Rheumatol. 2008;35:635–42.
45. Pouchot J, Kherani RB, Brant R, et al. Determination of the minimal clinically important difference for seven fatigue measures in rheumatoid arthritis. J Clin Epidemiol. 2008;61:705–13.
46. Smets EMA, Garssen B, Bonke B, De Haes JCJM. The Multidimensional Fatigue Inventory (MFI) psychometric qualities of an instrument to assess fatigue. J Psychosom Res. 1995;39:315–25.
47. Krupp LB, LaRocca NG, Muir J, Steinberg AD. A study of fatigue in systemic lupus erythematosus. J Rheumatol. 1990;17:1450–2.
48. Cauch-Dudek K, Abbey S, Steward DE, Heathcote EJ. Fatigue in primary biliary cirrhosis. Gut. 1998;43:705–10.
49. Flachenecker P, Kumpfel T, Kallmann B, et al. Fatigue in multiple sclerosis: a comparison of different rating scales and correlation to clinical parameters. Mult Scler. 2002;8:523–6.
50. Kleinman L, Zodet MW, Hakim Z, et al. Psychometric evaluation of the fatigue severity scale for use in chronic hepatitis C. Qual Life Res. 2000;9:499–508.
51. Keyser RE, Rus V, Cade WT, Kalappa N, Flores RH, Handwerger BS. Evidence for aerobic insufficiency in women with systemic lupus erythematosus. Arthritis Rheum. 2003;49:16–22.
52. Wolfe F, Hawley DJ, Wilson K. The prevalence and meaning of fatigue in rheumatic disease. J Rheumatol. 1996;23:1407–17.
53. Jump RL, Robinson ME, Armstrong AE, Barnes EV, Kilbourn KM, Richards HB. Fatigue in systemic lupus erythematosus: contributions of disease activity, pain, depression, and perceived social support. J Rheumatol. 2005;32:1699–705.
54. van der Werf SP, Evers A, Jongen PJ, Bleijenberg G. The role of helplessness as mediator between neurological disability, emotional instability, experienced fatigue and depression in patients with multiple sclerosis. Mult Scler. 2003;9:89–94.
55. Burgos PI, Alarcón GS, McGwin GJ, Crews KQ, Reveille JD, Vilá LM. Disease activity and damage are not associated with increased levels of fatigue in systemic lupus erythematosus patients from a multiethnic cohort: LXVII. Arthritis Rheum. 2009;61:1179–86.
56. Omdal R, Waterloo L, Koldingsnes W, Husby G, Mellgen SI. Fatigue in patients with systemic lupus erythematosus; the psychosocial aspects. J Rheumatol. 2003;30:283–7.
57. Wang B, Gladman DD, Urowitz MB. Fatigue in lupus is not correlated with disease activity. J Rheumatol. 1998;25:892–5.

58. Zonana-Nacach A, Roseman JM, McGwin Jr G, et al. Systemic lupus erythematosus in three ethnic groups. VI: factors associated with fatigue within 5 years of criteria diagnosis. LUMINA Study Group. Lupus in minority populations: nature vs nurture. Lupus. 2000;9:101–9.
59. Kant IJ, Bültmann U, Schröer KA, Beurskens AJ, van Amelsvoort LG, Swaen GM. An epidemiological approach to study fatigue in the working population: the Maastricht Cohort Study. Occup Environ Med. 2003;60(Suppl I):i32–9.
60. Ware JE, Sherbourne CD. The MOS 36-item short-form health survey(SF-36): conceptual framework and item selection. Med Care. 1992;30:473–83.
61. Anderson JJ, Ruwe M, Miller DR, Kazis L, Felson DT, Prashker M. Relative costs and effectiveness of specialist and general internist ambulatory care for patients with 2 chronic musculoskeletal conditions. J Rheumatol. 2002;29:1488–95.
62. Komaroff AL, Fagioli LR, Doolittle TH, et al. Health status in patients with chronic fatigue syndrome and in general population and disease comparison groups. Am J Med. 1996;101:281–90.
63. Fox PC, Bowman SJ, Segal B, et al. Oral involvement in primary Sjogren syndrome. J Am Dent Assoc. 2008;139:1592–601.
64. Wolfe F, Michaud K. Prevalence, risk, and risk factors for oral and ocular dryness with particular emphasis on rheumatoid arthritis. J Rheumatol. 2008;35:1023–30.
65. Wolfe F, Michaud K. Predicting depression in rheumatoid arthritis: the signal importance of pain extent and fatigue, and comorbidity. Arthritis Rheum. 2009;61:667–73.
66. Segal BM, Pogatchnik B, Holker E, et al. Primary Sjögren's syndrome: cognitive symptoms, mood and cognitive performance. Acta Neurol Scand. 2011. doi:10.1111/j.1600-0404.2011.01530x.
67. Le Guern V, Belin C, Henegar C, et al. Cognitive function and 99mTc-ECD brain SPECT are significantly correlated in patients with primary Sjogren's syndrome: a case-control study. Ann Rheum Dis. 2010;69:132–7.
68. Segal B, Mueller B, Zhu X, et al. Disruption of brain white matter microstructure in primary Sjögren's syndrome: evidence from diffusion tensor imaging. Rheumatology (Oxford). 2010;49(8):1530–9.
69. Price JL, Drevets WC. Neurocircuitry of mood disorders. Neuropsychopharmacology. 2010;35:192–216.
70. Arnsten FT. Stress signaling pathways that impair prefrontal cortex structure and function. Nat Rev Neurosci. 2009;10:410–20.
71. Dolcos F, Kragel P, Wang L, McCarthy G. Role of the inferior frontal cortex in coping with distracting emotions. Neuroreport. 2006;17:1591–4.
72. Harboe E, Tjensvoll AB, Vefring HK, Goransson LG, Kvaloy JT, Omdal R. Fatigue in primary Sjögren's syndrome – a link to sickness behaviour in animals? Brain Behav Immun. 2009;23:1104–8.
73. Sepulcre J, Masdeu JC, Goni J, et al. Fatigue in multiple sclerosis is associated with the disruption of frontal and parietal pathways. Mult Scler. 2009;15:337–44.
74. Harboe E, Greve OJ, Beyer M, et al. Fatigue is associated with cerebral white matter hyperintensities in patients with systemic lupus erythematosus. J Neurol Neurosurg Psychiatry. 2008;79:199–201.
75. Rocca MA, Agosta F, Colombo B, et al. FMRI changes in relapsing-remitting multiple sclerosis patients complaining of fatigue after IFN beta-1a injection. Hum Brain Mapp. 2007;28:373–82.
76. DeLuca J, Genova HM, Hillary FG, Wylie G. Neural correlates of cognitive fatigue in multiple sclerosis using functional MRI. J Neurol Sci. 2008;270:28–39.
77. Inglese M, Park S, Johnson G, et al. Deep gray matter perfusion in multiple sclerosis dynamic susceptibility contrast perfusion magnetic resonance imaging at 3T. Arch Neurol. 2007;64:196–202.
78. Tartaglia MC, Narayanan S, Francis S, et al. The relationship between diffuse axonal damage and fatigue in multiple sclerosis. Arch Neurol. 2004;61:201–7.

79. Segal B, Mueller BA, Pogatchnik BP, et al. Abnormalities in cerebral white matter microstructure correlate with cognitive function and psychological symptoms in patients with primary Sjogren's syndrome. Presented at the 10th international Sjogren's syndrome congress. Brest, France; 2009.

80. Tench C, Bentley D, Vleck V, McCurdie I, White P, D'Cruz D. Aerobic fitness, fatigue, and physical disability in systemic lupus erythematosus. J Rheumatol. 2002;29:474–81.

81. Gudbjornsson B, Broman JE, Hetta J, Halgren R. Sleep disturbances in patients with primary Sjogren's syndrome. Br J Rheumatol. 1993;32:1072–6.

82. Tishler M, Barak Y, Paran D, Yaron M. Sleep disturbances, fibromyalgia and primary Sjogren's syndrome. Clin Exp Rheumatol. 1997;15:71–4.

83. Chandrasekhara PK, Jayachandran NV, Rajasekhar L, Thomas J, Narsimulu G. The prevalence and associations of sleep disturbances in patients with systemic lupus erythematosus. Mod Rheumatol. 2009;19:407–15.

84. Tench CM, McCurdie I, White PD, D'Cruz DP. The prevalence and associations of fatigue in systemic erythematosus. Rheumatology (Oxford). 2000;39:1249–54.

85. Buysse DJ, Reynolds 3rd CF, Monk TH, Berman SR, Kupfer DJ. The Pittsburgh sleep quality index: a new instrument for psychiatric practice and research. Psychiatry Res. 1989;28:193–213.

86. Lichstein KL, Stone KC, Donaldson J, et al. Actigraphy validation with insomnia. Sleep. 2006;29:232–9.

87. Kapsimalis F, Basta M, Varouchakis G, Gourgoulianis K, Vgontzas A, Kryger M. Cytokines and pathological sleep. Sleep Med. 2008;9:603–14.

88. Johnson EO, Kostandi M, Moutsopoulos HM. Hypothalamic-pituitary-adrenal axis function in Sjogren's syndrome: mechanisms of neuroendocrine and immune system homeostasis. Ann N Y Acad Sci. 2006;1088:41–51.

89. Mandl T, Jacobsson L, Lilja B, Sundkvist G, Manthorpe R. Disturbances of autonomic nervous function in primary Sjogren's syndrome. Scand J Rheumatol. 1997;26:401–6.

90. Kovacs L, Paprika D, Takacs R, et al. Cardiovascular autonomic dysfunction in primary Sjogren's syndrome. Rheumatology (Oxford). 2004;43:95–9.

91. Barendregt PJ, Tulen JHM, van den Meiracker AH, Markusse HM. Spectral analysis of heart rate and blood pressure variability in primary Sjögren's syndrome. Ann Rheum Dis. 2002;61:232–6.

92. d'Elia HF, Rehnberg E, Kvist G, Ericsson A, Konttinen Y, Mannerkorpi K. Fatigue and blood pressure in primary Sjogren's syndrome. Scand J Rheumatol. 2008;37:284–92.

93. Konsman JP, Parnet P, Dantzer R. Cytokine-induced sickness behaviour: mechanisms and implications. Trends Neurosci. 2002;25:154–9.

94. Kelly KW, Bluthe R, Dantzer R, et al. Cytokine-induced sickness behavior. Brain Behav Immun. 2003;17:112–8.

95. Rothwell NJ. Functions and mechanisms of interleukin 1 in the brain. Trends Pharmacol Sci. 1991;12:43–436.

96. Santos RV, Tufik S, De Mello MT. Exercise, sleep and cytokines: is there a relation? Sleep Med Rev. 2007;11:231–9.

97. Valtysdottir ST, Wide L, Hallgren R. Mental wellbeing and quality of sexual life in women with primary Sjogren's syndrome are related to circulating dehydroepiandrosterone sulphate. Ann Rheum Dis. 2003;62:875–9.

98. Valtysdottir ST, Wide L, Hallgren R. Low serum dehydroepiandrosterone sulfate in women with primary Sjogren's syndrome as an isolated sign of impaired HPA axis function. J Rheumatol. 2001;28:1259–65.

99. Hartkamp A, Geenen R, Godaert GL, et al. Effect of dehydroepiandrosterone administration on fatigue, well-being, and functioning in women with primary Sjogren syndrome: a randomised controlled trial. Ann Rheum Dis. 2008;67:91–7.

100. Porola P, Virkki L, Przybyla BD, et al. Androgen deficiency and defective intracrine processing of dehydroepiandrosterone in salivary glands in Sjogren's syndrome. J Rheumatol. 2008;35:2229–35.
101. Wolfe F, Smythe HA, Yunus MB, Bennet RM, Bombardier C, Goldenberg DL. The American College of Rheumatology 1990 criteria for the classification of fibromyalgia: report of the multicenter criteria committee. Arthritis Rheum. 1990;33:160–72.
102. Bennett RM. Fibromyalgia: the commonest cause of widespread pain. Compr Ther. 1995;21:69–75.
103. Lorentzen F. Fibromyalgia: a clinical challenge. J Intern Med. 1994;235:199–203.
104. Arnold LM, Hudson JI, Keck PE, Auchenbach MB, Javaras KN, Hess EV. Comorbidity of fibromyalgia and psychiatric disorders. J Clin Psychiatry. 2006;67:1219–25.
105. Thieme K, Turk DC, Flor H. Comorbid depression and anxiety in fibromyalgia syndrome: relationship to somatic and psychosocial variables. Psychosom Med. 2004;66:837–44.
106. Wolfe F, Petri M, Alarcon GS, et al. Fibromyalgia, SLE and evaluation of SLE disease activity. J Rheumatol. 2009;36:82–8.
107. Wolfe F. Fibromyalgianess. Arthritis Rheum. 2009;61:715–6.
108. Ostuni P, Botsios C, Sfriso P, et al. Prevalence and clinical features of fibromyalgia in systemic lupus erythematosus, systemic sclerosis and Sjögren's syndrome. Minerva Med. 2002;93:203.
109. Giles I, Isenberg D. Fatigue in primary Sjogren's syndrome: is there a link with the fibromyalgia syndrome? Ann Rheum Dis. 2000;59:875–8.
110. McBeth J, Silman AJ, Gupta A, et al. Moderation of psychosocial risk factors through dysfunction of the hypothalamic-pituitary-adrenal stress axis in the onset of chronic widespread pain. Arthritis Rheum. 2007;56:360–71.
111. Staud R. Biology and therapy of fibromyalgia: pain in fibromyalgia syndrome. Arthritis Res Ther. 2006;8:208.
112. Van Houdenhove B. Central sensitivity syndromes: stress system failure may explain the whole picture. Semin Arthritis Rheum. 2009;39:218–9.
113. Gracely RH, Petzke F, Wolf JM, Clauw DJ. Functional magnetic resonance imaging evidence of augmented pain processing fibromyalgia. Arthritis Rheum. 2002;46:1333–43.
114. Segal B, Bowman SJ, Fox PC, et al. Prevalence of sensory symptoms in primary Sjogren's Syndrome (pSS) and relationship of neuropathic symptoms to depression and fibromyalgia. Arthritis Rheum. 2007;56(Supple):S448.
115. Giske L, Bautz-Holter E, Sandvik L, Roe C. Relationship between pain and neuropathic symptoms in chronic musculoskeletal pain. Pain Med. 2009;10:910–7.
116. Bjerrum K, Prause J. Primary Sjögren's syndrome: a subjective description of the disease. Clin Exp Rheumatol. 1990;8:283–8.
117. Al-Allaf AW, Ottewell L, Pullar T. The prevalence and significance of positive antinuclear antibodies in patients with fibromyalgia syndrome: 2–4 years' follow-up. Clin Rheumatol. 2002;21:472–7.
118. Rhodus NL, Fricton J, Carlson P, Messner R. Oral symptoms associated with fibromyalgia. J Rheumatol. 2003;30:1841–5.
119. Lopate G, Pestronk A, Al-Lozi M, et al. Peripheral neuropathy in an outpatient cohort of patients with Sjogren's syndrome. Muscle Nerve. 2006;33:672–6.
120. Batbayar B, Nagy G, Kovesi G, Zelles T, Feher E. Morphological basis of sensory neuropathy and neuroimmunomodulation in minor salivary glands of patients with Sjogren's syndrome. Arch Oral Biol. 2004;49:529–38.
121. Staud R. Pharmacological treatment of fibromyalgia syndrome: new developments. Drugs. 2010;70:1–14.
122. Neill J, Belan I, Ried K. Effectiveness of non-pharmacological interventions for fatigue in adults with multiple sclerosis, rheumatoid arthritis, or systemic lupus erythematosus: a systematic review. J Adv Nurs. 2006;56:617–35.

123. Dass S, Bowman SJ, Vital EM, et al. Reduction of fatigue in Sjogren syndrome with rituximab: results of a randomised, double-blind, placebo-controlled pilot study. Ann Rheum Dis. 2008;67:1541–4.
124. Meijer JM, Pijpe J, Vissink A, Kallenberg CG, Bootsma H. Treatment of primary Sjogren syndrome with rituximab: extended follow-up, safety and efficacy of retreatment. Ann Rheum Dis. 2009;68:284–5.
125. Karlson EW, Liang MH, Eaton H, et al. A randomized clinical trial of a psychoeducational intervention to improve outcomes in systemic lupus erythematosus. Arthritis Rheum. 2004;50:1832–41.
126. Strombeck BE, Theander E, Jacobsson LT. Effects of exercise on aerobic capacity and fatigue in women with primary Sjogren's syndrome. Rheumatology (Oxford). 2007;46:868–71.
127. Strömbeck B, Theander E, Jacobsson LT. Assessment of fatigue in primary Sjögren's syndrome: the Swedish version of the Profile of Fatigue. Scand J Rheumatol. 2005;34:455–9.

Chapter 10
Musculoskeletal Involvement

Guillermo J. Pons-Estel, Bernardo A. Pons-Estel, and Graciela S. Alarcón

Contents

G.J. Pons-Estel (✉)
Department of Autoimmune Diseases,
Institut Clínic de Medicina i Dermatologia, Hospital Clínic,
Barcelona, Catalonia, Spain

Division of Clinical Immunology and Rheumatology, Department of Medicine,
School of Medicine, The University of Alabama at Birmingham,
Birmingham, AL, USA
e-mail: gponsestel@hotmail.com

B.A. Pons-Estel
Department of Rheumatology,
Instituto Cardiovascular de Rosario,
Rosario, Argentina
e-mail: baponsestel@buenaventuraguarani.com.ar

G.S. Alarcón
Division of Clinical Immunology and Rheumatology, Department of Medicine,
School of Medicine, The University of Alabama at Birmingham,
Birmingham, AL, USA
e-mail: galarcon@uab.edu

M. Ramos-Casals et al. (eds.), *Sjögren's Syndrome*,
DOI 10.1007/978-0-85729-947-5_10, © Springer-Verlag London Limited 2012

10.1   Introduction

Musculoskeletal manifestations such as myalgias, arthralgias, an intermittent non-erosive mild polyarthritis affecting mainly small joints, are common in patients with primary Sjögren's syndrome. Myositis may also occur but much less frequently. The most important features of these manifestations are described in this chapter.

10.2   Arthralgias and Arthritis

Articular involvement is the most common extra-glandular manifestation of primary Sjögren's syndrome as noted by a number of different authors [1–5]. Arthralgias, with or without evidence of arthritis, may occur in 40–75% of patients and in about one third of them, they occur at presentation [1, 4–6]. Arthralgias, morning stiffness, and intermittent arthritis are frequent but chronic polyarthritis is not; when it occurs it is often non-erosive. It should be noted, however, that arthritis has not been universally reported in patients with primary Sjögren's syndrome; for example, Kruize et al. from the Netherlands followed 31 patients for 10–12 years and failed to observe arthritis in any of them [7]. This contrasts with another longitudinal study conducted in Finland in which arthritis developed in 24% of 110 patients diagnosed between 1977 and 1992 and reexamined between 1994 and 1997 [1]. Finally, it seems that arthritis occurs with comparable frequency in patients with early- vs. late-onset disease (12.5% vs. 9.8, respectively), as noted by Haga et al. from Denmark [8] and confirmed by Ramos-Casals et al. from Spain [9]; however, this is not always the case as articular involvement was reported in nearly 30% vs. 46% (not statistically significant) of primary Sjögren's syndrome patients older comparable to younger than 70 years of age [10].

10.3   Arthritis: Patterns of Expression

The arthropathy of primary Sjögren's syndrome is usually symmetric and intermittent, affecting shoulders, wrists, hands, knees, ankles, and feet; it is typically non-erosive and non-deforming. The patterns of arthritis in these patients and its associated immunological and clinical features have been recently described by Haga et al. [6]. These authors studied 102 patients and followed them for about 5 years; arthralgias occurred in nearly 75% of these patients whereas arthritis was demonstrated in about 18% of them. The most commonly affected joints were shoulders, wrists, MCP joints, ankles, and MTP joints. Symmetrical bilateral arthritis was most commonly observed in ankles, wrists, shoulders, and MTP joints and less so in the MCP joints. Five patients had longstanding persistent arthritis, and one developed seronegative rheumatoid arthritis (RA). The presence of arthralgias/arthritis was not correlated with any clinical or immunological feature, and erythrocyte sedimentation rate (ESR) and C-reactive protein (CRP) values were normal. This study demonstrated that the arthritis of primary Sjögren's syndrome is usually mild, self-limited, involving joints of various sizes, and not associated with other clinical and immunological features. A typical pattern is uni- or bilateral arthritis of the ankles, which in fact has been felt to be characteristic in patients with primary Sjögren's syndrome, [6] but other joints may also be affected. Involvement of the cricoarytenoid joints has been reported infrequently [11, 12].

Rheumatoid factor (IgM-RF) is reported in a variable proportion of patients with primary Sjogren's syndrome (32–74%) [1, 4–6, 13]. In the study by Garcia Carrasco et al., for example, IgM-RF was present in 38% of patients; these IgM-RF positive patients had articular involvement more often than the seronegative ones (45% vs. 33%, $p = 0.017$) [13]. Anti-cyclic citrullinated peptide (CCP) antibodies are much less common in patients with primary Sjogren's syndrome (4–10%) [6, 14, 15] but when present synovitis is much more likely to be present as well [15].

10.4 Differential Diagnosis: RA, SLE, and Other Arthropathies

Mild synovitis affecting mainly the small joints of the hands and feet is common in patients with primary Sjögren's syndrome, but also in those with RA and SLE. The presence of IgM-RF may not be helpful in distinguishing RA from primary Sjögren's syndrome since it is positive in both [16–18]; however, the presence of anti-CCP antibodies may favor the diagnosis of RA over primary Sjögren's syndrome [14, 19]. In fact anti-CCP antibody positivity has been reported only in a minority of patients with primary Sjögren's syndrome [20–22], who according to Atzeni et al. may later develop RA [15].

Joint involvement in SLE varies, ranging from non-erosive arthropathy (it is the most frequent form), erosive symmetrical polyarthritis with deformities similar to RA and mild deforming arthropathy (characterized as Jaccoud's); severe functional disability may occur. In general, arthritis is less frequent in patients with primary Sjögren's syndrome than in those with SLE [22]. Furthermore, the arthritis pattern of these patients is not directly comparable to those with SLE. In SLE, arthritis usually starts in the small hand joints (MCPs and PIPs) in a symmetrical fashion, and may be indistinguishable from early RA. The main distinguishing feature between the arthritis of primary Sjögren's syndrome and SLE is the high frequency of ankle arthritis and the lack of deformities in the first [6].

Sarcoidosis should also be considered in the differential diagnosis because of the presence of sicca symptoms and even a positive biopsy of the minor salivary glands in these patients. The presence of hilar adenopathy and erythema nodosum in conjunction with arthritis usually involving the knees and ankles in conjunction with granulomas in the minor labial salivary gland biopsy as well as absence of reactivity to Ro/SSA and La/SSB favors the diagnosis of sarcoidosis [23]. Chronic arthritis in sarcoidosis is usually non-deforming and non-erosive involving the ankle, knees, and hand joints but a Jaccoud's type arthritis has also been described. Finally, ankle

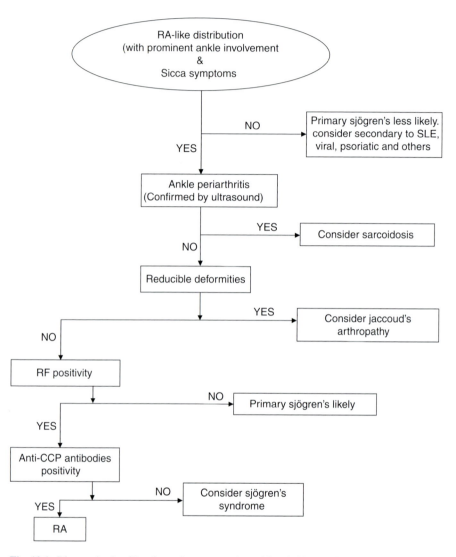

Fig. 10.1 Diagnostic algorithm for patients presenting with arthritis and sicca symptoms

periarthritis is a common manifestation of sarcoidosis, which has not been observed in patients with primary Sjögren's syndrome [6].

Arthritis and arthralgias are well recognized and occur relatively frequently in patients with viral infections. Patients with viral arthritis tend to present with symmetric polyarthralgias or arthritis; its abrupt onset, limited course, and lack of serological markers of inflammation are usually a clue to this diagnosis. Even in instances of persistent or recurrent symptoms, viral arthritis has not been shown to lead to chronic and destructive arthritis. Retrovirus may be associated with arthritis in knees, ankles, wrists, and occasionally small finger joints while infection with Epstein-Barr virus may be associated with monoarticular arthritis of the knees [24].

Both of these viruses have been associated with the pathogenesis of primary Sjögren's syndrome, although the evidence for this is circumstantial.

In conclusion, arthritis in primary Sjögren's syndrome is less common than in RA and in SLE, and is usually mild, resolving, and not associated to other clinical and immunological features. The arthritis pattern is more like the pattern found in retrovirus infections than in other inflammatory rheumatic diseases.

Figure 10.1 depicts such algorithm.

10.5 Myalgias and Myositis: Diagnosis, Classification, and Role of Muscular Biopsy

Fatigue and myalgias are common in patients with primary Sjögren's syndrome, although the underlying mechanisms are mainly unknown. A mild inflammatory myopathy of insidious onset and characterized by proximal muscle weakness has been described. Myalgias have been reported in 33% of patients with primary Sjögren's syndrome [25] whereas fibromyalgia (FM), characterized by widespread chronic muscle pain, stiffness, and fatigue, has been reported in 47–55% of these patients [26, 27]. An inflammatory cell infiltrate on muscle biopsy has been described in some patients without any muscle symptoms.

Subclinical myositis, with histopathological signs of myositis, is very common and has been reported in 72% of patients with primary Sjögren's syndrome [28] whereas clinically significant signs of polymyositis (PM) have been reported in 2.5–10% of these patients [29]. Inclusion body myositis (IBM)-like features have also been reported [30–32]. Most of the histopathological data in primary Sjögren's syndrome derive from reports of single patients or smaller series of cases [33–36]. Perivascular inflammation and interstitial myositis without involvement of muscle fibers have been described [33] but this picture is relatively common in several other rheumatological diseases and its clinical significance is uncertain [34, 37, 38].

More recently, Lindvall et al. [28] investigated all patients with primary Sjögren's syndrome registered at their rheumatology unit. The aim of the study was to relate light microscope and immunomorphological muscle biopsy findings to clinical symptoms, especially regarding pain in relation to inflammatory myopathy. They reported that histopathological signs of myositis, with or without degeneration, were present in 72% of muscle biopsies and the inflammation was always localized perivascularly; however, muscle symptoms were not related to histological signs of muscle inflammation. The criteria for FM were fulfilled by 27% of patients, whereas 17% had experienced muscle pain with no FM. The remaining 56% had not experienced muscle pain. None of the patients had clinical symptoms of IBM; however, 28% showed rimmed vacuoles in association with muscle fiber degeneration, and inflammation as well. The authors concluded that IBM-like findings may represent vacuolar myopathic degeneration due to previous subclinical muscle inflammation rather than a specific clinical entity.

To determine whether treatment of subclinical myositis can prevent the development of manifest degenerative changes, treatment trials are required. The presence of

Table 10.1 Classification of muscular involvement in primary Sjögren's syndrome

1. Myalgias (33%) [25]
2. Fibromyalgia (47–55%) [26, 27]
3. Subclinical myositis (72%) [28]
4. Myositis similar to PM (2.5–10%) [29]
5. Inclusion body myositis-like (22%) [28]

vacuolar changes is possibly related to the increased expression of membrane attack complex suggesting pathogenetic similarities to dermatomyositis. A classification of muscular involvement in primary Sjögren's syndrome is shown in Table 10.1.

Considering all these data together, muscle biopsy is not justified in patients with primary Sjögren's syndrome regardless of the presence or absence of muscle pain; however, the presence of FM does not rule out PM. Thus, biopsy should be considered in patients with primary Sjögren's syndrome who exhibit significant muscle weakness whether FM manifestations are present or not.

References

1. Pertovaara M, Pukkala E, Laippala P, et al. A longitudinal cohort study of Finnish patients with primary Sjögren's syndrome: clinical, immunological, and epidemiological aspects. Ann Rheum Dis. 2001;60:467–72.
2. Ioannidis J, Vassiliou V, Moutsopoulos H. Long-term risk of mortality and lymphoproliferative disease and predictive classification of primary Sjögren's syndrome. Arthritis Rheum. 2002;46:741–7.
3. Theander E, Manthorpe R, Jacobsson L. Mortality and causes of death in primary Sjögren's syndrome: a prospective cohort study. Arthritis Rheum. 2004;50:1262–9.
4. Alamanos Y, Tsifetaki N, Voulgari PV, Venetsanopoulou AI, et al. Epidemiology of primary Sjögren's syndrome in north-west Greece, 1982–2003. Rheumatology (Oxford). 2006;45:187–91.
5. Ramos-Casals M, Solans R, Rosas J, et al. Primary Sjögren syndrome in Spain: clinical and immunologic expression in 1010 patients. Medicine (Baltimore). 2008;87:210–9.
6. Haga HJ, Peen E. A study of the arthritis pattern in primary Sjögren's syndrome. Clin Exp Rheumatol. 2007;25:88–91.
7. Kruize AA, Hené RJ, Van Der Heide A, et al. Long-term followup of patients with Sjögren's syndrome. Arthritis Rheum. 1996;39:297–303.
8. Haga HJ, Jonsson R. The influence of age on disease manifestations and serological characteristics in primary Sjögren's syndrome. Scand J Rheumatol. 1999;28:227–32.
9. Ramos-Casals M, Cervera R, Font J, et al. Young onset of primary Sjögren's syndrome: clinical and immunological characteristics. Lupus. 1998;7:202–6.
10. García-Carrasco M, Cervera R, Rosas J, et al. Primary Sjögren's syndrome in the elderly: clinical and immunological characteristics. Lupus. 1999;8:20–3.
11. Barrs DM, McDonald TJ, Duffy J. Sjögren's syndrome involving the larynx: report of a case. J Laryngol Otol. 1979;93:933–6.
12. Sève P, Poupart M, Bui-Xuan C, et al. Cricoarytenoid arthritis in Sjögren's syndrome. Rheumatol Int. 2005;25:301–2.
13. García-Carrasco M, Ramos-Casals M, Rosas J, et al. Primary Sjögren syndrome: clinical and immunologic disease patterns in a cohort of 400 patients. Medicine (Baltimore). 2002;81:270–80.
14. Kamali S, Polat NG, Kasapoglu E, et al. Anti-CCP and antikeratin antibodies in rheumatoid arthritis, primary Sjögren's syndrome, and Wegener's granulomatosis. Clin Rheumatol. 2005;24:673–6.

15. Atzeni F, Sarzi-Puttini P, Lama N, et al. Anti-cyclic citrullinated peptide antibodies in primary Sjögren syndrome may be associated with non-erosive synovitis. Arthritis Res Ther. 2008;10:1–6.
16. Papiris SA, Tsonis IA, Moutsopoulos HM. Sjögren's syndrome. Semin Respir Crit Care Med. 2007;28:459–71.
17. Rehman HU. Sjögren's syndrome. Yonsei Med J. 2003;44:947–54.
18. Castro-Poltronieri A, Alarcón-Segovia D. Articular manifestations of primary Sjögren's syndrome. J Rheumatol. 1983;10:485–8.
19. Rantapaa-Dahlqvist SR, de Jong BA, Berglin E, et al. Antibodies against cyclic citrullinated peptides and IgA rheumatoid factor predict the development of rheumatoid arthritis. Arthritis Rheum. 2003;48:2741–9.
20. Gottenberg JE, Mignot S, Nicaise-Rolland P, et al. Prevalence of anti-cyclic citrullinated peptide and anti-keratin antibodies in patients with primary Sjögren's syndrome. Ann Rheum Dis. 2005;64:114–7.
21. Goëb V, Salle V, Duhaut P, et al. Clinical significance of autoantibodies recognizing Sjögren's syndrome A (SSA), SSB, calpastatin and alpha-fodrin in primary Sjögren's syndrome. Clin Exp Immunol. 2007;148:281–7.
22. Cervera R, Khamashta MA, Font J, et al. Systemic lupus erythematosus: clinical and immunologic patterns of disease expression in a cohort of 1,000 patients. The European working party on systemic lupus erythematosus. Medicine (Baltimore). 1993;72:113–24.
23. Spilberg I, Siltzbach LE, McEwen C. The arthritis of sarcoidosis. Arthritis Rheum. 1969;12:126–37.
24. Petri MA. In: Koopman WJ, editor. Arthritis and allied conditions – a textbook of rheumatology. 14th ed. Philadelphia: Lippincott Williams & Wilkin; 2001. p. 1455–79.
25. Martinez-Lavin M, Vaughan JH, Tan EM. Autoantibodies and the spectrum of Sjögren's syndrome. Ann Intern Med. 1979;91:185–90.
26. Vitali C, Tavoni A, Neri R, et al. Fibromyalgia features in patients with primary Sjögren's syndrome. Evidence of a relationship with psychological depression. Scand J Rheumatol. 1989;18:21–7.
27. Tishler M, Barak Y, Paran D, et al. Sleep disturbances, fibromyalgia and primary Sjögren's syndrome. Clin Exp Rheumatol. 1997;15:71–4.
28. Lindvall B, Bengtsson A, Ernerudh J, et al. Subclinical myositis is common in primary Sjögren's syndrome and is not related to muscle pain. J Rheumatol. 2002;29:717–25.
29. Alexander EL. Neuromuscular complications of primary Sjögren's syndrome. In: Talal N, Moutsopoulos HM, Kassan SS, editors. Sjögren's syndrome. Clinical and immunological aspects. Berlin: Springer; 1987. p. 61–82.
30. Chad D, Good P, Adelman L, et al. Inclusion body myositis associated with Sjögren's syndrome. Arch Neurol. 1982;39:186–8.
31. Gutmann L, Govindan S, Riggs JE, et al. Inclusion body myositis and Sjögren's syndrome. Arch Neurol. 1985;42:1021–2.
32. Khraishi MM, Jay V, Keystone EC. Inclusion body myositis in association with vitamin B12 deficiency and Sjögren's syndrome. J Rheumatol. 1992;19:306–9.
33. Vrethem M, Lindvall B, Holmgren H, et al. Neuropathy and myopathy in primary Sjögren's syndrome: neurophysiological, immunological and muscle biopsy results. Acta Neurol Scand. 1990;82:126–31.
34. Kraus A, Cifuentes M, Villa AR, et al. Myositis in primary Sjögren's syndrome. Report of 3 cases. J Rheumatol. 1994;21:649–53.
35. Molina R, Provost TT, Arnett FC, et al. Primary Sjögren's syndrome in men. Clinical, serologic, and immunogenetic features. Am J Med. 1986;80:23–31.
36. Ringel SP, Forstot JZ, Tan EM, et al. Sjögren's syndrome and polymyositis or dermatomyositis. Arch Neurol. 1982;39:157–63.
37. Layzer RB. Inflammatory and immune disorders. In: Layzer RB, editor. Neuromuscular manifestations of systemic disease. Philadelphia: Davis; 1985. p. 227–8.
38. Leroy JP, Drosos AA, Yiannopoulos DI, et al. Intravenous pulse cyclophosphamide therapy in myositis and Sjögren's syndrome. Arthritis Rheum. 1990;33:1579–81.

Chapter 11
Non-Vasculitic Cutaneous Involvement

Hobart W. Walling and Richard D. Sontheimer

Contents

11.1 Introduction

As with other clinically and genetically heterogeneous, multisystem autoimmune disorders, cutaneous abnormalities are frequently encountered in Sjogren's syndrome (SjS). Thus, it is important to have a rational framework for identifying and treating skin changes that can be encountered in SjS patients and to understand the relationships of key skin changes to the SjS systemic disease process.

H.W. Walling
Private Practice of Dermatology, Coralville, IA, USA

R.D. Sontheimer (✉)
Department of Dermatology, University of Utah School of Medicine, Salt Lake City, UT, USA

M. Ramos-Casals et al. (eds.), *Sjögren's Syndrome*,
DOI 10.1007/978-0-85729-947-5_11, © Springer-Verlag London Limited 2012

Table 11.1 A Classification framework for the various types of skin change that can be encountered in SjS patients

Skin changes that are thought to relate directly from the underlying systemic autoimmune abnormalities of SjS[a]

Dryness (syn. xerosis, astetosis)

    Skin changes associated with mucosal dryness

        Eyelid dermatitis

        Angular cheilitis

Pruritus

Annular erythema of Sjögren's syndrome

    Erythema multiforme-like lesions

    Doughnut-like lesions

    Sweet's syndrome-like lesions

    Erythema perstans-like lesions

Panniculitis

    Erythema nodosum

    Necrotizing lymphocytic panniculitis

    Granulomatous panniculitis

Primary nodular cutaneous amyloidosis

Cutaneous B cell lymphoma

Skin changes seen in other systemic autoimmune disorders that can overlap with SjS[a]

Rheumatoid arthritis

    Rheumatoid nodules

    Rheumatoid papules (syn. rheumatoid neutrophilic dermatosis, interstitial granulomatous dermatitis, palisading neutrophilic granulomatous dermatitis)

Lupus erythematosus

    Photosensitive malar rash of acute cutaneous LE

    Subacute cutaneous LE

    Classical discoid LE

    Chilblains LE (syn. perniotic LE, "perniosis")

    Neonatal LE skin lesions in infants of mothers with SjS

Systemic sclerosis

    Hand and finger changes

        Raynaud's phenomenon

        Sclerodactly

        Periungual nalilfold changes (capillary dropout, ectasia, and arborization; cuticular hemorrhages, ragged cuticles [Samitz sign])

    Proximal extremity, trunkal and facial scleroderma

    Cutaneous calcinosis

    Salt and pepper pattern of cutaneous dyspigmentation

Dermatomyositis

    Hallmark cutaneous manifestations of DM

        Periorbital heliotrope erythema

        Göttron's papules

        Göttron's sign of DM (violaceous erythema of the extensor surfaces of the upper and lower extremities, especially the elbows and knees)

        Violaceous erythema of the scalp

        Violaceous erythema over the nape of the neck and posterior upper shoulders (shawl sign)

        Violaceous erythema over the lateral trochanteric of the hips (holster sign)

    Cutaneous calcinosis

Table 11.1 (continued)

Skin changes associated with the 8.1 ancestral haplotype that can be fortituously encountered in SjS patients[b]

Alopecia areata

Vitiligo

Skin changes reported anecdotally in SjS patients for which a significant association has yet to be confirmed[b]

Amicrobial pustulosis

Cutaneous T cell lymphoma

Disseminated superficial actinic porokeratosis

Erythema elevatum diutinum

Erythema nodosum

Erythematous swelling of the lip mimicking cheilitis granulomatosa

Lichen planus

Livedoid vasculopathy

Multiple dermatofibromas

Painful indurated erythema (Kikuchi-Fujimoto disease)

Postmenopausal frontal fibrosing alopecia

Primary anetoderma

Psoriasis

Pyoderma gangrenosum

Subcorneal pustular dermatosis

Sweet's syndrome

Ulcerative lichen planus

Skin changes that can result from the treatment of SjS[b]

Corticosteroid-induced acne

Antimalarial-induced skin changes

    Hyperpigmentation

    Hypersensitivity reactions

        Acute generalized exanthematous pustulosis

        Eczematous reactions

        Exanthematous reactions

        Erythema multiforme reactions

        Lichenoid drug eruptions (including subacute cutaneous LE-like reactions)

[a]Listed in relative descending order of prevalence
[b]Listed in alphabetical order

The focus of this chapter will be on the cutaneous manifestations of primary SjS. However, a number of other types of skin change can be encountered in SjS patients (see Table 11.1). To better recognize and appreciate the skin disorders that are thought to relate directly to the systemic autoimmune process associated with SjS, one must be aware of the full spectrum of skin changes that can be encountered in SjS patients. We therefore have provided a framework for considering the entire spectrum of skin change that can be encountered in SjS patients (Table 11.1).

One such set of cutaneous changes that can be encountered in SjS are those that the overlapping autoimmune entities seen in secondary SjS patients can "bring along." Examples include subacute cutaneous lupus erythematosus (SCLE) and

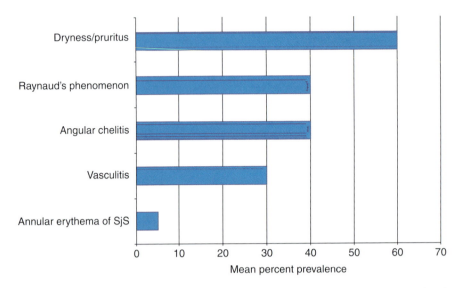

Fig. 11.1 Mean prevalence of skin disorders occurring in SjS. Summary data abstracted and compiled from several SjS patient study cohorts

Raynaud's phenomenon. In addition, SjS patients are at increased risk for developing skin disorders that, like SjS, occur in association with the 8.1 ancestral haplotype. Examples include vitiligo and alopecia areata. Also, certain skin changes can occur as a result of treatments that are given to SjS patients. Examples include steroid-induced acne and antimalarial hyperpigmentation. Finally, because of the tendency to ascribe anything that happens to an individual diagnosed with SJS to SjS itself, banal and unfamiliar dermatoses having no known relationship to SjS are attributed to this disorder.

This review focuses particularly on work reported since the year 2000. The literature on this subject prior to then can be found in earlier PubMed cited reviews and textbook chapters. Examples include references [1–6]. Please note that the various clinical manifestations of cutaneous vasculitis/vasculopathy are being addressed in a separate chapter in this book and will not be addressed here.

11.2   Epidemiology

SjS is among the most common rheumatologic disorders. Various epidemiological studies and reviews indicate that one-half of SjS patients have cutaneous changes thought to relate directly or indirectly to the SjS autoimmune process. Figure 11.1 presents a summary of the mean prevalences of various SjS-associated skin changes from several different SjS study cohorts. The rates at which these skin lesions can be encountered varies between primary and secondary SjS. In addition, there is significant ethnic variation in patterns of skin disease seen in SjS. For example, the autoimmune annular erythema seen in Japanese SjS patients is extremely rare in patients from North America. Similarly, SCLE, a common skin feature among North American SjS patients, is unusual in SjS patients from Japan.

11.3 Skin Changes Encountered in Primary SjS

Xerosis of both cutaneous and mucosal surfaces is a key manifestation of SjS [7]. Cutaneous xerosis may be characterized both on the basis of subjective symptoms (dryness, pinprick sensation) and objective findings (fine, dry scale; loss of light reflection from the skin surface; increased transepidermal water loss) [4]. Patients may report dryness and loss of luster of hair, as well as dryness and brittleness of the nails [1].

Cutaneous xerosis is generally reported in half to two-thirds of cases of SjS. In their classic paper, Bloch et al. [8] reported that 33/62 patients (53%) complained of dryness of the skin. Bernacchi et al. observed xerosis in 34/62 patients (55%) with primary SjS and found xerosis to be significantly higher in primary as opposed to secondary SjS [4]. In that study, patients with xerosis tended to be older (mean age 65 vs. 50) and were more likely to have circulating anti-Ro/SS-A or anti-La/SS-B antibodies [4]. Skin dryness and pruritus are very common among healthy senior and elderly individuals who do not have SjS. Because SjS patients are often older than the mean population age, data describing the prevalence of dryness and pruritus in SjS should be viewed in this context.

The pathogenesis of xerosis in SjS is not completely understood. Dysfunction of the sebaceous and eccrine glands has been suggested because these organs are responsible for intrinsic skin lubrication [1]. A lymphohistocystic infiltrate within the eccrine glands has been demonstrated in some cases [1], supporting the hypothesis of loss of function secondary to an immune-mediated inflammatory process. However, a quantitative study of 12 patients with SjS (3 primary, 9 secondary), including eight patients who complained specifically of xerosis, failed to show diminished pilocarpine-induced sweat production compared to controls [9].

Altered function of the autonomic nervous system, both sympathetic and parasympathic, has been reported in SjS. Kovacs et al. reported a blunted response to cholinergic stimulation in SjS patients [10]. Mandl et al. reported abnormal responses for cutaneous vasoconstriction, orthostatic blood pressure, and deep breathing in patients with SjS compared to controls [11]. Xerosis in SjS may also relate to alterations in barrier function of the stratum corneum and to an altered keratinocyte protein-expression profile [12].

The human stratum corneum plays a major role in limiting preventing transepidermal water loss and desiccation of the skin. However, there has been very little research on the biochemical integrity of the stratum corneum in SjS patients.

11.3.1 Pruritus

Xerosis is often accompanied by pruritus. Pruritus was reported in 26/62 patients (42%) with primary SjS and associated with xerosis in 19 (73%) of those with pruritus [4]. Chronic rubbing and scratching may lead to hyperpigmentation and lichenification [1, 7, 13]. When pruritus is particularly intense, other incidental causes should be addressed (e.g., dermatitis herpetiformis, dermatographic urticaria, prodromal pemphigoid, and eczematous drug eruptions) [1].

Treatment of xerosis and pruritus in SjS can be challenging [1]. For xerosis, limiting daily bathing to 5–10 min with lukewarm (rather than hot) water can be helpful. Heat tends to soften and liquefy the natural skin oils, making them more likely to be removed by soapy water while bathing. Mild soaps or soapless cleansers should be used to cleanse dry areas such as the arms and legs while bathing. Strong antibacterial soaps and surgical scrubs (chlorhexidine) should be reserved for cleansing the body fold areas. Liquid body scrubs should be avoided while bathing. Colloidal oatmeal added to bath water can be soothing for dry, itchy skin.

After bathing, the patient should be directed to gently pat off excess water with a towel and to apply a bland emollient cream or ointment to damp skin. The emollient should be reapplied during the day as often as necessary and practical. When significant pruritus is present, topical corticosteroids (e.g., hydrocortisone, triamcinolone, fluocinonide, or clobetasol, in increasing order of potency) may be applied in ointments or creams once or twice daily for up to 2-week intervals. Ointments are preferred to creams because they trap water in the skin more effectively and are therefore more moisturizing. Nonsteroidal topical immunomodulators (tacrolimus, pimecrolimus) may be useful [14]. Oral antihistamines may provide relief of pruritis for some patients.

Caution should be observed with over-the-counter products alleged to treat dry skin. Ingredients such as neomycin and diphenhydramine (in rub-on or spray-on itch relief products) can cause cutaneous allergic reactions, often resulting in worsening of the itching and confusion about the correct diagnosis.

Two manifestations of SjS merit particular attention: eyelid dermatitis and angular cheilitis. Both commonly occur in association with regional mucosal dryness, though the cutaneous findings may not be attributably only to the xerophthalmia and xerostomia.

11.3.2 Annular Erythema of SjS

Annular erythema of SjS is comprised of erythematous skin lesions with indurated borders. These generally occur on the upper body and display mononuclear infiltrates in perivascular and periappendageal regions on skin biopsy. Annular erythema was first linked with primary SjS in Japanese patients in the 1980s [15]. This skin lesion was associated with the presence of circulating anti-Ro/SS-A and anti-La/SS-B autoantibodies but lacked the prominent interface dermatitis usually demonstrated by

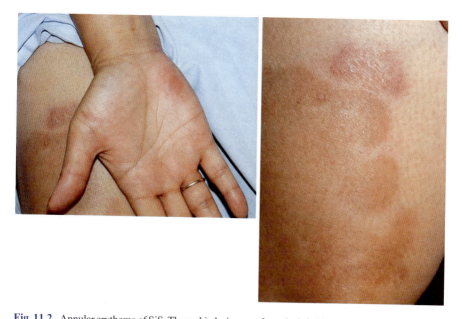

Fig. 11.2 Annular erythema of SjS. These skin lesions are from the left thigh and palm of a 40-year-old Filipino woman with a history of parotid swelling, sicca symptoms, and arthralgias. She had a positive antinuclear antibody assay (1:640, speckled pattern) and anti-Ro/SS-A and anti-La/SS-B autoantibodies were present. Double-stranded DNA antibody assay was negative. The recurrent annular skin lesions with overlying mild scale that are shown had skin biopsy findings that were consistent with annular erythema of SjS. A mild degree of interface dermatitis on biopsy was likely responsible for the mild clinical scaling shown in the photos (potassium hydroxide exam of scraped scale was negative for dermatophytes). In addition to the upper trunk, neck and face, annular erythema of SjS skin lesions have also been described on the palms and soles (Clinical images were kindly provided by Dr. Jan P. Dutz, Department of Dermatology, University of British Columbia, Canada)

subacute cutaneous lupus erythematosus (SCLE). Moreover, SCLE lesions are quite rare among Japanese individuals. Annular erythema occurs in Caucasian SjS patients only rarely. Debate has existed about a potential relationship between annular erythema of SjS and SCLE. Some authors have speculated that annular erythema of SjS is the Japanese equivalent of lupus tumidus skin lesions in Westerners.

Katayama et al. have recently analyzed the clinical and laboratory findings in 28 of their own SjS patients with annular erythema. These cases were identified from a Japanese Dermatology Department and combined with data abstracted from 92 previously published cases [15]. Three clinical types of annular erythema have been identified: a doughnut-shaped, ring-like erythema with elevated borders: an SCLE-like marginally scaled, polycyclic erythema; and a papular insect bite-like erythema. Each of the three morphologies displays the same set of histopathologic changes. In addition to the upper extremities and face, annular erythema has also been described on the soles of the feet (Fig. 11.2).

Three quarters of the annular erythema patients reported by Katayama et al. had circulating anti-Ro/SS-A and anti-La/SS-B autoantibodies. However, the presence of annular erythema did not portend the occurrence of any specific SjS manifestations or complications. Annular erythema is very sensitive to systemic glucocorticoids and is typically controlled effectively with prednisone 10 mg/day.

11.3.3 Eyelid Dermatitis

Eyelid dermatitis, common in SjS, can affect the upper or lower eyelids and is associated with pruritus or a foreign-body sensation. Three patterns of eyelid dermatitis are described: the slightly lichenified; the moderately lichenified and papular; and eyelid edema [13]. In a study of 52 Japanese patients with primary SjS, 22 (42%) had eyelid dermatitis. Patients with eyelid dermatitis tended to be older (mean age 61 vs. 49) and complain of ocular dryness (86% vs. 59%).

A study from Italy reported a somewhat lower prevalence of eyelid dermatitis among SjS patients [4]. Approximately equal percentages of primary and secondary SjS patients were described as having this condition: 15 of 62 patients (24%) and 8 of 31 (26%) patients, respectively. Of the patients with primary SjS, eyelid dermatitis was commonly associated with xerosis (13/15; 87%) and sicca symptoms (14/15; 93%). Only upper eyelid involvement was reported in this study.

Eyelid dermatitis may be managed with the intermittent use of low potency topical steroid creams (e.g., hydrocortisone, desonide). Nonsteroidal topical immunomodulators such as tacrolimus (0.03% or 0.1% ointment) and pimecrolimus (1% cream) are also useful.

Angular cheilitis. The xerostomia of SjS is associated with a number of intraoral consequences. These include a diminished rate of saliva secretion; a decreased buffering capacity of saliva; an increased risk of colonization by *Candida*, lactobacillus, or streptococcus species; and increased rates of dental caries [16, 17].

Angular cheilitis is a sign commonly associated with oral candidiasis. Both angular cheilitis and oral candidiasis have been correlated with the diminished salivary flow seen in SjS [17]. About a third of SjS patients will have difficulty with angular cheilitis.

A study from Italy found angular cheilitis to be more prevalent in patients with primary SjS (24/62; 39%) compared to secondary SjS (5/31; 16%). More than 95% of cases were associated with xerostomia [4].

Investigators from Sweden reported erythema or fissuring at the angles of the mouth in 28 (70%) of 40 patients with primary SjS and angular cheilitis in 14 (35%) of those same patients. In contrast, angular cheilitis is estimated to occur in about 3–5% of the general population [16].

In a study of 50 patients with SjS, three quarters were diagnosed with oral candidiasis and angular cheilitis was present in approximately one-fourth [18]. Oral candidiasis is more common in patients taking certain medicines such as prednisone or other immunosuppressives.

Angular cheilitis may be managed with topical antimycotic ointments (e.g., ketoconazole, miconazole, clotrimazole, or nystatin). Measures to increase salivary function such as the use of saliva substitutes, sugarless chewing gum, or systemic pilocarpine may be useful at addressing the underlying xerostomia [18].

11.3.4 Panniculitis

Various forms of panniculitis are reported in association with SjS including erythema nodosum [19], lobular plasma cell panniculitis [20], necrotizing lymphocytic panniculitis [21], and granulomatous panniculitis [21].

Yamamoto et al. reported four cases of erythema nodosum associated with SjS [19]. All four patients were women (age 27, 43, 65, and 77) and all had lower extremity involvement. One patient had erythema nodosum on the forearms, as well. The patients responded to nonsteroidal anti-inflammatory drug therapy in all cases [19]. However, the precise relationship between SjS and erythema nodosum – direct association or chance co-occurrence – is uncertain.

Granulomatous panniculitis is perhaps the most distinctive form of SjS-associated panniculitis. Five cases, all tending to affect the forearms and lower legs of women, have been reported [21, 22]. The histopathologic findings in these cases were mixed lobular and septal granulomatous inflammation in the subcuticular adipose tissue and prominent multinucleated giant cells [21].

Plasma cell panniculitis has been rarely associated with SjS. This pattern of panniculitis is also reported to occur in association with both lupus erythematosus (lupus profundus) [23] and scleroderma (morphea profundus)[24].

11.3.5 Primary Nodular Cutaneous Amyloidosis

Amyloidosis is characterized by the extracellular deposition of amyloid fibrils comprised of misfolded host proteins [25]. Primary cutaneous nodular amyloidosis (PCNA) is a rare condition characterized by cutaneous deposition of immunoglobin light chains produced by a clonal plasma cell population that infiltrates the skin (Fig. 11.3). The amyloid fibrils are of the same class (AL) as those found in primary systemic amyloidosis, but relate to a skin-limited plasma cell dyscrasia. At least 20 cases of PCNA – approximately a quarter of all reported patients with PCNA – have been reported in patients with SjS [25–30].

The typical clinical presentation of PCNA consists of waxy, red-to-yellow nodules located preferentially on the lower extremities, face, scalp, and genitals [27].

Histopathologic examination shows an amorphous eosinophilic material within the dermis that demonstrates apple-green birefringence upon Congo-red staining and visualization under polarized microscopy. Immunoblot analysis demonstrates immunoglobulin light chains. Monoclonal immunoglobulin is the more common pattern, though cases characterized by polyclonal immunoglobulin deposition have rarely been reported. Of 14 cases of SjS-associated PCNA for which positive

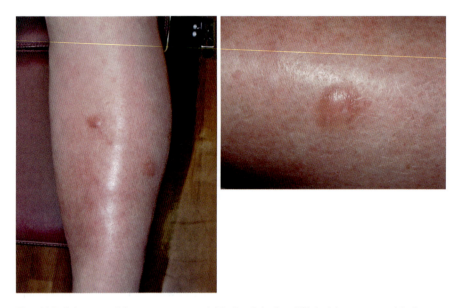

Fig. 11.3 Primary nodular cutaneous amyloidosis of the leg (Clinical images were kindly provided by Dr. Scott Florell, Department of Dermatology, University of Utah, USA)

immunoblotting was reported, 11 cases showed single class immunoglobulin staining and three cases showed staining with both anti-lambda- and anti-kappa-light-chain antibodies along with polyclonal gammaglobulinemia [25, 26, 28, 30–32]. Polyclonal immunoglobulin may be unique to PCNA associated with SjS, perhaps relating to development of polyclonal B cell proliferation in some SjS cases [26].

PCNA in SjS thus appears to result from a benign clonal proliferation of plasma cells that home to the skin, perhaps as part of the spectrum of SjS-related lymphoproliferative diseases [25]. The presence of PCNA warrants screening for lymphoproliferative disorders or systemic amyloidosis [27]. Systemic amyloidosis can also cause sicca syndrome through the deposition of amyloid fibrils within salivary glands [33].

11.3.6   B Cell Lymphoma

Patients with SjS have a 6.5–40-fold increased risk of lymphoma, most often extranodal B cell lymphomas of the non-Hodgkin's variety [34, 35]. The risk of non-Hodgkin's lymphoma may be somewhat higher in patients with secondary compared to primary SjS, though both have increased risk compared to the general population [35]. Indeed, a meta-analysis found the risk of non-Hodgkin's lymphoma to be higher among patients with SjS compared to patients with SLE [36]. A long-term study of 723 patients with primary SjS (mean follow-up 6 years) found that one in five deaths was attributable to lymphoma [37].

Fig. 11.4 Cutaneous large
B cell lymphoma of the leg
(Clinical images were kindly
provided by Dr. Glen Bowen,
Department of Dermatology,
University of Utah, USA)

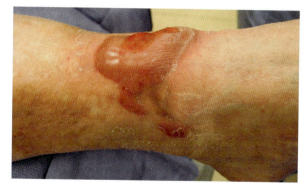

Approximately 4–7.5% of SjS patients develop lymphoma over time [38–40]. In a multicenter European study of 768 SjS patients, 33 (4.6%) developed non-Hodgkin's lymphoma [39]. Patients with severe parotid involvement by scintigraphy are more likely to develop lymphoma [41]. Other predictive factors for the development of lymphoma are splenomegaly, cryoglobulinemia, low C4 levels, neutropenia, and lymphadenopathy [40, 42]. Low serum C4 levels, presence of parotid enlargement, and presence of palpable purpura were independent predictors of eventual development of lymphoma [37]. Another study found the presence of vasculitis, low-grade fever, anemia, and peripheral nerve involvement to occur more frequently in SjS patients with lymphoma compared to SjS patients without lymphoma [39].

Marginal zone MALT-type (mucosa-associated lymphoid tissue) lymphoma is the most common type of non-Hodgkin's lymphoma seen in SjS. Many cases involve the major salivary glands, frequently the parotid glands. In a multicenter European study of 765 SS patients, 33 (4.3%) developed non-Hodgkin's lymphoma. The median age at lymphoma diagnosis was 58 years (range 33–82 years), and the median time from SjS diagnosis to lymphoma diagnosis was 7.5 years [39].

The skin, lungs, and stomach may also be sites of lymphoma involvement [43]. Bcl-2t(14;18) translocations may be present [1]. Markers for viruses associated with lymphoma (including Epstein-Barr virus, human T-leukotrophic virus, or human herpesvirus 8) are generally not present in biopsies of lymphomas from SjS patients [43].

Most cases of lymphoma in SjS patients are indolent and do not require aggressive chemotherapeutic regimens [39]. A small number of cases transform to high-grade lymphomas. Rituximab, a chimeric monoclonal antibody directed against the CD20 surface marker present on pre-B cells, is commonly employed as a therapy in this setting [44].

Other reported types of lymphoma in SS patients include follicle center lymphoma, lymphoplasmacytoid lymphoma, and diffuse, large B cell lymphomas [39] (Fig. 11.4). A large population-based from Sweden found the risk of lymphoplasmacytic lymphoma/Waldenström's macroglobulinemia to be increased in patients with SjS (odds ratio 12.1) [45]. A case of subcutaneous panniculitis-like T-cell lymphoma associated with SjS has been described [46]. At times, subcutaneous

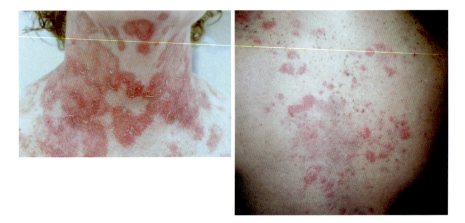

Fig. 11.5 Subacute cutaneous LE. *Left panel* – annular SCLE lesions on the neck of a patient with SjS. Note the polycyclic arrays produced by the merging of peripherally expanding lesions. *Right panel* – Papulosquamous SCLE lesions. A retiform array results from the merging of such lesions

panniculitis-like T-cell lymphoma can be difficult to distinguish both clinically and histopathologically from lupus panniculitis (lupus profundus), which can occur in overlap with SLE.

11.4 Skin Changes Encountered in Secondary SjS

11.4.1 Skin Changes Associated with Lupus Erythematosus

Subacute cutaneous lupus erythematosus (SCLE). SCLE is a photosensitive rash consisting of nonscarring, papulosquamous or annular skin lesions that occur over the back, trunk, and shoulders, typically sparing the face (Fig. 11.5). Skin biopsy shows characteristic features of LE-specific skin disease that are focused at the dermal-epidermal junction. On direct immunofluorescence microscopy, approximately 60% of SCLE lesions display a continuous, granular band of immunoglobulin and complement deposits at the dermal-epidermal junction. SCLE skin lesions mark the presence of homogenous immunogenetic subset of LE that typically enjoys a good prognosis with respect to SLE morbidity and mortality [47, 48].

Because of the shared 8.1 ancestral genotype and it serological correlates, anti-Ro/SS-A and anti-La/SS-B autoantibodies, a subgroup of the original cohort of 27 SCLE patients reported in 1979 was subsequently evaluated for evidence of SjS [47]. Only 2 of the 17 (12%) SCLE patients evaluated were found to have clinical and histopathologic evidence of SjS [49]. A question was then raised about the risk of SCLE patients developing SjS when observed over longer periods of time. Few primary data address this risk. However, it has been estimated that 20–40% of SCLE patients might develop features of SjS over long periods of follow-up. As an example, Black et al. reported that 33 (43%) of 76 SCLE patients followed for between 2 and 10 years had features of SjS as determined by physician assessment at the time of study analysis [50]. The rates at which SCLE develops in patients initially diagnosed as having SjS has not been examined thoroughly.

11.4.2 Skin Changes Associated with Rheumatoid Arthritis, Systemic Sclerosis, and the Idiopathic Inflammatory Myopathies

It is beyond the scope of this presentation to address each of the other autoimmune connective tissue diseases that can overlap with SjS. The more common skin findings that are found in these disorders are listed in the Table 11.1.

The reader is also referred to Table 11.1 for: (1) skin changes associated with the 8.1 ancestral haplotype that can be encountered in SjS patients; (2) skin changes reported anecdotally in SjS patients for which an association has yet to be confirmed; and (3) skin changes that can result from the treatment of SjS.

Acknowledgments There was no extramural support for this project. Dr. Sontheimer's effort on this project were facilitated by internal support from the University of Utah Department of Dermatology in return for his work in strengthening the departmental academic mission. We express our appreciation to the following individuals who generously provided clinical images to illustrate this chapter: Jan P. Dutz, M.D. (Department of Dermatology, University of British Columbia, Canada) as well as Glen M. Bowen, M.D. and Scott R. Florell, M.D. (Department of Dermatology, University of Utah School of Medicine, USA).

Conflicts of interest None to declare.

External funding sources None.

References

1. Flint SR, Watson R, Provost TT. Mucocutaneous manifestatons of Sjogren syndrome. In: Cutaneous manifestations of rheumatic diseases. 2 ed. Philadelphia: Lippincott Williams & Wilkins; 2004. p. 135–52.
2. Soy M, Piskin S. Cutaneous findings in patients with primary Sjögren's syndrome. Clin Rheumatol. 2007;26:1350–2.
3. Roguedas AM, Misery L, Sassolas B, Le MG, Pennec YL, Youinou P. Cutaneous manifestations of primary Sjögren's syndrome are underestimated. Clin Exp Rheumatol. 2004;22: 632–6.
4. Bernacchi E, Amato L, Parodi A, Cottoni F, Rubegni P, De PO, et al. Sjögren's syndrome: a retrospective review of the cutaneous features of 93 patients by the Italian Group of Immunodermatology. Clin Exp Rheumatol. 2004;22:55–62.
5. Connolly MK. Sjogern's syndrome. Semin Cutan Med Surg. 2001;20:46–52.
6. Fox RI, Liu AY. Sjögren's syndrome in dermatology. Clin Dermatol. 2006;24:393–413.

7. Provost TT, Watson R. Cutaneous manifestations of Sjögren's syndrome. Rheum Dis Clin North Am. 1992;18:609–16.

8. Bloch KJ, Buchanan WW, Wohl MJ, Bunim JJ. Sjögren's syndrome. A clinical, pathological, and serological study of sixty-two cases. 1965. Medicine (Baltimore). 1992 Nov;71(6):386-401; discussion 401-3. PubMed PMID: 1435231

9. Hart LE, Caspi D, Hull RG, Begant A, Beacham J, Hughes GR. Sweat gland function in Sjögren's syndrome. Ann Rheum Dis. 1986;45:350–1.

10. Kovács L, Török T, Bari F, Kéri Z, Kovács A, Makula E, et al. Impaired microvascular response to cholinergic stimuli in primary Sjögren's syndrome. Ann Rheum Dis. 2000;59:48–53.

11. Mandl T, Bornmyr SV, Castenfors J, Jacobsson LT, Manthorpe R, Wollmer P. Sympathetic dysfunction in patients with primary Sjögren's syndrome. J Rheumatol. 2001;28:296–301.

12. Bernacchi E, Bianchi B, Amato L, Giorgini S, Fabbri P, Tavoni A, et al. Xerosis in primary Sjögren syndrome: immunohistochemical and functional investigations. J Dermatol Sci. 2005;39:53–5.

13. Katayama I, Koyano T, Nishioka K. Prevalence of eyelid dermatitis in primary Sjögren's syndrome. Int J Dermatol. 1994;33:421–4.

14. Walling HW, Sontheimer RD. Cutaneous lupus erythematosus: issues in diagnosis and treatment. Am J Clin Dermatol. 2009;10:365–81.

15. Katayama I, Kotobuki Y, Kiyohara E, Murota H. Annular erythema associated with Sjögren's syndrome: review of the literature on the management and clinical analysis of skin lesions. Mod Rheumatol. 2010;20:123–9.

16. Lundström IM, Lindström FD. Subjective and clinical oral symptoms in patients with primary Sjögren's syndrome. Clin Exp Rheumatol. 1995;13:725–31.

17. Rhodus NL, Bloomquist C, Liljemark W, Bereuter J. Prevalence, density, and manifestations of oral Candida albicans in patients with Sjögren's syndrome. J Otolaryngol. 1997;26:300–5.

18. Soto-Rojas AE, Villa AR, Sifuentes-Osornio J, Alarcón-Segovia D, Kraus A. Oral candidiasis and Sjögren's syndrome. J Rheumatol. 1998;25:911–5.

19. Yamamoto T, Yokoyama A, Yamamoto Y, Mamada A. Erythema nodosum associated with Sjögren's syndrome. Br J Rheumatol. 1997;36:707–8.

20. McGovern TW, Erickson AR, Fitzpatrick JE. Sjögren's syndrome plasma cell panniculitis and hidradenitis. J Cutan Pathol. 1996;23:170–4.

21. Chandrupatla C, Xia L, Stratman EJ. Granulomatous panniculitis associated with Sjögren syndrome. Arch Dermatol. 2008;144:815–6.

22. Tait CP, Yu LL, Rohr J. Sjögren's syndrome and granulomatous panniculitis. Australas J Dermatol. 2000;41:187–9.

23. Massone C, Kodama K, Salmhofer W, Abe R, Shimizu H, Parodi A, et al. Lupus erythematosus panniculitis (lupus profundus): clinical, histopathological, and molecular analysis of nine cases. J Cutan Pathol. 2005;32:396–404.

24. Hamadah IR, Banka N. Autosomal recessive plasma cell panniculitis with morphea-like clinical manifestation. J Am Acad Dermatol. 2006;54(5 Suppl):S189–91.

25. Meijer JM, Schonland SO, Palladini G, Merlini G, Hegenbart U, Ciocca O, et al. Sjögren's syndrome and localized nodular cutaneous amyloidosis: coincidence or a distinct clinical entity? Arthritis Rheum. 2008;58:1992–9.

26. Yoneyama K, Tochigi N, Oikawa A, Shinkai H, Utani A. Primary localized cutaneous nodular amyloidosis in a patient with Sjögren's syndrome: a review of the literature. J Dermatol. 2005;32(2):120–3.

27. Schwendiman MN, Beachkofsky TM, Wisco OJ, Owens NM, Hodson DS. Primary cutaneous nodular amyloidosis: case report and review of the literature. Cutis. 2009;84:87–92.

28. Konishi A, Fukuoka M, Nishimura Y. Primary localized amyloidosis with unusual clinical features in a patient with Sjögren's syndrome. J Dermatol. 2007;34:394–6.

29. Srivastava M. Primary cutaneous nodular amyloidosis in a patient with Sjögren's syndrome. J Drugs Dermatol. 2006;5:279–80.

30. Kitajima Y, Seno J, Aoki S, Tada S, Yaoita H. Nodular primary cutaneous amyloidosis. Isolation and characterization of amyloid fibrils. Arch Dermatol. 1986;122:1425–30.

31. Inazumi T, Hakuno M, Yamada H, Tanaka M, Naka W, Tajima S, et al. Characterization of the amyloid fibril from primary localized cutaneous nodular amyloidosis associated with Sjögren's syndrome. Dermatology. 1994;189:125–8.
32. Aoki A, Ono S, Ueda A, Hagiwara E, Takashi T, Ideguchi H, et al. Two cases of limited cutaneous nodular amyloidosis with primary Sjögren's syndrome. Nihon Rinsho Meneki Gakkai Kaishi. 2002;25:205–11.
33. Richey TK, Bennion SD. Etiologies of the sicca syndrome: primary systemic amyloidosis and others. Int J Dermatol. 1996;35(8):553–7.
34. Kassan SS, Thomas TL, Moutsopoulos HM, Hoover R, Kimberly RP, Budman DR, et al. Increased risk of lymphoma in sicca syndrome. Ann Intern Med. 1978;89:888–92.
35. Ekström Smedby K, Vajdic CM, Falster M, Engels EA, Martínez-Maza O, Turner J, et al. Autoimmune disorders and risk of non-Hodgkin lymphoma subtypes: a pooled analysis within the InterLymph Consortium. Blood. 2008;111:4029–38.
36. Zintzaras E, Voulgarelis M, Moutsopoulos HM. The risk of lymphoma development in autoimmune diseases: a meta-analysis. Arch Intern Med. 2005;165:2337–44.
37. Ioannidis JP, Vassiliou VA, Moutsopoulos HM. Long-term risk of mortality and lymphoproliferative disease and predictive classification of primary Sjögren's syndrome. Arthritis Rheum. 2002;46:741–7.
38. Skopouli FN, Dafni U, Ioannidis JPA, Moutsopoulos HM. Clinical evolution, and morbidity and mortality of primary Sjögren's syndrome. Semin Arthritis Rheum. 2000;29:296–304.
39. Voulgarelis M, Dafni UG, Isenberg DA, Moutsopoulos HM. Malignant lymphoma in primary Sjögren's syndrome: a multicenter, retrospective, clinical study by the European Concerted Action on Sjögren's Syndrome. Arthritis Rheum. 1999;42:1765–72.
40. Baimpa E, Dahabreh IJ, Voulgarelis M, Moutsopoulos HM. Hematologic manifestations and predictors of lymphoma development in primary Sjögren syndrome: clinical and pathophysiologic aspects. Medicine (Baltimore). 2009;88:284–93.
41. Ramos-Casals M, Brito-Zerón P, Perez-DE-Lis M, Diaz-Lagares C, Bove A, Soto MJ, et al. Clinical and prognostic significance of parotid scintigraphy in 405 patients with primary Sjögren's syndrome. J Rheumatol. 2010;37:585–90.
42. Renic A, Nousari HC. Other rheumatologic diseases. In: Bolognia J, Jorizzo J, Rapini R, editors. Dermatology. Elsevier; Burlington, Massachusetts, USA 2003. p 636–8.
43. Royer B, Cazals-Hatem D, Sibilia J, Agbalika F, Cayuela JM, Soussi T, et al. Lymphomas in patients with Sjögren's syndrome are marginal zone B-cell neoplasms, arise in diverse extranodal and nodal sites, and are not associated with viruses. Blood. 1997;90:766–75.
44. Quartuccio L, Fabris M, Salvin S, Maset M, De Marchi G, De Vita S. Controversies on rituximab therapy in sjögren syndrome-associated lymphoproliferation. Int J Rheumatol. 2009;2009: 424935.
45. Kristinsson SY, Koshiol J, Björkholm M, Goldin LR, McMaster ML, Turesson I, et al. Immune-related and inflammatory conditions and risk of lymphoplasmacytic lymphoma or Waldenstrom macroglobulinemia. J Natl Cancer Inst. 2010;102(8):557–67.
46. Yokota K, Akiyama Y, Adachi D, Shindo Y, Yoshida Y, Miyoshi F, et al. Subcutaneous panniculitis-like T-cell lymphoma accompanied by Sjögren's syndrome. Scand J Rheumatol. 2009;38:494–5.
47. Sontheimer RD, Thomas JR, Gilliam JN. Subacute cutaneous lupus erythematosus: a cutaneous marker for a distinct lupus erythematosus subset. Arch Dermatol. 1979;115:1409–15.
48. Sontheimer RD. Subacute cutaneous lupus erythematosus: 25-year evolution of a prototypic subset (subphenotype) of lupus erythematosus defined by characteristic cutaneous, pathological, immunological, and genetic findings. Autoimmun Rev. 2005;4:253–63.
49. Sontheimer RD, Maddison PJ, Reichlin M, Jordan RE, Stastny P, Gilliam JN. Serologic and HLA associations in subacute cutaneous lupus erythematosus, a clinical subset of lupus erythematosus. Ann Intern Med. 1982;97:644–71.
50. Black DR, Hornung CA, Schneider PD, Callen JP. Frequency and severity of systemic disease in patients with subacute cutaneous lupus erythematosus. Arch Dermatol. 2002;138:1175–8.

Chapter 12
Vasculitis and Sjögren's Syndrome

George E. Fragoulis, Haralampos M. Moutsopoulos, and John H. Stone

Contents

12.1 Introduction

Sjögren's syndrome (SjS) is a chronic autoimmune disorder characterized by dysfunction and destruction of exocrine glands, principally the salivary and lacrimal glands. Vasculitis, one of the major extraglandular manifestations of SjS, frequently heralds the need for systemic therapy and serves as an indicator of a risk for poor outcomes in many patients. Poor outcomes associated with the development of vasculitis may include direct complications of the vascular inflammation, such as complications of cutaneous ulceration and vasculitic neuropathy, as well as the side

G.E. Fragoulis • H.M. Moutsopoulos
Department of Pathophysiology, School of Medicine,
National University of Athens, Athens, Greece

J.H. Stone (✉)
Division of Rheumatology, Allergy and Immunology, Massachusetts General Hospital,
Boston, MA, USA

M. Ramos-Casals et al. (eds.), *Sjögren's Syndrome*,
DOI 10.1007/978-0-85729-947-5_12, © Springer-Verlag London Limited 2012

Fig. 12.1 *Palpable purpura.*
Purpuric lesions are the most
common manifestation of
vasculitis in Sjögren's
syndrome. These lesions can
be either palpable or
non-palpable. Direct
immunofluorescence studies
on skin biopsies are usually
necessary to distinguish the
small-vessel vasculitis
associated with Sjögren's
syndrome from that of
Henoch-Schönlein purpura,
microscopic polyangiitis, and
other disorders that can cause
leukocytoclastic vasculitis

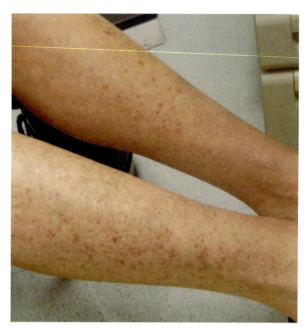

effects of the intensive treatment sometimes required to manage vasculitis. The occurrence of vasculitis along with certain other clinical and serologic features (e.g., salivary gland enlargement and low C4 levels) are markers for patients at increased risk for B cell lymphoma development.

12.2 Epidemiology

The prevalence of vasculitis among patients with primary SjS is estimated to be between 9% and 15%, based upon studies that have employed the new American-European criteria for the diagnosis of SjS [1, 2]. Approximately half of the cutaneous lesions associated with SjS are attributable to vasculitis [3]. Vasculitis is generally a late clinical complication of SjS, with a median time to appearance approximately 10 years after the diagnosis [4]. However, vasculitis is occasionally the presenting feature of SjS.

In the vast majority of SjS patients in whom vasculitis occurs, small-vessel disease predominates [3]. Small blood vessels include capillaries and post-capillary venules, and in SjS there is a major predilection for involvement of the skin (Fig. 12.1). In a significant minority of SjS patients – approximately 5% of those patients who develop vasculitis – the disease involves medium-sized blood vessels. The occurrence of medium-vessel disease (Fig. 12.2), which frequently resembles polyarteritis nodosa or rheumatoid vasculitis, signals a more serious development and the need for intensive therapy.

Fig. 12.2 *Cutaneous ulceration.* Sjögren's syndrome causes a medium-vessel vasculitis if approximately 5% of patients in whom vasculitis occurs. This medium-vessel vasculitis resembles polyarteritis nodosa. In addition to this cutaneous ulceration on the lower extremity, the patient also has a severe sensorimotor vasculitic neuropathy

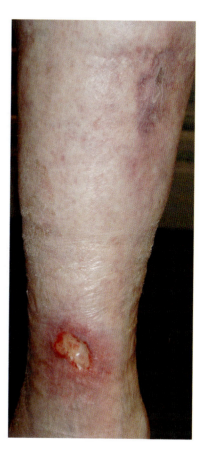

12.3   Histopathology

Several histopathologic types of vasculitis have been described in SjS. There is overlap among these types, and more than one type of histopathology can be found in the same patient. The four histopathologic types described are leukocytoclastic vasculitis, lymphocytic vasculitis, acute necrotizing vasculitis, and endarteritis obliterans.

Leukocytoclastic vasculitis is the most common pattern observed. This histopathology is characterized by infiltration of the blood vessel wall by polymorphonuclear leukocytes, fibrinoid necrosis, karyorrhexis (scattered nuclear debris; "nuclear dust"), and extravasation of erythrocytes (Fig. 12.3). Leukocytoclastic vasculitis is a non-specific finding that must be distinguished in SjS from other causes of small-vessel vasculitis that can cause identical histopathology on light microscopy. Other causes of this histopathology include the drug-induced ("hypersensitivity" vasculitis); the pauci-immune vasculitides (e.g., those associated with antineutrophil cytoplasmic antibodies [ANCA]); Henoch-Schönlein purpura; hypocomplementemic urticarial vasculitis; essential cryoglobulinemia; and others. The diagnosis

Fig. 12.3 *Histopathology of leukocytoclastic vasculitis.* The histopathology associated with most often with vasculitis in Sjögren's syndrome is leukocytoclastic vasculitis, characterized by neutrophilic invasion of blood vessel walls, degranulation, karyorrhexis, and red blood cell extravasation

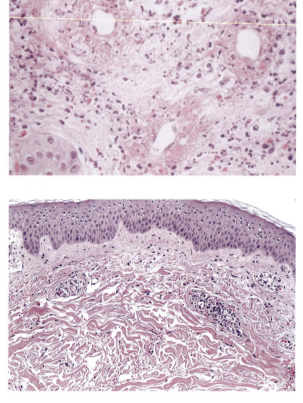

Fig. 12.4 *Lymphocytic vasculitis.* A small minority of patients Sjögren's syndrome have a lymphocytic vasculitis as opposed to a leukocytoclastic vasculitis. Lymphocytic vasculitis is generally less destructive of the blood vessel wall than is leukocytoclastic vasculitis

of SjS-associated vasculitis is rendered generally on the basis of the clinical context, the exclusion of mimickers through appropriate testing, and the performance of direct immunofluorescence on skin biopsies. Direct immunofluorescence on biopsies from patients with SjS-associated vasculitis generally shows signs of immune complex deposition.

In contrast to leukocytoclastic vasculitis, the infiltrates in lymphocytic vasculitis consist of lymphocytes and monocytes. Lymphocytic vasculitis, generally less destructive than leukocytoclastic vasculitis, does not usually cause vessel wall necrosis (Fig. 12.4). Lymphocytic vasculitis is far less common than the leukocytoclastic histopathology. In a study by Ramos-Casals et al. [3], only 1 of 52 patients with SjS had lymphocytic vasculitis. Lymphocytic vasculitis has been observed in tissues other than skin, such as peripheral nerves and muscles [4].

In the third type of histopathology, acute necrotizing vasculitis, the entire vascular wall is infiltrated by inflammatory cells and the degree of fibrinoid necrosis is profound [4] (Fig. 12.5). This form of vasculitis, although rare, is a very serious complication of SjS and is usually associated with internal organ involvement. Acute necrotizing vasculitis can affect medium-sized blood vessels as well as small blood vessels. In the study by Ramos-Casals et al. [3], acute necrotizing vasculitis resembling polyarteritis nodosa was reported in only 2 of 52 patients.

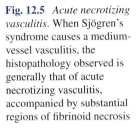

Fig. 12.5 *Acute necrotizing vasculitis.* When Sjögren's syndrome causes a medium-vessel vasculitis, the histopathology observed is generally that of acute necrotizing vasculitis, accompanied by substantial regions of fibrinoid necrosis

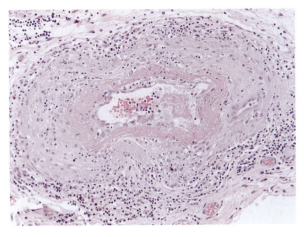

Endarteritis obliterans, the fourth type of histopathology observed in SjS, probably represents a healed or healing form of pre-existing acute vasculitis. This histopathology is a non-inflammatory, obstructive vasculitis that involves medium-sized vessels and is associated with fibrous thickening of the intima.

12.4 Laboratory Findings

The laboratory findings observed in SjS patients with vasculitis are those typically seen in the setting of systemic inflammatory illnesses; e.g., a normochromic, normocytic anemia, hypergammaglobulinemia, and elevated acute phase reactants. Other common findings in SjS include high titers of rheumatoid factor and antinuclear antibodies (ANA), low serum complement levels, and cryoglobulinemia [4]. The presence of cryoglobulins in SjS is an important prognostic factor. Cryoglobulinemia is associated with a higher risk or mortality and is a predictor for the development of lymphoproliferative disorders.

Some investigators have observed different serologic profiles corresponding to the leukocytoclastic and lymphocytic vasculitis subtypes [3]. Leukocytoclastic vasculitis is more likely to be associated with high levels of circulating immunoglobulins and immune complexes; high titers of rheumatoid factor; low complement levels; the presence of cryoglobulins; and anti-Ro/SS-A or anti-La/SS-B autoantibodies. In contrast, lymphocytic vasculitis is more likely to be associated with normocomplementemia and seronegativity for antibodies to the Ro/SS-A and La/SS-B antigens [5].

12.5 Pathogenesis

The exact mechanisms involved in the pathogenesis of vasculitis in SjS are largely unknown and the precise inflammatory pathways may differ to some degree according to the major histopathology subclass. Immune complexes appear to play a major role in the pathogenesis of vasculitis in SjS, but the inciting event(s) leading to immune complex deposition within blood vessel walls at a point years into the disease process remain unknown. B cell activation and the production of cryoglobulins also contribute in many cases of vasculitis, but the relationships of these and other immunologic events to the development of clinical vasculitis are not clear [6]. Type II cryoglobulins, generally monoclonal IgM-kappa immunoglobulins that possess rheumatoid factor activity, appear to participate directly in disease pathophysiology in many cases of SjS-associated vasculitis. However, these cryoglobulins are neither necessary nor sufficient to cause vasculitis in SjS.

12.6   Clinical Findings

Vasculitis is usually not a subtle event in SjS and can generally be suspected and recognized easily. The clues to the presence of vasculitis are found most often in the skin, but multiple organs and tissues can be involved. In addition to cutaneous involvement, vasculitis has been described in SjS in the peripheral nerves, muscles, kidneys, gallbladder, small and large bowel, liver, spleen, pancreas, salivary glands, central nervous system, and the organs of the reproductive tract. The discussion in this chapter focuses upon vasculitis in the skin and the peripheral nervous system, two organs in which vasculitis commonly occurs in SjS, and on the central nervous system, an organ system in which true vasculitis is rare.

12.7   Skin

Ramos-Casals et al. described the clinical, laboratory, and histological features of SjS patients with skin vasculitis, demonstrating that small-vessel involvement was the rule in 95% of cases and that only 5% of patients had medium-vessel involvement [3]. Small-vessel cutaneous vasculitis can be manifested by a host of skin findings, including purpura (both palpable and non-palpable) (Fig. 12.1), urticaria, pustules, vesicles, and flat, confluent patches [7]. In contrast, medium-vessel disease is associated with livedo reticularis (racemosa), nodules (Fig. 12.6), and ulcers (Fig. 12.2). Cutaneous vasculitis is occasionally the complaint that brings the patient's SjS to medical attention [8].

Approximately three quarters of SjS patients with vasculitis manifest palpable purpura. Purpura, which can be associated with stinging or pain, appears most commonly on the lower limbs. In extensive cases, the upper extremities, lower trunk, and even the face can be involved. Purpuric lesions tend to be exacerbated by dependency and activity and may leave residual hyperpigmentation (Fig. 12.7). Palpable purpura is closely associated with the presence of circulating cryoglobulins, but cryoglobulins are not necessary for vasculitis to occur.

Fig. 12.6 *Nodules.*
Medium-vessel vasculitis in
Sjögren's syndrome can be
manifested by cutaneous
nodules

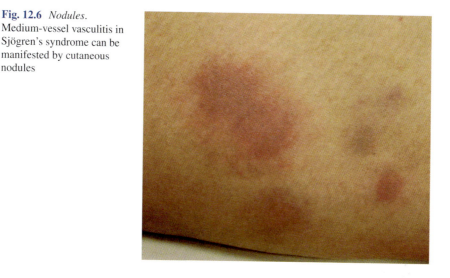

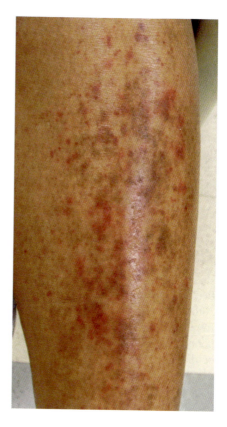

Fig. 12.7 *Palpable purpura with*
hyperpigmentation. The vasculitis in Sjögren's
syndrome is frequently recurrent, with repeated
bouts of purpura. This figure reveals acute
purpuric lesions superimposed upon older,
healed lesions that have left a residual
hyperpigmentation due to lipofuscin

Fig. 12.8 *Urticaria.* Sjögren's
syndrome-related vasculitis leads
occasionally to lesions that resemble
urticaria, although pruritus is often not
associated with these findings.
The lesions last for more than 24 h
permitting them to be distinguished
from common urticaria (which resolve
generally in 6–12 h). Koebner's
phenomenon, the purpuric streaks on
the skin, is also evident in this figure

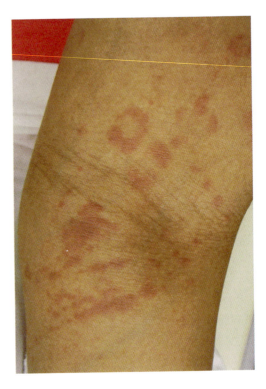

Erythematous macules and papules appear in a significant subset of patients with SjS-associated cutaneous vasculitis and may be termed urticaria with or without the presence of pruritus (Fig. 12.8). These lesions differ from the classic urticaria in that they last for longer than 24 h (classic urticaria generally resolve in 6–12 h). Other clinical findings in the cutaneous vasculitis of SjS include violaceous discoloration of fingers and toes, subcutaneous nodules (Fig. 12.6), and ulcerations caused by medium-vessel disease in the deep dermis or sub-cutis.

12.8   Peripheral and Central Nervous System

Peripheral neuropathy is a well-described manifestation of vasculitis in SjS patients. Although vasculitis is an important mechanism of peripheral neuropathy, it is far from the only cause of peripheral neuropathy in this disease. The prevalence of peripheral neuropathy in SjS is estimated to be about 2%, and the various causes can be dissected through electrophysiological studies and biopsies of skin, peripheral nerve, and muscle.

Among the multiple types of peripheral neuropathy, only sensorimotor neuropathies and mononeuritis multiplex are associated with vasculitis of the vasa nervosum. In contrast, pure sensory neuropathies, sensorimotor demyelinating polyneuropathies, and small fiber neuropathies occurring in the context of SjS appear to have other disease mechanisms. It is important to remember that most peripheral nerves are mixed nerves, containing both motor and sensory fibers. Thus, when vasculitis involves peripheral nerves, both motor and sensory findings are generally present.

Biopsy specimens from patients with moneuritis multiplex show fibrinoid necrosis in the vasa nervosum and infiltrates by T cells and macrophages. In a study of 40 patients with neuropathy secondary to SjS [9], the authors described 8 patients with lymphocytic vasculitis and 14 with necrotizing vasculitis. Comparing these two subgroups of SjS patients, no significant difference regarding the clinical or the biological picture has been revealed [9]. Patients with peripheral neuropathy occurring in the setting of SjS should be evaluated for the possibility of vasculitis, including perhaps biopsy of both nerve and muscle. The simultaneous biopsy of nerve and muscle is synergistic for the diagnosis of vasculitis and has an estimated sensitivity of 85% [10].

In contrast to peripheral nervous system vasculitis, the incidence of true CNS vasculitis in SjS appears to be very low [11, 12]. The diagnosis is difficult to make because of imperfect sensitivities of brain biopsy. High prevalences of CNS involvement (not necessarily vasculitis) have been reported in SjS in the past, but such reports likely represent substantial overestimates of the true prevalence of CNS disease. They are probably attributable to the fact that patients who did not strictly fulfilled the diagnostic criteria of SjS were included [12]. The enrichment of reported cases of CNS disease is likely due to the inclusion of patients with overlap syndromes of SLE and SjS rather than primary SjS.

12.9   Other Organs

Vasculitis that affects other organs in SjS such as the gastrointestinal tract, kidneys, and lungs is unusual but known to occur. In such cases, the vessels involved are usually medium-sized and the vascular inflammation in these vessels typically co-exists small-vessel vasculitis and cutaneous disease [4]. Vasculitis of internal organs can be life-threatening, especially if the physician is not familiar with the subtle clinical and laboratory findings accompanying this situation. Such findings include diarrhea, "intestinal angina" (post-prandial abdominal pain), clinical symptoms of appendicitis, hypertension with hematuria and proteinuria (mesangial proliferative glomerulonephritis) [13], myalgias (muscle involvement), and elevated acute phase reactants. Systemic vasculitis appears late in the natural history of SjS and is accompanied by cryoglobulinemia in about half of the cases.

12.10   Vasculitis and Mortality

The development of vasculitis constitutes an adverse prognostic sign in SjS. Ioannidis et al. [14] identified the fact that the combination of palpable purpura and low C4 serum levels correlate with the evolution of lymphoproliferative disorders in a substantial subset of patients, a finding confirmed by others [15]. Multivariate analyses have confirmed that vasculitis in SjS patients is associated not only with lymphoma development but also with mortality. A subgroup of SjS patients who have systemic vasculitis coupled with peripheral neuropathy or glomerulonephritis is at increased risk of lymphomagenesis. These patients possess distinct serological characteristics (e.g., low C4 complement levels, the presence of cryoglobulins) that correlate independently with the development of lymphoproliferative disease and increased mortality [16].

12.11   Treatment

Skin vasculitis characterized by mild, intermittent purpura may respond to local measures such as the avoidance of dependency (spending less time on one's feet) during periods of active disease and support stockings. Hydroxychloroquine (200 mg twice daily) has not been studied formally in the setting of SjS-related vasculitis but appears to be a reasonable intervention for patients with recurrent mild disease. More severe cases typically respond initially at least to modest doses of glucocorticoids.

For patients whose disease cannot be controlled during prednisone tapers or for those whose disease is refractory to glucocorticoids alone, rituximab (anti-CD20) (1 g times two, separated by 15 days) is increasingly the agent to which clinicians turn. Palpable purpura and cryoglobulins disappear while complement levels return to normal after anti-CD20 therapy [17–19]. This approach has never been subjected to a randomized clinical trial in SjS, but data extrapolated from such trials in other patients support this approach [20].

If rituximab is not available, is ineffective, or is not tolerated well by the patient, then a variety of conventional immunomodulating therapies can be employed. These include azathioprine (up to 2 mg/kg/day) and methotrexate (up to 25 mg/week) [21, 22]. Cyclophosphamide, a potentially life-saving therapy if employed in a timely and prudent way, should be reserved for patients in whom rituximab is not an option and have vital organ- or life-threatening disease. The avoidance of cyclophosphamide whenever possible is particularly important because the use of this medication might contribute further to the potential for lymphomagenesis in SjS. Plasma exchange is seldom required but does appear to be effective in cases of overwhelming immune complex-mediated disease.

References

1. Skopouli FN, Dafni U, Ioannidis JP, Moutsopoulos HM. Clinical evolution, and morbidity and mortality of primary Sjögren's syndrome. Semin Arthritis Rheum. 2000;29(5):296–304.
2. Brito-Zeron P, Ramos-Casals M, Bove A, Sentis J, Font J. Predicting adverse outcomes in primary Sjögren's syndrome: identification of prognostic factors. Rheumatology (Oxford). 2007;46(8): 1359–62.

3. Ramos-Casals M, Anaya JM, Garcia-Carrasco M, Rosas J, Bove A, Claver G, et al. Cutaneous vasculitis in primary Sjögren syndrome: classification and clinical significance of 52 patients. Medicine (Baltimore). 2004;83(2):96–106.

4. Tsokos M, Lazarou SA, Moutsopoulos HM. Vasculitis in primary Sjögren's syndrome. Histologic classification and clinical presentation. Am J Clin Pathol. 1987;88(1):26–31.

5. Alexander E, Provost TT. Sjögren's syndrome. Association of cutaneous vasculitis with central nervous system disease. Arch Dermatol. 1987;123(6):801–10.

6. Ferri C, Mascia MT. Cryoglobulinemic vasculitis. Curr Opin Rheumatol. 2006;18(1):54–63.

7. Stone JH, Nousari HC. "Essential" cutaneous vasculitis: what every rheumatologist should know about vasculitis of the skin. Curr Opin Rheumatol. 2001;13:23–34.

8. Markusse HM, Schoonbrood M, Oudkerk M, Henzen-Logmans SC. Leucocytoclastic vasculitis as presenting feature of primary Sjögren's syndrome. Clin Rheumatol. 1994;13(2):269–72.

9. Terrier B, Lacroix C, Guillevin L, Hatron PY, Dhote R, Maillot F, et al. Diagnostic and prognostic relevance of neuromuscular biopsy in primary Sjögren's syndrome-related neuropathy. Arthritis Rheum. 2007;57(8):1520–9.

10. Collins MP, Mendell JR, Periquet MI, Sahenk Z, Amato AA, Gronseth GS, et al. Superficial peroneal nerve/peroneus brevis muscle biopsy in vasculitic neuropathy. Neurology. 2000;55(5): 636–43.

11. Ramos-Casals M, Solans R, Rosas J, Camps MT, Gil A, Del Pino-Montes J, et al. Primary Sjögren syndrome in Spain: clinical and immunologic expression in 1010 patients. Medicine (Baltimore). 2008;87(4):210–9.

12. Ioannidis JP, Moutsopoulos HM. Sjögren's syndrome: too many associations, too limited evidence. The enigmatic example of CNS involvement. Semin Arthritis Rheum. 1999;29(1): 1–3.

13. Moutsopoulos HM, Balow JE, Lawley TJ, Stahl NI, Antonovych TT, Chused TM. Immune complex glomerulonephritis in sicca syndrome. Am J Med. 1978;64(6):955–60.

14. Ioannidis JP, Vassiliou VA, Moutsopoulos HM. Long-term risk of mortality and lymphoproliferative disease and predictive classification of primary Sjögren's syndrome. Arthritis Rheum. 2002;46(3):741–7.

15. Theander E, Henriksson G, Ljungberg O, Mandl T, Manthorpe R, Jacobsson LT. Lymphoma and other malignancies in primary Sjögren's syndrome: a cohort study on cancer incidence and lymphoma predictors. Ann Rheum Dis. 2006;65(6):796–803.

16. Voulgarelis M, Tzioufas AG. Pathogenetic mechanisms in the initiation and perpetuation of Sjögren's syndrome. Nat Rev Rheumatol. 2010;6(9):529–37.

17. Quartuccio L, Fabris M, Salvin S, Maset M, De Marchi G, De Vita S. Controversies on rituximab therapy in Sjögren syndrome-associated lymphoproliferation. Int J Rheumatol. 2009; 2009:424935.

18. Gottenberg JE, Guillevin L, Lambotte O, Combe B, Allanore Y, Cantagrel A, et al. Tolerance and short term efficacy of rituximab in 43 patients with systemic autoimmune diseases. Ann Rheum Dis. 2005;64(6):913–20.

19. Voulgarelis M, Giannouli S, Anagnostou D, Tzioufas AG. Combined therapy with rituximab plus cyclophosphamide/doxorubicin/vincristine/prednisone (CHOP) for Sjögren's syndrome-associated B-cell aggressive non-Hodgkin's lymphomas. Rheumatology (Oxford). 2004;43(8): 1050–3.

20. Stone JH, Merkel PA, Spiera R, et al. Rituximab compared with cyclophosphamide for remission induction in ANCA-associated vasculitis. N Engl J Med. 2010;363:221–32.

21. Jayne D, Rasmussen N, Andrassy K, Bacon P, Tervaert JW, Dadoniene J, et al. A randomized trial of maintenance therapy for vasculitis associated with antineutrophil cytoplasmic autoantibodies. N Engl J Med. 2003;349(1):36–44.

22. Pagnoux C, Mahr A, Hamidou MA, Boffa JJ, Ruivard M, Ducroix JP, et al. Azathioprine or methotrexate maintenance for ANCA-associated vasculitis. N Engl J Med. 2008;359(26): 2790–803.

Chapter 13
Cardiovascular Involvement

George E. Tzelepis, Clio P. Mavragani, and Haralampos M. Moutsopoulos

Contents

13.1 Introduction

Cardiac involvement occurs rarely in primary Sjögren's syndrome (pSS), with the majority of descriptions coming primarily from single case reports or small patient series. In this respect, pSS differs from other systemic autoimmune diseases such as systemic lupus erythematosus (SLE), rheumatoid arthritis, or systemic sclerosis, in which cardiac complications are quite common [1]. The rarity of clinically overt cardiac involvement in pSS should be kept in mind so that an exhaustive search for other autoimmune diseases, especially SLE with secondary Sjögren's syndrome, or diseases of non-immune etiology, should be first considered in the differential diagnosis. The spectrum of cardiovascular complications described in pSS includes

G.E. Tzelepis (✉) • C.P. Mavragani • H.M. Moutsopoulos
Department of Pathophysiology, University of Athens Medical School, Laiko University
Hospital, Athens, Greece

M. Ramos-Casals et al. (eds.), *Sjögren's Syndrome*,
DOI 10.1007/978-0-85729-947-5_13, © Springer-Verlag London Limited 2012

185

Table 13.1 Cardiovascular complications in primary Sjögren's syndrome

Pericarditis
Myocarditis
Valvular abnormalities
Diastolic dysfunction
Atrioventricular block
Subclinical atheromatosis
Raynaud's phenomenon
Pulmonary arterial hypertension
Autonomic cardiovascular dysfunction

pericarditis, myocarditis, valvular abnormalities, pulmonary arterial hypertension, left ventricular diastolic dysfunction, and autonomic dysfunction (Table 13.1).

13.2 Pericarditis

Acute pericarditis in pSS has been described in few reports in the literature [2–4], with only one reporting an exudative effusion [3]. In the remaining reports, acute pericarditis with pericardial effusion was reported in patients with renal or other system involvement, or in patients with features of mixed connective tissue disease [5]. In nine patients with pSS and pulmonary hypertension reported by Launey et al. [6], pericardial effusion was found in three patients. In contrast, more frequent is the echocardiographic finding of small, silent pericardial effusions or evidence of previous pericardial inflammation [3, 7]. The frequency of these echocardiographic findings in several studies involving pSS patients with no cardiac manifestations ranges from 8% to 33% [3, 7–10]. In an echocardiographic study that included more than 100 patients with pSS [7], clinically silent pericardial effusions were found in 8% of patients and were associated with the presence of cryoglobulinemia and primary biliary cirrhosis. The etiology of pericardial inflammation is poorly understood when one considers that pSS does not cause serositis. Pericardial effusion due to cardiac lymphoma is extremely rare in pSS [11].

13.3 Myocarditis

Autoimmune myocarditis is rare in pSS. Clinically, autoimmune myocarditis should be suspected in the setting of tachycardia out of proportion to fever, presence of a gallop rhythm, and suggestive ECG changes. In the English literature, there are few reports of pSS patients diagnosed with myocarditis. In all cases, patients presented with dyspnea, fever, increased inflammatory markers (erythrocyte sedimentation rate, C-reactive protein) and signs of dilated or restrictive cardiomyopathy [12–14]. In one patient, there was a unique uptake of gallium-67-labelled isotope by the myocardium [14]. In the absence of myocardial biopsies, the diagnosis of myocarditis was made by excluding other causes of cardiomyopathy, primarily of infectious etiology. Autoimmune myocarditis responded to augmented immunosuppression with glucocorticoids, cyclophosphamide, and azathioprine.

13.4 Valvular Abnormalities

Valvular abnormalities such as mild aortic or mitral regurgitation have been described with a greater frequency in asymptomatic patients with pSS than in healthy, age-matched controls [7]. Since these abnormalities were associated with low C4 values, the authors of the study [7] postulated that immune complexes and the activated classical complement pathway might be involved in the pathogenesis of these abnormalities. In most patients, these abnormalities have no clinical significance.

13.5 Diastolic Dysfunction

A relatively high prevalence of left ventricular diastolic dysfunction and increased left ventricular mass has been reported by echocardiographic studies in pSS patients [3, 7, 8]. Because these patients had no cardiac symptoms, the etiology and clinical significance of these findings remain unknown at present [3, 7, 8].

13.6 Atrioventricular Block

Complete heart block has been described in two patients with pSS and anti-SS-A/anti-SS-B antibodies [15, 16]. Another ECG study [17] reported a prevalence of first degree atrioventricular block of about 10% in pSS patients. The finding of first-degree heart block was associated with disease activity and anti-SSB antibodies [17]. In contrast to the neonatal heart, which is susceptible to conduction abnormalities such as congenital heart block caused by maternal anti-SS-A/anti-SS-B autoantibodies, the adult atrioventricular node is generally thought to be resistant to the damaging effects of anti-SSA/anti-SSB antibodies.

13.7 Subclinical Atherosclerosis

Although mortality data in pSS show no excess in cardiovascular mortality [18, 19], the possibility of accelerated atherosclerosis in these patients has recently been raised [20–22]. Premature atherosclerosis is known to occur in rheumatoid arthritis and systemic lupus erythematosus. Although the precise etiology of accelerated atherosclerosis in rheumatologic diseases has not been elucidated completely, there is evidence that inflammation plays a pivotal role in the atherosclerotic process [23]. In a small cohort of patients with pSS, Vaudo et al. described greater intima-media thickness of the carotid and femoral arteries in women with pSS than in healthy controls [22]. Furthermore, the association of artery thickening with anti-SSA antibodies and leucopenia raises the possibility that immune dysregulation contributes to early atheromatosis [22]. Greater frequencies of hypercholesterolemia, hypertriglyceridemia, diabetes mellitus, and hyperuricemia have recently been described in patients with pSS compared to healthy controls [20, 24, 25]. The question of premature atherosclerosis in pSS requires further investigation.

13.8 Pulmonary Arterial Hypertension

Pulmonary arterial hypertension (PAH) occurs rarely in pSS, which contrasts with the relatively high prevalence of PAH in SSc, MCTD, or SLE [6, 26–28]. Although various studies based exclusively on Doppler echocardiography have reported a relatively high frequency of pulmonary hypertension in pSS [3, 7], the only study that used hemodynamic measurements to establish the diagnosis of PAH in patients with pSS is by Launey et al. [6]. These authors described nine cases of pSS associated PAH with a complete clinical assessment including hemodynamic evaluation, type of PAH as well as outcome.

Based on findings of nine pSS patients with PAH and a review of additional 19 cases of PAH reported in the literature, it has been suggested [6] that there is a true cause and effect relationship between PAH and pSS. This is supported by the data of Launey et al., who showed that PAH occurs in pSS patients with laboratory markers of intense B-cell activation, such as antinuclear antibodies, anti-Ro/SSA or anti-RNP antibodies, and hypergammaglobulinemia [6]. In addition, immunofluorescence studies have revealed deposits by immunoglobulin and complement in the pulmonary arterial walls of pSS patients with PAH. In the nine pSS patients reported by Lanuey et al. [6], Raynaud's phenomenon occurred in 67%, cutaneous vasculitis in 33%, and interstitial lung disease in 44%. Thromboembolic lung disease was the underlying cause of PAH in two patients [6]. Additional risk factors for development of PAH in pSS such as portal hypertension and interstitial lung disease are present in some patients [6].

The pathogenesis of PAH in pSS is unknown. The higher frequency of Raynaud's phenomenon, cutaneous vasculitis, and various antibodies detected in these patients, points towards a pulmonary vasculopathy and B-cell activation playing a role in the pathophysiology of PAH [6]. The efficacy of standard PAH and immunosuppressive therapy lends further support to the notion of an underlying vasculopathy [6].

In most cases, the PAH was severe at presentation, with the mean pulmonary artery pressure being 47 mmHg (±10 mmHg). Exertional dyspnea was the initial symptom in the majority of patients whereas a delay in diagnosis of more than a year was also common. The reported survival in the cohort reviewed by Launey et al. was overall poor, being 73% and 66% at 1 and 3 years, respectively [6].

Table 13.2 Clinical features in pSS-associated cardiovascular autonomic dysfunction

Orthostatic hypotension
Syncope
Hypohidrosis/anidrosis
Diarrhea
Constipation
Vomiting
Urinary disturbance
Abnormal cardiovascular reflexes
Decreased uptake of ^{123}I-MIBG

13.9   Autonomic Cardiovascular Dysfunction

Symptomatic autonomic cardiovascular neuropathy is rare in pSS [29–36]. Symptomatic patients with autonomic neuropathy typically present with symptoms of orthostatic hypotension, with or without syncope [29–36]. Other manifestations (Table 13.2) such as anhidrosis, constipation, diarrhea, or presence of Adie's pupil frequently accompany postural hypotension [37]. Although signs of autonomic dysfunction are often present in pSS patients with sensory neuropathy, predominant autonomic neuropathy is less common. Generally, in pSS-associated neuropathy, autonomic symptoms are mild in comparison with the sensory symptoms [36]. In the series of patients reported by Mori et al., pure autonomic cardiovascular neuropathy accounted for about 3% of all pSS-associated neuropathies [37]. Antibodies to ganglionic acetylcholine receptor (AChR) were reported in one patient with pSS and autonomic cardiovascular neuropathy [32].

In asymptomatic patients, studies employing specific tests of cardiovascular autonomic function including Valsalva maneuvers, deep breathing tests, and heart rate response to standing have reported abnormal responses suggestive of autonomic dysfunction in a significant percentage of patients [38–43]. In a small group of patients with pSS, Andonopoulos et al. reported symptoms of autonomic dysfunction in approximately half of patients specifically asked for symptoms, while specific testing revealed abnormal results in about two-thirds of patients [44]. In contrast, other studies reported no differences in the prevalence of autonomic dysfunction in these patients and in healthy controls [45–47].

The autonomic cardiovascular dysfunction in pSS has been linked to immunological factors including anti-muscarine-3 (M3)-receptor antibodies, cytokines interfering with nerve function, and inflammation of autonomic nerves or ganglia [37, 44, 48–50]. Autopsy reports of patients with autonomic dysfunction showed loss of sympathetic ganglion neurons associated with T-cell invasion, supporting involvement of autonomic ganglion cells [37].

13.10   Therapeutic Management

Because of the rarity of cardiac complications in pSS, the recommended treatment is based on expert opinion rather than on information derived from clinically validated data. For autoimmune myocarditis, intense immunosuppression with glucocorticoids and intravenous pulses of cyclophosphamide are often administered [51]. Maintenance immunosuppression with glucocorticoids and azathioprine or mycophenolate mofetil is continued for a period of months. Congestive heart failure due to myocarditis is treated similarly to heart failure of all causes with afterload-reducing agents, diuretics, and beta-blockers. In the symptomatic pSS patient with congestive heart failure of paramount importance is to exclude other causes before attributing the cardiac manifestations to primary autoimmune myocarditis.

The best management of PAH in pSS and particularly the role of immunosuppression as a first-line therapy remains to be defined. On the basis of uncontrolled

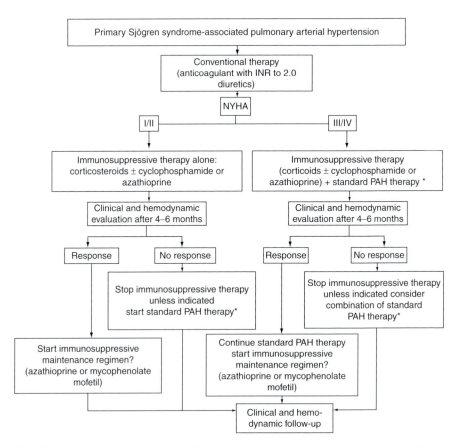

Fig. 13.1 Treatment algorithm for pSS associated pulmonary arterial hypertension (From Launey et al. [6]) (*) Standard PAH therapy: endothelin receptor antagonists, phosphodiesterase type-5 inhibitors or prostanoids.

data derived from patients with lupus or mixed connective tissue disease [52, 53], it has been suggested that patients with pSS-associated PAH and NYHA class I and II should be initially considered for treatment with immunosuppressants alone, such as glucocorticoids with or without cyclophosphamide or azathioprine for a period of 4–6 months [6]. If response is documented on hemodynamic evaluation, a maintenance regimen consisting of azathioprine or mycophenolate mofetil should then be continued [6]. Patients not responding to a trial of immunosuppressants should be switched to standard PAH therapy. For patients in NYHA class III or IV, a regimen consisting of both immunosuppressant and standard PAH medications is recommended for a period of 4–6 months. Maintenance immunosuppressant therapy is then continued when on hemodynamic evaluation response is documented; if there is no response, immunosuppression is replaced with combined standard PAH therapy (Fig. 13.1).

In the patient with symptoms of cardiac autonomic neuropathy, exclusion of potentially reversible causes of orthostatic hypotension is the first and most important management step. Non-pharmacological therapy such as use of elastic stockings or elevation of the head of the bed, avoiding hypotensive drugs (e.g., diuretics, vasodilators) and a high-salt high-fluid diet may be useful. A synthetic mineralocorticoid, 9-α-fluorohydrocortisone, should be considered in patients not responding to non-pharmacological treatment. A sympathomimetic agent, such as midodrine, can be added to fludrocortisone acetate if the patient remains symptomatic. The role of immunosuppression in treating pure autonomic neuropathy is entirely unknown [37].

13.11 Conclusion

Symptomatic cardiovascular involvement occurs rarely in primary Sjögren's syndrome. Cardiovascular complications that may occasionally require clinical attention include myocarditis, pulmonary arterial hypertension, pericarditis, and autonomic cardiovascular dysfunction manifested primarily with orthostatic hypotension and/or syncope. Equally rare are other abnormalities, which are mostly asymptomatic and include left ventricular diastolic dysfunction and mild valvular abnormalities. Management of cardiovascular complications in these patients is based on clinical knowledge acquired from treating similar complications in other autoimmune diseases.

References

1. Riboldi P, Gerosa M, Luzzana C, et al. Cardiac involvement in systemic autoimmune diseases. Clin Rev Allergy Immunol. 2002;23:247–61.
2. Chen HA, Chen CH, Cheng HH. Hemolytic uremic syndrome and pericarditis as early manifestations of primary Sjogren's syndrome. Clin Rheumatol. 2009;28 Suppl 1:S43–6.
3. Gyongyosi M, Pokorny G, Jambrik Z, et al. Cardiac manifestations in primary Sjogren's syndrome. Ann Rheum Dis. 1996;55:450–4.

4. Suzuki H, Hickling P, Lyons CB. A case of primary Sjogren's syndrome, complicated by cryoglobulinaemic glomerulonephritis, pericardial and pleural effusions. Br J Rheumatol. 1996;35:72–5.

5. Mohri H, Kimura M, Ieki R, et al. Cardiac tamponade in Sjogren's syndrome. J Rheumatol. 1986;13:830–1.

6. Launay D, Hachulla E, Hatron PY, et al. Pulmonary arterial hypertension: a rare complication of primary Sjogren syndrome: report of 9 new cases and review of the literature. Medicine (Baltimore). 2007;86:299–315.

7. Vassiliou VA, Moyssakis I, Boki KA, et al. Is the heart affected in primary Sjogren's syndrome? An echocardiographic study. Clin Exp Rheumatol. 2008;26:109–12.

8. Manganelli P, Bernardi P, Taliani U, et al. Echocardiographic findings in primary Sjogren's syndrome. Ann Rheum Dis. 1997;56:568.

9. Mita S, Akizuki S, Koido N, et al. Cardiac involvement in Sjögren's syndrome detected by two dimensional ultrasonic cardiography. In: Homma M et al., editors. Sjögren's syndrome – state of the art. Amsterdam: Kugler; 1994. p. 427–30.

10. Rantapaa-Dahlqvist S, Backman C, Sandgren H, et al. Echocardiographic findings in patients with primary Sjogren's syndrome. Clin Rheumatol. 1993;12:214–8.

11. Yoong JK, Chew LC, Quek R, et al. Cardiac lymphoma in primary Sjogren syndrome: a novel case established by targeted imaging and pericardial window. J Thorac Cardiovasc Surg. 2007;134:513–4.

12. Kau CK, Hu JC, Lu LY, et al. Primary Sjogren's syndrome complicated with cryoglobulinemic glomerulonephritis, myocarditis, and multi-organ involvement. J Formos Med Assoc. 2004;103:707–10.

13. Levin MD, Zoet-Nugteren SK, Markusse HM. Myocarditis and primary Sjogren's syndrome. Lancet. 1999;354:128–9.

14. Yoshioka K, Tegoshi H, Yoshida T, et al. Myocarditis and primary Sjogren's syndrome. Lancet. 1999;354:1996.

15. Baumgart DC, Gerl H, Dorner T. Complete heart block caused by primary Sjogren's syndrome and hypopituitarism. Ann Rheum Dis. 1998;57:635.

16. Lee LA, Pickrell MB, Reichlin M. Development of complete heart block in an adult patient with Sjogren's syndrome and anti-Ro/SS-A autoantibodies. Arthritis Rheum. 1996;39:1427–9.

17. Lodde BM, Sankar V, Kok MR, et al. Adult heart block is associated with disease activity in primary Sjogren's syndrome. Scand J Rheumatol. 2005;34:383–6.

18. Skopouli FN, Dafni U, Ioannidis JP, et al. Clinical evolution, and morbidity and mortality of primary Sjogren's syndrome. Semin Arthritis Rheum. 2000;29:296–304.

19. Theander E, Manthorpe R, Jacobsson LT. Mortality and causes of death in primary Sjogren's syndrome: a prospective cohort study. Arthritis Rheum. 2004;50:1262–9.

20. Gerli R, Bartoloni BE, Vaudo G, et al. Traditional cardiovascular risk factors in primary Sjogren's syndrome–role of dyslipidaemia. Rheumatology (Oxford). 2006;45:1580–1.

21. Gerli R, Vaudo G, Bocci EB, et al. Functional impairment of arterial wall in primary Sjogren's syndrome: combined action of immunological and inflammatory factors. Arthritis Care Res (Hoboken). 2010;62:712–8.

22. Vaudo G, Bocci EB, Shoenfeld Y, et al. Precocious intima-media thickening in patients with primary Sjogren's syndrome. Arthritis Rheum. 2005;52:3890–7.

23. Abou-Raya A, Abou-Raya S. Inflammation: a pivotal link between autoimmune diseases and atherosclerosis. Autoimmun Rev. 2006;5:331–7.

24. Lodde BM, Sankar V, Kok MR, et al. Serum lipid levels in Sjogren's syndrome. Rheumatology (Oxford). 2006;45:481–4.

25. Ramos-Casals M, Brito-Zeron P, Siso A, et al. High prevalence of serum metabolic alterations in primary Sjogren's syndrome: influence on clinical and immunological expression. J Rheumatol. 2007;34:754–61.

26. Asherson RA, Hughes GR. Pulmonary hypertension in Sjogren's syndrome. Ann Rheum Dis. 1988;47:703–4.

27. Bertoni M, Niccoli L, Porciello G, et al. Pulmonary hypertension in primary Sjogren's syndrome: report of a case and review of the literature. Clin Rheumatol. 2005;24:431–4.
28. Sato T, Matsubara O, Tanaka Y, et al. Association of Sjogren's syndrome with pulmonary hypertension: report of two cases and review of the literature. Hum Pathol. 1993;24:199–205.
29. Andonopoulos AP, Ballas C. Autonomic cardiovascular neuropathy in primary Sjogren's syndrome. Rheumatol Int. 1995;15:127–9.
30. Barendregt PJ, Markusse HM, Man In't Veld AJ. Primary Sjogren's syndrome presenting as autonomic neuropathy. Case report. Neth J Med. 1998;53:196–200.
31. Goto H, Matsuo H, Fukudome T, et al. Chronic autonomic neuropathy in a patient with primary Sjogren's syndrome. J Neurol Neurosurg Psychiatry. 2000;69:135.
32. Kondo T, Inoue H, Usui T, et al. Autoimmune autonomic ganglionopathy with Sjogren's syndrome: significance of ganglionic acetylcholine receptor antibody and therapeutic approach. Auton Neurosci. 2009;146:33–5.
33. Sakakibara R, Hirano S, Asahina M, et al. Primary Sjogren's syndrome presenting with generalized autonomic failure. Eur J Neurol. 2004;11:635–8.
34. Shimoyama M, Ohtahara A, Okamura T, et al. Isolated autonomic cardiovascular neuropathy in a patient with primary Sjogren syndrome: a case of successful treatment with glucocorticoid. Am J Med Sci. 2002;324:170–2.
35. Sorajja P, Poirier MK, Bundrick JB, et al. Autonomic failure and proximal skeletal myopathy in a patient with primary Sjogren syndrome. Mayo Clin Proc. 1999;74:695–7.
36. Wright RA, Grant IA, Low PA. Autonomic neuropathy associated with sicca complex. J Auton Nerv Syst. 1999;75:70–6.
37. Mori K, Iijima M, Koike H, et al. The wide spectrum of clinical manifestations in Sjogren's syndrome-associated neuropathy. Brain. 2005;128:2518–34.
38. Andonopoulos AP, Christodoulou J, Ballas C, et al. Autonomic cardiovascular neuropathy in Sjogren's syndrome. A controlled study. J Rheumatol. 1998;25:2385–8.
39. Mandl T, Bornmyr SV, Castenfors J, et al. Sympathetic dysfunction in patients with primary Sjogren's syndrome. J Rheumatol. 2001;28:296–301.
40. Mandl T, Wollmer P, Manthorpe R, et al. Autonomic and orthostatic dysfunction in primary Sjogren's syndrome. J Rheumatol. 2007;34:1869–74.
41. Mandl T, Granberg V, Apelqvist J, et al. Autonomic nervous symptoms in primary Sjogren's syndrome. Rheumatology (Oxford). 2008;47:914–9.
42. Stojanovich L, Milovanovich B, de Luka SR, et al. Cardiovascular autonomic dysfunction in systemic lupus, rheumatoid arthritis, primary Sjogren syndrome and other autoimmune diseases. Lupus. 2007;16:181–5.
43. Tumiati B, Perazzoli F, Negro A, et al. Heart rate variability in patients with Sjogren's syndrome. Clin Rheumatol. 2000;19:477–80.
44. Goldstein DS, Holmes C, Imrich R. Clinical laboratory evaluation of autoimmune autonomic ganglionopathy: preliminary observations. Auton Neurosci. 2009;146:18–21.
45. Barendregt PJ, van den Bent MJ, van Raaij-van den Aarssen VJ, et al. Involvement of the peripheral nervous system in primary Sjogren's syndrome. Ann Rheum Dis. 2001;60:876–81.
46. Niemela RK, Pikkujamsa SM, Hakala M, et al. No signs of autonomic nervous system dysfunction in primary Sjogren's syndrome evaluated by 24 hour heart rate variability. J Rheumatol. 2000;27:2605–10.
47. Niemela RK, Hakala M, Huikuri HV, et al. Comprehensive study of autonomic function in a population with primary Sjogren's syndrome. No evidence of autonomic involvement. J Rheumatol. 2003;30:74–9.
48. Fox RI, Stern M. Sjogren's syndrome: mechanisms of pathogenesis involve interaction of immune and neurosecretory systems. Scand J Rheumatol Suppl. 2002;116:3–13.
49. Gordon TP, Bolstad AI, Rischmueller M, et al. Autoantibodies in primary Sjogren's syndrome: new insights into mechanisms of autoantibody diversification and disease pathogenesis. Autoimmunity. 2001;34:123–32.

50. Stojanovich L. Autonomic dysfunction in autoimmune rheumatic disease. Autoimmun Rev. 2009;8:569–72.
51. Law WG, Thong BY, Lian TY, et al. Acute lupus myocarditis: clinical features and outcome of an oriental case series. Lupus. 2005;14:827–31.
52. Jais X, Launay D, Yaici A, et al. Immunosuppressive therapy in lupus- and mixed connective tissue disease-associated pulmonary arterial hypertension: a retrospective analysis of twenty-three cases. Arthritis Rheum. 2008;58:521–31.
53. Sanchez O, Sitbon O, Jais X, et al. Immunosuppressive therapy in connective tissue diseases-associated pulmonary arterial hypertension. Chest. 2006;130:182–9.

Chapter 14
Pulmonary Involvement

Clio P. Mavragani, George E. Tzelepis, and Haralampos M. Moutsopoulos

Contents

C.P. Mavragani (✉)
Department of Experimental Physiology,
School of Medicine, University of Athens, Athens, Greece

G.E. Tzelepis • H.M. Moutsopoulos
Department of Pathophysiology, School of Medicine, University of Athens, Athens, Greece

M. Ramos-Casals et al. (eds.), *Sjögren's Syndrome*,
DOI 10.1007/978-0-85729-947-5_14, © Springer-Verlag London Limited 2012

Table 14.1 Type of respiratory system involvement in Sjögren's syndrome (SS) (lymphoproliferative disorders are not included)

Upper airway disease	Rhina sicca
	Recurrent sinusitis
	Xerotrachea
Lower airway disease	Lymphocytic bronchitis/bronchiolitis
	Bronchial hyperresponsiveness
	Diffuse panbronchiolitis
Interstitial lung disease	Non specific interstitial pneumonia (NSIP)
	Usual interstitial pneumonia (UIP)
	Cryptogenic organizing pneumonia (COP)
	Follicular bronchiolitis/cysts/bullae
	Lymphocytic interstitial pneumonia (LIP)
Pleural disease	Mainly in SS associated with other autoimmune diseases

14.1 Introduction

Isolated cases of lung involvement in Sjögren's syndrome (SS) were first reported in the early 60s [1]. Since then an extensive number of reports have attempted to characterize lung involvement, often with conflicting data. Principally interstitial [2–5] to mixed [6, 7] or purely obstructive respiratory patterns [8] have been described, with frequencies that range from 9% to 75% [3, 4]. The observed variability partly reflects differences in definitions and varying applications of diagnostic criteria among studies, the sensitivity of modalities employed for the detection of lung abnormalities, and the inclusion of patients with concomitant pulmonary disease such as that resulting from smoking or other primary autoimmune conditions. Despite the differences observed across studies, one consistent theme is that the pulmonary manifestations of patients with primary SS differ from those associated with secondary SS. As examples, pleural effusions and fibrosis, found commonly in patients with secondary SS, rarely occur in pSS [9, 10]. Such manifestations are generally attributed most appropriately to the underlying primary connective tissue disease (CTD) [11].

In this chapter, we focus on pulmonary involvement in pSS, with particular attention to the two major clinicopathological disease phenotypes: airway and interstitial lung disease (ILD) (Table 14.1). Pulmonary arterial hypertension and bronchus-associated lung lymphoma (BALT) are discussed elsewhere in this book (Chaps. 13 and 33, respectively).

14.2 Airway Disease

14.2.1 Overview

Mucus secretion from the lining epithelial cells of the upper respiratory tract is one of the major innate natural barriers against inhaled pathogens. In the context of an autoimmune exocrinopathy, impaired secretions from the epithelial cells can result in reduced moistening, nasal crusting, epistaxis, and recurrent episodes of sinusitis. Furthermore, dryness of the throat, persistent hoarseness, and foreign body sensation presumably due to lymphoid infiltration of the nasal cavity and pharynx can also occur [3, 12]. Lymphocytic infiltration of the laryngeal, tracheal, and bronchial exocrine glands in a similar way to that observed in the salivary and lachrymal exocrine glands of pSS patients results in desiccation of the respiratory tree and is mainly manifested by a commonly persistent and irritating dry cough.

Isolated dry cough, described first by Henrik Sjögren in his original report, is a frequent complaint in pSS, reported in up to 50% of patients [3], even in those without radiographic findings or pulmonary function impairment [13]. Although the origin of cough was attributed to desiccation of the mucosa of the tracheobronchial tree (xerotrachea) [3, 4], identifiable abnormalities by means of rhinoscopy or indirect laryngoscopy are detected in only 20% of patients [14, 15]. In the absence of concomitant features, incorrect diagnoses such as asthma or bronchitis are often made prior to the diagnosis of pSS [3].

Although some reports have suggested increased prevalence of bronchiectasis in pSS [16–18], presumably resulting from plugging of the respiratory tract by inspissated secretions [4, 12], the majority of studies failed to document such an association [3, 13, 19, 20].

14.2.2 Pathology

The principal histopathological abnormality of airways is a peribronchial and/or peribronchiolar infiltration by CD4-positive T-lymphocytes, leading to small airway obstruction. These cells are predominant in the lamina propria outside the bronchial submucosal glands [21]. Hyperplasia of goblet cells and bronchial glands by morphometric analysis was also disclosed in autopsies from six patients with pSS [22].

14.2.3 Imaging Studies

Radiological studies in patients with pSS revealed the presence of reticular and reticulonodular abnormalities, reminiscent of an interstitial disorder [3, 4]. However, on the basis of high-resolution CT (HRCT) lung findings, Papiris et al. have suggested that this pattern actually corresponds to thickened bronchioles probably resulting from peribronchial and/or peribronchiolar mononuclear inflammation [13]. Predominant bronchiolar abnormalities have also been reported in studies involving non-smoking pSS patients by Franquet et al. and Taouli et al., with frequencies ranging from 32% to 65%, respectively [18, 23]. A mosaic pattern of lung attenuation or air trapping was identified on expiratory HRCT scans, corresponding to bronchiolar disease [23]. Finally, evidence of bronchiectasis on HRCT has been reported in up to 38% of patients with pSS in the study of Koyama et al. [16].

14.2.4   Pulmonary Function Tests in pSS-Associated Airway Disease

Pulmonary function tests in most patients with lung involvement in pSS reveal small airway involvement, with maximal mid-expiratory flows (MMEF) markedly reduced compared to controls. Concomitant impairment in diffusing capacity for carbon monoxide (DLCO) has also been reported [3, 6]. Although the extent of air trapping on expiratory CT scans was found to be increased in non-smoking pSS patients compared to healthy controls, correlation with pulmonary function parameters was found in some but not all studies [19, 24].

Bronchial hyperresponsiveness (BHR) to inhaled aerosolised methacholine was described by a study in a substantial portion (60%) of patients with pSS, in contrast to only 10% of the control population [25]. In the same study, BHR was highly prevalent in patients with small airway disease on spirometry and correlated strongly with subjective symptoms of xerotracheitis. Although the mechanism underlying BHR in pSS is unknown, it may be associated with increased osmolarity in the bronchial mucosa secondary to dryness in the airways or with bronchial or tracheal inflammation [25]. The latter possibility is supported by findings of increased levels of nitric oxide in the exhaled air of patients with pSS, similar to that described in asthma [26]. However, the BHR in pSS, unlike BHR associated with asthma, appears to be resistant to inhaled corticosteroids and sodium cromoglycate [27].

14.3   Interstitial Lung Disease

14.3.1   Overview

Over the last decade, ILD and especially nonspecific interstitial pneumonia has been recognized as an important subset of ILD associated with CTD. In some cases, clinically evident pulmonary disease precedes the diagnosis of CTD [28, 29]. Initial and retrospective studies have suggested a predominance of ILD in pSS patients [3, 4], but subsequent studies disclosed with larger numbers of pSS patients disclosed a much lower prevalence (<5%) [reviewed in 28]. Primary SS patients occasionally present with radiological and pulmonary function abnormalities suggestive of ILD, but without prominent self-reported sicca symptoms [28, 30]. Careful questioning for sicca symptoms is essential and if pSS is suspected on this basis, minor salivary gland biopsy and serological testing for specific autoantibodies including anti-SSA/Ro and anti-SSB/La should be performed. One study of minor salivary gland biopsy in a cohort of 38 ILD reported positive findings (defined as focus score >1) in 8% of patients [30].

Early studies showed that ILD was more prevalent in pSS patients with extraglandular features [31]. In addition, patients with ILD were more likely to have

Table 14.2 Frequency (n, %) of various histopathological patterns in primary Sjogren's syndrome related lung involvement

		Histopathological pattern					
		NSIP	LIP	UIP	COP	Lymphoma	Other[b]
Study	Patients	n (%)					
Strimlan et al. [4]	13	0 (0)	3 (23)[a]	2 (15)	4 (31)	3 (23)	1 (8)
Gardiner et al. [15]	14	0 (0)	0 (0)	6 (43)	0 (0)	0 (0)	8 (57)
Yamadori et al. [40]	9	3 (33)	0 (0)	6 (67)	0 (0)	0 (0)	0 (0)
Ito et al. [35]	33	20 (61)	0 (0)	1 (3)	0 (0)	4 (12)	6 (18)
Parambil et al. [36]	18	5 (28)	3 (17)	3 (17)	4 (22)	2 (11)	1 (5.5)
Shi et al. [34]	14	5 (36)	2 (14)	0 (0)	4 (28)	0	6 (43)

NSIP non specific interstitial pneumonia, *LIP* lymphocytic interstitial pneumonia, *UIP* usual interstitial pneumonia, *COP* cryptogenic organizing pneumonia"
[a]Two patients had associated amyloidosis
[b]Include non caseating granulomas, amyloidosis, pleural thickening, pseudolymphoma, follicular bronchiolitis, chronic bronciolitis and constrictive bronchiolitis (isolated or in association with other histological patterns)

rheumatoid factor (RF), anti-Ro/SSA and anti-La/SSB antibodies, and lymphopenia [32]. However, the presence of these autoantibodies was associated with the "intensity" of alveolitis, as graded by cellularity in the bronchoalvelolar lavage (BAL) [33].

14.3.2   Pathology

Video-assisted thoracoscopic (VATS) lung biopsy is the preferred method for obtaining multiple lung tissue samples for histopathological analysis. The small size of transbronchial biopsies limits the specific pathological diagnosis of ILD and also may miss small airway abnormalities [34]. The main histopathological patterns detected in lung biopsies from pSS patients with ILD include non-specific interstitial pneumonia (NSIP), usual interstitial pneumonitis (UIP), follicular bronchiolitis, lymphocytic interstitial pneumonia (LIP), and cryptogenic organizing pneumonia (COP) [34–37] (details in Table 14.2).

14.3.3   Non-Specific Interstitial Pneumonia

NSIP is characterized histopathologically by a uniform interstitial involvement of varying degrees of chronic inflammation or fibrosis [38, 39]. On high-resolution computed tomography (HRCT) studies, the most frequent finding is ground-glass opacities with reticulation, traction bronchiectasis, and little or no honeycombing. In addition to collagen vascular diseases, NSIP may be idiopathic or seen in other settings such as hypersensitivity pneumonitis, drug-induced lung disease, infection, or immunodeficiency [39].

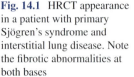

Fig. 14.1 HRCT appearance in a patient with primary Sjögren's syndrome and interstitial lung disease. Note the fibrotic abnormalities at both bases

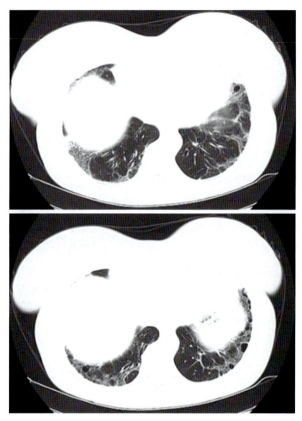

NSIP was the most common histological pattern, found in 60% of patients with pSS and ILD reported by Ito et al. [35]. NSIP, followed by UIP and LIP, was also the predominant histopathological type in another study involving 18 patients with pSS and ILD [36]. According to the findings of Ito et al., the NSIP pattern on HRCT had a high positive predictive value for the histological diagnosis of NSIP [35].

14.3.4 Usual Interstitial Pneumonia

UIP is characterized histopathologically by a variable distribution of patchy interstitial fibrosis, inflammation, honeycombing, and normal lung. The presence of small aggregates of fibroblasts and myofibroblasts, termed fibroblast foci, is necessary for the diagnosis [38]. UIP in the setting of pSS is rather rare. In the series of 343 patients reported by Strimlan et al., including cases of both pSS and secondary SS, UIP was histopathologically diagnosed in only two patients [4]. Since then most reports of UIP have been found in patients with SS associated with another CTD. Reporting on 18 pSS patients with ILD and available histopathological findings,

Fig. 14.2 Representative HRCT lung findings in a patient with primary Sjögren's syndrome and a biopsy-proven lymphocytic interstitial pneumonia. Note the bilateral symmetric diffuse micronodular pattern, with a predominantly centrilobular distribution

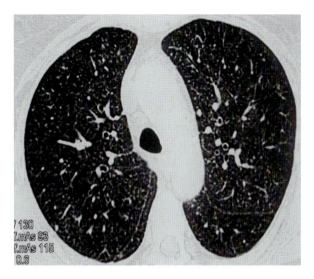

Parambil et al. described three patients with UIP and demonstrated signs of progression [36]. UIP cases have also been reported in the studies of Deheinzelin and Yamadori by surgical biopsies [37, 40]. In the latter, UIP histology was detected in 6 out of 9 patients tested [40] (Fig. 14.1).

14.3.5 Follicular Bronchiolitis

Follicular bronchiolitis is characterized by proliferation of peribronchial lymphoid follicles leading to obliteration of the airway lumen, which in turn through a valve phenomenon can lead to bullae formation. It may present either alone or most commonly in the context of another autoimmune disease such as rheumatoid arthritis or a viral infection, including HIV. Follicular bronchitis usually coexists with LIP in the context of pSS [41, 42].

14.3.6 Lymphocytic Interstitial Pneumonia

LIP, first described by Liebow and Carrington [43], is characterized by a diffuse, polyclonal lymphoid cell infiltrate surrounding airways and expanding into the lung interstitium (Fig. 14.2). LIP has been classically associated with underlying autoimmune disorders, including systemic lupus erythematosus and pSS [44].

Early studies suggested that LIP and primary pulmonary lymphoma were the most common forms of parenchymal lung disease in pSS. In the initial report of Strimlan et al., among 13 patients in whom histopathological findings were available, three patients with LIP, three with malignant lymphoma, and one with pseudolymphoma were described [4]. The natural history of LIP is variable, ranging from a benign course (stabilization or improvement) to the evolution of BALT lymphoma [10, 44].

14.3.7 Cryptogenic Organizing Pneumonia

COP is a pathological subtype of ILD characterized by intra-alveolar buds of connective tissue. Typical radiologic findings include bilateral patchy alveolar opacities with air-bronchograms and normal lung volumes [45]. While COP has been described previously in the setting of several autoimmune disorders – mainly rheumatoid arthritis – it occurs quite rarely in pSS [45]. Since the clinical and radiological features of COP are reminiscent of those of community acquired pneumonia, diagnosis is often delayed, usually after one or more failed courses of antibiotics [46, 47].

14.3.8 Clinical Features

Patients with pSS and ILD typically present with dyspnea and cough [36]. On physical examination, bibasilar crackles are often present. However, the absence of symptoms does not preclude subclinical respiratory involvement, which is detected most effectively by HRCT and pulmonary function tests [11, 19].

14.3.9 Imaging Studies

HRCT is more sensitive in detecting parenchymal lung abnormalities than is chest radiography and provides important information regarding the pattern of pulmonary involvement [18, 23, 48]. Franquet et al. reported HRCT abnormalities in 34% of patients with pSS compared to 14% of those who underwent plain radiographs [18]. Similar findings were described by Uffmann et al., who reported abnormal HRCT findings in more than 60% of asymptomatic pSS patients with normal radiographs [19].

The most common findings on chest radiographs in pSS patients with ILD are linear, reticular, and reticulonodular opacities, predominantly seen in the lower lung zones [3, 37, 49]. Bullae and pleural abnormalities are detected occasionally. HRCT patterns suggestive of ILD include ground-glass attenuation [13, 16, 18], subpleural small nodules, non-septal linear opacities, interlobular septal thickening, and honeycombing in subpleural areas [16, 19, 49] (Table 14.3). In the series of Franquet et al., honeycombing was detected in 8% of patients, always in as bilateral, asymmetric, peripheral lower lung distribution [18]. The corresponding figure in the study by Uffmann et al. was 24% [19]. In the study of Papiris et al., interstitial

Table 14.3 Frequency of specific HRCT patterns of respiratory involvement in primary Sjögren's syndrome

Study	Abnormal HRCT's	Ground glass	Honey-combing	Interlobular septal thickening	Small nodules (<10 mm)	Parenchymal opacities[a]	Thickened bronchioles/air trapping	Bronchiectasies	Bullae/cysts	Other[b]
					Frequency (n, %) of HRCT findings					
Franquet et al. [18]	17	7 (41)	4 (23.5)	0 (0)	4 (23.5)	5 (29)	5 (29)	6 (35)	0 (0)	1 (6)
Salaffi et al. [20]	5	2 (40)	0 (0)	4 (80)	0 (0)	0 (0)	0 (0)	0 (0)	0 (0)	0 (0)
Papiris et al. [13]	10	3 (30)	0 (0)	0 (0)	1 (10)	0 (0)	7 (70)	0 (0)	3 (30)	0 (0)
Koyama et al. [15]	60	55 (92)	6 (10)	33 (55)	26 (44)	6 (10)	13 (22)	23 (38)	18 (30)	18 (30)
Uffmann et al. [19]	24	4 (17)	3 (12.5)	9 (37.5)	9 (37.5)	3 (12.5)	3 (12.5)	1 (4)	5 (21)	1 (4)
Matsuyama et al. [49]	15	12 (80)	3 (20)	9 (60)	3 (20)	10 (67)	10 (67)	8 (53)[c]	4 (27)	1 (7)
Shi et al. [34]	14	7 (50)	0 (0)	7 (50)	1 (7)	0 (0)	1 (7)	2 (14)[c]	2 (14)	3 (21)
Parambil et al. [36]	18	16 (89)	3 (17)	1 (6)	8 (44)	2 (11)	0 (0)	4 (22)[c]	3 (17)	10 (56)
Lohrmann et al. [59]	19	9 (47)	6 (31.5)	7 (37)	11 (58)	2 (10.5)	5 (26)	11 (58)	11 (58)	3 (16)

[a] Include masses and large nodules (>10 mm)
[b] Includes pleural irregularities, air space consolidation
[c] Traction

involvement consisted mainly of ground-glass appearance or fine nodular pattern distributed in a predominantly peribronchial pattern. Both honeycombing and peripheral and lower lobe findings typical of fibrosing alveolitis were absent [13].

Parenchymal bullae and cysts are often seen in pSS patients. They are most likely related to a check-valve mechanism due to peribronchiolar mononuclear cell infiltration or amyloid deposition [50, 51]. In pSS patients with abnormal HRCT findings, the presence of bullae or cysts ranged from 20% to 30% [16, 19]. In some early reports, lung cysts coexisted with amyloidosis [41, 52, 53]. In a recent study, lung cysts were associated with anti-SSB/La seropositivity and occurrence of lymphoproliferative disease [9].

14.3.10 Pulmonary Function Tests in pSS-Associated ILD

In pSS-associated ILD, a restrictive pattern with impairment of diffusing capacity for carbon monoxide (DLCO) is usually found [2, 6, 31, 35, 54]. Evidence of small airway dysfunction is also typically present [4–6]. Ito et al. reported that the vital capacity was lower in patients with an ILD pattern on HRCT than in patients with a different pattern (i.e., bronchiolar). In contrast, the FEV1/FVC ratio was lower in patients with a bronchiolar pattern [35]. HRCT and pulmonary function testing appear to be sensitive for detecting early lung involvement in asymptomatic patients with pSS, but abnormalities detected by HRCT do not necessarily connote significant functional impairment [19].

Although pulmonary function in most patients with pSS remains stable [20, 55], this is not always true for the subset of patients with ILD. In the largest study on pSS-associated ILD, Ito et al. reported that a low PaO_2 at baseline and the presence of microscopic honeycombing on HRCT were associated with reduced survival [35].

14.4 Pleuritis

Isolated pleuritis in pSS is very rare and is mainly linked to the underlying causes. Thus, patients with SS and pleuritis should be carefully investigated for the presence of a concomitant autoimmune disease, such as systemic lupus erythematosus or rheumatoid arthritis [10].

14.5 Diagnosis and Management

The diagnostic approach to a pSS patient with respiratory complaints is, in general, similar to that used for patients with other connective tissue diseases and same symptoms. Following a detailed history and physical examination, pulmonary function studies and HRCT testing are required in most patients. If HRCT features are compatible with NSIP or UIP, lung biopsy is not usually necessary, given the high correlation between HRCT and pathological findings for these two forms of ILD. In contrast, in the setting of non-specific CT patterns or suspicion for malignancy, open lung biopsy should be performed.

Because lung involvement can precede the onset of respiratory symptoms, we recommend complete pulmonary function tests and/or HRCT scanning at baseline. These studies may require repeating at various intervals depending upon the functional status and clinical manifestations of the individual patient.

Therapy of pSS-related pulmonary involvement is mainly empirical. Sinusitis in the context of upper respiratory involvement should be treated with antibiotics and, when indicated, surgical drainage. Dry cough related to "xerotrachea" can be alleviated in some cases with normal saline nebulizers and high doses of bromhexine. β-agonists and corticosteroids are of little benefit for patients with lower airway disease. For ILD, a rational approach is to establish therapies primarily upon evidence derived from the idiopathic interstitial pneumonitis literature. The standard treatment for patients with pSS and ILD (e.g., NSIP, COP) is prednisone at a dose of 1 mg/kg per day with subsequent tapering [56]. Only limited evidence supports the addition of a second immunosuppressive agent, but this is often suggested in severe cases. In a nonrandomized study of 20 patients, treatment with azathioprine led to substantial improvement in the FVC at 6 months compared to untreated patients [37]. Cyclophosphamide and cyclosporine have been also employed in small numbers of reported patients [57, 58]. B-cell depletion therapies appear to be a promising option, but definitive data from well controlled studies are needed.

References

1. Bucher U, Hadorn W. Chronic bronchitis: the significance of sputum examination for diagnosis and therapy. Med Klin. 1960;55:688–92.
2. Fairfax AJ, Haslam PL, Pavia D, Sheahan NF, Bateman JR, Agnew JE, et al. Pulmonary disorders associated with Sjögren's syndrome. Q J Med. 1981;50:279–95.
3. Constantopoulos SH, Papadimitriou CS, Moutsopoulos HM. Respiratory manifestations in primary Sjögren's syndrome. A clinical, functional, and histologic study. Chest. 1985;88:226–9.
4. Strimlan CV, Rosenow 3rd EC, Divertie MB, Harrison Jr EG. Pulmonary manifestations of Sjögren's syndrome. Chest. 1976;70:354–61.
5. Oxholm P. Primary Sjögren's syndrome–clinical and laboratory markers of disease activity. Semin Arthritis Rheum. 1992;22:114–26.
6. Vitali C, Tavoni A, Viegi G, Begliomini E, Agnesi A, Bombardieri S. Lung involvement in Sjögren's syndrome: a comparison between patients with primary and with secondary syndrome. Ann Rheum Dis. 1985;44:455–61.
7. Segal I, Fink G, Machtey I, Gura V, Spitzer SA. Pulmonary function abnormalities in Sjögren's syndrome and the sicca complex. Thorax. 1981;36:286–9.
8. Newball HH, Brahim SA. Chronic obstructive airway disease in patients with Sjögren's syndrome. Am Rev Respir Dis. 1977;115:295–304.
9. Watanabe M, Naniwa T, Hara M, Arakawa T. Maeda T. Pulmonary manifestations in Sjögren's syndrome: correlation analysis between chest computed tomographic findings and clinical subsets with poor prognosis in 80 patients. J Rheumatol. 2010;37:365–73.

10. Papiris SA, Tsonis IA, Moutsopoulos HM. Sjögren's syndrome. Semin Respir Crit Care Med. 2007;28:459–71.
11. Vitali C, Viegi G, Tassoni S, Tavoni A, Paoletti P, Bibolotti E, et al. Lung function abnormalities in different connective tissue diseases. Clin Rheumatol. 1986;5:181–8.
12. Bloch KJ, Buchanan WW, Wohl MJ, Bunim JJ. Sjoegren's syndrome. A clinical, pathological, and serological study of sixty-two cases. Medicine (Baltimore). 1965;44:187–231.
13. Papiris SA, Maniati M, Constantopoulos SH, Roussos C, Moutsopoulos HM, Skopouli FN. Lung involvement in primary Sjögren's syndrome is mainly related to the small airway disease. Ann Rheum Dis. 1999;58:61–4.
14. Bariffi F, Pesci A, Bertorelli G, Manganelli P, Ambanelli U. Pulmonary involvement in Sjögren's syndrome. Respiration. 1984;46:82–7.
15. Gardiner P, Ward C, Allison A, Ashcroft T, Simpson W, Walters H, et al. Pleuropulmonary abnormalities in primary Sjögren's syndrome. J Rheumatol. 1993;20:831–7.
16. Koyama M, Johkoh T, Honda O, Mihara N, Kozuka T, Tomiyama N, et al. Pulmonary involvement in primary Sjögren's syndrome: spectrum of pulmonary abnormalities and computed tomography findings in 60 patients. J Thorac Imaging. 2001;16:290–6.
17. Robinson DA, Meyer CF. Primary Sjögren's syndrome associated with recurrent sinopulmonary infections and bronchiectasis. J Allergy Clin Immunol. 1994;94:263–4.
18. Franquet T, Gimenez A, Monill JM, Diaz C, Geli C. Primary Sjögren's syndrome and associated lung disease: CT findings in 50 patients. AJR Am J Roentgenol. 1997;169:655–8.
19. Uffmann M, Kiener HP, Bankier AA, Baldt MM, Zontsich T, Herold CJ. Lung manifestation in asymptomatic patients with primary Sjögren syndrome: assessment with high resolution CT and pulmonary function tests. J Thorac Imaging. 2001;16:282–9.
20. Salaffi F, Manganelli P, Carotti M, Baldelli S, Blasetti P, Subiaco S, et al. A longitudinal study of pulmonary involvement in primary Sjögren's syndrome: relationship between alveolitis and subsequent lung changes on high-resolution computed tomography. Br J Rheumatol. 1998;37:263–9.
21. Papiris SA, Saetta M, Turato G, La Corte R, Trevisani L, Mapp CE, et al. CD4-positive T-lymphocytes infiltrate the bronchial mucosa of patients with Sjögren's syndrome. Am J Respir Crit Care Med. 1997;156:637–41.
22. Andoh Y, Shimura S, Sawai T, Sasaki H, Takishima T, Shirato K. Morphometric analysis of airways in Sjögren's syndrome. Am Rev Respir Dis. 1993;148:1358–62.
23. Taouli B, Brauner MW, Mourey I, Lemouchi D, Grenier PA. Thin-section chest CT findings of primary Sjögren's syndrome: correlation with pulmonary function. Eur Radiol. 2002;12:1504–11.
24. Franquet T, Diaz C, Domingo P, Gimenez A, Geli C. Air trapping in primary Sjögren syndrome: correlation of expiratory CT with pulmonary function tests. J Comput Assist Tomogr. 1999;23:169–73.
25. Gudbjornsson B, Hedenstrom H, Stalenheim G, Hallgren R. Bronchial hyperresponsiveness to methacholine in patients with primary Sjögren's syndrome. Ann Rheum Dis. 1991;50:36–40.
26. Ludviksdottir D, Janson C, Hogman M, Gudbjornsson B, Bjornsson E, Valtysdottir S, et al. Increased nitric oxide in expired air in patients with Sjögren's syndrome. BHR study group. Bronchial hyperresponsiveness. Eur Respir J. 1999;13:739–43.
27. Stalenheim G, Gudbjornsson B. Anti-inflammatory drugs do not alleviate bronchial hyperreactivity in Sjögren's syndrome. Allergy. 1997;52:423–7.
28. Tzelepis GE, Toya SP, Moutsopoulos HM. Occult connective tissue diseases mimicking idiopathic interstitial pneumonias. Eur Respir J. 2008;31:11–20.
29. Strange C, Highland KB. Interstitial lung disease in the patient who has connective tissue disease. Clin Chest Med. 2004;25:549–59, vii.
30. Fischer A, Swigris JJ, du Bois RM, Groshong SD, Cool CD, Sahin H, et al. Minor salivary gland biopsy to detect primary Sjögren syndrome in patients with interstitial lung disease. Chest. 2009;136:1072–8.
31. Papathanasiou MP, Constantopoulos SH, Tsampoulas C, Drosos AA, Moutsopoulos HM. Reappraisal of respiratory abnormalities in primary and secondary Sjögren's syndrome. A controlled study. Chest. 1986;90:370–4.

32. Yazisiz V, Arslan G, Ozbudak IH, Turker S, Erbasan F, Avci AB, et al. Lung involvement in patients with primary Sjögren's syndrome: what are the predictors? Rheumatol Int. 2010;30: 1317–24.

33. Dalavanga YA, Constantopoulos SH, Galanopoulou V, Zerva L, Moutsopoulos HM. Alveolitis correlates with clinical pulmonary involvement in primary Sjögren's syndrome. Chest. 1991;99:1394–7.

34. Shi JH, Liu HR, Xu WB, Feng RE, Zhang ZH, Tian XL, et al. Pulmonary manifestations of Sjögren's syndrome. Respiration. 2009;78:377–86.

35. Ito I, Nagai S, Kitaichi M, Nicholson AG, Johkoh T, Noma S, et al. Pulmonary manifestations of primary Sjögren's syndrome: a clinical, radiologic, and pathologic study. Am J Respir Crit Care Med. 2005;171:632–8.

36. Parambil JG, Myers JL, Lindell RM, Matteson EL, Ryu JH. Interstitial lung disease in primary Sjögren syndrome. Chest. 2006;130:1489–95.

37. Deheinzelin D, Capelozzi VL, Kairalla RA, Barbas Filho JV, Saldiva PH, de Carvalho CR. Interstitial lung disease in primary Sjögren's syndrome. Clinical-pathological evaluation and response to treatment. Am J Respir Crit Care Med. 1996;154:794–9.

38. American Thoracic Society; European Respiratory Society International. American Thoracic Society/European Respiratory Society International Multidisciplinary Consensus Classification of the Idiopathic Interstitial Pneumonias. This joint statement of the American Thoracic Society (ATS), and the European Respiratory Society (ERS) was adopted by the ATS board of directors and by the ERS Executive Committee, June 2001. Am J Respir Crit Care Med. 2001;165:277–304.

39. Travis WD, Hunninghake G, King Jr TE, Lynch DA, Colby TV, Galvin JR, et al. Idiopathic nonspecific interstitial pneumonia: report of an American Thoracic Society project. Am J Respir Crit Care Med. 2008;177:1338–47.

40. Yamadori I, Fujita J, Bandoh S, Tokuda M, Tanimoto Y, Kataoka M, et al. Nonspecific interstitial pneumonia as pulmonary involvement of primary Sjögren's syndrome. Rheumatol Int. 2002;22:89–92.

41. Kobayashi H, Matsuoka R, Kitamura S, Tsunoda N, Saito K. Sjögren's syndrome with multiple bullae and pulmonary nodular amyloidosis. Chest. 1988;94:438–40.

42. Yousem SA, Colby TV, Carrington CB. Follicular bronchitis/bronchiolitis. Hum Pathol. 1985;16:700–6.

43. Liebow AA, Carrington CB. Diffuse pulmonary lymphoreticular infiltrations associated with dysproteinemia. Med Clin North Am. 1973;57:809–43.

44. Parke AL. Pulmonary manifestations of primary Sjögren's syndrome. Rheum Dis Clin North Am. 2008;34:907–20, viii.

45. Ioannou S, Toya SP, Tomos P, Tzelepis GE. Cryptogenic organizing pneumonia associated with primary Sjögren's syndrome. Rheumatol Int. 2008;28:1053–5.

46. Cordier JF. Update on cryptogenic organising pneumonia (idiopathic bronchiolitis obliterans organising pneumonia). Swiss Med Wkly. 2002;132:588–91.

47. Myers JL, Colby TV. Pathologic manifestations of bronchiolitis, constrictive bronchiolitis, cryptogenic organizing pneumonia, and diffuse panbronchiolitis. Clin Chest Med. 1993;14:611–22.

48. Lynch DA. Lung disease related to collagen vascular disease. J Thorac Imaging. 2009;24: 299–309.

49. Matsuyama N, Ashizawa K, Okimoto T, Kadota J, Amano H, Hayashi K. Pulmonary lesions associated with Sjögren's syndrome: radiographic and CT findings. Br J Radiol. 2003;76:880–4.

50. Sakamoto O, Saita N, Ando M, Kohrogi H, Suga M, Ando M. Two cases of Sjögren's syndrome with multiple bullae. Intern Med. 2002;41:124–8.

51. Hubscher O, Re R, Iotti R. Cystic lung disease in Sjögren's syndrome. J Rheumatol. 2002;29:2235–6.

52. Schlegel J, Kienast K, Storkel S, Ferlinz R. Primary pulmonary nodular amyloidosis and multiple emphysematous bullae in Sjögren syndrome. Pneumologie. 1992;46:634–7.

53. Bonner Jr H, Ennis RS, Geelhoed GW, Tarpley Jr TM. Lymphoid infiltration and amyloidosis of lung in Sjögren's syndrome. Arch Pathol. 1973;95:42–4.

54. Kelly C, Gardiner P, Pal B, Griffiths I. Lung function in primary Sjögren's syndrome: a cross sectional and longitudinal study. Thorax. 1991;46:180–3.
55. Davidson BK, Kelly CA, Griffiths ID. Ten year follow up of pulmonary function in patients with primary Sjögren's syndrome. Ann Rheum Dis. 2000;59:709–12.
56. Mavragani CP, Moutsopoulos NM, Moutsopoulos HM. The management of Sjögren's syndrome. Nat Clin Pract Rheumatol. 2006;2:252–61.
57. Ogasawara H, Sekiya M, Murashima A, Hishikawa T, Tokano Y, Sekigawa I, et al. Very low-dose cyclosporin treatment of steroid-resistant interstitial pneumonitis associated with Sjögren's syndrome. Clin Rheumatol. 1998;17:160–2.
58. Schnabel A, Reuter M, Gross WL. Intravenous pulse cyclophosphamide in the treatment of interstitial lung disease due to collagen vascular diseases. Arthritis Rheum. 1998;41: 1215–20.
59. Lohrmann C, Uhl M, Warnatz K, Ghanem N, Kotter E, Schaefer O, et al. High-resolution CT imaging of the lung for patients with primary Sjögren's syndrome. Eur J Radiol. 2004;52: 137–43.

Chapter 15
Raynaud's Phenomenon and Sjögren's Syndrome

Fredrick M. Wigley

Contents

In 1862, Maurice Raynaud published his medical school thesis in which he argued that some people have transient digital ischemia when exposed to cold temperatures. It is now recognized that skin blood flow in humans provides an important mechanism for normal thermoregulation. In fact, a normal response to cold exposure is vasoconstriction of the cutaneous blood vessels, leading to a decrease in heat loss from the body and protection against hypothermia [1]. Human cutaneous vessels are innervated by the sympathetic adrenergic vasoconstrictor nerves that initiate thermoregulatory responses to cold [2]. This accounts, in part, for the clinical connection between emotional stress and vasoconstriction in the skin.

The term "Raynaud's phenomenon" (RP) is now used to describe an exaggerated response in the skin thermoregulatory vessels to exposure to cold and/or emotional

F.M. Wigley
Johns Hopkins University, Department of Medicine, Division of Rheumatology, Baltimore, MD, USA

M. Ramos-Casals et al. (eds.), *Sjögren's Syndrome*,
DOI 10.1007/978-0-85729-947-5_15, © Springer-Verlag London Limited 2012

Table 15.1 Primary
Raynaud's phenomenon
(Raynaud's disease)

- Vasospastic attacks precipitated by cold or emotional stress
- Symmetric attacks in both hands
- Absence of tissue necrosis or gangrene
- No history or physical findings suggestive of secondary cause
- Normal nailfold capillaries
- Normal erythrocyte sedimentation rate (ESR)
- Negative serologic findings

Source: Modified with permission from LeRoy et al. [7]

stress. These episodic events sometimes involve the superficial thermoregulatory vessels alone and present as cold skin that has a cyanotic, mottled appearance. In contrast, in other cases, the vasoconstriction is more intense and extends to involve the digital arteries, precapillary arterioles, and cutaneous thermoregulatory arteriovenous shunts. These more intense episodes, which represent true ischemia, present clinically with pallor of the skin. The white appearance of the digital skin results from the absence of blood flow to the skin and deeper tissues.

Raynaud's phenomenon is characterized by episodic tissue ischemia that most commonly involves the digits of the hands and feet and sometimes affects the ears, nose, face, tongue, or nipples. Either dual (white/pallor [no flow] and blue/cyanosis [reduced flow]) or tricolor skin color changes (pallor, cyanosis, and erythema) can occur. When erythema is present, this color phase represents the recovery and rebound of blood flow to the skin. Patients with RP often experience numbness and paresthesias during the ischemic phase that involves digital vessel vasospasm. True pain is a symptom of deprived tissue nutrition and constitutes a warning of potential tissue injury. Uncomplicated ischemic events are typically over about 15 min after relief from the cold exposure and the occurrence of rewarming.

The index and middle fingers tend to be more sensitive to cold exposure while the thumb is often spared [3]. However, severe RP can involve all fingers with demarcation of the ischemia, leading to pallor from the fingertip to the proximal digit. A history of typical cold sensitivity with blue or white color changes is adequate to make a diagnosis of Raynaud's phenomenon. Provocative testing with cold exposure (e.g., immersion of the hand in ice water) are important research tools but are not needed to confirm the diagnosis made by a good clinical history.

RP can be simply the manifestation of a normal (but exaggerated) response of the cutaneous thermoregulatory vessels and digital arteries to cold, stress, or trauma (primary Raynaud's phenomenon). However, RP can also be associated with a disease state such as Sjögren's syndrome (SS), in which case the digital ischemia is termed secondary RP. Primary RP is characterized by the absence of an underlying systemic disorder and represents a common symptom in the general population; it is observed in approximately 3–5% of individuals in the USA [4–6]. Criteria for making a diagnosis of primary RP include considerations of clinical features, physical examination, and laboratory testing (see Table 15.1) [7]. A frequent cause of secondary RP is an underlying systemic rheumatic disease. The highest prevalence of RP among patients with a rheumatic disease is observed in systemic sclerosis (scleroderma) or in mixed connective tissue disease (MCTD), approaching 90% or greater in most studies [8–11]. It is estimated that approximately 21–44% of patients who have SLE [12, 13], up to 17% of patients who have rheumatoid arthritis [14], and approximately 10% of patients who have polymyositis suffer from Raynaud's phenomenon. Furthermore, patients who have undifferentiated connective tissue disease (UCTD) demonstrate a high prevalence (~50%) of RP [15, 16].

The reported prevalence of RP in primary SS varies from 13% to 33% of patients [17–20]. The true prevalence of RP in primary Sjögren's is not well defined because studies have employed varying definitions of primary SS. In addition, most studies have been retrospective and therefore have contained substantial potential for errors in the detection of true RP. Investigations also suggest that the prevalence of RP varies depending on regional ambient temperature of the study population [21]. In addition, RP often (reportedly 40–50% of the time) precedes the onset of sicca symptoms and may be an early manifestation of SS [18, 20]. A longitudinal study in northern England involving 100 patients with primary SS found 81% of patients had RP that did not associate with systemic disease or the presence or absence of anti-Ro/SSA antibodies [22]. Although both RP and primary SS are both more common among women, one survey of 521 females and 28 males found no statistical difference in the presence of RP between men and women with primary SS [23].

In the author's experience, RP in SS varies in intensity. Most SS patients with RP have mild expressions of digital ischemia that are similar in severity to that of individuals with primary RP. In fact, given the common occurrence of both primary RP and SS, it is possible that some patients who have primary RP develop SS and that the two problems are independent of each other. Some investigators have reported that the clinical course of RP is generally benign and not associated with vascular sequelae such as digital ulcers or amputation [17, 20].

Although RP appeared to be a common manifestation (33%) in patients with primary SS in one study, the symptom of RP disappeared in 14% and decreased in severity in 30% over the course of follow-up [18]. Other studies indicate that vascular complications of RP in SS are unusual. In one series of 40 patients with primary SS and RP, there were no vascular complications and only 40% were treated with vasodilatory drugs [20]. These findings, confirmed by others [19], pose a striking contrast to patients with scleroderma, who tend to have severe RP and digital ulcers or vascular complications in approximately 30% of cases [24]. Thus, when one encounters a patient with SS and severe RP, especially with critical ischemia and painful attacks associated with tissue injury (ulcerations, gangrene, or amputation); a secondary disease process associated with SS must be considered (Table 15.2).

The significance of RP in a patient with SS is not fully defined but studies suggest that its presence may associate with unique clinical features and pathological risks. A large cohort study of 1,010 patients found that the subset of SS patients with antiRo/La antibodies had the highest frequency of RP, altered parotid scintigraphy, positive salivary gland biopsy, peripheral neuropathy, thrombocytopenia, and positive rheumatoid factor [25]. Although these single-center observations are interesting, they do not identify clinical associations that are consistent between published surveys. For example, a survey of 320 patients with primary SS reported that RP

Table 15.2 Secondary causes of
Raynaud's phenomenon

- Immune: Autoimmune disease
- Trauma: Hand-arm vibration syndrome
- Mechanical: Thoracic outlet syndrome
- Proteins: Cryoglobulins; cryofibrinogens
- Neurogenic: Carpal tunnel syndrome
- Hormones: Hypothyroid
- Toxins/drugs/vasoconstrictors: smoking
- Vascular disease: Vasculitis, atherosclerosis

was present in 40 (13%) of patients [20]. Compared to patients without RP, those with RP showed a higher prevalence of articular involvement, cutaneous vasculitis, antinuclear antibodies, anti-Ro/SSA and anti-La/SSB patients. Kraus et al. suggested that patients with primary SS and RP are significantly more likely to have nonerosive arthritis, vasculitis, and pulmonary fibrosis compared to those without RP [19]. Skopouli suggested that patients with primary SS and RP develop glomerulonephritis, myositis, and peripheral neuropathy more often than patients without RP, but the differences did not achieve statistical significance [18]. Another study found that 36 of 108 patients with RP and primary SS were more likely to have leukopenia, thyroiditis, and low complement (C3) than primary SS patients without RP [26]. Foster et al. and Youinou et al. reported a higher frequency of arthritis among SS patients with RP and suggested that the symptom of RP was a marker for secondary SS [17, 27].

A survey of 402 patients with primary SS found that 20% had autoantibodies characteristic of another autoimmune disease (anti-DNA, anti-Sm, anti-RNP, anti-topoisomerase, anticentromere, anti-Jo1, antineutrophil cytoplasmic antibodies, and anticardiolipin antibodies) [28]. RP was more frequent among the patients with one of these autoantibodies (28% vs 7%, $p = 0.001$), which are not typical for SS alone. A MEDLINE search for articles published between January 1966 and December 2005 that specifically analyzed the overlap between SS and other systemic autoimmune disease identified a list of diagnostic problems in patients with primary SS who had features considered typical of other diseases including arthritis, Raynaud's phenomenon, cutaneous features, interstitial pulmonary disease, cytopenias, and autoantibodies [29]. It is important to recognize that RP and a variety of other clinical and immunological manifestations can be seen in patients who are considered to have a diagnosis of primary SS. These patients with clinical features that overlap with other rheumatic diseases make it challenging to associate some of these features as secondary to SS alone. For example, SS was identified in 26 of 283 systemic lupus erythematosus (SLE) patients who had a higher frequency of RP than those without SS; the SS syndrome preceded the diagnosis of SLE in 69%, again suggesting that the presence of RP in a patient with SS indicates an increased risk for another autoimmune disease [30]. Another example is the fact that antineutrophil cytoplasmic antibodies (ANCA) can be found in patients with primary SS and they associate with the presence of cutaneous vasculitis, peripheral neuropathy, and Raynaud's phenomenon, features that can be seen in primary vasculitis [31]. A recent survey to define the clinical characteristics of primary and secondary SS found that RP was more common in those with secondary SS (pSS 16% vs secondary SS 41%, $p = 0.001$) [32].

In the general population, the presence of anticentromere antibodies (ACA) in a patient presenting with RP is of value in predicting systemic disease or possible future development of distinct clinical manifestations, especially scleroderma [33, 34]. Gelber et al. compared 45 patients with primary SS with 33 patients with limited cutaneous scleroderma and found that 29% of the patients with primary SS had RP compared to 100% of the limited scleroderma patients [35]. An interesting finding pertained to the fact that 10 of 45 patients (22%) with primary SS and 18 of 33 (55%) with scleroderma had antibodies directed against centromere proteins. Although the CENP-positive patients with primary SS recognize predominantly CENP C alone, this pattern was very uncommon among CENP-positive patients with scleroderma. In contrast, dual recognition of CENP B and CENP C was a feature found exclusively in patients with limited scleroderma and was absent in those with primary SS [35].

Other surveys find a high frequency of RP among primary SS who have a positive test for ACA [25, 36–40]. This suggests that the presence RP associates with ACA in primary SS and identifies a unique subset of patients who are at risk for developing another rheumatic disease, especially scleroderma. In a study of patients with ACA, Miyawaki et al. found SS in 40 of 108 patients (37%) examined, including 10 with primary SS and 30 with secondary SS (27 with scleroderma and 3 with other diseases) [41]. Patients who have ACA and present with "primary" SS may develop scleroderma several years later [25, 39, 41]. Moreover, careful examination in prospective studies of SS patients with ACA often find subtle features of limited scleroderma [41], suggesting that retrospective surveys may overestimate the prevalence of primary SS in patients with ACA and RP and miss the presence of another disease process.

Other surveys support the idea that the presence of both ACA and RP identifies patients with primary SS who also have an associated overlap syndrome [36, 42]. For example, a recent survey of 212 patients with primary SS found 4.7% had ACA [36]. Patients with ACA and SS were found to have a greater frequency of RP, objective xerophthalmia, peripheral neuropathy, and evidence of another autoimmune disorder, such as biliary cirrhosis [36]. SS is known to complicate the course of patients with primary biliary cirrhosis and CREST syndrome [43, 44]. However, Caramaschi et al. found that while the ACA positive SS patients were more likely to have RP, they were less likely to have leucopenia, polyclonal hypergammaglobulinemia, rheumatoid factor, and antibodies to the SSA/Ro antigen [39]. The take-home message from these studies is that a SS patient who presents with RP should be examined carefully for clinical and serological evidence of another rheumatic disease. In addition, the presence of ACA should make one think of scleroderma and its associated features.

RP is associated with migraine headaches in the general population [45]. An association between migraine headaches and RP in patients with primary SS has been suggested but not confirmed [46, 47]. Pulmonary arterial hypertension (PAH), a major complication of the rheumatic diseases, is reported to occur in primary SS [48, 49]. The presence of PAH is associated with a poor prognosis in patients with SS. One report suggests that a subset of primary SS patients are at added risk in that the presence of RP, cutaneous vasculitis, and interstitial lung disease is more commonly seen when compared to patients with primary SS without PAH [49]. The presence of a positive anti-Ro/SSA, anti-RNP, rheumatoid factor or hypergammaglobulinemia in a patient with SS syndrome may also increase the risk for PAH [49]. When confronted with this subset of patients, it justifies a careful evaluation for underlying PAH with noninvasive screening by echocardiography and, if suspected, a right-heart catheterization to validate the diagnosis. Another report suggests that screening by echocardiography is warranted in primary SS patients when palpable purpura, antibody reactivity to Ro/SSA, and low C4 levels are present in that this subset of patients had increased risk for pericardial effusion and pulmonary hypertension [50]. There are now several therapeutic options for patients with PAH associated with a connective tissue disease that may improve outcome if not quality of life [51, 52].

The biological mechanism of what might link RP to primary SS is unknown. Very few studies have been done to investigate the causes of RP in primary SS and thus it is difficult to make any conclusions. Endothelium-dependent vasodilation using brachial artery responses measured by ultrasonography was reported to be impaired in patients with primary SS and RP when compared to healthy controls [53]. However, this study was small and remains unconfirmed. One theory is that interactions between blood vessels and activated lymphocytes might disturb endothelial function and cause abnormal vascular reactivity. Willeke et al. [26] reported that an increase in the number of interferon-gamma secreting peripheral blood mononuclear cells was seen in primary SS patients with RP compared to normal controls and to patients with primary SS without RP. The authors speculated there might be a pathological role of this subpopulation of interferon secreting T-lymphocyte that mediates vasospasm in these patients. The presence of RP has been associated with higher concentrations of circulating sL-selectin (CD62L) in the serum of patients with primary SS, suggesting that L-selectin is released from activated cells and may indicate a mechanism for vascular perturbation [54]. This study requires further confirmation but its results are consistent with a report that serum sL-selectin levels are elevated in patients with scleroderma [55].

15.1 Evaluation of the Sjögren's Syndrome and Raynaud's Phenomenon

Most patients with primary SS will have relatively mild RP without digital ulceration or critical ischemia that threatens loss of the digit. The presence of severe RP and ischemic lesions should make the physician suspicious of a complicating secondary process or underlying associated rheumatic disease, especially scleroderma or lupus. Each patient should be fully evaluated for major or macrovascular disease that may be causing or aggravating the digital events. This begins with a good bedside examination including a palpation of all pulses, bilateral arm blood pressures, and use of an Allen's test at the wrist to assess for ulnar, radial artery, or palmar arch occlusion. Squeezing and releasing the distal digit provides a view of nutritional blood flow in that a rapid return of a blush to the skin should be observed, even if the surface skin is cold to touch or cyanotic in color. A lack of return or persistent pallor is an indication of poor nutritional blood flow and associated structural vascular disease rather than vasospasm alone. Lace-like mottling of the skin of the limbs due to vasoconstriction of thermoregulatory vessels is common in primary RP and is quickly reversible with rewarming. Fixed or impressive irreversible mottling (livedo racemosa) would be suggestive of antiphospholipid syndrome, while petechiae and/or purpura is suggestive of an inflammatory or occlusive process. Underlying associated macrovascular disease may occur due to vasculitis, proximal atherosclerosis, embolic disease, thrombotic or extrinsic vascular obstruction. Splinter hemorrhages under the nail are not seen secondary to RP alone and suggest an inflammatory or embolic process; while digital ulcers or deep areas of gangrene point toward digital artery and/or associated macrovascular disease.

Noninvasive assessment of the peripheral circulation will supplement the physical examination and may provide clues as to the cause and size of the vessels involved. Doppler ultrasound is a useful noninvasive test that can quickly give evidence for larger vessel disease [56]. Arteriography is recommended in specific cases with digital ischemia when the underlying cause is in question or the option of surgery is considered. Magnetic resonance angiography (MRA) is a fast, noninvasive method that can visualize vessel in the hand and digits. MRA studies in patients with scleroderma found substantial arterial and venous damage in the hands and could correlate these changes with clinical severity [57].

15.2   Management of Raynaud's Phenomenon

RP associated with primary SS is generally mild without vascular complications and therefore, like primary RP, conservative management is appropriate. The use of nondrug modalities are often very effective and may be all that is needed. An interaction between both cold sensitivity and emotional stress exists such that the intensity of the RP events becomes more severe if both cold exposure and the patient's emotional state are not addressed. Treatment begins with education. Patients need to have a clear understanding of the causes, consequences, and factors triggering the RP attacks. Education reduces fear and tension about the disease process and offers strategies for the patient in avoiding triggering factors. Patients need to know that the events are an exaggeration of a normal response to cold and emotional stress and, in uncomplicated cases, these events are not harmful even if they are uncomfortable. Treatment of anxiety/depression with medication may help the RP [58]. Cold exposures, especially shifting temperatures (e.g., going to the frozen food section of the grocery store) and situations such as sitting in a cold breeze without body movement, are best avoided. Keeping the whole body warm by wearing layered clothing and good head coverage will reduce the severity of attacks. Chemical warmers placed in gloves, stockings, or pockets can provide local heat in an ambulatory setting. Biofeedback and other forms of cognitive training are reported helpful, but a controlled trial of biofeedback compared with a sham procedure found no measurable benefit [59]. Treatment of both primary and secondary RP should always start with a foundation of nondrug methods.

15.2.1 Vasodilator Therapy

Whenever deciding on which type of vasodilator therapy to use for RP, one must look critically at the evidence for their benefit. RP varies greatly with weather conditions, activity, and stress; thus, drug interventions may appear helpful when in fact these other issues are influencing the outcome. The placebo effect in RP is robust, as documented in clinical trials where a 20–40% reduction in the severity of RP is reported [60]. Many agents are used with enthusiasm to treat RP but few have been formally studied to provide solid guidelines for their use.

15.2.2 Calcium Channel Blockers

Calcium channel blockers are the best studied and are still the most widely used agents for the treatment of RP. They continue to be both reasonable and safe as first-line drug therapy [61, 62]. It is recommended that a calcium channel blocker be used alone as initial therapy, titrating the medication to the maximal tolerated dose and then assessing its impact on the severity and frequency of RP by clinical follow-up. This titration should be done before changing therapy or adding other agents to the calcium channel blocker. The dihydropyridine calcium channel blockers (e.g., nifedipine, amlodipine) are more potent peripheral vasodilators than other calcium channel blockers (e.g., verapamil) but studies show that diltiazem, a benzothiazepine, is also effective [63]. Adverse effects such as hypotension, dizziness, flushing, dependent edema, and headaches are fairly common with these agents but usually mild. In cases of severe RP, the addition of a second vasodilator to a calcium channel is commonly done, but this approach is not evidence based.

15.2.3 Adrenergic Blockers

Studies of the cutaneous blood vessels demonstrate that while some alpha-1 adrenoreceptors are present on vessel, the alpha-2 adrenoreceptors are dominant and play a significant role in cutaneous thermoregulation [64]. Prazosin, an alpha-1 inhibitor is modestly effective in treating RP secondary to scleroderma, but side effects often limit tolerability [65]. Although a good alpha-2 inhibitor is not yet available, a study of a selective alpha (2C)-adrenergic receptor blocker in scleroderma patients with vasospasm found potential for therapeutic efficacy in a laboratory-based study [66]. From a practical viewpoint, alpha-adrenergic blocking agents are not the first-line therapy for critical ischemia but there is the theoretical potential for selective new agents to prevent vasospasm in the digital and thermoregulatory circulation.

Botulinum toxin type A (botox) injected into the base of the finger to block release of neuropeptides from cutaneous nerves is reported in uncontrolled case series to improve RP and digital ulcer healing [67, 68]. While interesting, these findings need to be confirmed in controlled trials before botox therapy can be recommended. In fact, sensory nerves also release vasodilatory neuropeptides (e.g., calcitonin-related polypeptide) and like topical lidocaine, botox in theory or other inhibitors of nerve function may have a negative effect by inhibiting the release of these beneficial vasodilators [69].

15.2.4 Nitrates

Topical nitrates can improve cutaneous blood flow [70]. Topical nitrates at full dose have limited practical use in that they require repeated application and side effects, particularly headache, are common. Newer formulations in development may also be of benefit [71]. It is the author's practice to use topical nitrates in the 2% ointment preparation in small amounts on single or few problem digits, usually in conjunction with another vasodilator such as a calcium channel blocker.

15.2.5 Phosphodiesterase Inhibitors

Several phosphodiesterase inhibitors have been used in the treatment of RP, including cilostazol, pentoxifylline, sildenafil, tadalafil, and vardenafil [72–75]. Sildenafil improved frequency and severity of RP in a relatively small placebo-controlled trial, but a similar trial in scleroderma patients found that tadalafil was not significantly better than placebo [76, 77]. In the author's anecdotal experience, these agents may improve RP when used alone in mild RP and can be helpful when added to a calcium channel blocker in patients with severe secondary RP. Topical nitrates cannot be used with the phosphodiesterase inhibitors due to the added risk of hypotension. Few studies are yet done to provide solid guidelines for the use of these agents in the management of RP.

15.2.6 Prostacyclins

Prostacyclins are potentially helpful in both pulmonary and peripheral vascular disease because they induce vasodilation by increasing intracellular cAMP. They may also prevent smooth muscle proliferation. Intravenous iloprost, a prostacyclin

analog, decreases the frequency and severity of RP attacks and improves healing
of digital ulcers [78, 79]. Low dose (0.5 ng/kg to 2 ng/kg body weight per minute) iloprost or epoprostenol is now used for severe RP and critical digital ischemia, primarily in patients with scleroderma by short term (several days) or
intermittent intravenous infusion via peripheral vein [80]. Intravenous treprostinil may also be effective [81]. Studies of oral prostacyclins (beraprost, iloprost,
and cisaprost) have variable and generally disappointing results, but a new formulation of oral treprostinil is now under study. Other prostaglandins (PGE1)
have also shown benefit when delivered intravenously and are an alternative to
prostacyclins [82].

15.2.7   Other Agents

Angiotensin converting enzyme (ACE) inhibitors were thought to have some benefit for RP but a multicenter, randomized, double-blind, placebo-controlled study
evaluating quinapril in over 200 patients with RP found no benefit in limiting the
occurrence of digital ulcers or influencing the frequency or severity of the RP episodes [83]. ACE inhibitors are not recommended for the treatment of RP. A relatively small study suggested that losartan, an angiotensin receptor blocker (ARB),
offered benefits that were similar to those of low-dose nifedipine [84]. ARBs may
provide some minor benefits in the relief of RP, although no definite evidence
exists to suggest that they are superior to traditionally used treatments such as
calcium-channel blockers. Larger, randomized controlled trials of longer duration
are needed [85].

A study of the selective serotonin reuptake inhibitor (SSRI) fluoxetine also found
comparable benefit to low-dose nifedipine [86]. More studies are needed, but SSRIs
have the potential to induce vasodilation by blocking uptake of the vasoconstrictor
serotonin. The use of these agents is particularly attractive for mild RP in patients
with low blood pressure.

Endothelins, released from the endothelial layer of blood vessels, act as potent
vasoconstrictors. Two placebo-controlled trials of bosentan, a endothelin receptor
inhibitor, demonstrated a reduction of new digital ulcers compared to placebo but
no change in the frequency or severity of RP [87, 88]. This suggests that bosentan
have vasoprotective properties that may help prevent ischemic ulcers but is insufficient for RP alone.

Statins demonstrate vasculoprotective effects by improving lipid profiles,
decreasing free radicals, coagulation, and blood viscosity, decreasing matrix metalloproteases, and increasing platelet function [89]. A placebo-controlled trial of ator-
vastatin in patients with scleroderma and RP demonstrated fewer digital ulcers and
a reduction in the severity of RP in the treated group [90]. This study sets the scene
for further investigations into the role of statins in patients with RP associated with
rheumatic diseases when there is associated peripheral vascular disease and digital
ischemia.

There is evidence of a defect in natural antioxidants and an increase in oxidative stress in patients with scleroderma, thus justifying trials or empiric use of antioxidant therapies [91]. Benefits of antioxidants remain to be demonstrated in clinical trials, but studies of N-acetylcysteine and probucol suggest that antioxidant therapy decreases the severity and consequences of RP [92, 93].

A variety of agents have the potential to prevent digital ischemia indirectly by their vasoprotective properties. These include antiplatelet agents, statins, prostaglandins, thrombolytics, anticoagulation, antithrombin agents, rho kinase inhibitors, and antioxidants. At this time, few formal studies are available to inform guidelines about their use. The author regularly uses low-dose aspirin therapy (81 mg) in scleroderma patients with significant vascular disease because there is evidence of platelet activation in those patients. The indications for using aspirin in SS are less clear.

15.3 Surgical Options

15.3.1 Sympathectomies

The thermoregulatory vessels in cold temperatures are normally under increased sympathetic tone. Thus, the disruption of sympathetic nerves to the limbs or fingers should result in vasodilatation and improve local blood flow. Both proximal and digital sympathectomies are used for the treatment of RP and are reported in uncontrolled case series to be effective [94–97]. Long-term follow-up of patients who have undergone sympathectomies suggests that the RP eventually returns but the severity is improved and subsequent digital ulcers are less likely. The author typically employs digital sympathectomies in patients who have failed medical therapy, who have evidence of critical digital ischemia, or are in an urgent situation of acute digital ischemia that threatens the viability of the digit. Surgical sympathectomy is not recommended for RP alone.

15.3.2 Management of Critical Digital Ischemia

Digit-threatening ischemia should be considered a medical emergency that requires hospitalization. In patients with SS, a careful investigation of a secondary process causing micro- and macrovascular disease is essential in that a reversible disease process is often causing the ischemic event (Table 15.3). Deeper tissue ischemia with infarction is usually associated with structural disease of larger vessels, inflammatory damage to vessels, and/or acute thrombosis. When persistent ischemia is clinically present (i.e., a painful, pale digit), then vasospasm of the superficial thermoregulatory vessels is usually coupled with occlusion of small nutritional vessels or larger proximal vessels, leading to low blood flow and critical tissue ischemia.

Table 15.3 Workup
for digital ischemia

- Nailfold capillary microscopy
- Examination: BP, pulses, bruits, Allen's test, provocative testing
- Comprehensive laboratory data
- Arterial Doppler
- Radiology
  - Conventional angiography: Lumen
  - MR-angiography: Lumen, vessel, and tissue
  - CT-angiography: 3 dimensional

Table 15.4 Managing acute
digital ischemia

- Rest and warm
- Control pain
  - Local digital block
- Start vasodilator:
  - Calcium channel blocker
  - If no response add a second vasodilator agent:
    - PDE-5 inhibitor
    - IV prostaglandins
- Novel preventive therapy
  - Statins
  - Antiplatelet: ASA 81 mg
  - Antioxidant therapy
- Surgery
  - Digital sympathectomy
  - Vascular repair

A rapid therapeutic intervention to prevent tissue infarction is required. This can be started by placing the patient in a warm ambient temperature, providing bed rest to decrease trauma and activity of the involved limb, and instituting appropriate pain control. Although systemic narcotics are known to be vasoconstrictors, their use may be necessary to control pain while other therapy to reverse the event is started. A local injection of lidocaine or bupivicaine at the base of a finger with critical ischemia can give rapid improvement, both in terms of pain and occasionally with improved blood flow by reducing sympathetic tone. Repeat injections or a local regional block can be done while waiting for other vasodilator therapy to take full effect. Vasodilator therapy should be started immediately and maximized rapidly (Table 15.4). A short-acting calcium channel blocker (e.g., nifedipine) is an appropriate choice, and it should be titrated to the highest tolerable dose. In cases of rapidly progressing ischemia that fails to respond to standard oral vasodilatory therapy, intravenous iloprost, alprostadil, or epoprostenol can be given. For patients who have rapidly advancing ischemic tissue, anticoagulant therapy is initiated. Although no formal studies exist, the use of heparin for 24–72 h during an acute crisis makes sense. Chronic anticoagulation is not recommended unless an associated hypercoagulable state is discovered. When medical therapy fails, several surgical interventions can be considered. These include proximal or distal (digital) sympathectomy and arterial reconstruction. Distal sympathectomy is associated with a lower complication rate than proximal sympathectomy, but long-term outcomes have not been documented thoroughly. Angiography should be performed if macrovascular or larger-vessel occlusive disease amenable to revascularization appears to be an issue.

References

1. Charkoudian N. Skin blood flow in adult human thermoregulation: how it works, when it does not, and why. Mayo Clin Proc. 2003;78:603–12.
2. Thompson-Torgerson CS, Holowatz LA, Kenney WL. Altered mechanisms of thermoregulatory vasoconstriction in aged human skin. Exerc Sport Sci Rev. 2008;36:122–7.
3. Chikura B, Moore TL, Manning JB, et al. Sparing of the thumb in Raynaud's phenomenon. Rheumatology (Oxford). 2008;47:219–21.
4. Gelber AC, Wigley FM, Stallings RY, et al. Symptoms of Raynaud's phenomenon in an inner city African-American community: prevalence and self-reported cardiovascular comorbidity. J Clin Epidemiol. 1999;52:441–6.
5. Block JA, Sequeira W. Raynaud's phenomenon. Lancet. 2001;357:2042–8.
6. Maricq HR, Carpentier PH, Weinrich MC, et al. Geographic variation in the prevalence of Raynaud's phenomenon: Charleston, SC, USA, vs. Tarentaise, Savoie, France. J Rheumatol. 1993;20:70–6.
7. LeRoy EC, Medsger Jr TA. Raynaud's phenomenon: a proposal for classification. Clin Exp Rheumatol. 1992;10:485–8.
8. Sharp GC, Irvin WS, May CM, et al. Association of antibodies to ribonucleoprotein and Sm antigens with mixed connective-tissue disease, systematic lupus erythematosus and other rheumatic diseases. N Engl J Med. 1976;295:1149–54.
9. Tuffanelli DL, Winkelmann RK. Systemic scleroderma, a clinical study of 727 cases. Arch Dermatol. 1961;84:359–71.
10. Parker MD. Ribonucleoprotein antibodies: frequency and clinical significance in systemic lupus erythematosus, scleroderma, and mixed connective tissue disease. J Lab Clin Med. 1973;82:769–75.
11. Cohen ML, Dawkins B, Dawkins RL, et al. Clinical significance of antibodies to ribonucleoprotein. Ann Rheum Dis. 1979;38:74–8.
12. Estes D, Christian CL. The natural history of systemic lupus erythematosus by prospective analysis. Medicine (Baltimore). 1971;50:85–95.
13. Hochberg MC, Boyd RE, Ahearn JM, et al. Systemic lupus erythematosus: a review of clinicolaboratory features and immunogenetic markers in 150 patients with emphasis on demographic subsets. Medicine (Baltimore). 1985;64:285–95.
14. Saraux A, Allain J, Guedes C, et al. Raynaud's phenomenon in rheumatoid arthritis. Br J Rheumatol. 1996;35:752–4.
15. De Angelis R, Cerioni A, Del Medico P, et al. Raynaud's phenomenon in undifferentiated connective tissue disease (UCTD). Clin Rheumatol. 2005;24:145–51.
16. Mosca M, Neri R, Bencivelli W, et al. Undifferentiated connective tissue disease: analysis of 83 patients with a minimum followup of 5 years. J Rheumatol. 2002;29:2345–9.
17. Youinou P, Pennec YL, Katsikis P, et al. Raynaud's phenomenon in primary Sjögren's syndrome. Br J Rheumatol. 1990;29:205–7.
18. Skopouli FN, Talal A, Galanopoulou V, et al. Raynaud's phenomenon in primary Sjögren's syndrome. J Rheumatol. 1990;17:618–20.
19. Kraus A, Caballero-Uribe C, Jakez J, et al. Raynaud's phenomenon in primary Sjögren's syndrome. Association with other extraglandular manifestations. J Rheumatol. 1992;19:1572–4.

20. Garcia-Carrasco M, Sisó A, Ramos-Casals M, et al. Raynaud's phenomenon in primary Sjögren's syndrome. Prevalence and clinical characteristics in a series of 320 patients. J Rheumatol. 2002;29:726–30.
21. Maricq HR, Carpentier PH, Weinrich MC, et al. Geographic variation in the prevalence of Raynaud's phenomenon: a 5 region comparison. J Rheumatol. 1997;24:879–89.
22. Kraus A, Guerra-Bautista G, Espinoza G, et al. Defects of the retinal pigment epithelium in scleroderma. Br J Rheumatol. 1991;30:112–4.
23. Diaz-López C, Geli C, Corominas H, et al. Are there clinical or serological differences between male and female patients with primary Sjögren's syndrome? J Rheumatol. 2004;31:1352–5.
24. Steen V, Denton CP, Pope JE, et al. Digital ulcers: overt vascular disease in systemic sclerosis. Rheumatology (Oxford). 2009;48:iii19–24.
25. Ramos-Casals M, Solans R, Rosas J, et al. Primary Sjögren syndrome in Spain: clinical and immunologic expression in 1010 patients. Medicine (Baltimore). 2008;87:210–9.
26. Willeke P, Schlüter B, Schotte H, et al. Interferon-gamma is increased in patients with primary Sjögren's syndrome and Raynaud's phenomenon. Semin Arthritis Rheum. 2009;39:197–202.
27. Foster H, Kelly C, Griffiths I. Raynaud's phenomenon and primary Sjögren's syndrome. Br J Rheumatol. 1990;29:493–4.
28. Ramos-Casals M, Nardi N, Brito-Zerón P, et al. Atypical autoantibodies in patients with primary Sjögren syndrome: clinical characteristics and follow-up of 82 cases. Semin Arthritis Rheum. 2006;35:312–21.
29. Ramos-Casals M, Brito-Zerón P, Font J. The overlap of Sjögren's syndrome with other systemic autoimmune diseases. Semin Arthritis Rheum. 2007;36:246–55.
30. Manoussakis MN, Georgopoulou C, Zintzaras E, et al. Sjögren's syndrome associated with systemic lupus erythematosus: clinical and laboratory profiles and comparison with primary Sjögren's syndrome. Arthritis Rheum. 2004;50:882–91.
31. Font J, Ramos-Casals M, Cervera R, et al. Antineutrophil cytoplasmic antibodies in primary Sjögren's syndrome: prevalence and clinical significance. Br J Rheumatol. 1998;37:1287–91.
32. Hernandez-Molina G, Avila-Casado C, Cardenas-Velazquez F, et al. Similarities and differences between primary and secondary Sjögren's syndrome. J Rheumatol. 2010;37(4):800–8.
33. Kallenberg CG, Pastoor GW, Wouda AA. Antinuclear antibodies in patients with Raynaud's phenomenon: clinical significance of anticentromere antibodies. Ann Rheum Dis. 1982;41:382–7.
34. Koenig M, Joyal F, Fritzler MJ, et al. Autoantibodies and microvascular damage are independent predictive factors for the progression of Raynaud's phenomenon to systemic sclerosis: a twenty-year prospective study of 586 patients, with validation of proposed criteria for early systemic sclerosis. Arthritis Rheum. 2008;58:3902–12.
35. Gelber AC, Pillemer SR, Baum BJ, et al. Distinct recognition of antibodies to centromere proteins in primary Sjögren's syndrome compared with limited scleroderma. Ann Rheum Dis. 2006;65:1028–32.
36. Salliot C, Gottenberg JE, Bengoufa D, et al. Anticentromere antibodies identify patients with Sjögren's syndrome and autoimmune overlap syndrome. J Rheumatol. 2007;34:2253–8.
37. Katano K, Kawano M, Koni I, et al. Clinical and laboratory features of anticentromere antibody positive primary Sjögren's syndrome. J Rheumatol. 2001;28:2238–44.
38. Tektonidou M, Kaskani E, Skopouli FN, et al. Microvascular abnormalities in Sjögren's syndrome: nailfold capillaroscopy. Rheumatology. 1999;38:826–30.
39. Caramaschi P, Biasi D, Carletto A, et al. Sjögren's syndrome with anticentromere antibodies. Rev Rhum Engl Ed. 1997;64:785–8.
40. Bournia VK, Diamanti KD, Vlachoyiannopoulos PG, et al. Anticentromere antibody positive Sjogren's syndrome: a retrospective descriptive analysis. Arthritis Res Ther. 2010;12(2):R47.
41. Miyawaki S, Asanuma H, Nishiyama S, et al. Clinical and serological heterogeneity in patients with anticentromere antibodies. J Rheumatol. 2005;32:1488–94.
42. Vlachoyiannopoulos PG, Drosos AA, Wiik A, et al. Patients with anticentromere antibodies, clinical features, diagnoses and evolution. Br J Rheumatol. 1993;32:297–301.

43. Masayuki I, Kojima T, Miyata M, et al. Primary biliary cirrhosis (PBC)-CREST (Calcinosis, Raynaud's phenomenon, esophageal dysfunction, Sclerodactyly and telangiectasia) overlap syndrome complicated by Sjögren's syndrome and arthritis. Intern Med. 1995;34:451–4.
44. Nakamura T, Higashi S, Tomoda K, et al. Primary biliary cirrhosis (PBC)-CREST overlap syndrome with coexistence of Sjögren's syndrome and thyroid dysfunction. Clin Rheumatol. 2007;26:596–600.
45. O'Keefe ST, Tsapatsaris NP, Beetham Jr WP. Association between Raynaud's phenomenon and migraine in a random population of hospital employees. J Rheumatol. 1993;20:1187–8.
46. Pal B, Gibson C, Passmore J, et al. A study of headaches and migraine in Sjögren's syndrome and other rheumatic disorders. Ann Rheum Dis. 1989;48:312–6.
47. Gökçay F, Öder G, Çelebisoy N, et al. Headache in primary Sjögren's syndrome: a prevalence study. Acta Neurol Scand. 2008;118:189–92.
48. Hassoun PM. Pulmonary arterial hypertension complicating connective tissue diseases. Semin Respir Crit Care Med. 2009;30:429–39.
49. Launay D, Hachulla E, Hatron PY, et al. Pulmonary arterial hypertension: a rare complication of primary Sjögren syndrome: report of 9 new cases and review of the literature. Medicine (Baltimore). 2007;86:299–315.
50. Vassilliou VA, Moyssakis I, Boki KA, et al. Is the heart affected in primary Sjögren's syndrome? An echocardiographic study. Clin Exp Rheumatol. 2008;26:109–12.
51. Hassoun PM. Therapies for scleroderma-related pulmonary arterial hypertension. Expert Rev Respir Med. 2009;3:187–96.
52. Abdelhady K, Gramling-Babb P, Awad S, et al. Current and future therapy for pulmonary hypertension in patients with right and left heart failure. Expert Rev Cardiovasc Ther. 2010;8: 241–50.
53. Pirildar T, Tikiz C, Ozkaya S, et al. Endothelial dysfunction in patients with primary Sjögren's syndrome. Rheumatol Int. 2005;25:536–9.
54. Garcia-Carrasco M, Pizcueta P, Cervera R, et al. Circulating concentrations of soluble L-selectin (CD62L) in patients with primary Sjögren's syndrome. Ann Rheum Dis. 2000;59: 297–9.
55. Inaoki M, Sato S, Shimada Y, et al. Elevated serum levels of soluble L-selectin in patients with systemic sclerosis declined after intravenous injection of lipo-prostaglandin E1. J Dermatol Sci. 2001;25:78–82.
56. Stafford L, Englert H, Gover J, et al. Distribution of macrovascular disease in scleroderma. Ann Rheum Dis. 1998;57:476–9.
57. Allanore Y, Seror R, Chevrot A, et al. Hand vascular involvement assessed by magnetic resonance angiography in systemic sclerosis. Arthritis Rheum. 2007;56:2747–54.
58. Colakoğu M, Cobankara V, Akpolat T. Effect of clonazepam on Raynaud's phenomenon and fingertip ulcers in scleroderma. Ann Pharmacother. 2007;41:1544–7.
59. Raynaud's Treatment Study Investigators. Comparison of sustained-release nifedipine and temperature biofeedback for treatment of primary Raynaud phenomenon. Results from a randomized clinical trial with 1-year follow-up. Arch Intern Med. 2000;160:1101–8.
60. Wigley FM, Korn JH, Csuka ME. Oral iloprost treatment in patients with Raynaud's phenomenon secondary to systemic sclerosis: a multicenter, placebo-controlled, double-blind study. Arthritis Rheum. 1998;41:670–7.
61. Thompson AE, Shea B, Welch V, et al. Calcium-channel blockers for Raynaud's phenomenon in systemic sclerosis. Arthritis Rheum. 2001;44:1841–7.
62. Thompson AE, Pope JE. Calcium channel blockers for primary Raynaud's phenomenon: a meta-analysis. Rheumatology (Oxford). 2005;44:145–50.
63. Rhedda A, McCans J, Willan AR, et al. A double blind placebo controlled crossover randomized trial of diltiazem in Raynaud's phenomenon. J Rheumatol. 1985;12:724–7.
64. Wigley FM, Flavahan NA. Raynaud's phenomenon. Rheum Dis Clin North Am. 1996;22:765–81.
65. Harding SE, Tingey PC, Pope J, et al. Prazosin for Raynaud's phenomenon in progressive systemic sclerosis. Cochrane Database Syst Rev 1998;(2):CD000956.

66. Wise RA, Wigley FM, White B, et al. Efficacy and tolerability of a selective alpha(2C)-adrenergic receptor blocker in recovery from cold-induced vasospasm in scleroderma patients: a single-center, double-blind, placebo-controlled, randomized crossover study. Arthritis Rheum. 2004; 50:3994–4001.

67. Fregene A, Ditmars D, Siddiqui A. Botulinum toxin type A: a treatment option for digital ischemia in patients with Raynaud's phenomenon. J Hand Surg Am. 2009;34:446–52.

68. Van Beek AL, Lim PK, Gear AJ, et al. Management of vasospastic disorders with Botulinum toxin A. Plast Reconstr Surg. 2007;119:217–26.

69. Generini S, Seibold JR, Matucci-Cerinic M. Estrogens and neuropeptides in Raynaud's phenomenon. Rheum Dis Clin North Am. 2005;31:177–86.

70. Anderson ME, Moore TL, Hollis S, et al. Digital vascular response to topical glyceryl trinitrate, as measured by laser Doppler imaging, in primary Raynaud's phenomenon and systemic sclerosis. Rheumatology (Oxford). 2002;41:324–8.

71. Chung L, Shapiro L, Fiorentino D, et al. MQX-503, a novel formulation of nitroglycerin, improves the severity of Raynaud's phenomenon: a randomized, controlled trial. Arthritis Rheum. 2009;60:870–7.

72. Rajagopalan S, Pfenninger D, Somers E, et al. Effects of cilostazol in patients with Raynaud's syndrome. Am J Cardiol. 2003;92:1310–5.

73. Goldberg J, Diesk A. Successful treatment of Raynaud's phenomenon with pentoxifylline. Arthritis Rheum. 1986;29:1055–6.

74. Levien TL. Phosphodiesterase inhibitors in Raynaud's phenomenon. Ann Pharmacother. 2006;40:1388–93.

75. Caglayan E, Huntgeburth M, Karasch T, et al. Phosphodiesterase Type 5 inhibition is a novel therapeutic option in Raynaud disease. Arch Intern Med. 2006;166:231–3.

76. Fries R, Shariat K, von Wilmowsky H, et al. Sildenafil in the treatment of Raynaud's phenomenon resistant to vasodilatory therapy. Circulation. 2005;112:2980–5.

77. Schiopu E, Hsu VM, Impens AJ, et al. Randomized placebo-controlled crossover trial of tadalafil in Raynaud's phenomenon secondary to systemic sclerosis. J Rheumatol. 2009;36: 2264–8.

78. Wigley FM, Wise RA, Seibold JR, et al. Intravenous iloprost infusion in patients with Raynaud phenomenon secondary to systemic sclerosis. Ann Intern Med. 1994;120:199–206.

79. Pope J, Fenlon D, Thompson A, et al. Iloprost and cisaprost for Raynaud's phenomenon in progressive systemic sclerosis. Cochrane Database Syst Rev 1998;(2):CD000953.

80. Bettoni L, Geri A, Airò P, et al. Systemic sclerosis therapy with iloprost: a prospective observational study of 30 patients treated for a median of 3 years. Clin Rheumatol. 2002;21: 244–50.

81. Chung L, Fiorentino D. A pilot trial of Treprostinil for the treatment and prevention of digital ulcers in patients with systemic sclerosis. J Am Acad Dermatol. 2006;54:880–2.

82. Marasini B, Massarotti M, Bottasso B, et al. Comparison between iloprost and alprostadil in the treatment of Raynaud's phenomenon. Scand J Rheumatol. 2004;33:253–6.

83. Gliddon AE, Doré CJ, Black CM, et al. Prevention of vascular damage in scleroderma and autoimmune Raynaud's phenomenon. A multicenter, randomized, double-blind, placebo-controlled trial of the angiotensin-converting enzyme inhibitor quinapril. Arthritis Rheum. 2007;56:3837–46.

84. Dziadzio M, Denton CP, Smith R, et al. Losartan therapy for Raynaud's phenomenon and scleroderma. Clinical and biochemical findings in a fifteen-week, randomized, parallel-group, controlled trial. Arthritis Rheum. 1999;42:2646–55.

85. Wood HM, Ernst ME. Renin-angiotensin system mediators and Raynaud's phenomenon. Ann Pharmacother. 2006;40:1998–2002.

86. Coleiro B, Marshall SE, Denton CP, et al. Treatment of Raynaud's phenomenon with the selective serotonin reuptake inhibitor fluoxetine. Rheumatology (Oxford). 2001;40:1038–43.

87. Korn JH, Mayes M, Matucci Cerinic M, et al. Digital ulcers in systemic sclerosis: prevention by treatment with bosentan, an oral endothelin receptor antagonist. Arthritis Rheum. 2004;50: 3985–93.

88. Matucci-Cerinic M, Seibold JR. Digital ulcers and outcomes assessment in scleroderma. Rheumatology (Oxford). 2008;47 Suppl 5:v46–7.
89. Kuwana M. Potential benefit of statins for vascular disease in systemic sclerosis. Curr Opin Rheumatol. 2006;18:594–600.
90. Abou-Raya A, Abou-Raya S, Helmii M. Statins: potentially useful in therapy of systemic sclerosis-related Raynaud's phenomenon and digital ulcers. J Rheumatol. 2008;35:1801–8.
91. Herrick AL, Matucci Cerinic M. The emerging problem of oxidative stress and the role of antioxidants in systemic sclerosis. Clin Exp Rheumatol. 2001;19:4–8.
92. Rosato E, Borghese F, Pisarri S, et al. The treatment with N-acetylcysteine of Raynaud's phenomenon and ischemic ulcers therapy in sclerodermic patients: a prospective observational study of 50 patients. Clin Rheumatol. 2009;28:1379–84.
93. Denton CP, Bunce TD, Dorado MB, et al. Probucol improves symptoms and reduces lipoprotein oxidation susceptibility in patients with Raynaud's phenomenon. Rheumatology (Oxford). 1999;38:309–15.
94. Matsumoto Y, Ueyama T, Endo M, et al. Endoscopic thoracic sympathicotomy for Raynaud's phenomenon. J Vasc Surg. 2002;36:57–61.
95. Yee AM, Hotchkiss RN, Paget SA. Adventitial stripping: a digit saving procedure in refractory Raynaud's phenomenon. J Rheumatol. 1998;25:269–76.
96. Kotsis SV, Chung KC. A systematic review of the outcomes of digital sympathectomy for treatment of chronic digital ischemia. J Rheumatol. 2003;30:1788–92.
97. Hartzell TL, Makhni EC, Sampson C. Long-term results of periarterial sympathectomy. J Hand Surg Am. 2009;34:1454–60.

Chapter 16
Gastrointestinal Involvement in Primary Sjögren's Syndrome

Manuel Ramos-Casals, José Rosas, Roser Solans, Margit Zeher, and Peter Szodoray

Contents

M. Ramos-Casals (✉)
Spanish Group of Autoimmune Diseases (GEAS), Spanish Society of Internal Medicine (SEMI), Sjögren Syndrome Research Group (AGAUR), Laboratory of Autoimmune Diseases Josep Font, Institut d'Investigacions Biomèdiques August Pi i Sunyer (IDIBAPS), Department of Autoimmune Diseases, ICMD Hospital Clínic, Barcelona, Spain

J. Rosas
Department of Rheumatology, Hospital de la Vila-Joiosa, Alicante, Spain

R. Solans
Department of Internal Medicine, Hospital Vall d'Hebron, Barcelona, Spain

M. Zeher • P. Szodoray
Medical and Health Science Center, Clinical Immunology Division, University of Debrecen, Debrecen, Hungary

M. Ramos-Casals et al. (eds.), *Sjögren's Syndrome*,
DOI 10.1007/978-0-85729-947-5_16, © Springer-Verlag London Limited 2012

Table 16.1 Gastrointestinal diseases described in patients with primary SS	• Esophageal motor dysfunction • Upper esophageal webs • Decreased esophageal peristalsis • Gastroesophageal reflux • Chronic gastritis • Atrophic gastritis • *Helicobacter pylori* infection • Gastric lymphoma • Celiac disease • Intestinal vasculitis • Sensitivity to cow's milk protein

Gastrointestinal involvement in primary Sjögren's syndrome (pSS) may include altered esophageal motility, gastroesophageal reflux, chronic gastritis and, less frequently, intestinal malabsorption [1–3] (Table 16.1).

16.1 Dysphagia

Recent studies have analyzed esophageal involvement in patients with primary SS. Decreased saliva production in SS might contribute to the development of dysphagia, because adequate pharyngoesophageal transfer of the alimentary bolus requires saliva [4]. However, Anselmino et al. observed no differences in salivary flow rates of primary SS patients with and without dysphagia, and Grande et al. found no relationship between dysphagia and the parotid saliva flow rate [5, 6].

Dysphagia has also been associated with esophageal motor dysfunction and upper esophageal webs [7]. Thus, Rosztoczy et al. [8] described decreased peristaltic velocity in the esophageal body of 11 (44%) out of 25 patients with primary SS. However, the majority of studies have found that SS patients with and without dysphagia have similar function [5–7, 9], and that dysphagia is independent of esophageal motility [6, 10, 11]. Although patients with primary SS may have altered manometric studies, to date, studies have failed to describe any consistent pattern of esophageal dysfunction. Moreover, the motor disorders that some patients have correlate poorly with dysphagia [12]. Esophageal candidiasis is very infrequent (Fig. 16.1).

16.2 Gastroesophageal Reflux

A recent study investigated the prevalence and clinical significance of gastroesophageal reflux (GER) in patients with primary SS, and its possible association with esophageal dysmotility [7], and found abnormalities in motility in 21 patients with SS,

Fig. 16.1 Esophageal candidiasis in a 53-year-old woman with Sjögren's syndrome, limited systemic sclerosis, and primary biliary cirrhosis (Reynolds' syndrome)

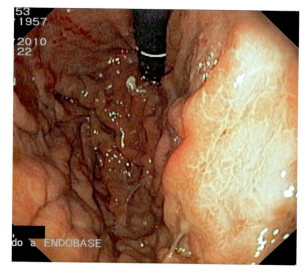

which was associated with GER. The study found slow acid clearance in the esophagus of SS patients with GER suggesting a prolonged duration of reflux. This extended exposure of the esophagus to refluxed acid may result either from defective acid neutralization by salivary bicarbonates or to altered esophageal motility [13–16]. Ho et al. [17] described a high frequency of tertiary waves in patients with markedly abnormal pH that correlated with the total reflux time, suggesting a relationship between these contractions and prolonged exposure of the esophageal mucosa to low pH values.

16.3 Chronic Gastritis

Although earlier reports described chronic gastric inflammation with mucosal atrophy in nearly 80% of patients with SS [18–20], the prevalence of chronic gastritis has not been evaluated in recent series. In clinical practice, patients frequently complain of gastric pain, but gastroscopic studies generally reveal only mild abnormalities such as mild atrophic changes in the antrum [21].

Two recent studies have analyzed the prevalence and clinical significance of anti-parietal cell gastric antibodies (anti-PCA) in primary SS. Nardi et al. [22] found positive anti-PCA antibodies in 90 (27%) out of 335 patients. These patients showed a higher prevalence of thyroiditis and autoimmune liver involvement, but not gastrointestinal involvement. El Miedany et al. [23] found anti-PCA antibodies in one third of SS patients and controls. However, all SS patients with anti-PCA antibodies had *Helicobacter pylori* infection, in comparison with less than half of the autoantibody positive controls. Likewise, only 22% of the autoantibody positive controls

Fig. 16.2 Gastritis (*H. pylori* infection+) in a patient with primary SS with dyspepsia

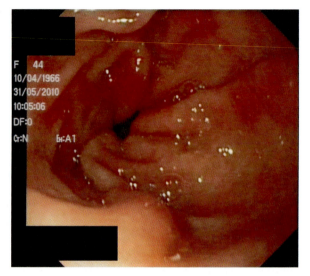

had atrophic changes in gastric mucosa compared with 86% of those with SS. This study found a close association between anti-PCA antibodies and *H. pylori* infection, suggesting that this bacterium may induce a local hyperreactive/autoimmune response that facilitates the induction of autoantibodies against the gastric mucosa of SS patients.

Although anti-PCA antibodies have been associated with chronic atrophic gastritis and pernicious anemia, the two processes are only rarely described in patients with primary SS. Two cases were described in a recent review of hematologic manifestations in a cohort of 380 SS patients [24], with only four additional cases being reported [25–27], suggesting that chronic atrophic gastritis and pernicious anemia are very infrequent in primary SS.

16.4 *Helicobacter pylori* Infection

A number of studies have analyzed the prevalence and clinical significance of *H. Pylori* infection in primary SS, searching for a possible association with dyspepsia, gastritis (Fig. 16.2), gastric ulcers, or lymphoma, with controversial results. Sorrentino et al. [28] and Theander et al. [29] found that SS patients have *H. pylori* seroprevalence rates that are similar to those of controls, while Collin et al. [21] found that the seroprevalence of *H. pylori* infection in dyspeptic SS patients was similar to that of dyspeptic patients without SS. In contrast, other studies have described a higher prevalence of *H. pylori* antibodies in primary SS compared with controls [30–32]. El Miedany et al. [23] found both a significantly higher prevalence and higher serum titers of IgG and IgM anti-*H. pylori* antibodies in SS patients compared with both patients with other autoimmune diseases without sicca syndrome and healthy controls. This might reflect geographical differences in the prevalence of *H. pylori* infection, which is reported to be lower in Sweden than in other countries. Moreover, a recent study has shown that *H. pylori* was detected in gastric biopsies in 71% of Italian SS patients in comparison with 31% of Scandinavian patients [29].

The histological severity of gastritis has been associated closely with the presence of *H. pylori* in primary SS. However, a recent study showed that eradication of *H. pylori* caused a significant regression of gastric MALT and atrophy in controls but not in SS patients [33]. In addition, dyspepsia did not improve following bacterial eradication in the majority of SS patients, suggesting that *H. pylori* does not play a role in the dyspeptic symptoms found in SS.

A possible relationship between *H. pylori* and gastric lymphomagenesis in SS has recently been postulated. Lymphoid accumulation in the gastric mucosa is common in SS but full evidence for an antigen-driven B-cell expansion has not been demonstrated. De Vita et al. [30] described a low-grade gastric lymphoma concomitantly with *H. pylori* infection in a patient with SS. After *H. pylori* eradication, a dramatic regression of gastric lymphoma into chronic gastritis was observed, but no amelioration occurred in the parotid and nodal involvement. Multiple molecular analyses showed the expansion of the same B-cell clone in synchronous and metachronous lymph node, parotid, and gastric lesions before and after *H. pylori* eradication. Ferraccioli et al. [34], who studied the gastric tissue in SS in order to define whether the presence of MALT in the stomach is associated with several infectious agents, showed that *H. pylori* infection is not more frequent among patient with SS than in controls, and that the abnormal accumulation of MALT may occur in the stomach even in the absence of *H. pylori* infection. Other studies performed on a limited number of SS patients with simple dyspepsia indicate that clonality may persist for up to 6 months after the eradication of *H. pylori* [35]. Thus, although *H. pylori* may play a crucial role in the local boosting of B-cell lymphoproliferation, the underlying B-cell disorder seems to be a nonmalignant process [30].

16.5   Association with Celiac Disease

Recent studies have analyzed the potential association between primary SS and celiac disease in small series of patients. In the general population, the prevalence of celiac disease is estimated to be 0.45%. Iltanen et al. [36] found that 5 (15%) out of 34 SS patients had celiac disease, while Szodoray et al. [37] diagnosed celiac disease in 5 (4.5%) out of 111 patients with SS. In contrast, Lazarus and Isenberg [38] found 1 (0.9%) patient with celiac disease out of 114 individuals with primary SS, and another series of 400 SS patients detected not a single celiac disease case [39].

Table 16.2 Previous reported cases of biopsy-proven vasculitis involving the gastrointestinal tract in patients with primary Sjögren syndrome [41]

Number of cases	Gastrointestinal vasculitic involvement	Type of vasculitis
1	Gastrointestinal (NS)	Necrotizing
2	Gastrointestinal (NS)	Necrotizing
3	Ileum	Necrotizing
4	Ileum	Leukocytoclastic
5	Bowel	Necrotizing
6	Bowel	Necrotizing
7	Bowel	Leukocytoclastic
8	Bowel	Leukocytoclastic
9	Colon	Necrotizing
10	Colon	Necrotizing
11	Rectum	Leukocytoclastic
12	Gallbladder	Necrotizing
13	Gallbladder	Leukocytoclastic

These latter studies conflict with the notion that patients with primary SS should be evaluated routinely for celiac disease [40].

16.6   Intestinal Vasculitis

Among patients with primary SS, systemic vasculitis only rarely involves the gastrointestinal tract. Of the 19 reports of SS patients with systemic necrotizing vasculitis [41], 13 had gastrointestinal tract involvement (Table 16.2). In addition, of the 19 reported deaths of SS patients due to vasculitis, the two main causes were CNS involvement in 6 and gastrointestinal perforation in 5. Cryoglobulins were determined in 12 of these patients and were positive in 10 (83%) cases. In spite of its rarity, gastrointestinal vasculitis, often related to cryoglobulinemia, should be considered as a life-threatening situation in patients with primary SS.

16.7   Other Intestinal Diseases

Recent studies have described other intestinal diseases in patients with primary SS. Lidén et al. [42] found an inflammatory mucosal response after rectal exposure to cow's milk protein in 38% of patients with primary SS. The same authors also found [43] a similar reaction after gluten exposure in 20% of patients. However, the two studies found no correlation between sensitivity to gluten or cow's milk protein with food intolerance or gastrointestinal symptoms.

16.8 Conclusion

A number of studies have analyzed the prevalence and clinical significance of gastrointestinal diseases in patients with primary SS, including esophageal dysfunction, gastritis, *H. pylori* infection, and intestinal malabsorption, with differing results. Esophageal and gastric diseases are frequent in primary SS, but it is not clear whether they are etiopathogenically related to SS. In contrast, intestinal involvement should be considered as one of the less-frequent extraglandular manifestations of primary SS, with isolated cases of malabsorption or vasculitis being reported. Some issues remain unresolved, including the prevalence of celiac disease in patients with primary SS and the possible role of hypersensitivity to cow's milk protein in irritable bowel syndrome, which is often presented by patients with primary SS. However, current knowledge suggests that the majority of gastrointestinal diseases diagnosed in patients with primary SS have a similar prevalence to that found in nonautoimmune patients with a similar epidemiological profile.

References

1. Fox RI. Sjogren's syndrome. Lancet. 2005;366:321–31.
2. Kassan SS, Moutsopoulos HM. Clinical manifestations and early diagnosis of Sjogren syndrome. Arch Intern Med. 2004;164:1275–84.
3. Ramos-Casals M, Tzioufas AG, Font J. Primary Sjogren's syndrome: new clinical and therapeutic concepts. Ann Rheum Dis. 2005;64:347–54.
4. Helm JF. Role of saliva in esophageal function and disease. Dysphagia. 1989;4:76–84.
5. Anselmino M, Zaninotto G, Costantini M, Ostuni P, Ianniello A, Boccu C, et al. Esophageal motor function in primary Sjogren's syndrome: correlation with dysphagia and xerostomia. Dig Dis Sci. 1997;42:113–8.
6. Grande L, Lacima G, Ros E, Font J, Pera C. Esophageal motor function in primary Sjogren's syndrome. Am J Gastroenterol. 1993;88:378–81.
7. Volter F, Fain O, Mathieu E, Thomas M. Esophageal function and Sjogren's syndrome. Dig Dis Sci. 2004;49:248–53.
8. Rosztoczy A, Kovacs L, Wittmann T, Lonovics J, Pokorny G. Manometric assessment of impaired esophageal motor function in primary Sjogren's syndrome. Clin Exp Rheumatol. 2001;19:147–52.
9. Tsianos EB, Chiras CD, Drosos AA, Moutsopoulos HM. Esophageal dysfunction in patients with primary Sjögren's syndrome. Ann Rheum Dis. 1998;544:610–3.
10. Kjellen G, Fransson SG, Lindstrom F, Sokjer H, Tibbling L. Esophageal function, radiography and dysphagia in Sjögren's syndrome. Dig Dis Sci. 1986;31:225–9.
11. Palma R, Freire A, Freitas J, Morbey A, Costa T, Saraiva F, et al. Esophageal motility disorders in patients with Sjogren's syndrome. Dig Dis Sci. 1994;39:758–61.
12. Mandl T, Ekberg O, Wollmer P, Manthorpe R, Jacobsson LT. Dysphagia and dysmotility of the pharynx and oesophagus in patients with primary Sjögren's syndrome. Scand J Rheumatol. 2007;36:394–401.
13. Kahrilas PJ, Dodds WJ, Hogan WJ, Kern M, Arndorfer RC, Reece A. Esophageal peristaltic dysfunction in peptic esophagitis. Gastroenterology. 1986;91:897–904.
14. Schowengerdt CG. Standard acid reflux testing revisited. Dig Dis Sci. 2001;46:603–5.

15. Geatti O, Shapiro B, Fig LM, Fossaluzza V, Franzon R, De Vita S. Radiolabelled semisolid test meal clearance in the evaluation of esophageal involvement in scleroderma and Sjögren's syndrome. Am J Physiol Imaging. 1991;6:65–73.
16. Fitzgerald RC, Triadafilopoulos G. Esophageal manifestations of rheumatic disorders. Semin Arthritis Rheum. 1997;26:641–66.
17. Ho SC, Chang CS, Wu CY, Chen GH. Ineffective esophageal motility is a primary motility disorder in gastroesophageal reflux disease. Dig Dis Sci. 2002;47:652–7.
18. Buchanan WW, Cox AG, McG Harden R, Glen AIM, Gray KG. Gastric studies in Sjogren's syndrome. Gut. 1966;7:351–4.
19. Kilpi A, Bergroth V, Konttinen YT, Maury CPJ, Reitamo S, Wegelius O. Lymphocyte infiltration of the gastric mucosa in Sjogren's syndrome. Arthritis Rheum. 1983;26:1196–200.
20. Maury CPJ, Tornroth T, Teppo AM. Atrophic gastritis in Sjogren's syndrome. Arthritis Rheum. 1985;28:388–94.
21. Collin P, Karvonen AL, Korpela M, Laippala P, Helin H. Gastritis classified in accordance with the Sydney system in patients with primary Sjögren's syndrome. Scand J Gastroenterol. 1997;32:108–11.
22. Nardi N, Brito-Zeron P, Ramos-Casals M, Aguilo S, Cervera R, Ingelmo M, et al. Circulating auto-antibodies against nuclear and non-nuclear antigens in primary Sjogren's syndrome: prevalence and clinical significance in 335 patients. Clin Rheumatol. 2006;25:341–6.
23. El Miedany YM, Baddour M, Ahmed I, Fahmy H. Sjogren's syndrome: concomitant H pylori infection and possible correlation with clinical parameters. Joint Bone Spine. 2005;72: 135–41.
24. Ramos-Casals M, Font J, Garcia-Carrasco M, Brito MP, Rosas J, Calvo-Alen J, et al. Primary Sjogren syndrome: hematologic patterns of disease expression. Medicine (Baltimore). 2002;81:281–92.
25. Pedro-Botet J, Coll J, Tomás S, Soriano JC, Gutiérrez Cebollado J. Primary Sjogren's syndrome associated with chronic atrophic gastritis and pernicious anemia. J Clin Gastroenterol. 1993;16:146–8.
26. Wegelious O, Fyhrquist F, Adner PL. Sjogren's syndrome associated with vitamin B12 deficiency. Acta Rheumatol Scand. 1970;16:184–90.
27. Williamson J, Paterson RW, McGavin DD, Greig WR, Whaley K. Sjogren's syndrome in relation to pernicious anaemia and idiophatic Addison's disease. Br J Ophthalmol. 1970;54: 31–6.
28. Sorrentino D, Faller G, DeVita S, Avellini C, Labombarda A, Ferraccioli G, et al. Helicobacter pylori associated antigastric autoantibodies: role in Sjögren's syndrome gastritis. Helicobacter. 2004;9:46–53.
29. Theander E, Nilsson I, Manthorpe R, Jacobsson LT, Wadstrom T. Seroprevalence of Helicobacter pylori in primary Sjogren's syndrome. Clin Exp Rheumatol. 2001;19:633–8.
30. De Vita S, Ferraccioli G, Avellini C. Widerspread clonal B-cell disorder in Sjogren's syndrome predisposing to H. pylori related gastric lymphoma. Gastroenterology. 1996;110:1969–74.
31. Ostuni PA, Germana B, DiMario F, Rugge M, Plebani M, DeZambiasi P. Gastric involvement in primary Sjogren's syndrome. Clin Exp Rheumatol. 1993;11:21–5.
32. Sugaya T, Sakai H, Sugiyama T, Imai K. Atrophic gastritis in Sjogren's syndrome. Nippon Rinsho. 1995;53:2540–4.
33. Witteman EM, Mravunac M, Becx MJ, Hopman WP, Verschoor JS, Tytgat GN, et al. Improvement of gastric inflammation and resolution of epithelial damage one year after eradication of Helicobacter pylori. J Clin Pathol. 1995;48:250–6.
34. Ferraccioli GF, Sorrentino D, De Vita S, et al. B cell clonality in gastric lymphoid tissues of patients with Sjogren's syndrome. Ann Rheum Dis. 1996;55:311–6.
35. Illes A, Varoczy L, Papp G, et al. Aspects of B-cell non-Hodgkin's lymphoma development: a transition from immune-reactivity to malignancy. Scand J Immunol. 2009;69:387–400.

36. Iltanen S, Collin P, Korpela M, Holm K, Partanen J, Polvi A, et al. Celiac disease and markers of celiac disease latency in patients with primary Sjogren's syndrome. Am J Gastroenterol. 1999;94:1042–6.
37. Szodoray P, Barta Z, Lakos G, Szakall S, Zeher M. Coeliac disease in Sjogren's syndrome – a study of 111 Hungarian patients. Rheumatol Int. 2004;24:278–82.
38. Lazarus MN, Isenberg DA. Development of additional autoimmune diseases in a population of patients with primary Sjogren's syndrome. Ann Rheum Dis. 2005;64:1062–4.
39. Garcia-Carrasco M, Ramos-Casals M, Rosas J, et al. Primary Sjogren syndrome: clinical and immunologic disease patterns in a cohort of 400 patients. Medicine (Baltimore). 2002;81: 270–80.
40. Roblin X, Helluwaert F, Bonaz B. Celiac disease must be evaluated in patients with Sjogren syndrome. Arch Intern Med. 2004;164:2387.
41. Ramos-Casals M, Anaya JM, Garcia-Carrasco M, et al. Cutaneous vasculitis in primary Sjogren syndrome: classification and clinical significance of 52 patients. Medicine (Baltimore). 2004;83:96–106.
42. Lidén M, Kristjánsson G, Valtysdottir S, Venge P, Hällgren R. Cow's milk protein sensitivity assessed by the mucosal patch technique is related to irritable bowel syndrome in patients with primary Sjögren's syndrome. Clin Exp Allergy. 2008;38:929–35.
43. Lidén M, Kristjánsson G, Valtýsdóttir S, Hällgren R. Gluten sensitivity in patients with primary Sjögren's syndrome. Scand J Gastroenterol. 2007;42:962–7.

Chapter 17
Liver Involvement in Sjögren's Syndrome

George E. Fragoulis, Fotini N. Skopouli, Carlo Selmi, and M. Eric Gershwin

Contents

G.E. Fragoulis (✉)
Department of Pathophysiology, School of Medicine,
National University of Athens, Athens, Greece

F.N. Skopouli
Department of Dietetics and Nutritional Science,
Harokopio University of Athens, Athens, Greece

C. Selmi
Division of Rheumatology, Allergy and Clinical Immunology,
University of California at Davis, Davis, CA, USA

Department of Translational Medicine, IRCCS Istituto Clinico Humanitas,
University of Milan, Rozzano (MI), Italy

M.E. Gershwin
Division of Rheumatology, Allergy and Clinical Immunology,
Genome and Biomedical Sciences Facility, University of California at Davis, Davis, CA, USA

M. Ramos-Casals et al. (eds.), *Sjögren's Syndrome*,
DOI 10.1007/978-0-85729-947-5_17, © Springer-Verlag London Limited 2012

17.1 Introduction

Liver involvement in Sjögren's syndrome (SS) is commonly subclinical and almost never appears as the first manifestation of the disease. The prevalence of liver involvement in SS varies among series and depends on the diagnostic criteria used. Studies conducted in the 1960s, based on clinical (i.e., liver enlargement) and serological (i.e., elevated alkaline phosphatase) findings estimated the SS liver involvement as high as 20% [1]. A somewhat lower prevalence of liver disease has been reported in more recent studies, with estimates ranging from 2% to 20% of SS patients [2–6].

Because the predominant markers of SS liver involvement are altered liver function tests (LFT), most studies of hepatic dysfunction in SS are based on these laboratory parameters. LFT are elevated in 5–49% of SS cases [2–6] and this wide variability may be secondary to different criteria used for the diagnosis of SS, the different population examined, and the inclusion of hepatitis C virus (HCV)-positive SS patients by some investigators. Analyzing the results of studies with larger populations of well-documented patients with SS [2, 3, 6], the occurrence of elevated LFT probably does not exceed 10%. The majority of such patients manifest a cholestatic pattern of LFT abnormality and a preserved liver function.

The association of liver involvement in SS with serum antimitochondrial antibodies (AMA) was first reported in 1970 [7] with studies on well-documented SS patient populations, observing a 5–10% antibody prevalence. Approximately, half of such patients have elevated LFT. However, LFT can be elevated in SS patients in the absence of AMA.

A 1994 study evaluated the histological features of SS patients with liver involvement [2]. Patients with elevated LFT or AMA in their sera underwent a liver biopsy. The typical histopathology observed was liver injury in a pericholangial pattern, similar to that detected in primary biliary cirrhosis at early stages. Another study also demonstrated that the main histological finding in the liver was that of cholangitis of variable severity [5]. More recently, Hatzis et al. examined the natural history of SS-associated cholangitis. Out of 410 SS patients, 36 (9%) had elevated LFT suggestive of cholestasis, among whom 21 (5%) had AMA, consistent with the presence of primary biliary cirrhosis (PBC). In addition, 6 patients were negative for AMA but their histological picture in liver biopsy was compatible with cholangitis. During a mean follow-up of 66 months, most individuals had stable liver disease but 27% experienced worsening of their LFT abnormalities and 4% had clinically relevant deterioration in hepatic function. The comparison of histology in five paired liver biopsies taken at a mean interval of 46 months showed no significant change [6].

The literature also includes sporadic cases of coexisting SS and autoimmune hepatitis or primary sclerosing cholangitis [8]. These comorbidities are rare and usually diagnosed on the basis of the autoantibody profile. All such putative cases require histological confirmation by an experienced pathologist.

17.2 Primary Biliary Cirrhosis (PBC)

17.2.1 Definition and Diagnosis

PBC is a chronic autoimmune liver disease that has a striking female predominance (9:1). The condition is characterized by progressive bile duct destruction that leads eventually to cirrhosis and liver failure. PBC is characterized histopathologically by portal inflammation and immune-mediated destruction of the intrahepatic bile ducts. The serologic hallmark of the disease is the presence of serum AMA, which are found in 90–95% of cases. AMA are directed against components of the 2-oxoacid dehydrogenase complex (2-OADC) family, including the E2 subunit of the pyruvate dehydrogenase complex (PDC-E2), the branched chain 2-oxo-acid dehydrogenase complex (BCOADC-E2), and the oxoglutarate dehydrogenase complex (OGDC-E2), as well as the dihydrolipoamide dehydrogenase (E3)-binding protein (E3BP) [9].

The 5–10% of patients with PBC who are AMA negative are referred as having autoimmune cholangitis (AIC). AMA-negative PBC or AIC manifests clinical features that are similar to those of AMA-positive PBC [10]. No clinical, biochemical, or histological differences exist between AMA-positive PBC and AIC. In the same studies, despite the AMA negativity by indirect immunofluorescence (IIF) in the sera from AIC patients, in some cases there was evident reactivity by immunoblotting with the E2 subunits of the 2-OADC enzymes, and particularly with the lower molecular weight E2 subunits [10].

17.2.2 Similarities, Differences, and Overlap Among SS and PBC

PBC and SS share several clinical, histological, and serological features, as well as pathogenetic mechanisms. Symptoms that are characteristic of SS – for example, dry mouth or dry eyes – are also found commonly in PBC (47–73%). In addition, objective findings of dry eyes or dry mouth (such as abnormal Schirmer test, or diminished salivary flow rate) are also found in 30–50% of patients with PBC while radiological findings of sialectasia were demonstrated in 25% of PBC cases. Furthermore, such PBC patients often manifest histological changes compatible with the diagnosis of SS at salivary gland biopsies (4) [11, 12].

Despite these similarities, patients with PBC differ from those with primary SS. They rarely have serious sequelae and their serological and immunogenetic features are not identical to those observed in patients with primary SS. Anti-Ro autoantibodies are rarely observed in PBC and the frequency of HLA-B8, -DR3, and DRW52 is lower compared to patients with primary SS. Thus, the association of SS with PBC is considered to be similar to that of secondary SS that complicates RA [13].

PBC has also been described to overlap with other diseases such as systemic sclerosis (SSc). Interestingly, the majority of the PBC-SSc patients suffer from the limited cutaneous form of the disease and are positive for anticentromere antibodies. Their clinical course and natural history of the disease seems to be milder than those of patients with PBC [14].

17.2.3   Epithelium Involvement

In both PBC and SS, the autoantibody targets (AMA, anti-Ro, and anti-La antibodies) are ubiquitous proteins expressed in all nucleated cells. Nevertheless, PBC and, to a lesser degree, SS are organ-specific diseases, indicating that epithelia (biliary epithelial cells and salivary gland epithelial cells for PBC and SS, respectively) are unlikely to be innocent victims but rather are active participants in disease pathogenesis. In agreement with the notion that epithelia play a major role are the kidney findings in SS. Indeed, the renal histopathological lesions in SS patients resemble those of the salivary glands (focal infiltrates around tubular epithelium that extend into and occupy the interstitium, resulting in tubular dysfunction) [15].

Several lines of evidence support the major role of epithelium for both PBC and SS. Biliary epithelial cells (BEC, i.e., cholangiocytes) express cell surface adhesion molecules that permit adhesion and recognition of lymphocytes. In addition, BECs of healthy as well as diseased liver have the capacity to increase the expression of adhesion molecules, MHC class I and II molecules, TNF-alpha, interferon (IFN)-gamma, and IL-1 upon stimulation with proinflammatory cytokines [16]. Most recently, a solid theory based on the unique apoptosis features in bile duct cells has been proposed [17]. It was first demonstrated that PDC-E2 remains intact and retains its immunogenicity during cholangiocyte apoptosis, secondary to a cell-specific lack of glutathionylation of BECs [18]. The intact PDC-E2 in apoptotic blebs (i.e., apotopes) could be then taken up by local antigen-presenting cells and transferred to regional lymph nodes for priming of cognate T cells, thereby initiating PBC [19].

17.2.4   Animal Models

The animal models for PBC and SS affirm that these two diseases share many common pathogenetic mechanisms. More specifically, one of the recently proposed mouse models for PBC is the NOD.c3c4 mouse where insulin-dependent diabetes (*Idd*) resistance loci from chromosomes 3 and 4 (including Idd3) were modified on the NOD background. These mice were diabetes resistant, yet developed extensive peribiliary lymphocytic infiltrates, granuloma-like lesions, and chronic nonsuppurative destructive cholangitis in the liver resembling PBC. Furthermore, 50–60% of the NOD.c3c4 mice produce AMA that react with the inner lipoyl domain of PDC-E2 and inhibit PDC enzyme function [20]. However, it is known that NOD strains manifest autoimmune diabetes and autoimmune exocrinopathy. More interestingly, Idd3 seems to be necessary for the manifestation of autoimmune exocrinopathy [21].

Other murine models have been described for PBC. Two animal models, that is, dnTGFβRII and IL-2Rα knockout mouse, point out the possible crucial role of Treg cell deficiency in the loss of immune tolerance with consequent development of autoimmune response against PDC-E2 in PBC. A mouse with dominant negative form of transforming growth factor β (TGFβ) receptor II, (dnTGFβRII) showed PBC-like liver disease, for example, 100% AMA positivity against PDC-E2 [22]. Of note, the depletion of B cells worsens liver disease in this model [23]. On the other hand, a mouse deficient for IL2 receptor α (IL-2Rα), which is highly expressed on Treg cells developed 100% AMA positivity against PDC-E2, 80% ANA positivity, and lymphocyte infiltration around the portal tracts associated with cholangiocyte injury [24].

Other animal models strongly support the hypothesis that xenobiotics can induce autoimmunity. Among these, the induction of PBC-like lesions was obtained in a NOD background by Wakabayashi et al. and in guinea pigs by Leung et al. exposed to xenobiotic immunization [20, 25] with halogenated compounds. Finally, the induction of a PBC-like phenotype following *N. aromaticivorans* immunization [26] has important potential implications.

17.2.5 Histology and Serology

Both SS and PBC are characterized by infiltrates developing around ducts, with CD4+ T cells predominating in the tissue lesions [27] (liver and minor salivary gland for PBC and SS, respectively) and NK cells being absent in lesions from PBC and very rare in those from SS [28]. In addition, T regulatory cells are found to be reduced in the peripheral blood of patients with PBC as well as of patients with SS compared to healthy controls [29].

The autoantibody profiles in PBC and SS are different, although the same wide spectrum of autoantibodies is present in both PBC and SS. Patients with SS have significantly higher frequencies of anti-Ro/SSA, anti-La/SSB, and anti-U1RNP, while patients with PBC have significantly higher frequencies of antibodies to PDC (i.e., AMA), Sm, Jo-1, collagen, and MPO [30].

The prevalence of serum ANA is higher in SS patients compared to PBC patients. In PBC, autoantibodies against nuclear antigens are found in the sera of about half of patients and are thought to be more prevalent among AMA-negative PBC patients [31]. Two patterns are highly specific for PBC: the multiple nuclear dot (MND) and rim-like/membranous (RL/M) immunofluorescence patterns. The first pattern is produced by autoantibodies against gp210 and nucleoporin 62 within the nucleopore complex and the second pattern by autoantibodies against sp100, promyelocytic leukemia (PML), and small ubiquitin-like modifier (SUMO) proteins.

Anti-pyruvate dehydrogenase complex (anti-PDC) antibodies, which are the hallmark of PBC, have been detected in other autoimmune rheumatic diseases by immunofluorescence. In a multicenter study, Zurgil et al. [32] examined sera from 1,400 patients with autoimmune rheumatic diseases and showed that anti-PDC antibodies detected by ELISA were present in 22% of SS patients, 17% of SLE patients, 10% of rheumatoid arthritis patients, and 10% of scleroderma patients. The prevalence of anti-PDH was higher among patients with coexistent SS and either SLE or RA compared to patients with only SLE or RA [32].

17.3   Autoimmune Hepatitis (AIH)

AIH is a chronic autoimmune liver disease of unknown etiology that can progress to cirrhosis. It is characterized histologically by an interface hepatitis, biochemically by elevated transaminase levels, and serologically by the presence of autoantibodies and increased levels of immunoglobulin G. Seropositivity for smooth muscle and/or antinuclear antibodies defines type 1 AIH, while positivity for liver kidney microsomal type 1 antibodies defines type 2 AIH, more common in pediatric ages [33, 34]. Anti-inflammatory/immunosuppressive treatment usually induce remission, since amelioration of symptoms is observed along with improvement in biochemical markers (aminotransferases, bilirubin, gamma globulin levels) and histological findings [35].

AIH and SS are rarely observed together. Until 2009, 56 cases of coexistence of AIH with SS had been described (all of them were of type 1 AIH) [20]. Of note, there are overlapping cases of AIH-PBC as up to 8% of AIH patients have autoantibodies against PDC. These individuals have histological features compatible with both AIH and PBC and a cholestatic biochemical pattern [36]. Indeed, many of the cases described with coexistence of SS with AIH manifested characteristics that were not typical for AIH but were consistent with the diagnosis of an overlapping syndrome of AIH-PBC.

17.4   Hepatitis C Virus (HCV) Infection and Sicca Syndrome

Viral infection has been considered for a long time as a putative trigger for SS. A possible association between HCV (found in the saliva) and SS was reported for the first time by Haddad in 1992 [37], who found that histological changes characteristic of SS were significantly more common in anti-HCV positive patients (57%) compared to controls (5%). From these patients, less than half complained of dry mouth and none reported dry eyes. Only later, Pawlotsky et al. examined 61 labial minor salivary gland biopsies of anti-HCV positive patients and reported that 49% had lymphocytic capillaritis. However, these patients did not have any *sicca* features or positive anti-Ro/SSA antibodies [38]. Scott et al., comparing salivary gland biopsies from 22 HCV patients and 10 SS patients, showed that there was similar degree of tissue damage but a lesser extent of inflammation in samples from HCV patients compared with those from SS patients [39]. Koike et al. reported that transgenic mice expressing HCV envelope genes developed exocrinopathy of lacrimal and salivary glands, which resembled SS [40].

HCV infection can produce a clinical picture that is very similar to SS. Comparing SS patients with and without HCV infection, SS patients with chronic HCV infections manifest a higher frequency of cryoglobulinemia and rheumatoid factor positivity compared to SS patients who do not have HCV, but the prevalence of anti-Ro/SSA and anti-La/SSB is lower. Extraglandular manifestations such as pulmonary, renal, or joint involvement are less common among HCV-infected SS patients [41–44]. In 2006, Ramos-Casals et al. compared SS patients who had autoimmune liver involvement with SS patients who had viral liver involvement. They reported that liver tests were elevated in the same pattern in the two groups, but the patients with autoimmune liver involvement had higher mean values of sedimentation rate, circulating gamma-globulins, and higher prevalence of serum ANA, AMA, anti-SMA, and anti-Ro/SSA and anti-La/SSB, while patients with chronic viral hepatitits had a higher frequency of cryoglobulinemia and hypocomplementemia [45].

Considering all these findings, HCV infection appears to be able to cause a clinical picture that is very similar, but not identical, to SS. In addition, there are histological and serological differences between these two clinical entities. Thus, a term that may be appropriate to describe this situation is "sicca syndrome associated with HCV infection."

17.5 Algorithm for the Diagnosis of Liver Involvement in SS

Taking into account all the above, we propose the following algorithm for patients with SS who have altered liver function tests (Fig. 17.1). First, hepatic steatosis, drug-induced liver injury, and metabolic and lymphoproliferative disorders that can affect the liver need to be excluded. Second, HCV infection must be excluded. Third, the serological and immunological profiles of the patient must be characterized. SS cases with a cholestatic pattern may have PBC (most of them are AMA positive). SS patients who have a hepatocellular biochemical pattern and are ANA or anti-SMA positive may have autoimmune hepatitis. Liver biopsy is reserved for cases in which the diagnosis cannot be made on the basis of serological or immunological profiles, or when histological data are required for staging purposes.

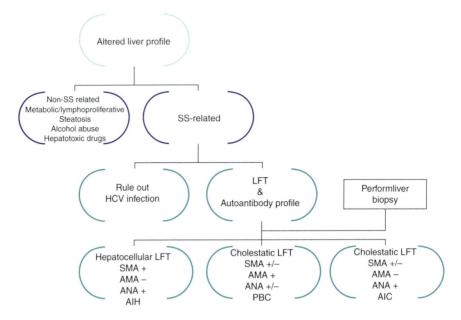

Fig. 17.1 Diagnostic algorithm for a SS patient with liver involvement. *LFT* liver function tests, *AIH* autoimmune hepatitis, *PBC* primary biliary cirrhosis, *AIC* autoimmune cholangitis

References

1. Bloch KJ, Buchanan WW, Wohl MJ, et al. Sjoegren's syndrome. A clinical, pathological and serological study of sixty-two cases. Medicine (Baltimore). 1965;44:187–231.
2. Skopouli FN, Barbatis C, Moutsopoulos HM. Liver involvement in primary Sjögren's syndrome. Br J Rheumatol. 1994;33(8):745–8.
3. Csepregi A, Szodoray P, Zeher M. Do autoantibodies predict autoimmune liver disease in primary Sjögren's syndrome? Data of 180 patients upon a 5 year follow-up. Scand J Immunol. 2002;56(6):623–9.
4. Kaplan MJ, Ike RW. The liver is a common non-exocrine target in primary Sjögren's syndrome: a retrospective review. BMC Gastroenterol. 2002;2:21.
5. Lindgren S, Manthorpe R, Eriksson S. Autoimmune liver disease in patients with primary Sjögren's syndrome. J Hepatol. 1994;20(3):354–8.
6. Hatzis GS, Fragoulis GE, Karatzaferis A, et al. Prevalence and longterm course of primary biliary cirrhosis in primary Sjögren's syndrome. J Rheumatol. 2008;35(10):2012–6.
7. Whaley K, Goudie RB, Williamson J, et al. Liver disease in Sjögren's syndrome and rheumatoid arthritis. Lancet. 1970;1(7652):861–3.
8. Zeher M, Szodoray P. Sjogren's syndrome and associated disorders. Published by Research Signpost, 2009.
9. Kaplan MM, Gershwin ME. Primary biliary cirrhosis. N Engl J Med. 2005;353(12):1261–73.
10. Invernizzi P, Crosignani A, Battezzati PM, et al. Comparison of the clinical features and clinical course of antimitochondrial antibody-positive and -negative primary biliary cirrhosis. Hepatology. 1997;25(5):1090–5.
11. Tsianos EV, Hoofnagle JH, Fox PC, et al. Sjögren's syndrome in patients with primary biliary cirrhosis. Hepatology. 1990;11(5):730–4.

12. Uddenfeldt P, Danielsson A, Forssell A, et al. Features of Sjögren's syndrome in patients with primary biliary cirrhosis. J Intern Med. 1991;230(5):443–8.
13. Andonopoulos AP, Drosos AA, Skopouli FN, et al. Secondary Sjögren's syndrome in rheumatoid arthritis. J Rheumatol. 1987;14(6):1098–103.
14. Rigamonti C, Shand LM, Feudjo M, et al. Clinical features and prognosis of primary biliary cirrhosis associated with systemic sclerosis. Gut. 2006;55(3):388–94.
15. Moutsopoulos HM, Kordossis T. Sjögren's syndrome revisited: autoimmune epithelitis. Br J Rheumatol. 1996;35(3):204–6.
16. Shimoda S, Harada K, Niiro H, et al. Biliary epithelial cells and primary biliary cirrhosis: the role of liver-infiltrating mononuclear cells. Hepatology. 2008;47:958–65.
17. Lleo A, Selmi C, Invernizzi P, et al. The consequences of apoptosis in autoimmunity. J Autoimmun. 2008;31:257–62.
18. Odin JA, Huebert RC, Casciola-Rosen L, et al. Bcl-2-dependent oxidation of pyruvate dehydrogenase-e2, a primary biliary cirrhosis autoantigen, during apoptosis. J Clin Invest. 2001;108:223–32.
19. Lleo A, Selmi C, Invernizzi P, et al. Apotopes and the biliary specificity of primary biliary cirrhosis. Hepatology. 2009;49:871–9.
20. Wakabayashi K, Yoshida K, Leung PS, et al. Induction of autoimmune cholangitis in non-obese diabetic (NOD).1101 mice following a chemical xenobiotic immunization. Clin Exp Immunol. 2009;155(3):577–86.
21. Cha S, Nagashima H, Brown VB, et al. Two NOD Idd-associated intervals contribute synergistically to the development of autoimmune exocrinopathy (Sjögren's syndrome) on a healthy murine background. Arthritis Rheum. 2002;46(5):1390–8.
22. Oertelt S, Lian ZX, Cheng CM, et al. Anti-mitochondrial antibodies and primary biliary cirrhosis in tgf-beta receptor ii dominant-negative mice. J Immunol. 2006;177:1655–60.
23. Moritoki Y, Zhang W, Tsuneyama K, et al. B cells suppress the inflammatory response in a mouse model of primary biliary cirrhosis. Gastroenterology. 2009;136:1037–47.
24. Wakabayashi K, Lian ZX, Moritoki Y, et al. Il-2 receptor alpha(−/−) mice and the development of primary biliary cirrhosis. Hepatology. 2006;44:1240–9.
25. Wakabayashi K, Lian ZX, Leung PS, et al. Loss of tolerance in c57bl/6 mice to the autoantigen e2 subunit of pyruvate dehydrogenase by a xenobiotic with ensuing biliary ductular disease. Hepatology. 2008;48:531–40.
26. Mattner J, Savage PB, Leung P, et al. Liver autoimmunity triggered by microbial activation of natural killer T cells. Cell Host Microbe. 2008;3:304–15.
27. Abraham S, Begum S, Isenberg D. Hepatic manifestations of autoimmune rheumatic diseases. Ann Rheum Dis. 2004;63(2):123–9.
28. Christodoulou MI, Kapsogeorgou EK, Moutsopoulos HM. Characteristics of the minor salivary gland infiltrates in Sjögren's syndrome. J Autoimmun. 2010;34(4):400–7.
29. Christodoulou MI, Kapsogeorgou EK, Moutsopoulos NM, et al. Foxp3+ T-regulatory cells in Sjogren's syndrome: correlation with the grade of the autoimmune lesion and certain adverse prognostic factors. Am J Pathol. 2008;173(5):1389–96.
30. Tishler M, Alosachie I, Barka N, et al. Primary Sjögren's syndrome and primary biliary cirrhosis: differences and similarities in the autoantibody profile. Clin Exp Rheumatol. 1995;13(4):497–500.
31. Invernizzi P, Selmi C, Ranftler C, et al. Antinuclear antibodies in primary biliary cirrhosis. Semin Liver Dis. 2005;25:298–310.
32. Zurgil N, Bakimer R, Moutsopoulos HM, et al. Antimitochondrial (pyruvate dehydrogenase) autoantibodies in autoimmune rheumatic diseases. J Clin Immunol. 1992;12(3):201–9.
33. Vergani D, Longhi MS, Bogdanos DP, et al. Autoimmune hepatitis. Semin Immunopathol. 2009;31(3):421–35. Epub 2009 Jun 17.
34. Krawitt EL. Clinical features and management of autoimmune hepatitis. World J Gastroenterol. 2008;14(21):3301–5.
35. Ishibashi H, Komori A, Shimoda S, et al. Guidelines for therapy of autoimmune liver disease. Semin Liver Dis. 2007;27(2):214–26.

36. Chazouilleres O, Wendum D, Serfaty L, Montembault S, Rosmorduc O, Poupon R. Primary biliary cirrhosis-autoimmune hepatitis overlap syndrome: clinical features and response to therapy. Hepatology. 1998;28:296–301.
37. Haddad J, Deny P, Munz-Gotheil C, et al. Lymphocytic sialadenitis of Sjögren's syndrome associated with chronic hepatitis C virus liver disease. Lancet. 1992;339(8789):321–3.
38. Pawlotsky JM, Ben Yahia M, Andre C, et al. Immunological disorders in C virus chronic active hepatitis: a prospective case-control study. Hepatology. 1994;19(4):841–8.
39. Scott CA, Avellini C, Desinan L, et al. Chronic lymphocytic sialoadenitis in HCV-related chronic liver disease: comparison of Sjögren's syndrome. Histopathology. 1997;30(1):41–8.
40. Koike K, Moriya K, Ishibashi K, et al. Sialadenitis histologically resembling Sjogren syndrome in mice transgenic for hepatitis C virus envelope genes. Proc Natl Acad Sci USA. 1997;94(1):233–6.
41. Loustaud-Ratti V, Riche A, Liozon E, et al. Prevalence and characteristics of Sjögren's syndrome or Sicca syndrome in chronic hepatitis C virus infection: a prospective study. J Rheumatol. 2001;28(10):2245–51.
42. García-Carrasco M, Ramos M, Cervera R, et al. Hepatitis C virus infection in 'primary' Sjögren's syndrome: prevalence and clinical significance in a series of 90 patients. Ann Rheum Dis. 1997;56(3):173–5.
43. Jorgensen C, Legouffe MC, Perney P, et al. Sicca syndrome associated with hepatitis C virus infection. Arthritis Rheum. 1996;39(7):1166–71.
44. Ramos-Casals M, García-Carrasco M, Cervera R, et al. Hepatitis C virus infection mimicking primary Sjögren syndrome. A clinical and immunologic description of 35 cases. Medicine (Baltimore). 2001;80(1):1–8.
45. Ramos-Casals M, Sánchez-Tapias JM, Parés A, et al. Characterization and differentiation of autoimmune versus viral liver involvement in patients with Sjögren's syndrome. J Rheumatol. 2006;33(8):1593–9.

Chapter 18
Pancreatic Disease in Sjögren's Syndrome and IgG4-Related Disease

Arezou Khosroshahi, John H. Stone, and Vikram Deshpande

Contents

A. Khosroshahi (✉) • J.H. Stone
Division of Rheumatology, Allergy and Immunology, Massachusetts General Hospital, Boston, MA, USA

V. Deshpande
Department of Pathology, Massachusetts General Hospital, Boston, MA, USA

M. Ramos-Casals et al. (eds.), *Sjögren's Syndrome*,
DOI 10.1007/978-0-85729-947-5_18, © Springer-Verlag London Limited 2012

18.1   Introduction

The pancreas is a compound tubular-alveolar gland composed of an exocrine portion (serous acini) and an endocrine portion (islets of Langerhans). The islet cells make up only 1% of the total pancreatic mass.

Chronic inflammation of the salivary and lacrimal glands in Sjögren's syndrome (SjS) results in xerostomia and keratoconjunctivitis sicca in 95% of patients [1]. The pancreas, an exocrine gland with some functional, anatomical, and histological similarities to salivary glands, has been thought to be involved in SjS. Investigators have assessed pancreatic involvement of SjS by analyzing the histopathological changes, evaluating the pancreatic endocrine and exocrine function, interrogating specific pancreatic antibodies, and applying radiological techniques such as endoscopic retrograde cholangiopancreatography (ERCP), computed tomography, and ultrasonography. There still remains significant uncertainty regarding the true prevalence of pancreatic involvement in SjS, largely because of the realization recently that substantial overlap exists between SjS and IgG4-related disease (IgG4-RD).

18.2   The Overlap Between SjS and IgG4-Related Disease

The concept of chronic pancreatitis associated with or caused by an autoimmune mechanism was outlined first in the early 1960s [2–5]. In 1975, Waldram et al. [6] described what they believed to be a new syndrome of chronic pancreatitis, sclerosing cholangitis, and sicca complex in two siblings. A subsequent case with pancreas and salivary gland involvement was reported by Sjögren et al. [7] in 1979. Those authors indicated that this syndrome might represent a distinct disease entity with a common pathogenic mechanism. Subsequent reports alluded to the coexistence of SjS with pancreatitis, pulmonary infiltrates or fibrosis, retroperitoneal fibrosis, sclerosing cholangitis, and pancreatic pseudotumors [8–11]. Successful glucocorticoid therapy for pancreatitis associated with SjS was documented in 1976 [12].

In 1995, the concept of autoimmune pancreatitis (AIP) was introduced to the medical literature [13] and as the knowledge about this condition grew, it was realized that many of the cases previously regarded as SjS are actually part of the IgG4-RD spectrum. It is worth noting that the association of SjS with fibroinflammatory manifestations has not been reported since the recognition of IgG4-RD. One can justifiably speculate that many of the reported cases of pancreatitis cases in patients with SjS had IgG4-related sialadenitis and not SjS.

Most studies evaluating patients with SjS have included some cases of IgG4-related sialadenitis with negative Sjögren's autoantibodies. Consequently, the literature on "SjS" and pancreatitis is riddled with potential inaccuracies and interpreting the true association between SjS and pancreatitis is complex. Table 18.1 summarizes the characteristics that help distinguish SjS from IgG4-related sialadenitis and IgG4-related dacryoadenitis.

Table 18.1 Clinical characteristics of Sjögren's syndrome and IgG4-related disease (IgG4-RD)

	Sjögren syndrome	IgG4-RD
Sex predominance	Female	Male
Gland swelling	Recurrent	Persistent
Keratoconjunctivitis sicca	Mild to severe	None to slight
Gland function	Impaired	Normal
Response to glucocorticoid	Not significant	Significant
Antinuclear antibody	Positive, high titer	Positive, low titer
Anti-Ro/La antibodies	Present	Not present
Elevated serum IgG4	None	Most cases
Gland pathology	Presence of severe lymphocytic infiltration with no IgG4+ plasma cells	Infiltration of abundant IgG4+ plasma cells and fibrosis

18.3 Involvement of the Pancreas in SjS

18.3.1 Clinical Presentation

The pancreas secretes approximately 1.5 L of enzyme-rich fluid every day for the digestion of fats, carbohydrates, and protein. Advanced pancreatic exocrine insufficiency results in maldigestion of fat and protein leading to steatorrhea and weight loss. Although subtle changes in exocrine function can be detected in patients with early pancreatic disease, overt steatorrhea does not occur until approximately 90% of glandular function has been lost [14]. Patients with mild pancreatic exocrine insufficiency may have subclinical maldigestion and normal appearing bowel movements, although latent fat-soluble vitamin deficiencies may be detected.

Pancreatic manifestations in patients with SjS are diverse. In a large series of patients with primary SjS, the prevalence of acute pancreatitis of any etiology was reported to be 0.5% [15]. Acute pancreatitis is reported less frequently than chronic pancreatitis in the medical literature [2], but there is no information available on the prevalence of chronic pancreatitis in these patients. The clinical presentation of acute pancreatitis, associated with abdominal pain, nausea, and vomiting, is uncommon in SjS patients.

Abnormal exocrine pancreatic function has been documented in up to one third of patients with SjS [16], but this usually remains subclinical. Patients with SjS rarely suffer from maldigestion or steatorrhea. Several studies have investigated pancreatic exocrine function in SjS [5, 17–23]. In these studies, various diagnostic tests have been used to evaluate pancreatic exocrine function. The results of these tests are variable and are mainly useful for detecting cases of advanced pancreatic failure, not subtle dysfunction. The pancreatic function studies in SjS have shown variable and sometimes discordant results. The findings have varied from an absence of involvement [5], to minimum involvement [19] or involvement in up to 30% of patients [16, 18].

One recent study performed in the post-IgG4-RD era evaluated pancreatic function of 12 SjS patients combining the secretin test and magnetic resonance cholangiography (MRCP). This study showed up to 80% of patients had normal exocrine function and 100% had normal duodenal filling [24].

The endocrine function of the pancreas seems to be unaffected by SjS. The frequency of type 2 diabetes mellitus in patients with primary SjS is higher than in age-matched controls, but this may be a function of several factors, particularly increased glucocorticoid use, decreased antimalarial use, and higher body mass index among patients with both SjS and type 2 diabetes compared to those with SjS alone [24, 25]. In summary, slightly reduced exocrine function is the most common pancreatic abnormality in patients with SjS, but this finding has little clinical consequence for patients in most cases.

18.3.2 Autoantibodies

The presence of antibodies to pancreatic antigen and pancreatic duct cells has been demonstrated in patients with SjS [16, 26]. Pancreatic duct autoantibodies were detected in the sera of patients with SjS who had abnormal exocrine pancreatic function [27]. One study showed that the sera from patients with SjS who had antibodies against salivary duct epithelial cells also had a positive intra- and interlobular immunofluorescence reaction to human and monkey pancreatic duct cells. These sera also demonstrated positive staining in parotid, submandibular, and lacrimal tissue from healthy controls, suggesting the presence of a common antigen in the studied organs [28]. The presence of these antibodies and autoreactivity does not imply that they are pathogenic. In theory, chronic glandular inflammation and antigen exposure may lead to the production of nonspecific antibodies that react to similar exocrine gland tissues, namely, the salivary gland and pancreas.

18.3.3 Pancreatic Enzymes

Patients with systemic lupus erythematosus and SjS are known to have elevated pancreatic enzymes in some cases. One study showed that 24% of patients with SjS had hyperamylasemia of isotypes P and S. However, these patients did not have any clinical symptoms of pancreatitis [29]. Higher values of trypsinogen have also been documented in these patients [17]. On the other hand there are reports of reduced amylase and/or lipase in the pancreatic juice in patients with SjS, which is consistent with exocrine hypofunction [24].

18.3.4 Pathology

There are few pathologic descriptions of pancreatic pathology in SjS. Furthermore, as alluded to earlier in this chapter, it is likely that many of the reports that document involvement of the pancreas in SjS, in hindsight, actually represent IgG4-RD.

Pathological changes of the pancreas in autopsied patients with SjS who had no pancreatic symptoms during life have been described. These changes include moderate levels of chronic pancreatitis, atrophy, replacement of pancreatic tissue by vascular connective tissue, and lymphocytic infiltration [5, 30, 31]. Autopsy of patients with SjS who had known pancreatic dysfunction showed similar histopathological findings to those reported previously in cases of asymptomatic patients [18].

18.3.5 Imaging Studies of the Pancreas

Evaluation of a group of patients with SjS and elevated pancreatic enzymes revealed no specific alteration in the morphology of the pancreas as assessed by computed tomography [17]. Magnetic resonance cholangiopancreatography of asymptomatic patients with SjS showed chronic pancreatitis-like changes in 2 out of 12 patients. None of these patients had radiologic changes characteristic of autoimmune pancreatitis (AIP) [32].

18.4 Autoimmune Pancreatitis

18.4.1 Introduction

AIP is a fibroinflammatory disease of the pancreas. Although this disease was described initially by Sarles and colleagues in the early 1960s, wider recognition took another 50 years [33]. The revival of interest in this disease was triggered by a case report from Japan [13]. In addition to reporting their case, the authors identified a cohort of previously published reports that describe patients with enlarged pancreata, many of which were responsive to glucocorticoids. We now believe that these cases were examples of AIP. In a landmark paper, Hamano and coworkers identified serum IgG4 as a biomarker of AIP [34].

Following the observation by Hamano and colleagues in serum, investigators demonstrated that the diseased pancreas in AIP is infiltrated with large numbers of IgG4-positive plasma cells [35, 36]. It is likely but unproven that the intrapancreatic IgG4-bearing plasma cells are the source of elevated serum IgG4 concentration. Another potential contributor to serum IgG4 elevation is IgG4-producing plasma cells infiltrating other organs as part of systemic IgG4-RD. Immunohistochemical detection of IgG4-positive plasma cells in pancreatic tissue is now widely regarded as a robust marker of AIP [35–37].

As pathologists examined their archived cases of pancreatitis, it became apparent that not all cases of AIP were associated with elevated serum and tissue levels of IgG4. It is now accepted that there are two forms of the disease "autoimmune-mediated" pancreatic inflammation, currently termed type 1 and type 2 AIP. Of these two

Table 18.2 List of conditions believed to be part of IgG4-RD spectrum

Previous name	Target organ(s)
Mikulicz's disease	Salivary and lacrimal glands
Küttner's tumor	Submandibular glands
Riedel's thyroiditis	Thyroid
Chronic sclerosing aortitis	Aorta
Inflammatory abdominal aortitis	Abdominal aorta
Retroperitoneal fibrosis	Retroperitoneum
Autoimmune pancreatitis	Pancreas
Sclerosing cholangitis	Biliary tree
Orbital pseudotumor	Orbital adnexa
Eosinophilic angiocentric fibrosis	Sinuses and nasal cavities
Multifocal fibrosclerosis	Various organs
Interstitial nephritis	Kidney

disease subsets, type 1 AIP is now viewed as being part of the IgG4-RD spectrum [36, 38]. Types 1 and 2 AIP have overlapping clinical and radiological features, but distinct differences exist between the two groups with regard to histopathologic features and relapse rates. Type 2 AIP may in fact be a novel form of chronic pancreatitis that should be considered an entirely separate category of disease [38].

18.4.2 Clinical Features

The type 1 variant of AIP typically affects elderly males in their 60s and 70s [36, 38]. The prototypical patient is an elderly man who presents with painless obstructive jaundice and weight loss. These patients show little overlap with other forms of chronic pancreatitis. Specifically, they do not report episodes of acute pancreatitis, although some complain of mild abdominal pain.

Patients with type 2 AIP are younger, with a mean age of 52 years [36]. Moreover, in contrast to type 1 AIP, which affects male patients almost exclusively, the male:female ratio in type 2 disease is approximately 1:1. At presentation, patients with type 2 AIP also show overlap with other forms of chronic pancreatitis. In one series, two thirds of patients had abdominal pain. In rare patients, more overt overlaps between acute and chronic pancreatitis are observed, with recurrent attacks of pancreatitis and pseudocyst formation.

Type 1 AIP is a systemic disease even though the pancreas may appear to be the sole manifestation of the disease at presentation. The presence of tumefactive lesions in other organ, either synchronously or metachronously, often clinch the diagnosis of AIP (see Table 18.2). For example, the finding of such extrapancreatic disease as tumefactive enlargement of the submandibular glands in an elderly male with obstructive jaundice strongly favors the diagnosis of AIP over that of pancreatic carcinoma. Type 2 AIP is less likely to have extrapancreatic manifestations, but there does appear to be a connection between type 2 AIP and inflammatory bowel disease.

In contrast to SjS, AIP can have profound effects on both the exocrine and endocrine function of the pancreas. Up to 80% of patients with AIP demonstrate laboratory evidence of exocrine dysfunction and diabetes [39].

18.4.3 Imaging

Two major radiologic abnormalities are observed in AIP: a diffuse enlargement of the pancreas and a focal tumefactive lesion [40]. Tumefactive lesions can bear close resemblance to pancreatic malignancies. CT imaging in AIP demonstrates an enlarged pancreas with a distinctive delay in the pattern of contrast enhancement [41, 42]. In addition, another highly suggestive sign of AIP is a capsule-like rim on the periphery of the pancreas. Pancreatograms in AIP typically show diffuse narrowings of the pancreatic duct, with ductal irregularities but without significant dilatation [43]. These characteristic imaging features, in conjunction with an elevated serum IgG4, often permit reliable diagnoses of AIP without the need for invasive testing. However, these criteria are not infallible and a pancreatic biopsy is often required, both to exclude carcinoma and provide confirmatory evidence of AIP (see Sect. 18.5.6).

18.4.4 Serology

Serum IgG4 remains the most reliable biomarker of AIP [38, 44, 45]. However, while the significant majority of cases of type 1 disease show an elevated serum IgG4 (normal serum IgG4 <140 mg/dL), those with type 2 AIP do not [38]. The overall reported sensitivities of elevated serum IgG4 concentrations for the diagnosis of AIP vary from 68% to 95%, but this is likely affected by the stage of disease and the fact that some studies have included patients with type 2 AIP [44]. An extensive array of other antibodies have been associated with AIP including anti-lactoferrin, anti-carbonic anhydrase II, anti-carbonic anhydrase-IV, anti-pancreatic secretory trypsin inhibitor, anti-amylase-alpha, anti-HSP-10, and antiplasminogen-binding protein (PBP) peptide autoantibodies [44, 46–48]. However, none of these antibodies have been validated, and the few studies available suggest that they are inferior to the serum IgG4 concentration as a disease biomarker. Of note, serum IgG4 levels are elevated in 10% of pancreatic adenocarcinomas [44]. Thus, no single serological test is diagnostic for AIP. IgG4 has also been suggested to be a potential biomarker for monitoring the disease recurrence. The search for a robust serological marker remains a major goal in AIP and IgG4-RD research (see below).

18.4.5 Pathology

There are significant differences in the histopathology of the two forms of AIP. In fact the only consistent feature shared by the two forms of the disease is the

Fig. 18.1 Fibroinflammatory infiltrate organized in a storiform pattern. This pattern of inflammation is seen both within the pancreas (autoimmune pancreatitis) and with IgG4-RD. Hematoxylin and Eosin stain

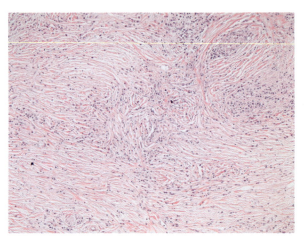

Fig. 18.2 Type 2 autoimmune pancreatitis. Note the periductal chronic inflammatory infiltrate (*arrow head*) and intraductal neutrophilic infiltrate (*arrow*). Hematoxylin and Eosin stain

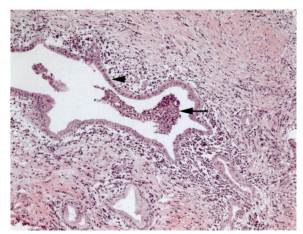

presence of periductal inflammation. Type 1 AIP is characterized by a storiform fibroinflammatory infiltrate, obliterative phlebitis, and occasionally obliterative arteritis (however, necrotizing features are absent) [36] (Fig. 18.1). In contrast, type 2 AIP shows a ductal pattern of injury, the most characteristic features of which are intraductal neutrophilic infiltrates, with microabscesses [36] (Fig. 18.2). More severe forms of ductal injury are also seen – ulceration and total loss of epithelial cells. These findings can be detected on needle biopsy specimens, enabling nonoperative management in many cases. Tissue immunostains for IgG4 have proven to be robust ancillary markers for the diagnosis of AIP. The presence of greater than 50 IgG4-positive plasma cells per high power field and an IgG4:IgG ratio of >50% is virtually diagnostic of type 1 AIP. Biopsies from patients with type 2 AIP lack this feature.

18.4.6   Diagnostic Criteria

The principle differential diagnosis remains pancreatic carcinoma, although AIP also shows overlapping features with other forms of chronic pancreatitis. AIP is significantly less common than pancreatic carcinoma. The low pretest probability of AIP and the significant overlap with pancreatic cancer invariably makes this a diagnostic challenge. In an attempt to facilitate the diagnosis of AIP, a plethora of diagnostic criteria have been proposed, the majority of which have been developed in Japan [49–52]. These algorithms rely on imaging, elevated serum IgG4, supportive biopsy findings and the presence of extrapancreatic disease. In addition, a clinical and radiological response to glucocorticoids is a component of some diagnostic algorithms, although the Japanese algorithms caution against using this parameter [39].

18.5   The Concept of IgG4-RD

18.5.1   Introduction

In 2000, Kamisawa and coworkers identified patients of AIP with extrapancreatic disease and proposed the concept of a systemic disease [53]. Over the next few years, it became apparent that the extrapancreatic forms of the disease can occur in the absence of pancreatic disease, and this realization transformed a relatively exotic pancreatic disease into a systemic disease that could be encountered by virtually every medical and surgical subspecialty. The pancreatic manifestation of this disease, type 1 AIP, now constitutes only a minority of IgG4-RD patients seen at the Massachusetts General Hospital. The two features that unify these apparently disparate diseases are elevated serum/tissue levels of IgG4 and characteristic histopathologic features [35, 54–56]. IgG4-RD joins that list of systemic diseases that are unified by histopathologic features, the prototype being sarcoidosis.

18.5.2   Nomenclature

The lack of a uniformly accepted name has been one of the factors that has stymied progress in this field. The following terms have been used commonly to describe this disease: IgG4-related autoimmune disease, IgG4-related sclerosing disease, systemic IgG4-related plasmacytic syndrome (SIPS), and IgG4+ positive multiorgan lymphoproliferative syndrome (MOLPS), IgG4-related systemic disease [39]. A study group in Japan proposed the term IgG4-RD, and we use this term to designate this multiorgan condition [57]. However, it must be acknowledged that the precise role played by IgG4 in this disorder is poorly understood. The term "IgG4-related" conveys our fundamental lack of understanding of this disease.

Table 18.3 Organs affected by IgG4-related disease	Pancreas
	Liver
	Bile duct
	Gallbladder
	Gastrointestinal tract
	Salivary and lacrimal glands
	Kidney
	Retroperitoneum and mesentery
	Lung
	Thyroid
	Aorta
	Orbit
	Mediastinum
	Prostate
	Breast
	Pituitary gland
	Meningitis
	Lymph nodes
	Skin

18.5.3   Clinical Manifestations

IgG4-RD involves virtually every organ in the body (Table 18.3). In the majority of cases, the disease manifests as a tumefactive lesion that has the potential to mimic a malignancy. Such is the case with involvement of the submandibular, parotid, and lacrimal glands (Fig. 18.3) [54, 58, 59]. Similar tumefactive lesions have been recognized in the meninges, lung, liver, retroperitoneum, kidney, breast, prostate, and other organs [60–63]. In fact, a significant proportion of cases previously classified as inflammatory pseudotumors belong to the IgG4-RD spectrum. A variety of disorders previously viewed as unrelated are now classified under the rubric of IgG4-RD, including Mikulicz's disease, Küttner tumor, and Riedel's thyroiditis (Table 18.2) [58, 64]. Patients with IgG4-RD often have multiorgan disease features, but the full extent of organ involvement may be either not present or not obvious at one particular time. A significant number of cases previously classified as "multifocal fibrosclerosis" actually represent IgG4-RD [65].

However, the spectrum of IgG4-RD also includes conditions that do not form tumefactive lesions. The prototypical example of this class is IgG4-related cholangitis [54, 66]. This disease mimics primary sclerosing cholangitis (PSC) but unlike PSC, IgG4-related cholangitis is a glucocorticoid-responsive disorder. IgG4-related aortitis, defined by lymphoplasmacytic infiltrates within the thoracic or abdominal aorta, generally presents with aneurysm or dissection rather than a tumefactive lesion (Fig. 18.4) [67].

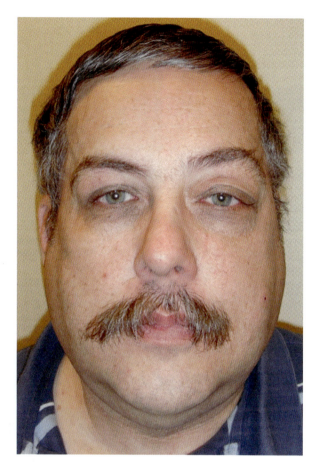

Fig. 18.3 A patient with IgG4-RD with tumefactive swelling of his parotids and lacrimal glands who was initially misdiagnosed with Sjögren's syndrome

18.5.4   Serological Issues

Patients with IgG4-RD may have polyclonal elevations of serum IgG4 concentrations up to 25 times the upper limit of normal [68]. Elevated serum concentrations of IgG4 are helpful in suggesting IgG4-RD but neither necessary nor sufficient for the diagnosis. Serum IgG4 concentrations tend to be higher in patients with multiple organ involvement.

18.5.5   Pathology

A lymphoplasmacytic infiltrate is observed in the great majority of cases, the only possible exceptions being the late phase of disease in which only acellular fibrosis maybe apparent (e.g., retroperitoneal fibrosis, Riedel's thyroiditis). A cuff of

Fig. 18.4 (**a**) Computed
tomographic angiogram
imaging of an aortic
aneurysm in a patient with
IgG4-related aortitis. (**b**) CT
imaging of a thoracic aortic
dissection in another patient
with IgG4-related aortitis

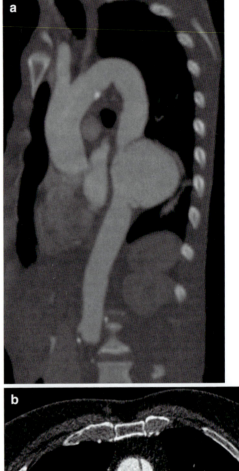

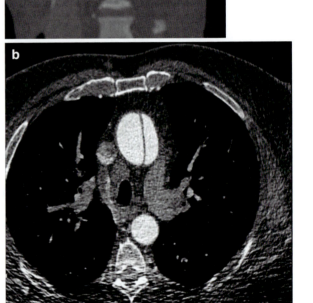

Fig. 18.5 (**a**) This biopsy from the lacrimal gland shows a dense lymphoplasmacytic infiltrate (Hematoxylin and Eosin stain); (**b**) Immunoperoxidase stain show large numbers of IgG4 positive plasma cells (Immunoperoxidase stain)

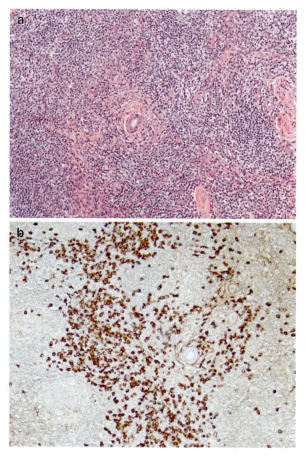

lymphocytes and plasma cells surrounding ducts tends to be present when the disease involves glands such as the pancreas or submandibular glands, but the lymphoplasmacytic infiltrate is also scattered throughout the tissue [36]. Eosinophils are often present and may be numerous [35].

The lymphoplasmacytic infiltrate and eosinophils are associated with fibrosis that generally occurs in a storiform pattern. In contrast, inflammatory pathology unrelated to IgG4-RD typically shows a "pattern-less" fibrosis [56]. Obliterative phlebitis is seen in most cases [69]. Granulomatous inflammation, necrosis, or fibrinoid necrosis of vessels argue strongly against the diagnosis of IgG4-RD. Neutrophils, particularly neutrophilic microabscesses are distinctly uncommon in IgG4-RD.

Positive staining for IgG4-bearing plasma cells can clinch the diagnosis in the appropriate clinical setting, but it is also essential that the IgG4-staining plasma cells be accompanied by histopathologic findings that are consistent with this diagnosis [56] (Fig. 18.5a, b). There remains no consensus on the minimum requirements for

IgG4-staining plasma cells within a pathologic sample and the numbers and percentages of IgG4-positive cells probably vary from tissue to tissue and stage of the disease. In general, however, one can feel comfortable about the diagnosis in the setting of ≥30 IgG4-positive plasma cells per high-power field and an IgG4:total IgG ratio of >50%.

18.5.6 Diagnostic Criteria

There are no widely accepted criteria for the diagnosis of IgG4-RD. Three key features are required for an unequivocal diagnosis of IgG4-RD, although it is not essential for all three are not present in all cases. These are either tumefactive organ enlargement or a destructive inflammatory infiltrate; an elevated serum IgG4 concentration; and pathologic features that include elevated numbers of IgG4-positive plasma cells and elevated IgG4:IgG ratios. A careful evaluation to exclude the diagnosis of lymphoma is required prior to rendering a diagnosis of IgG4-RD.

18.5.7 Pathogenesis of IgG4-RD

Despite the remarkable advances achieved in the clinical realm, much remains to be understood about the pathogenesis of IgG4-RD. Several lines of evidence are consistent with an autoimmune hypothesis, but an equally plausible alternate is that IgG4-RD is a chronic allergic reaction. Several human leukocyte antigen (HLA) (DRB1_0405 and DQB1_0401) and non-HLA haplotypes/genotypes have been associated with susceptibility to IgG4-related disease or to disease relapse after glucocorticoid therapy [70, 71].

The disease is typically associated with a T-helper 2 immune reaction, which may explain the robust IgG4 response in these individuals [72, 73]. But it is not certain that IgG4 antibody plays a direct pathogenetic role. Specific, target-directed autoantibodies of the IgG4 subclass have not been detected in IgG4-RD. Some studies have suggested that IgG4 suppresses the immune response, thereby fulfilling a protective role [74].

18.6 Conclusions

Pancreatic injury and exocrine dysfunction is a feature of SjS, but the true incidence of pancreatic dysfunction in this condition is difficult to assess. In contrast to AIP, a condition in which the exocrine dysfunction is often profound, the pancreatic involvement in SjS is relatively mild. IgG4-RD affects virtually the same organs as SjS including the salivary and lacrimal glands, pancreas, biliary tree, kidney, the lung, and skin. It is thus not surprising that many reports on SjS published prior to the recognition of IgG4-RD almost certainly represent the latter entity. The presence of elevated serum IgG4 and characteristic histological features further aided by IgG4 immunoperoxidase stain clinches diagnosis of IgG4-RD and excludes SjS.

References

1. Meijer JM, Meiners PM, Huddleston Slater JJ, Spijkervet FK, Kallenberg CG, Vissink A, et al. Health-related quality of life, employment and disability in patients with Sjogren's syndrome. Rheumatology (Oxford). 2009;48(9):1077–82.
2. Cardell BS, Gurling KJ. Observations on the pathology of Sjögren's syndrome. J Pathol Bacteriol. 1964;68:137–46.
3. Bloch KJ, Buchanan WW, Wohl MJ, Bunim JJ. Sjoegren's syndrome. A clinical, pathological, and serological study of sixty-two cases. Medicine (Baltimore). 1965;44:187–231.
4. Sarles H, Sarles JC, Muratore R, Guien C. Chronic inflammatory sclerosis of the pancreas – an autonomous pancreatic disease? Am J Dig Dis. 1961;6:688–98.
5. Fenster F, Buchanan WW, Laster L, Bunim J. Studies of pancreatic function in Sjögren's syndrome. Ann Intern Med. 1964;61:498–508.
6. Wakfram R, Kopelman H, Tsantoufas D, Williams Ft. Chronic pancreatitis, sclerosing cholangitis, and sicca complex in two siblings. Lancet. 1975;1:550–2.
7. Sjogren I, Wengle B, Korsgren M. Primary sclerosing cholangitis associated with fibrosis of the submandibular glands and the pancreas. Acta Med Scand. 1979;205(1–2):139–41.
8. Nieminen U, Koivisto T, Kahri A, Farkkila M. Sjögren's syndrome with chronic pancreatitis, sclerosing cholangitis, and pulmonary infiltrations. Am J Gastroenterol. 1997;92(1):139–42.
9. Fukui T, Okazaki K, Yoshizawa H, Ohashi S, Tamaki H, Kawasaki K, et al. A case of autoimmune pancreatitis associated with sclerosing cholangitis, retroperitoneal fibrosis and Sjögren's syndrome. Pancreatology. 2005;5(1):86–91.
10. Pickartz T, Pickartz H, Lochs H, Ockenga J. Overlap syndrome of autoimmune pancreatitis and cholangitis associated with secondary Sjogren's syndrome. Eur J Gastroenterol Hepatol. 2004;16(12):1295–9.
11. Eckstein RP, Hollings RM, Martin PA, Katelaris CH. Pancreatic pseudotumor arising in association with Sjogren's syndrome. Pathology. 1995;27(3):284–8.
12. Nakamura M, Okumura N, Sakakibara A, Kawai H, Takeichi M, Kanzaki M. A case of Sjögren's syndrome presenting pancreatitis symptoms which responded to steroid therapy. Proc Jpn Pancreas Soc. 1976;6:135–6.
13. Yoshida K, Toki F, Takeuchi T, Watanabe S, Shiratori K, Hayashi N. Chronic pancreatitis caused by an autoimmune abnormality. Proposal of the concept of autoimmune pancreatitis. Dig Dis Sci. 1995;40(7):1561–8.
14. DiMagno EP, Go VL, Summerskill WH. Relations between pancreatic enzyme and malabsorption in severe pancreatic insufficiency. N Engl J Med. 1973;288(16):813–5.
15. Ramos-Casals M, Solans R, Rosas J, Camps MT, Gil A, Del Pino-Montes J, et al. Primary Sjogren syndrome in Spain: clinical and immunologic expression in 1010 patients. Medicine (Baltimore). 2008;87(4):210–9.
16. Sheikh SH, Shaw-Stiffel TA. The gastrointestinal manifestations of Sjogren's syndrome. Am J Gastroenterol. 1995;90(1):9–14.
17. Ostuni PA, Gazzetto G, Chieco-Bianchi F, Riga B, Plebani M, Betterle C, et al. Pancreatic exocrine involvement in primary Sjogren's syndrome. Scand J Rheumatol. 1996;25(1):47–51.

18. Coll J, Navarro S, Tomas R, Elena M, Martinez E. Exocrine pancreatic function in Sjogren's syndrome. Arch Intern Med. 1989;149(4):848–52.
19. Nishimori I, Morita M, Kino J, Onodera M, Nakazawa Y, Okazaki K, et al. Pancreatic involvement in patients with Sjogren's syndrome and primary biliary cirrhosis. Int J Pancreatol. 1995;17(1):47–54.
20. Hradsky M, Bartos V, Keller O. Pancreatic function in Sjogren's syndrome. Gastroenterologia. 1967;108(5):252–60.
21. Lankishc PG, Arglebe C, Chilla R. Pancreatic function in Sjogren's syndrome. Dig Dis Sci. 1988;33:11.
22. Gobelet C, Gerster JC, Rappoport G, Hiroz CA, Maeder E. A controlled study of the exocrine pancreatic function in Sjogren's syndrome and rheumatoid arthritis. Clin Rheumatol. 1983;2(2):139–43.
23. Kelly CA, Katrak A, Griffiths ID. Pancreatic function in patients with primary Sjogren's syndrome. Br J Rheumatol. 1993;32(2):169.
24. Afzelius P, Fallentin EM, Larsen S, Moller S, Schiodt M. Pancreatic function and morphology in Sjogren's syndrome. Scand J Gastroenterol. 2010;45(6):752–8.
25. Ramos-Casals M, Brito-Zeron P, Siso A, Vargas A, Ros E, Bove A, et al. High prevalence of serum metabolic alterations in primary Sjogren's syndrome: influence on clinical and immunological expression. J Rheumatol. 2007;34(4):754–61.
26. Onodera M, Okazaki K, Morita M, Nishimori I, Yamamoto Y. Immune complex specific for the pancreatic duct antigen in patients with idiopathic chronic pancreatitis and Sjogren's syndrome. Autoimmunity. 1994;19(1):23–9.
27. Sundkvist G, Lindahlg G, Koskinene P, Bolinder J. Pancreatic autoantibodies and pancreatic function in Sjögreńs syndrome. Int J Pancreatol. 1991;8:141–9.
28. Ludwig H, Schernthaner G, Scherak O, Kolarz G. Antibodies to pancreatic duct cells in Sjögren's syndrome and rheumatoid arthritis. Gut. 1977;18:311–5.
29. Tsianos EB, Tzioufas AG, Kita MD, Tsolas O, Moutsopoulos HM. Serum isoamylases in patients with autoimmune rheumatic diseases. Clin Exp Rheumatol. 1984;2(3):235–8.
30. Szanto L, Farkas K, Gyulai E. On Sjogren's disease. Rheumatism. 1957;13(3):60–3.
31. Bucher UG, Reid L. Sjogren's syndrome: report of a fatal case with pulmonary and renal lesions. Br J Dis Chest. 1959;53:237–52.
32. Kamisawa T, Tu Y, Egawa N, Tsuruta K, Okamoto A, Kodama M, et al. Can MRCP replace ERCP for the diagnosis of autoimmune pancreatitis? Abdom Imaging. 2009;34(3):381–4.
33. Camatte R, Sarles H. Treatment of digestive disorders of allergic origin with prothipendyl hydrochloride (Dominal). Sem Hop. 1961;37:2989–94.
34. Hamano H, Kawa S, Horiuchi A, Unno H, Furuya N, Akamatsu T, et al. High serum IgG4 concentrations in patients with sclerosing pancreatitis. N Engl J Med. 2001;344(10):732–8.
35. Deshpande V, Chicano S, Finkelberg D, Selig MK, Mino-Kenudson M, Brugge WR, et al. Autoimmune pancreatitis: a systemic immune complex mediated disease. Am J Surg Pathol. 2006;30(12):1537–45.
36. Deshpande V, Gupta R, Sainani NI, Sahani DV, Virk R, Ferrone CR, et al. Subclassification of autoimmune pancreatitis: a histologic classification with clinical significance. Am J Surg Pathol. 2011;35:26–35.
37. Zhang L, Notohara K, Levy MJ, Chari ST, Smyrk TC. IgG4-positive plasma cell infiltration in the diagnosis of autoimmune pancreatitis. Mod Pathol. 2007;20(1):23–8.
38. Sah RP, Chari ST, Pannala R, Sugumar A, Clain JE, Levy MJ, et al. Differences in clinical profile and relapse rate of type 1 versus type 2 autoimmune pancreatitis. Gastroenterology. 2010;139(1):140–8; quiz e12–3.
39. Okazaki K, Kawa S, Kamisawa T, Shimosegawa T, Tanaka M. Japanese consensus guidelines for management of autoimmune pancreatitis: I. Concept and diagnosis of autoimmune pancreatitis. J Gastroenterol. 2010;45(3):249–65.
40. Frulloni L, Scattolini C, Falconi M, Zamboni G, Capelli P, Manfredi R, et al. Autoimmune pancreatitis: differences between the focal and diffuse forms in 87 patients. Am J Gastroenterol. 2009;104(9):2288–94.

41. Sahani DV, Kalva SP, Farrell J, Maher MM, Saini S, Mueller PR, et al. Autoimmune pancreatitis: imaging features. Radiology. 2004;233(2):345–52.
42. Irie H, Honda H, Baba S, Kuroiwa T, Yoshimitsu K, Tajima T, et al. Autoimmune pancreatitis: CT and MR characteristics. AJR Am J Roentgenol. 1998;170(5):1323–7.
43. Sugumar A, Levy MJ, Kamisawa T, JM Webster G, Kim MH, Enders F, et al. Endoscopic retrograde pancreatography criteria to diagnose autoimmune pancreatitis: an international multicentre study. Gut. 2011;60(5):666–70.
44. Sah RP, Chari ST. Serologic issues in IgG4-related systemic disease and autoimmune pancreatitis. Curr Opin Rheumatol. 2011;23(1):108–13.
45. Ghazale A, Chari ST, Smyrk TC, Levy MJ, Topazian MD, Takahashi N, et al. Value of serum IgG4 in the diagnosis of autoimmune pancreatitis and in distinguishing it from pancreatic cancer. Am J Gastroenterol. 2007;102(8):1646–53.
46. Raina A, Greer JB, Whitcomb DC. Serology in autoimmune pancreatitis. Minerva Gastroenterol Dietol. 2008;54(4):375–87.
47. Finkelberg DL, Sahani D, Deshpande V, Brugge WR. Autoimmune pancreatitis. N Engl J Med. 2006;355(25):2670–6.
48. Frulloni L, Lunardi C, Simone R, Dolcino M, Scattolini C, Falconi M, et al. Identification of a novel antibody associated with autoimmune pancreatitis. N Engl J Med. 2009;361(22): 2135–42.
49. Okazaki K, Kawa S, Kamisawa T, Naruse S, Tanaka S, Nishimori I, et al. Clinical diagnostic criteria of autoimmune pancreatitis: revised proposal. J Gastroenterol. 2006;41(7):626–31.
50. Kasai T, Miyauchi K, Kurata T, Satoh H, Ohta H, Tanimoto K, et al. Long-term (11-year) statin therapy following percutaneous coronary intervention improves clinical outcome and is not associated with increased malignancy. Int J Cardiol. 2007;114(2):210–7.
51. Chari ST. Diagnosis of autoimmune pancreatitis using its five cardinal features: introducing the Mayo Clinic's HISORt criteria. J Gastroenterol. 2007;42 Suppl 18:39–41.
52. Otsuki M, Chung JB, Okazaki K, Kim MH, Kamisawa T, Kawa S, et al. Asian diagnostic criteria for autoimmune pancreatitis: consensus of the Japan-Korea Symposium on Autoimmune Pancreatitis. J Gastroenterol. 2008;43(6):403–8.
53. Kamisawa T, Egawa N, Nakajima H. Autoimmune pancreatitis is a systemic autoimmune disease. Am J Gastroenterol. 2003;98(12):2811–2.
54. Deshpande V, Sainani NI, Chung RT, Pratt DS, Mentha G, Rubbia-Brandt L, et al. IgG4-associated cholangitis: a comparative histological and immunophenotypic study with primary sclerosing cholangitis on liver biopsy material. Mod Pathol. 2009;22(10):1287–95.
55. Deshpande V, Mino-Kenudson M, Brugge W, Lauwers GY. Autoimmune pancreatitis: more than just a pancreatic disease? A contemporary review of its pathology. Arch Pathol Lab Med. 2005;129(9):1148–54.
56. Cheuk W, Chan JK. IgG4-related sclerosing disease: a critical appraisal of an evolving clinico-pathologic entity. Adv Anat Pathol. 2010;17(5):303–32.
57. Okazaki K, Uchida K, Miyoshi H, Ikeura T, Takaoka M, Nishio A. Recent concepts of autoimmune pancreatitis and IgG4-related disease. Clin Rev Allergy Immunol. 2011;41:126–38.
58. Geyer JT, Deshpande V. IgG4-associated sialadenitis. Curr Opin Rheumatol. 2011;23(1): 95–101.
59. Geyer JT, Ferry JA, Harris NL, Stone JH, Zukerberg LR, Lauwers GY, et al. Chronic sclerosing sialadenitis (Kuttner tumor) is an IgG4-associated disease. Am J Surg Pathol. 2010;34(2):202–10.
60. Zen Y, Kitagawa S, Minato H, Kurumaya H, Katayanagi K, Masuda S, et al. IgG4-positive plasma cells in inflammatory pseudotumor (plasma cell granuloma) of the lung. Hum Pathol. 2005;36(7):710–7.
61. Cornell LD, Chicano SL, Deshpande V, Collins AB, Selig MK, Lauwers GY, et al. Pseudotumors due to IgG4 immune-complex tubulointerstitial nephritis associated with autoimmune pancreatocentric disease. Am J Surg Pathol. 2007;31(10):1586–97.
62. Lindstrom KM, Cousar JB, Lopes MB. IgG4-related meningeal disease: clinico-pathological features and proposal for diagnostic criteria. Acta Neuropathol. 2010;120(6):765–76.

63. Zen Y, Onodera M, Inoue D, Kitao A, Matsui O, Nohara T, et al. Retroperitoneal fibrosis: a clinicopathologic study with respect to immunoglobulin G4. Am J Surg Pathol. 2009;33(12):1833–9.
64. Movitz C, Brive L, Hellstrand K, Rabiet MJ, Dahlgren C. The annexin I sequence gln(9)-ala(10)-trp(11)-phe(12) is a core structure for interaction with the formyl peptide receptor 1. J Biol Chem. 2010;285(19):14338–45.
65. Bartholomew LG, Cain JC, Woolner LB, Utz DC, Ferris DO. Sclerosing cholangitis: its possible association with Riedel's struma and fibrous retroperitonitis. Report of two cases. N Engl J Med. 1963;269:8–12.
66. Ghazale A, Chari ST, Zhang L, Smyrk TC, Takahashi N, Levy MJ, et al. Immunoglobulin G4-associated cholangitis: clinical profile and response to therapy. Gastroenterology. 2008;134(3):706–15.
67. Stone JR. Aortitis, periaortitis, and retroperitoneal fibrosis, as manifestations of IgG4-related systemic disease. Curr Opin Rheumatol. 2011;23(1):88–94.
68. Khosroshahi A, Stone JR, Pratt DS, Deshpande V, Stone JH. Painless jaundice with serial multi-organ dysfunction. Lancet. 2009;373(9673):1494.
69. Zen Y, Nakanuma Y. IgG4-related disease: a cross-sectional study of 114 cases. Am J Surg Pathol. 2010;34(12):1812–9.
70. Kawa S, Ota M, Yoshizawa K, Horiuchi A, Hamano H, Ochi Y, et al. HLA DRB10405-DQB10401 haplotype is associated with autoimmune pancreatitis in the Japanese population. Gastroenterology. 2002;122(5):1264–9.
71. Zen Y, Nakanuma Y. Pathogenesis of IgG4-related disease. Curr Opin Rheumatol. 2011;23(1): 114–8.
72. Zen Y, Fujii T, Harada K, Kawano M, Yamada K, Takahira M, et al. Th2 and regulatory immune reactions are increased in immunoglobin G4-related sclerosing pancreatitis and cholangitis. Hepatology. 2007;45(6):1538–46.
73. Okazaki K, Uchida K, Ohana M, Nakase H, Uose S, Inai M, et al. Autoimmune-related pancreatitis is associated with autoantibodies and a Th1/Th2-type cellular immune response. Gastroenterology. 2000;118(3):573–81.
74. Aalberse RC, Schuurman J. IgG4 breaking the rules. Immunology. 2002;105(1):9–19.

Chapter 19
Nephro-Urological Involvement

Andreas V. Goules and Haralampos M. Moutsopoulos

Contents

A.V. Goules (✉) • H.M. Moutsopoulos
Department of Pathophysiology, School of Medicine, University of Athens, Athens, Greece

M. Ramos-Casals et al. (eds.), *Sjögren's Syndrome*,
DOI 10.1007/978-0-85729-947-5_19, © Springer-Verlag London Limited 2012

19.1   Introduction

One of the parenchymal organs that can be affected in patients with Sjögren's syndrome (SS) is the kidney [1]. Kidneys in primary SS (pSS) can be a target of the immune system either by activated lymphocytes that infiltrate the renal interstitium resulting in interstitial nephritis (IN) or by an immune complex mediated process appearing as glomerulonephritis (GN). Furthermore, epidemiologic and immunologic data suggest an association between SS and painful bladder syndrome/interstitial cystitis (PBS/IC), a chronic pelvic pain syndrome that produces lower urinary symptoms such as discomfort related to bladder, nocturia, frequency, and urge to void [1]. The term interstitial cystitis is reserved for patients with specific histologic lesions including lymphocytic inflammatory infiltrate of the submucosa and detrusor mastocytosis.

19.2   Interstitial Nephritis in Primary Sjögren's Syndrome

19.2.1   Historical Aspects

IN is by far the most common type of renal involvement in pSS. In 1962, Kahn et al. performed renal function studies in eight SS patients and found that half had persistent hyposthenuria, suggesting a primary concentrating defect due to impaired water permeability of the distal convoluted tubules and collecting ducts [2]. Shearn et al. described a patient with SS who presented with nephrogenic diabetes insipidus, renal tubular acidosis (RTA), and Fanconi syndrome and proposed that SS could be a cause of acquired Fanconi syndrome due to renal tubular dysfunction [3]. Nephrogenic diabetes insipidus has been reported to occur in pSS patients with IN and was clinically expressed by polydipsia and polyuria as a result of inadequate response of the distal renal tubules to the action of vasopressin [4]. Latent distal RTA (dRTA) in SS, manifested by an inability to lower urinary pH below 5.5 after an acid loading test (i.e., administration of ammonium chloride), was first described by Shearn and Tu [5]. Subsequently, Tu et al. reported histologic features of IN in six out of eight patients with SS [6]. Talal et al. demonstrated that the major histologic finding in patients with SS and dRTA was a chronic lymphocytic infiltration of interstitium, strongly supporting that these periepithelial lesions could be the cause of renal tubular defects [7]. These data were then confirmed by Shioji et al., who described similar histologic findings in SS patients with dRTA but not in SS patients without this complication [8]. Hence, the clinical manifestations and urinary abnormalities of IN in pSS were pathogenetically associated with periepithelial lymphocytic infiltration of renal tubules.

19.2.2   Clinical Features

IN is an early complication of pSS, and dRTA may be present many years before disease onset. Eriksson et al. after evaluating ten patients with dRTA and urolithiasis without subjective sicca symptoms, found that eight of them had anti-Ro/SSA and anti-La/SSB autoantibodies and seven of them developed SS after a mean of 15 years [9]. Pertovaara et al. reported that high serum levels of gammaglobulin, total serum protein, and beta-2 microglobulin were the best predictors of dRTA in pSS [10] but these findings have not been confirmed by other investigators.

In large series, the prevalence of dRTA and IN among pSS patients ranges from 11% to 48% [11–16]. Although IN occurs in almost one third of patients with pSS, it usually remains asymptomatic [17]. Most of these patients may present with complete or incomplete dRTA. Latent dRTA is characterized by impaired urinary acidification and evolves subclinically. This specific disorder seems to represent an incomplete form of dRTA that remains clinically silent but can be revealed after an acid loading test. Patients with latent dRTA are able to maintain normal acid–base balance with the usual dietary and endogenous hydrogen ion quantities, but exhibit an impaired urinary acidification under conditions of acid excess. On the other hand, complete dRTA constitutes the clinically apparent form of IN and may present with persistent alkaline urinary pH and hyposthenuria, hyperchloremic metabolic acidosis with an anion gap, hypokalemia, and hypercalciuria [18]. Longstanding dRTA, complete or incomplete, can lead to nephrolithiasis/nephrocalcinosis, renal colics and renal insufficiency (Fig. 19.1).

Hypercalciuria due to chronic acidosis, alkaline urine, and low levels of urine citrate contribute to renal stone formation. In some cases, hypokalemia is severe enough to cause muscular weakness expressed by periodic paralysis [12, 19–23]. Nephrogenic diabetes insipidus is centered in this particular spectrum of complete dRTA since inadequate response to vasopressin represents a tubular defect at this specific portion of the nephron. Some pSS patients may present with type 2 RTA and Fanconi syndrome rather than dRTA [3, 23–25]. Proximal renal tubule, although less frequently, can also be affected in pSS leading to impaired reabsorption of various nutrients and minerals. Fanconi syndrome is characterized by glucosuria, phosphaturia, aminoaciduria and tubular proteinuria but the complete form of the syndrome is rarely observed in pSS. In Table 19.1, the major clinical and laboratory findings of IN are presented.

Severe renal involvement due to IN is rare and has a good prognosis at least for several years. In a study of 471 pSS patients who were followed up from 1 to 15 years, 20 (4.2%) patients presented overt renal disease that was severe enough to warrant a kidney biopsy [26]. Ten patients were diagnosed as having IN, eight with GN, and two fulfilled criteria for both entities. Clinically significant IN was manifested by renal colics, polydipsia, polyuria, and nocturia. The major urinary abnormalities were persistently low specific gravity and alkaline urinary pH.

Fig. 19.1 Plain abdominal film of a patient with primary Sjögren's syndrome and nephrocalcinosis due to renal tubular acidosis

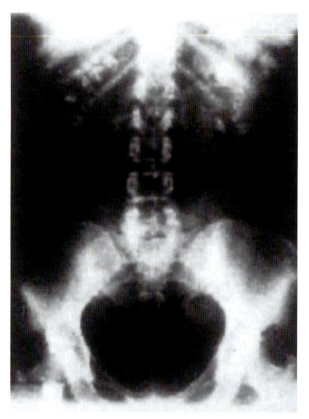

Table 19.1 The major clinical and laboratory findings of IN in pSS

Type of involvement	Clinical and laboratory findings
Latent distal RTA	Impaired urinary acidification after acid loading test
Complete distal RTA	Persistent alkaline urinary pH, hyposthenuria, hyperchloremic hypokalemic metabolic acidosis with anion gap
Nephrogenic diabetes insipidus	Polydipsia, polyuria
Proximal RTA	Fanconi syndrome (proteinuria, aminoaciduria, glucosuria, phosphaturia)
Nephrocalcinosis	Renal colics, renal insufficiency

Abbreviations: *IN* interstitial nephritis, *pSS* primary Sjögren's syndrome, *RTA* renal tubular acidosis

These data suggest that most cases of IN are asymptomatic and may escape clinical attention. Thus, the prevalence of severe IN in pSS is low and does not exceed 2.5% of pSS population. In addition, IN follows a rather benign course in pSS and has a favorable outcome, since none of the patients developed end-stage renal failure.

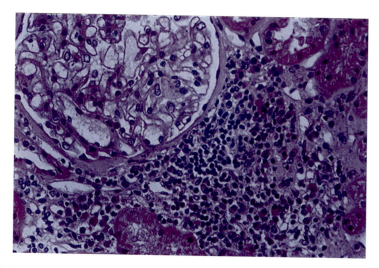

Fig. 19.2 Focal lymphocytic infiltration of kidney interstitium in a patient with primary Sjögren's syndrome and interstitial nephritis (Hematoxylin and eosin × 200)

19.2.3 Histology

The histologic hallmark of IN is periepithelial lymphocytic infiltration of renal tubules (Fig. 19.2) similar to that observed around the epithelium of salivary and lacrimal glands. This fact implies a common immunological process that occurs early in the disease course. The inflammatory infiltrate consists mainly of mature lymphocytes; plasma cells and monocytes participate to a lesser extent [7, 8, 27, 28]. Variable degree of interstitial fibrosis and tubular atrophy, along with hyaline casts and degeneration of tubular epithelial cells, can be also observed [7, 8]. Another histologic feature is the presence of a subset of lymphocytes that invades the epithelium and produces the histologic picture of tubulitis [27]. Immunofluorescence studies rarely reveal trace staining of the interstitium and the tubular basement membrane with immunoglobulins and C3 [28].

19.2.4 Pathogenesis

Almost 50% of the infiltrating cells bear the CD4 phenotype, while CD8-positive cells account for 25% of the total population [27]. This increased CD4/CD8 ratio is similar to that observed in the salivary gland lesion. However, the majority of these T lymphocytes express a restricted repertoire of TCR Vβ genes compared to that of salivary glands, suggesting that T cells that infiltrate the kidney of SS patient with IN, might recognize different autoantigens than those that infiltrate the salivary glands [29]. On the contrary, monocytes and B cells comprise only minor components of the infiltrating cell population [27].

The invading cells consist exclusively of CD8-positive cells that exhibit cytotoxic properties and may participate in tissue damage [27]. On the other hand, epithelial cells seem to play a central role in the pathogenesis of IN. Renal tubular epithelium has been found to express adhesion molecules such as ICAM-1 in and around the foci of cellular infiltration, implying that tubular epithelial cells contribute to the induction and maintenance of lymphocytic infiltrates of IN [30]. Furthermore, it has been demonstrated that tubular epithelial cells from SS patients with IN express the CD86 costimulatory molecule, activating the adjacent CD28 positive T cells [31]. Finally, Fas-FasL-mediated apoptotic changes of tubular epithelial cells have been observed in patients with SS and IN [32]. The above data confirm the notion that extraglandular manifestations share common immunopathological features with the primary glandular lesion and justify the term autoimmune epithelitis for SS.

Considering the pathogenesis of dRTA in pSS, antibodies against carbonic anhydrase (CA) II are implied to be involved. Anti-CA II autoantibodies have been found to induce autoimmune sialadenitis in experimental animal models [33] and have been detected in the serum of pSS patients [34–36]. In this context, Takemoto et al. measured the levels of anti-CA II in 46 subjects with pSS from whom 16 had been diagnosed with dRTA [37]. Antibody levels were found significantly higher in pSS patients with dRTA than those without, and correlated with increased $\beta2$ micro-globulin in the urine and disease duration. Furthermore, anti-CA II antibodies have been shown to induce RTA in a mouse model of SS [38]. Whether anti-CA II anti-bodies are produced in response to tubular damage or are pathogenetically associated with dRTA in pSS remains to be elucidated.

19.2.5   Differential Diagnosis

The other most important medical conditions that lead to dRTA (type 1 RTA) are drugs such as lithium and ifosfamide and hereditary forms of dRTA that most commonly affect children [39]. A careful family and personal history along with clinical evaluation will differentiate SS from other causes of dRTA. In SS patients with dRTA, the clinical picture is dominated by sicca symptoms and autoantibodies such as antinuclear antibodies (ANA), anti-Ro/SSA, and/or anti-La/SSB antibodies are usually present. In idiopathic cases of dRTA and nephrolithiasis, the patients should be evaluated for SS because these complications may precede the main disease by many years. The differential diagnosis of type 2 RTA and Fanconi syndrome includes various types of familial disorders, drugs (e.g., acetazolamide, a carbonic anhydrase inhibitor), toxins such as heavy metals, and multiple myeloma [39, 40]. Thus, before proximal RTA is attributed to SS, these entities should be excluded.

19.2.6   Treatment

Alkali supplements are the cornerstone of therapy for the management of patients with dRTA to control acidosis and prevent renal stone formation. The dose ranges from 1 to 2 mEq/kg body weight divided in four doses per day and is gradually raised until hypercalciuria and acidosis are both eliminated [39]. Potassium alkali salts are indicated if persistent hypokalemia is present. For patients with proximal RTA, alkali salts of 10–15 mEq/kg body weight per day may be required to compensate for renal losses [39]. Alkali replacement must be administered as potassium salts because of increased renal loss of potassium due to bicarbonaturia. The addition of a thiazide diuretic may reduce the amounts of alkali salts requirements [41]. Although in one study, steroid administration was beneficial [42], the role of immunosuppressive agents in the treatment of IN has not been addressed yet.

19.3 Glomerulonephritis in Primary Sjögren's Syndrome

19.3.1 Historical Aspects

GN can occur in pSS, but relatively few cases have been reported in the literature. In 1966, Meltzer et al. described an SS patient with proliferative GN related to type II mixed cryoglobulinemia who presented with facial edema, increased arterial pressure, hematuria, and proteinuria [43]. Similarly, in a series of 86 patients with cryoglobulinemia, 3 had SS and signs of glomerular disease, although not biopsy proven [44]. Moutsopoulos et al. described three cases of pSS with GN [45]. The clinical picture of GN included typically hypertension and pitting edema. The major laboratory findings were renal insufficiency and active urine sediment accompanied by proteinuria. Circulating immune complexes were detected in all three patients and cryoglobulinemia was found in two of them. Thus, GN was associated with cryoglobulinemia and an immune complex mediated process.

19.3.2 Clinical Features

GN occurs later during the disease course of pSS compared to IN [26]. Hypertension, periorbital or facial pitting edema, and renal insufficiency due to decreased glomerular filtration rate (GFR) are the presenting features [26, 43, 45]. Some patients may also present with other extraepithelial manifestations such as purpura, peripheral neuropathy, and necrotizing vasculitis [44]. GN has also been observed as a part of systemic vasculitis, resulting from deposition of immune complexes at various sites. A patient with pSS and focal cresentic GN in the setting of necrotizing vasculitis affecting the central nervous system, the gastrointestinal tract, the pancreas, and the lungs was reported by Sato et al. [46]. Similarly, Tsokos et al. described three pSS patients with small and/or medium vessel vasculitis, without aneurysmal formation, resembling polyarteritis nodosa who had evidence of glomerular disease [47].

The most common urinary abnormalities are hematuria of glomerular origin with or without red blood cell casts and proteinuria of more than 500 mg/day [26, 43, 45]. Proteinuria of nephrotic range and full-blown nephrotic syndrome have been also

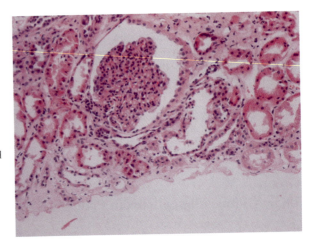

Fig. 19.3 Mesangial proliferation of glomerulus in a patient with primary Sjögren's syndrome and glomerulonephritis (Hematoxylin and eosin × 400) (Image kindly provided by Dr. Hariklia Gakiopoulou, Lecturer in Pathology, First Department of Pathology, Medical School of Athens)

reported but are not common manifestations among pSS patients with GN [12, 13, 17, 23]. Almost half of pSS patients with GN may develop non-Hodgkin's lymphoma of B cell origin during follow-up [26]. This observation has also been reported in the past by Bruet et al [44]. GN, purpura, and peripheral neuropathy are extraepithelial manifestations that arise from an underlying immune complex-mediated process and define a distinct subset of patients who have a tendency to develop lymphomas.

The largest series of pSS patients with biopsy documented GN has been published from our department [26]. Among 471 pSS patients, 20 had overt renal involvement and 10 had clinical and laboratory findings indicative of glomerular disease, suggesting that severe renal impairment due to GN occurs in approximately 2.5% of pSS population. Two patients from the GN group required hemodialysis because of end-stage renal failure, implying that GN carries a less favorable prognosis.

19.3.3   Histology

The most common histologic types of GN in pSS are membranoproliferative, membranous, and mesangial GN. Membranoproliferative GN is characterized by diffuse proliferation of mesangial cells and infiltration of glomeruli by macrophages, increased mesangial matrix, and thickening along with reduplication of the glomerular basement membrane [12, 17, 23, 26, 45]. In most cases, C3 and IgM deposits are observed on immunofluorescence microscopy [12, 26]. In membranous GN, the major histologic findings are diffuse thickening of the glomerular basement membrane and subepithelial electron dense deposits [12, 17, 23, 45]. Mesangial proliferative GN is characterized by proliferation of mesangial cells and matrix, and probably represents an early stage of the disease that may evolve into more aggressive forms (Fig. 19.3) [12, 13, 23, 26]. Other rare forms of GN include focal segmental glomerulosclerosis [23, 42], cresentic GN [46], and proliferative GN [13, 43]. The limited

Table 19.2 Biopsy documented cases of glomerulonephritis in pSS

First author of the study [reference number]	Year of publication	Number of cases	Type of GN (number of cases)	Indication for renal biopsy
Meltzer [43]	1966	1	Proliferative (1)	Hypertension, edema, proteinuria, red blood cell casts
Moutsopoulos [45]	1978	3	Membranoproliferative (2), membranous (1)	Hypertension, edema, renal impairment, proteinuria, hematuria
Siamopoulos [17]	1986	2	Membranoproliferative (1), membranous (1)	Nephrotic range proteinuria
Sato [46]	1987	1	Focal cresentic (1)	Active urine sediment
Pertovaara [13]	1999	2	Mesangial (1), proliferative (1)	Proteinuria, hematuria, renal impairment
Goules [26]	2000	9	Membranoproliferative (5), mesangial (4)	Edema, hypertension, proteinuria, hematuria, active urine sediment
Bossini [12]	2001	3	Membranoproliferative (1), membranous (1), mesangial (1)	Proteinuria >2 g/day
Ren [23]	2008	8	Membranoproliferative (2) membranous (1), mesangial (3) FSGS (2)	Not mentioned
Maripuri [42]	2009	4	Cryoglobulinemic (2), FSGS(2)	Renal impairment

Abbreviations: *FSGS* focal segmental glomerulosclerosis, *pSS* primary Sjögren's syndrome

number of cases and the lack of relevant data do not allow any correlation between a particular histologic type of GN and the severity of renal involvement in GN of pSS. However, it seems that patients with histologic lesions of membranous or membranoproliferative GN are more likely to develop nephrotic range proteinuria while mesangial GN is associated with mild proteinuria [12, 13, 26]. Table 19.2 summarizes all the biopsy documented cases of GN in pSS as well as the major clinical and laboratory findings that led to kidney biopsy.

19.3.4 *Pathogenesis*

The pathogenesis of GN in pSS is closely related to type II mixed cryoglobulinemia. This association connotes an underlying oligoclonal or monoclonal B cell activation that becomes clinically apparent late in the disease course as a result of the ongoing antigenic stimulation of B lymphocytes. Cryoglobulins are serum immunoglobulins, which precipitate at temperatures below 37°C and redissolve after rewarming. According to the Brout classification, type II cryoglobulins are composed of IgG and an IgM of monoclonal origin with rheumatoid factor activity (anti IgG-RF) [48].

Type II cryoglobulinemia has been described in association with chronic infections, autoimmune diseases, and lymphoproliferative disorders. IgM-kappa cryoglobulins are detected in the majority of pSS patients with GN [26]. Low C4 complement levels is another common finding, indicative of complement activation in these patients [26]. These data, in combination with the presence of C3 and IgM deposits in biopsy specimens, suggest an immune complex-mediated process as a possible pathogenetic mechanism of GN in pSS [12, 26].

19.3.5 Differential Diagnosis

The differential diagnosis of GN in pSS includes those diseases that can cause type II cryoglobulinemia and similar clinical manifestations. The most important are chronic HCV infection, HIV infection, and lymphoproliferative disorders [48, 49]. Patients with HCV infection may present with chronic sialadenitis, purpura, peripheral neuropathy, and glomerulonephritis due to cryoglobulinemia. However, in these patients, liver involvement is more common than in pSS patients and the prevalence of parotid enlargement is lower. In addition, the frequency of anti-HCV antibodies among patients with SS is low [50]. HIV infection may produce sicca manifestations, parotid swelling, lymphadenopathy, and rarely type II cryoglobulinemia [49]. SS can be distinguished from HIV infection serologically, since HIV patients generally lack anti-Ro/SSA and anti-La/SSB antibodies but they have anti-HIV antibodies. In a patient with pSS who presents with low C4 complement levels, cryoglobulinemia, purpura, and GN, an underlying lymphoproliferative disorder should be excluded, particularly if generalized lymphadenopathy is apparent. Systemic lupus erythematosus (SLE) should be also included in the differential diagnosis of a patient with cryoglobulinemic GN. Lupus nephritis may present with either nephritic or nephrotic syndrome and is usually accompanied by low C4 complement levels and elevated titers of anti-dsDNA antibodies. The presence of lupus-specific skin lesions, serositis, and hematologic abnormalities such as leukopenia, hemolytic anemia, or thrombocytopenia can distinguish lupus nephritis from GN of pSS.

19.3.6 Treatment

Management of pSS patients with GN is based on clinical judgment since no clinical trials have been conducted to address this issue. In our series, six patients with membranoproliferative or mesangial GN and proteinuria with an active urine sediment received a combination of methylprednisolone and intravenous pulses of cyclophosphamide [26]. The fact that this combination has been proven beneficial in other types of immune complex-mediated glomerulonephritides such as lupus nephritis makes it a reasonable option for aggressive forms of pSS GN. Despite this regimen, two of the six patients developed end-stage renal failure and required hemodialysis after 1 year of follow-up. For mild forms of GN without active urine sediment and stable renal function, a watchful waiting policy and close monitoring is another proposal. The role of other immunosuppressive agents such as azathioprine or B cell depletion is unclear.

19.4 Painful Bladder Syndrome/Interstitial Cystitis and Primary Sjögren's Syndrome

19.4.1 Historical Aspects

Painful bladder syndrome/interstitial cystitis (PBS/IC) is a chronic pelvic pain syndrome [51–54] that has been associated with SS. IC with the characteristic cytoscopic finding of Hunner's ulcer was originally described by Hanash and Pool [55]. Subsequently, Messing and Samey described the more frequent nonulcerative form of IC [56]. Since then, many definitions of IC have been used but the European Society for the study of IC (ESSIC) proposed a convenient system for nomenclature and classification based upon the presence of chronic pelvic pain, which is related to the urinary bladder [54]. In 1993, Van de Merve et al. evaluated ten patients with IC and diagnosed focal lymphocytic sialadenitis and keratoconjuctivitis in almost half of them, implying an association between SS and IC [57].

19.4.2 Clinical, Cytoscopic, and Histologic Features

Painful bladder syndrome/interstitial cystitis (PBS/IC) presents with chronic pelvic pain, pressure, or discomfort related to the urinary bladder [54]. Pain, a fundamental feature of the syndrome, is usually accompanied by other urinary symptoms such as frequency, urge to void, and nocturia. Some patients also experience dyspareunia [58]. There is a considerable overlap between PBS/IC and other painful conditions including irritable bowel syndrome, fibromyalgia, and various chronic pelvic pain syndromes [58, 59]. Urodynamics may reveal abnormal uroflow and lower median volumes for certain urodynamic parameters [60, 61]. Cytoscopy is usually normal but Hunner's ulcers may be observed. Hunner's lesion is an inflammatory and reddened area of the mucosa that becomes apparent only after hydrodistention during cytoscopy [54]. Although biopsy is not always indicated, the most common histologic features are inflammatory infiltrates, granulation tissue, detrusor mastocytosis, and intrafascicular fibrosis [54]. Although pain or equivalent pressure/discomfort related to the bladder is a prerequisite of PBS/IC the typical cytoscopic or histologic features are not always present. Thus, the term IC is reserved for such cases [54].

19.4.3   Pathogenesis and Association with Sjögren's Syndrome

The etiology of PBS/IC remains obscure, but neurogenic inflammation mediated by mast cells, epithelial permeability due to disruption of the glycosaminoglycan (GAG) layer, and autoimmunity have been proposed to play a role in the pathogenesis of the syndrome [62]. Several findings though support the autoimmunity theory. Antinuclear antibodies have been detected in 36% of patients with PBS/IC [63] and immune deposits have been found in the urinary bladder vessel wall of patients with IC [64]. In addition, HLA class I molecules seem to be overexpressed by most cells of the urinary bladder of patients with IC and along with the increased number of CD8, suggest a direct CD8 cytotoxicity [65, 66]. On the other hand, the increased number of CD4 lymphocytes and the expression of HLA-DR molecules within the bladder of patients with IC may contribute to disease pathogenesis [65, 66].

Two recent studies further support the association between SS and PBS/IC. In a study from Finland, 36 SS patients were included and the frequency of lower urinary tract problems was found significantly higher compared to normal individuals [67]. Leppilahti et al. recruited 870 SS patients from the Finnish SS organization and 1,304 normal controls and tried to estimate the prevalence of IC by using a specific questionnaire [68]. Forty-five SS patients (5%) versus four controls (0.3%) fulfilled the criteria for probable IC and the prevalence rate ratio was 15 (95% CI: 4.8–50). Although epidemiologic data clearly point out an association between SS and IC, the possible underlying pathogenetic mechanisms have not been elucidated yet. Autoantibodies against muscarinic M3 receptors have been detected in patients with SS and these antibodies have been proposed in the literature to play a role in the pathogenesis of IC by affecting the muscarinic receptors of the bladder [69]. However, this hypothesis needs further investigation to be confirmed.

19.4.4   Differential Diagnosis

Differential diagnosis of PBS/IC includes all the so-called "confusable diseases" as defined by the ESSIC [54]. These entities may produce overlap symptoms with PBS/IC and must be excluded before the diagnosis of PBS/IC is established. The most important are infections, urogenital prolapse, bladder stone, carcinoma of the urinary bladder, and overactive bladder (OAB). The majority of these conditions can be easily distinguished from PBS/IC by medical history, physical examination, and simple routine tests such as urinalysis, urine cultures, and ultrasound [54]. If there is a high suspicion for carcinoma, cytoscopy and biopsy should be performed. Overactive bladder is more common than PBS/IC and may present with urgency and frequency with or without incontinence. However, these patients are usually males and they experience urgency as a needing action rather than a strong desire to void like IC patients who urinate to alleviate pain. In difficult cases, urodynamic studies can differentiate the two conditions. Because SS affects mainly females, the confusable diseases that concern the prostate are of low clinical significance.

19.4.5 Treatment

Management of patients with PBS/IC is difficult and several therapeutic modalities have been tested. Evidence-based recommendations were made after analyzing a large number of studies [70]. The basic therapeutic strategies include medical (oral) treatment, intravesical drug instillation, and surgical intervention. The following drugs reached a high recommendation degree for the treatment of PBS/IC: (a) pentosan polysulfate sodium (PPS), a polysaccharide used to replenish the GAG layer of urothelium; (b) amitriptyline, a tricyclic antidepressant, which can alleviate symptoms of IC probably by blocking the acetylcholine receptors or by inhibiting the reuptake of serotonin and norepinephrine; (c) hydroxyzine, an H1-receptor antagonist that can block neuronal activation of mast cells by inhibiting serotonin secretion from thalamic mast cells; and (d) cyclosporine at a dose of 1.5 mg/kg twice daily. Regarding the intravesical instillation, only PPS and dimethyl sulfoxide (DMSO), a chemical solvent that penetrates cell membranes and exhibits analgesic and anti-inflammatory properties, have been found efficacious. Finally, surgical treatment such as transurethral resection and coagulation and major reconstructive surgery are reserved for patients with Hunner's ulcer or visible lesions.

References

1. Tzioufas G, Mitsias D, Moutsopoulos H. Sjogren's syndrome. In: Hochberg M, Smolen J, Weinblatt M, Weisman M, editors. Rheumatology. 4th ed. Mosby: Elsevier; 2008. p. 1341.
2. Kahn M, Merritt AD, Wohl MJ, et al. Renal concentrating defect in Sjogren's syndrome. Ann Intern Med. 1962;56:883–95.
3. Shearn MA, Tu WH. Nephrogenic diabetic insipidus and other defects of renal tubular function in Sjoergren's syndrome. Am J Med. 1965;39:312–8.
4. Bloch KJ, Buchanan WW, Wohl MJ, et al. Sjogren's syndrome. A clinical, pathological, and serological study of sixty-two cases. Medicine (Baltimore). 1965;44:187–231.
5. Shearn MA, Tu WH. Latent renal tubular acidosis in Sjogren's syndrome. Ann Rheum Dis. 1968;27:27–32.
6. Tu WH, Shearn MA, Lee JC, et al. Interstitial nephritis in Sjogren's syndrome. Ann Intern Med. 1968;69:1163–70.
7. Talal N, Zisman E, Schur PH. Renal tubular acidosis, glomerulonephritis and immunologic factors in Sjogren's syndrome. Arthritis Rheum. 1968;11:774–86.
8. Shioji R, Furuyama T, Onodera S, et al. Sjogren's syndrome and renal tubular acidosis. Am J Med. 1970;48:456–63.
9. Eriksson P, Denneberg T, Enestrom S, et al. Urolithiasis and distal renal tubular acidosis preceding primary Sjogren's syndrome: a retrospective study 5–53 years after the presentation of urolithiasis. J Intern Med. 1996;239:483–8.
10. Pertovaara M, Korpela M, Pasternack A. Factors predictive of renal involvement in patients with primary Sjogren's syndrome. Clin Nephrol. 2001;56:10–8.
11. Aasarod K, Haga HJ, Berg KJ, et al. Renal involvement in primary Sjogren's syndrome. QJM. 2000;93:297–304.
12. Bossini N, Savoldi S, Franceschini F, et al. Clinical and morphological features of kidney involvement in primary Sjogren's syndrome. Nephrol Dial Transplant. 2001;16:2328–36.

13. Pertovaara M, Korpela M, Kouri T, et al. The occurrence of renal involvement in primary Sjogren's syndrome: a study of 78 patients. Rheumatology (Oxford). 1999;38:1113–20.
14. Pokorny G, Sonkodi S, Ivanyi B, et al. Renal involvement in patients with primary Sjogren's syndrome. Scand J Rheumatol. 1989;18:231–4.
15. Viergever PP, Swaak TJ. Renal tubular dysfunction in primary Sjogren's syndrome: clinical studies in 27 patients. Clin Rheumatol. 1991;10:23–7.
16. Vitali C, Tavoni A, Sciuto M, et al. Renal involvement in primary Sjogren's syndrome: a retrospective-prospective study. Scand J Rheumatol. 1991;20:132–6.
17. Siamopoulos KC, Mavridis AK, Elisaf M, et al. Kidney involvement in primary Sjogren's syndrome. Scand J Rheumatol Suppl. 1986;61:156–60.
18. Moutsopoulos HM, Cledes J, Skopouli FN, et al. Nephrocalcinosis in Sjogren's syndrome: a late sequela of renal tubular acidosis. J Intern Med. 1991;230:187–91.
19. Aygen B, Dursun FE, Dogukan A, et al. Hypokalemic quadriparesis associated with renal tubular acidosis in a patient with Sjogren's syndrome. Clin Nephrol. 2008;69:306–9.
20. Dowd JE, Lipsky PE. Sjogren's syndrome presenting as hypokalemic periodic paralysis. Arthritis Rheum. 1993;36:1735–8.
21. Soy M, Pamuk ON, Gerenli M, et al. A primary Sjogren's syndrome patient with distal renal tubular acidosis, who presented with symptoms of hypokalemic periodic paralysis: report of a case study and review of the literature. Rheumatol Int. 2005;26:86–9.
22. Zimhony O, Sthoeger Z, Ben David D, et al. Sjogren's syndrome presenting as hypokalemic paralysis due to distal renal tubular acidosis. J Rheumatol. 1995;22:2366–8.
23. Ren H, Wang WM, Chen XN, et al. Renal involvement and follow-up of 130 patients with primary Sjogren's syndrome. J Rheumatol. 2008;35:278–84.
24. Kobayashi T, Muto S, Nemoto J, et al. Fanconi's syndrome and distal (type 1) renal tubular acidosis in a patient with primary Sjogren's syndrome with monoclonal gammopathy of undetermined significance. Clin Nephrol. 2006;65:427–32.
25. Yang Y, Kuang Y, Montes De Oca R. Targeted disruption of the murine Fanconi anemia gene, Fancg/Xrcc9. Blood. 2001;98:3435–40.
26. Goules A, Masouridi S, Tzioufas AG, et al. Clinically significant and biopsy-documented renal involvement in primary Sjogren syndrome. Medicine (Baltimore). 2000;79:241–9.
27. Matsumura R, Kondo Y, Sugiyama T, et al. Immunohistochemical identification of infiltrating mononuclear cells in tubulointerstitial nephritis associated with Sjogren's syndrome. Clin Nephrol. 1988;30:335–40.
28. Rosenberg ME, Schendel PB, McCurdy FA, et al. Characterization of immune cells in kidneys from patients with Sjogren's syndrome. Am J Kidney Dis. 1988;11:20–2.
29. Murata H, Kita Y, Sakamoto A, et al. Limited TCR repertoire of infiltrating T cells in the kidneys of Sjogren's syndrome patients with interstitial nephritis. J Immunol. 1995;155:4084–9.
30. Matsumura R, Umemiya K, Nakazawa T, et al. Expression of cell adhesion molecules in tubulointerstitial nephritis associated with Sjogren's syndrome. Clin Nephrol. 1998;49:74–81.
31. Matsumura R, Umemiya K, Goto T, et al. Glandular and extraglandular expression of costimulatory molecules in patients with Sjogren's syndrome. Ann Rheum Dis. 2001;60:473–82.
32. Matsumura R, Umemiya K, Kagami M, et al. Glandular and extraglandular expression of the Fas-Fas ligand and apoptosis in patients with Sjogren's syndrome. Clin Exp Rheumatol. 2001;16:561–8.
33. Nishimori I, Bratanova T, Toshkov I, et al. Induction of experimental autoimmune sialoadenitis by immunization of PL/J mice with carbonic anhydrase II. J Immunol. 1995;154:4865–73.
34. Inagaki Y, Jinno-Yoshida Y, Hamasaki Y, et al. A novel autoantibody reactive with carbonic anhydrase in sera from patients with systemic lupus erythematosus and Sjogren's syndrome. J Dermatol Sci. 1991;2:147–54.
35. Itoh Y, Reichlin M. Antibodies to carbonic anhydrase in systemic lupus erythematosus and other rheumatic diseases. Arthritis Rheum. 1992;35:73–82.
36. Kino-Ohsaki J, Nishimori I, Morita M, et al. Serum antibodies to carbonic anhydrase I and II in patients with idiopathic chronic pancreatitis and Sjogren's syndrome. Gastroenterology. 1996;110:1579–86.

37. Takemoto F, Hoshino J, Sawa N, et al. Autoantibodies against carbonic anhydrase II are increased in renal tubular acidosis associated with Sjogren syndrome. Am J Med. 2005;118:181–4.
38. Takemoto F, Katori H, Sawa N, et al. Induction of anti-carbonic-anhydrase-II antibody causes renal tubular acidosis in a mouse model of Sjogren's syndrome. Nephron Physiol. 2007;106: p63–8.
39. Rodriguez Soriano J. Renal tubular acidosis: the clinical entity. J Am Soc Nephrol. 2002;13: 2160–70.
40. Maldonado JE, Velosa JA, Kyle RA, et al. Fanconi syndrome in adults. A manifestation of a latent form of myeloma. Am J Med. 1975;58:354–64.
41. Donckerwolcke RA, van Stekelenburg GJ, Tiddens HA. Therapy of bicarbonate-losing renal tubular acidosis. Arch Dis Child. 1970;45:774–9.
42. Maripuri S, Grande JP, Osborn TG, et al. Renal involvement in primary Sjogren's syndrome: a clinicopathologic study. Clin J Am Soc Nephrol. 2009;4:1423–31.
43. Meltzer M, Franklin EC, Elias K, et al. Cryoglobulinemia – a clinical and laboratory study. II. Cryoglobulins with rheumatoid factor activity. Am J Med. 1966;40:837–56.
44. Brouet JC, Clauvel JP, Danon F, et al. Biologic and clinical significance of cryoglobulins. A report of 86 cases. Am J Med. 1974;57:775–88.
45. Moutsopoulos HM, Balow JE, Lawley TJ, et al. Immune complex glomerulonephritis in sicca syndrome. Am J Med. 1978;64:955–60.
46. Sato K, Miyasaka N, Nishioka K, et al. Primary Sjogren's syndrome associated with systemic necrotizing vasculitis: a fatal case. Arthritis Rheum. 1987;30:717–8.
47. Tsokos M, Lazarou SA, Moutsopoulos HM. Vasculitis in primary Sjogren's syndrome. Histologic classification and clinical presentation. Am J Clin Pathol. 1987;88:26–31.
48. Ferri C, Zignego AL, Pileri SA. Cryoglobulins. J Clin Pathol. 2002;55:4–13.
49. Dimitrakopoulos AN, Kordossis T, Hatzakis A, et al. Mixed cryoglobulinemia in HIV-1 infection: the role of HIV-1. Ann Intern Med. 1999;130:226–30.
50. Vitali C, Sciuto M, Neri R, et al. Anti-hepatitis C virus antibodies in primary Sjogren's syndrome: false positive results are related to hyper-gamma-globulinemia. Clin Exp Rheumatol. 1992;10:103–4.
51. Abrams P, Baranowski A, Berger RE, et al. A new classification is needed for pelvic pain syndromes – are existing terminologies of spurious diagnostic authority bad for patients? J Urol. 2006;175:1989–90.
52. Fall M, Baranowski AP, Fowler CJ, et al. EAU guidelines on chronic pelvic pain. Eur Urol. 2004;46:681–9.
53. Janicki TI. Chronic pelvic pain as a form of complex regional pain syndrome. Clin Obstet Gynecol. 2003;46:797–803.
54. van de Merwe JP, Nordling J, Bouchelouche P, et al. Diagnostic criteria, classification, and nomenclature for painful bladder syndrome/interstitial cystitis: an ESSIC proposal. Eur Urol. 2008;53:60–7.
55. Hanash KA, Pool TL. Interstitial cystitis in men. J Urol. 1969;102:427–8.
56. Messing EM, Stamey TA. Interstitial cystitis: early diagnosis, pathology, and treatment. Urology. 1978;12:381–92.
57. Van de Merwe J, Kamerling R, Arendsen E, et al. Sjogren's syndrome in patients with interstitial cystitis. J Rheumatol. 1993;20:962–6.
58. Ustinova EE, Fraser MO, Pezzone MA. Cross-talk and sensitization of bladder afferent nerves. Neurourol Urodyn. 2010;29:77–81.
59. Rodriguez MA, Afari N, Buchwald DS. Evidence for overlap between urological and nonurological unexplained clinical conditions. J Urol. 2009;182:2123–31.
60. Butrick CW, Sanford D, Hou Q, et al. Chronic pelvic pain syndromes: clinical, urodynamic, and urothelial observations. Int Urogynecol J Pelvic Floor Dysfunct. 2009;20:1047–53.
61. Sastry DN, Hunter KM, Whitmore KE. Urodynamic testing and interstitial cystitis/painful bladder syndrome. Int Urogynecol J Pelvic Floor Dysfunct. 2010;21:157–61.
62. Dasgupta J, Tincello DG. Interstitial cystitis/bladder pain syndrome: an update. Maturitas. 2009;64:212–7.

63. Ochs RL, Stein Jr TW, Peebles CL, et al. Autoantibodies in interstitial cystitis. J Urol. 1994;151: 587–92.
64. Helin H, Mattila J, Rantala I, et al. In vivo binding of immunoglobulin and complement to elastic structures in urinary bladder vascular walls in interstitial cystitis: demonstration by immunoelectron microscopy. Clin Immunol Immunopathol. 1987;43:88–96.
65. Christmas TJ, Bottazzo GF. Abnormal urothelial HLA-DR expression in interstitial cystitis. Clin Exp Immunol. 1992;87:450–4.
66. Christmas TJ. Lymphocyte sub-populations in the bladder wall in normal bladder, bacterial cystitis and interstitial cystitis. Br J Urol. 1994;73:508–15.
67. Haarala M, Alanen A, Hietarinta M, et al. Lower urinary tract symptoms in patients with Sjogren's syndrome and systemic lupus erythematosus. Int Urogynecol J Pelvic Floor Dysfunct. 2000;11:84–6.
68. Leppilahti M, Tammela TL, Huhtala H, et al. Interstitial cystitis-like urinary symptoms among patients with Sjogren's syndrome: a population-based study in Finland. Am J Med. 2003;115:62–5.
69. van de Merwe JP. Interstitial cystitis and systemic autoimmune diseases. Nat Clin Pract Urol. 2007;4:484–91.
70. Fall M, Oberpenning F, Peeker R. Treatment of bladder pain syndrome/interstitial cystitis 2008: can we make evidence-based decisions? Eur Urol. 2008;54:65–75.

Chapter 20
Central Nervous System Involvement

Stanley R. Pillemer, Aaron B. Mendelsohn, and Katrin E. Morgen

Contents

20.1 Prevalence and Classification

Neurologic signs and symptoms have been recognized in the setting of Sjögren's syndrome (SS) since the syndrome was first described by Sjögren in 1935 [1]. In particular, peripheral nervous system involvement in primary SS (pSS) has been well characterized and is believed to affect approximately 10–20% of SS patients [2]. The frequency of central nervous system (CNS) involvement is less clear, however, as controversy exists regarding the frequency and type of CNS manifestations in pSS.

S.R. Pillemer (✉)
American Biopharma Corporation, Gaithersburg, MD, USA

A.B. Mendelsohn
School of Health Sciences, Walden University, Minneapolis, MN, USA

K.E. Morgen
Department of Psychiatry, Central Institute of Mental Health (CIMH), Mannheim, Germany

M. Ramos-Casals et al. (eds.), *Sjögren's Syndrome*,
DOI 10.1007/978-0-85729-947-5_20, © Springer-Verlag London Limited 2012

In general, the prevalence of CNS involvement in pSS varies widely across studies, ranging from 0% to 62% [3]. Several theories have been proposed to explain the variability in these studies, including:

1. Lack of a standardized definition for SS diagnosis across studies [4]. Indeed, some investigators have included persons with secondary SS [4, 5], and it is likely that some of these patients may have lupus with CNS dysfunction [5]. In addition, misdiagnosis of SS may occur; for example, persons with multiple sclerosis presenting with sicca symptoms and possessing positive antinuclear antibodies.
2. Varying definitions of CNS disorders have been employed. As reviewed by Soliotis et al. [5], several studies [6–9] have classified psychiatric and/or cognitive diseases in their definitions of CNS disorders, thus raising the prevalence estimates, sometimes dramatically. The inclusion of mild symptoms such as headache or mood disturbances [4] would also impact prevalence estimates.
3. Generalizability of patient populations also may be an issue, that is, the patient groups investigated may not be directly comparable to one another, and potential confounding factors for cerebrovascular disease are not uniformly addressed [4]. Furthermore, data are often based upon single case reports or small cases series [2]. Finally, referral bias may be present if pSS patients with CNS disease are differentially referred to certain institutions for care compared with pSS patients without CNS disease [5].

According to Govoni et al. [2], the spectrum of CNS involvement in pSS is diverse and involves several major categories of disorders: focal symptoms (e.g., aphasia, seizure disorders); movement disorders/pyramidal tract signs (e.g., brain stem syndrome); diffuse nonfocal symptoms (e.g., acute/subacute encephalopathy, aseptic meningoencephalitis); spinal cord involvement (e.g., transverse myelitis); and other disorders such as optic neuropathy, mood disorders, and MS-like disease. The data on the prevalence of nervous system involvement among patients with SS mirror the experience of other autoimmune disorders [10]. Reliable predictors of CNS dysfunction in patients with pSS do not exist.

20.2 Cerebral Lesions

The frequency of cerebral MRI changes varies considerably in studies of pSS patients [8, 11–15]. Populations that include a high proportion of individuals with neurological impairments often display marked abnormalities on MRI, mostly in the periventricular and subcortical white matter [12].

The types of CNS abnormalities reported in patients with pSS vary substantially. MRI studies have revealed a wide spectrum of structural CNS changes, ranging from nonspecific disseminated white matter lesions [1, 6, 13, 16] to pseudotumoral brain lesions [16, 17], extensive spinal cord lesions [6, 16–18], subarachnoid hemorrhage, and brain atrophy [14, 19]. Moreover, correlations between CNS symptoms and abnormalities on MRI have been weak, providing further evidence for the heterogeneity of the underlying pathology [6, 18].

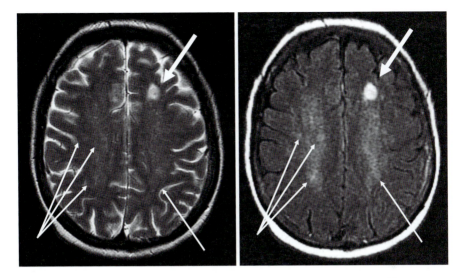

Fig. 20.1 White matter damage in a patient with primary Sjögren's syndrome. Large lesion on T2-weighted MRI (**a**) and FLAIR (**b**, *wide arrow*) as well as patchy hyperintensities more apparent on FLAIR (**b**, *thin arrows*). Because of strong tissue contrast, subtle tissue damage is more clearly revealed on FLAIR (**b**) than on conventional T2-weighted MRI (**a**) (With kind permission from Morgen [20], Fig. 1)

Most commonly, pSS patients have been found to exhibit nonspecific disseminated white matter lesions on MRI [1, 13, 16] (Fig. 20.1). These may occur in the absence of focal neurological deficits and be associated with psychiatric disturbances (anxiety and depression) and neuropsychological deficits, predominantly affecting attention, visuospatial abilities, and executive function [6, 16, 19].

Small white matter lesions on T2-weighted MRI have also been detected in pSS patients without measurable CNS symptoms [13]. Because such lesions are common among elderly subjects and pSS tends to occur relatively late in life, their true significance has been difficult to interpret. The risk of white matter damage is increased by factors such as hypertension, diabetes, and hyperlipidemia, which are frequently elevated in the elderly [21]. A controlled investigation would require a large sample size [3].

There is some evidence that pSS patients with nonspecific white matter lesions or without apparent white matter damage on conventional MRI may develop brain atrophy [14, 19]. However, the disease specificity of correlations between cognitive performance and MRI measures of atrophy remains unclear [19].

Another approach to detecting subtle structural CNS abnormalities in pSS patients has been to analyze regional cerebral blood flow with single emission photon emission tomography (SPECT). In a recent case-control study, 99mTc-ECD brain SPECT revealed hypoperfusion predominantly in parietal and temporal cortex in pSS patients compared to control subjects, which in turn was associated with executive dysfunction [22].

Less frequently, pSS patients develop extensive CNS lesions, generally associated with focal neurological deficits. Studies, predominantly of patients recruited in tertiary referral centers, have reported CNS involvement characterized by relapsing-remitting neurological deficits and white matter lesions mimicking multiple sclerosis (MS), an autoimmune demyelinating disease [1, 16, 23]. However, cases of focal CNS damage atypical of MS have also been described, for example, a patient with lethal subarachnoid hemorrhage resulting from spinal necrotizing vasculitis [24] or a patient with stroke-like onset of aphasia, anarthria, and hemiparesis caused by a pseudotumoral inflammatory white matter lesion with mass effect [16].

Some pSS patients with recurrent CNS deficits and positive anti-aquaporin 4-antibodies show a characteristic pattern of structural abnormalities on MRI reminiscent of neuromyelitis optica (NMO). Aside from spinal cord and optic nerve lesions, these patients appear to develop brain lesions in specific locations; that is, diencephalic and brainstem lesions adjacent to the third and fourth ventricles, longitudinal lesions of the internal capsule, and large cerebral lesions with a tendency toward cavity formation. The results suggest the importance of testing pSS patients with CNS disease for a possible coexistence of NMO [17, 25].

The pathology of CNS damage in pSS remains elusive and is likely to be heterogeneous. Subtle structural abnormalities indicated by punctate lesions on T2-weighted MRI and regional hypoperfusion in patients with or without discrete abnormalities on MRI presumably involve the dysfunction of small blood vessels [18, 22]. Feasible mechanisms of CNS involvement include different forms of vasculitis (small, medium, or large vessel; antibody or cell mediated, possibly immune complex deposition) and demyelinating inflammatory disease [3, 23, 26]. Whether specific immunological factors indicate a risk of developing CNS lesions has also not been resolved. Investigations of Anti-Ro (SSA) and anti-La (SSB) antibodies, antiphospholipid-antibodies, and rheumatoid factor have yielded inconclusive results [3]. The recently discovered evidence of aquaporin-4 antibodies as a risk factor for severe CNS involvement needs to be confirmed in larger studies [17].

Other autoimmune immune diseases associated with CNS tissue damage include MS and SLE. In these diseases, MRI studies can demonstrate clinical and subclinical tissue damage [27–29]. For example, only 5–10% of contrast-enhancing lesions observed on monthly MRI in MS patients are associated with neurological symptoms [27]. MS patients develop progressive cerebral atrophy early in the course of the disease [30]. In SLE, white matter lesions are associated with higher overall disease activity [29].

In pSS, CNS involvement is generally less marked than in MS and SLE, and MRI lesions often more discrete and interpretation more challenging. In the general population, most individuals over the age of 60 years have at least one white matter hyperintensity on T2-weighted MRI [31]. Since a high proportion of pSS cases have onset between the ages of 40 and 50 [6], it can be difficult to distinguish MRI-abnormalities associated with pSS from changes related to age and cerebrovascular risk factors.

20.3 Differential Diagnosis with Multiple Sclerosis, Neuromyelitis Optica, and Antiphospholipid Syndrome

MS is a major cause of disability in young adults that generally presents in those aged 20–40 years [32]. In contrast, SS and its CNS manifestations tend to have onset in later years. The course of MS is variable, but it most often presents with a relapsing, remitting disorder that gradually becomes progressive, leading to an accumulation of disability. MS has been categorized as having the following courses: relapsing remitting, secondary progressive, primary progressive, and relapsing progressive. Common presenting symptoms for MS are vision impairment (specifically, reduced color perception and/or blurred vision resulting from optic neuritis) and sensory abnormalities, for example, the loss of sensation, paresthesias, and dysesthesias of variable distribution. Motor symptoms resulting from pyramidal tract dysfunction and cerebellar involvement may also occur initially and increase over the course of the disease, leading to weakness, loss of dexterity, and spasticity.

Optic neuritis, which eventually involves about half of all patients with MS, can also occur in SS. Typically, visual loss occurs in one eye over a few days. Ocular pain may occur before or during the attack. Significant visual recovery usually occurs over 2 weeks.

In addition to visual loss, diplopia may occur in MS and is most commonly caused by internuclear ophthalmoplegia.

Cerebellar involvement is common in MS but rare in SS. In addition, the urinary tract symptoms differ between these two diseases. In MS, urinary frequency, urgency, and incontinence frequently occur. Urinary incontinence is rare in SS but may result from myelitis. More commonly, SS patients develop irritable bladder symptoms as a result of interstitial cystitis [33].

Up to 70% of MS patients develop cognitive disorders, which may be missed on a standard mental status evaluation [34]. Cognitive disorders have been little studied in SS. MS patients typically develop declines in their ability to deal with complex concepts, impairment of complex reasoning, decreased verbal fluency and processing speed, and decline in episodic memory. Affective disorders are common, and almost three fourths of MS patients experience depression. In SS, the prevalence of depression is about 30% [35]. Both MS and SS patients often have debilitating fatigue. Uhtoff's phenomenon, a temporary exacerbation of MS manifestations following exercise or body temperature elevation, is not a feature of SS, SLE, or antiphospholipid syndrome.

The diagnosis of MS requires evidence that white matter lesions are distributed in time and space, and the disease cannot be otherwise explained. The McDonald criteria are currently applied for the diagnosis of MS [36]. The diagnosis can be made on clinical grounds alone provided that two or more attacks have occurred and there is objective evidence that two or more areas of the CNS are involved. If objective evidence of MS is lacking or only a single attack has occurred, then investigations are required to substantiate the diagnosis. Relevant tests include MRI, cerebrospinal fluid (CSF) examinations, and visual evoked potentials (VEPs).

Typical MS lesions visualized on MRI are larger than 6 mm in diameter, ovoid, and tend to be oriented perpendicular to the lateral ventricles [37]. T1-weighted images of new lesions enhance with gadolinium initially, reflecting disruption of the blood–brain barrier. The inflammation and edema, which disrupt the blood–brain barrier and produce gadolinium enhancement, resolve within 1 or 2 months. At this stage, T1-weighted images may show low-attention signals known as "T1 black holes" that are thought to represent tissue loss. The CNS lesions on MRI may be indistinguishable from those seen in SS.

The CSF in MS shows a lymphocytic pleocytosis that generally is not more than 50 cells per deciliter. Generally, most of the immunoglobulin is IgG and discrete monoclonal bands of immunoglobulin (oligoclonal bands), not present in the serum, are detected in the CSF of approximately 90% of patients. Such bands may also occur in SLE and SS. An increased CSF IgG index can also be noted in both MS and SS.

VEPs measure sensory conduction velocity within the visual system. The great majority of MS patients, even those without a history of optic neuritis, have abnormal VEPs. Evoked response abnormalities may also occur in SS.

The distinction between SS and MS is accomplished most effectively through a careful history to identify features of SS such as symptoms of oral and ocular dryness, a search for evidence of dry mouth and dry eyes, serological testing for anti-Ro and anti-La antibodies, and pursuit of biopsy evidence of sialadenitis. CNS SS may be difficult to distinguish from relapsing-remitting MS using the symptoms and signs associated with and the investigations typically performed for relapsing-remitting MS.

Neuromyelitis optica (NMO), an autoimmune disease considered to be a subtype of MS in the past but recently classified as separate disease, is characterized by a single event or relapsing attacks of optic neuritis and myelitis. The finding that aquaporin4-antibodies constitute a biomarker of NMO has permitted the definition of additional variants. These include optic neuritis or myelitis associated with lesions in specific brain areas such as the hypothalamus, periventricular nucleus, and brainstem; Asian optic neuritis and/or myelitis with MS-like cerebral involvement; longitudinally extensive myelitis; and optic neuritis associated with systemic autoimmune disease [17, 38]. Contrary to MS, NMO tends to be associated with a pronounced CSF pleocytosis and a lower frequency of oligoclonal band (15–30% vs 85% in MS [38]). A recent case series of pSS patients who developed NMO suggests that there may be a subgroup of SS patients with a disposition toward developing NMO and that a test for aquaporin4-antibodies may help identify these patients even at early stages of CNS involvement [17].

Antiphospholipid syndrome (APS) requires a clinical event (thrombosis or pregnancy loss) and the presence of antiphospholipid antibody [39]. The presence of such antibodies can be documented as anticardiolipin antibodies, anti-β_2-glycoprotein-I antibodies, or by an inhibitor of phospholipid-dependent clotting (i.e., a lupus anticoagulant test). The antibodies must be persistently positive at high levels for 12 weeks or more. A number of features common to patients with the antiphospholipid syndrome are not part of the criteria for diagnosis, namely, livedo reticularis, valvular heart disease, and thrombocytopenia [40].

MRI studies in the antiphospholipid syndrome may show evidence of vascular occlusion [41]. Multiple hyperintense, periventricular white matter lesions may be seen. Multiple unexplained infarctions in young individuals are suggestive of antiphospholipid syndrome. Locations in the cerebral white matter, internal capsule, corpus callosum, optic nerves (optic neuritis), middle cerebellar peduncles, brainstem, and spinal cord (transverse myelitis) may be affected. Antiphospholipid syndrome may be difficult to distinguish from MS or SS. However, a history of thrombosis or fetal loss, the presence of livedo reticularis, MRI findings that show an atypical distribution for MS, high levels of antiphospholipid antibodies, and response to anticoagulants point to the antiphospholipid syndrome. In addition, the presence of serological features of SLE suggest lupus or a lupus-like disorder with an associated antiphospholipid syndrome.

Progressive multifocal leukoencephalopathy (PML) is a rare and serious viral neurologic disease that occurs in the context of immunosuppression [42]. Although PML is not currently a problem in SS, the use of immunosuppressive and immuno-modulatory treatments in SS is on the rise. PML has occurred in SLE and rheumatoid arthritis [42]. PML is caused by the JC virus, a polyoma DNA virus that commonly infects the general population. PML occurred during clinical trials of natalizumab for MS, a monoclonal antibody, in 2005. Subsequently, two cases of PML occurred in SLE patients who received off-label rituximab, a monoclonal antibody directed against CD20 that causes B cell depletion. Some trials of rituximab are ongoing in SS. The experience in SLE and MS suggests that concomitant immunosuppression may contribute to or be necessary for PML. PML tends to have a subacute onset over a period of weeks and a progressive course associated with an extremely high mortality. Unlike MS, PML does not respond to immunosuppressive treatment. Features of MS include optic neuritis, diplopia, paresthesia, paraparesis, and myelopathy, while those of PML include subacute cortical signs and symptoms, bilateral visual defects (cortical blindness), hemiparesis, and behavioral and neuropsychiatric manifestations. Both MS and PML may show cerebellar dysfunction. In SS, as treatments become more aggressive and increasingly directed toward controlling the underlying autoimmune disease as opposed to controlling symptoms, more adverse events and complications of treatment related to immunomodulatory and immunosuppressive therapies are likely to be seen, including the possibility of PML. In the context of immune-based therapies, cases PML are likely to be missed unless there is a high index of suspicion.

20.4   Cranial Nerve Involvement

Dysfunction of the optic nerve, cranial nerve two, has been discussed above. Sense of smell and taste can also be impaired in SS [43]. It is not clear to what extent this relates to decreased secretions or neuropathy in the nasal passages and oral cavity. The olfactory nerve, cranial nerve one, mediates the sense of smell. Taste sensation in the anterior two thirds of the tongue is supplied by the facial nerve, cranial nerve seven. Taste in the posterior third of the tongue is supplied by the glossopharyngeal nerve, cranial nerve nine. Decrease in salivary and tear secretions may relate in part to neuropathy or blockade of nerve action in the salivary and lacrimal glands. Parasympathetic innervation is supplied to the salivary glands via cranial nerves. The ninth cranial nerve supplies the parotid glands but the submandibular glands are innervated by cranial nerve seven. Trigeminal nerve neuropathy reflects, in most cases, sensory ganglionitis [35]. Sensorineural hearing loss has been reported in SS [44]. An early study noted that the majority of SS patients with hearing loss had anticardiolipin antibodies [45].

20.5   Diagnostic Algorithm of SS Patient with CNS Lesions, Myelitis, Meningitis

A description of the approach to CNS lesions in SS patients presenting with features similar to MS has been included earlier. However, patients may present with features of aseptic meningitis or myelitis. Aseptic meningitis refers to meningeal inflammation in which there is no identifiable bacterial pathogen in the CSF [46]. Aseptic meningitis is distinct from encephalitis, in which the brain parenchyma is affected, and from myelitis, which involves the spinal cord. The infectious causes of aseptic meningitis and meningoencephalitis overlap and must be excluded. Aseptic meningitis occurs in the setting of autoimmune diseases (e.g., SLE and SS), other systemic diseases such as vasculitides (e.g., Behcet's syndrome and Wegener's granulomatosis), and granulomatous disorders such as sarcoidosis and malignancies. Aseptic meningitis may also occur in association with vaccines and exposure to certain drugs, such as nonsteroidal anti-inflammatory drugs, and intravenous immunoglobulins. CSF shows mononuclear or polymorphonuclear pleocytosis, negative bacterial smears and cultures, normal to mildly elevated protein, and normal to slightly low glucose.

Viruses may cause acute myelitis [46]. Gray matter involvement results in acute flaccid paralysis without autonomic disturbances of bowel and bladder. This can be seen in West Nile virus infection. Involvement of the spinal white matter results in acute transverse myelitis. CSF should be tested to rule out viral, bacterial, and fungal causes. The differential diagnosis for myelitis includes SS, SLE, and antiphospholipid syndrome, vasculitides such as Behcet's disease, granulomatous conditions such as sarcoidosis, and demyelinating diseases such as MS and NMO. In addition, metabolic derangements such as vitamin E or vitamin B12 deficiency and hereditary disorders such as Friedrich's ataxia can present with features of chronic myelitis.

For rapidly progressing symptoms and signs of myelopathy, the presence of conditions requiring emergency surgical treatment, such as epidural metastasis or abscess, should be excluded by performing MRI of the entire spine [47]. If such lesions are identified, surgery is required to relieve the compression and prevent progression of the symptoms. For noncompressive causes, about half will represent inflammatory or demyelinating disorders. The most common disorders are demyelinating diseases (MS NMO), spinal cord infarction, parainfectious myelitis, and inflammatory disorders that include SS. Parainfectious myelitis is diagnosed when an infection occurs in close temporal relationship to myelitis. Infectious causes for myelopathy include Herpes zoster, enteroviruses, Chlamydia, Mycoplasma, Lyme disease, tuberculosis, and parasitic infestations such as schistosomiasis. A history of fever, rash, meningismus, and recent travel may suggest infectious causes. Treatable conditions such as syphilis, HIV, tuberculosis, herpes viruses, and Lyme disease must be considered. Serologic testing and CSF polymerase chain reaction (PCR) studies can help to identify specific organisms. Cytology may help to identify malignant tumors.

The overall approach to a patient with SS with CNS manifestations includes the performance of an MRI examination and laboratory tests to establish the nature of the CNS lesions. If the patient presents solely with symptoms of myelitis, an MRI of the spine and of the brain should be performed to exclude CNS lesions. A sample of CSF should be obtained to evaluate whether pleocytosis is present and to determine protein and glucose levels. These may be helpful in some cases of aseptic meningitis caused by viruses. For SS, the IgG index may be elevated and oligoclonal bands may be present. However, these findings could also be present in SLE and MS. If the patient appears to have aseptic meningitis, a careful history should be taken to identify possible causes other than SS, including viral, bacterial or fungal infections and appropriate samples of body fluids, including serum and CSF should be sent for tests. Cultures, PCR, and other tests should be performed to rule out infectious causes. Serological testing to exclude SLE and the antiphospholipid syndrome is essential.

References

1. Delalande S, de Seze J, Fauchais AL, et al. Neurologic manifestations in primary Sjogren's syndrome: a study of 82 patients. Medicine (Baltimore). 2004;83:280–91.
2. Govoni M, Padovan M, Rizzo N, Trotta F. CNS involvement in primary Sjogren's syndrome: prevalence, clinical aspects, diagnostic assessment and therapeutic approach. CNS Drugs. 2001;15:597–607.
3. Morgen K, McFarland HF, Pillemer SR. Central nervous system disease in primary Sjogren's syndrome: the role of magnetic resonance imaging. Semin Arthritis Rheum. 2004;34:623–30.
4. Ozgocmen S, Gur A. Treatment of central nervous system involvement associated with primary Sjogren's syndrome. Curr Pharm Des. 2008;14:1270–3.
5. Soliotis FC, Mavragani CP, Moutsopoulos HM. Central nervous system involvement in Sjogren's syndrome. Ann Rheum Dis. 2004;63:616–20.
6. Lafitte C, Amoura Z, Cacoub P, et al. Neurological complications of primary Sjogren's syndrome. J Neurol. 2001;248:577–84.
7. Belin C, Moroni C, Caillat-Vigneron N, et al. Central nervous system involvement in Sjogren's syndrome: evidence from neuropsychological testing and HMPAO-SPECT. Ann Med Interne (Paris). 1999;150:598–604.
8. Escudero D, Latorre P, Codina M, et al. Central nervous system disease in Sjogren's syndrome. Ann Med Interne (Parris). 1995;146:239–42.
9. Mauch E, Volk C, Kratzsch G, et al. Neurological and neuropsychiatric dysfunction in primary Sjogren's syndrome. Acta Neurol Scand. 1994;89:31–5.
10. Hietaharju A, Jannti V, Korpela M, Frey H. Nervous system involvement in systemic lupus erythematosus, Sjogren syndrome's and scleroderma. Acta Neurol Scand. 1993;88:299–308.
11. Andonopoulos AP, Lagos G, Drosos AA, Moutsopoulos HM. The spectrum of neurological involvement in Sjogren's syndrome. Br J Rheumatol. 1990;29:21–3.

12. Alexander EL, Beall SS, Gordon B, Selnes OA, Yannakakis GD, Patronas N, et al. Magnetic resonance imaging of cerebral lesions in patients with the Sjogren syndrome. Ann Intern Med. 1988;108:815–23.

13. Coates T, Slavotinek JP, Rischmueller M, Schultz D, Anderson C, Dellamelva M, et al. Cerebral white matter lesions in primary Sjogren's syndrome: a controlled study. J Rheumatol. 1999;26:1301–5.

14. Pierot L, Sauve C, Leger JM, Martin N, Koeger AC, Wechsler B, et al. Asymptomatic cerebral involvement in Sjogren's syndrome: MRI findings of 15 cases. Neuroradiology. 1993;35: 378–80.

15. Alexander EL, Ranzenbach MR, Kumar AJ, Kozachuk WE, Rosenbaum AE, Patronas N, et al. Anti-Ro(SS-A) autoantibodies in central nervous system disease associated with Sjogren's syndrome (CNS-SS): clinical, neuroimaging, and angiographic correlates. Neurology. 1994;44: 899–908.

16. Michel L, Toulgoat F, Desal H, et al. Atypical neurologic complications in patients with primary Sjogren's syndrome: report of 4 cases. Semin Arthritis Rheum. 2011;40(4):338–42.

17. Min JH, Kim SH, Park MS, Kim BJ, Lee KH. Brain MRI lesions characteristic of neuromyelitis optica and positive anti-aquaporin 4-antibody may predict longitudinal extensive myelitis and optic neuritis in Sjogren's syndrome. Mult Scler. 2010;16(6):762–4.

18. Alexander EL. Neurologic disease in Sjogren's syndrome: mononuclear inflammatory vasculopathy affecting central/peripheral nervous system and muscle. A clinical review and update of immunopathogenesis. Rheum Dis Clin North Am. 1993;19(4):869–908.

19. Mataro M, Escudero D, Ariza M, et al. Magnetic resonance abnormalities associated with cognitive dysfunction in primary Sjogren syndrome. J Neurol. 2003;250(9):1070–6.

20. Morgen KE. Central nervous system disease in primary Sjögren's syndrome. In: Binder M, Hirokawa N, Windhorst U, editors. Encyclopedia of neuroscience, vol. 3. New York: Springer-Verlag Berlin Heidelberg; 2009. p. 632.

21. Awad IA, Spetzler RF, Hodak JA, Awad CA, Carey R. Incidental subcortical lesions identified on magnetic resonance imaging in the elderly. I. Correlation with age and cerebrovascular risk factors. Stroke. 1986;17(6):1084–9.

22. Le Guern V, Belin C, Henegar C, et al. Cognitive function and 99mTc-ECD brain SPECT are significantly correlated in patients with primary Sjogren syndrome: a case-control study. Ann Rheum Dis. 2010;69(1):132–7.

23. Alexander EL, Craft C, Dorsch C, Moser RL, Provost TT, Alexander GE. Necrotizing arteritis and spinal subarachnoid hemorrhage in Sjogren syndrome. Ann Neurol. 1982;11(6):632–5.

24. Alexander MS, Dias PS, Uttley D. Spontaneous subarachnoid hemorrhage and negative cerebral panangiography. Review of 140 cases. J Neurosurg. 1986;64(4):537–42.

25. Marignier R, Giaudon P, Vukusic S, Confavreux C, Honnorat J. Anti-aquaporin-4 antibodies in Devic's neuromyelitis optica: therapeutic implications. Ther Adv Neurol Disord. 2010;3:311–21.

26. Malinow KL, Molina R, Gordon B, Selnes OA, Provost TT, Alexander EL. Neuropsychiatric dysfunction in primary Sjogren's syndrome. Ann Intern Med. 1985;103(3):344–50.

27. McFarland HF, Stone LA, Calabresi PA, Maloni H, Bash CN, Frank JA. MRI studies of multiple sclerosis: implications for the natural history of the disease and for monitoring effectiveness of experimental therapies. Mult Scler. 1996;2:198–205.

28. Simon JH, Jacobs LD, Campion M, Wende K, Simonian N, Cookfair DL, et al. Magnetic resonance studies of intramuscular interferon beta-1a for relapsing multiple sclerosis. The Multiple Sclerosis Collaborative Research Group. Ann Neurol. 1998;43:79–87.

29. Nomura K, Yamano S, Ikeda Y, Yamada H, Fujimoto T, Minami S, et al. Asymptomatic cerebrovascular lesions detected by magnetic resonance imaging in patients with systemic lupus erythematosus lacking a history of neuropsychiatric events. Intern Med. 1999;38:785–95.

30. Luks TL, Goodkin DE, Nelson SJ, Majumdar S, Bacchetti P, Portnoy D, et al. A longitudinal study of ventricular volume in early relapsing-remitting multiple sclerosis. Mult Scler. 2000;6:332–7.

31. de Leeuw FE, de Groot JC, Achten E, Oudkerk M, Ramos LM, Heijboer R, et al. Prevalence of cerebral white matter lesions in elderly people: a population based magnetic resonance imaging study. The Rotterdam Scan Study. J Neurol Neurosurg Psychiatry. 2001;70:9–14.

32. Cortese I, MacFarland HF. Multiple sclerosis. In: Rich RR, Fleisher TA, Shearer WT, Schroeder Jr HW, Frew AJ, Weyand CM, editors. Clinical immunology: principles and practice. 3rd ed. Mosby: Elsevier; 2008.

33. Van de Merve JP, Yamada T, Sakamoto Y. Systemic aspects of interstitial cystitis, immunology and linkage with autoimmune disorders. Int J Urol. 2003;10(Suppl):S35–8.

34. Achiron A, Polliack M, Rao SM, Barak Y, Lavie M, Appelboim N, et al. Cognitive patterns and progression in multiple sclerosis: construction and validation of percentile curves. J Neurol Neurosurg Psychiatry. 2005;76:744–9.

35. Segal B, Carpenter A, Walk D. Involvement of nervous system pathways in primary Sjogren's syndrome. Rheum Dis Clin North Am. 2008;34:885–906.

36. Polman CH, Reingold SC, Edan G, Filippi M, Hartung HP, Kappos L, et al. Diagnostic criteria for multiple sclerosis: 2005 revisions to the "McDonald Criteria". Ann Neurol. 2005;58(6): 840–6.

37. Napoli SQ, Bakshi R. Magnetic resonance imaging in multiple sclerosis. Rev Neurol Dis. 2005;2(3):109–16; Summer.

38. Wingerchuk MD. Neuromyelitis optica (Devic's syndrome). Accessed 2006. http://www.myelitis.org/rnds2006/Wingerchuk_NMO_Rare_Neuroimm_062406_final.pdf

39. Miyakis S, Lockshin MD, Atsumi T, Branch DW, Brey RL, Cervera R, et al. International consensus statement on an update of the classification criteria for definite antiphospholipid syndrome (APS). J Thromb Haemost. 2006;4:295–306.

40. Cervera R, Piette J-C, Font J, Mhamashta MA, Shoenfeld Y, Camps MT, et al. Antiphospholipid syndrome: clinical and immunologic manifestations and patterns of disease expression in a cohort of 1,000 patients. Arthritis Rheum. 2002;46:1019–27.

41. Cuadrado MJ, Khamashta MA, Ballesteros A, Godfrey T, Simon MJ, Hughes GRV. Can neurologic manifestations of Hughes (antiphospholipid) syndrome be distinguished from multiple sclerosis? Analysis of 27 patients and review of the literature. Medicine (Baltimore). 2000;79: 57–68.

42. Molloy ES, Calabrese LH. Progressive multifocal leukoencephalopathy. Arthritis Rheum. 2009;60:3761–5.

43. Weiffenbach JM, Fox PC. Odor identification ability among patients with Sjogren's syndrome. Arthritis Rheum. 1993;36:1752–4.

44. Boki KA, Ioannidis JP, Segas JV, Maragkoudakis PV, Petrou D, Adamopoulos GK, et al. How significant is sensorineural hearing loss in primary Sjögren's syndrome? An individually matched case-control study. J Rheumatol. 2001;28(4):798–801.

45. Tumiati B, Casoli P, Permeggiani A. Hearing loss in the Sjogren syndrome. Ann Intern Med. 1997;126:450–3.

46. Irani D. Aseptic meningitis and viral myelitis. Neurol Clin. 2008;26:635–55.

47. Schmalstieg WF, Weishenker BG. Approach to acute or subacute myelopathy. Neurol Clin Pract. 2010;75:S2–8.

Chapter 21
Peripheral Neuropathy

Pantelis P. Pavlakis and Marinos C. Dalakas

Contents

21.1   Prevalence and Classification

The prevalence of peripheral neuropathy among Sjögren's syndrome patients varies greatly between different published studies, with numbers ranging between 2% and 60% [1–14]. Such a large disparity is due to: (a) the use of different criteria for the diagnosis of Sjögren's syndrome, and (b) the varying definition of peripheral neuropathy with inconsistent application of objective clinical or electrodiagnostic criteria. An example of the problem is one recent report, based on a large population of Sjögren's syndrome patients, which estimates the frequency of peripheral neuropathy at 10% [5], without providing details on how the neuropathy was diagnosed.

P.P. Pavlakis • M.C. Dalakas (✉)
Neuroimmunology Unit, Department of Pathophysiology,
Medical School, University of Athens, Athens, Greece

M. Ramos-Casals et al. (eds.), *Sjögren's Syndrome*,
DOI 10.1007/978-0-85729-947-5_21, © Springer-Verlag London Limited 2012

Table 21.1 Patterns of peripheral neurologic involvement in Sjögren's syndrome

More common
Small fiber painful sensory neuropathy
Sensory polyneuropathy
Sensorimotor polyneuropathy
Less common
Cranial neuropathy
Mononeuropathy multiplex
Sensory ataxic neuronopathy (ganglionopathy)
Demyelinating polyradiculoneuropathy (CIDP)
Autonomic neuropathy

The clinical spectrum of peripheral neurologic involvement in Sjögren's syndrome is broad (Table 21.1) [15–17]. Sensory neuropathies, the most frequently encountered types, include three discrete subsets: (a) an axonal sensory polyneuropathy, which typically presents with distal symmetric sensory deficits and absent or reduced sensory potentials on nerve conduction studies; (b) a painful sensory neuropathy, due to involvement of the small unmyelinated fibers, which presents with painful paresthesias but lacks objective clinical and electrodiagnostic findings; and (c) a severe, disabling sensory ataxic neuropathy ("neuronopathy"), due to dorsal root ganglion involvement. Other types of peripheral neuropathies include: axonal sensorimotor polyneuropathy; various cranial neuropathies, with trigeminal neuralgia being the most common; mononeuropathy or mononeuropathy multiplex, probably related to vasculitis; demyelinating sensorimotor polyradiculoneuropathy; and autonomic neuropathy. Some of these neuropathies overlap within a single patient, necessitating correlations between clinical, electrophysiological, and histopathological findings to define the precise diagnosis.

The evidence regarding the temporal association of neuropathy with stage-specific disease state or disease severity of Sjögren's syndrome is conflicting. Some studies suggest that peripheral neuropathy is a late event in the course of the disease [1, 5], occurring when specific clinical and laboratory manifestations are prominent, such as palpable purpura, low C4 complement factor, cryoglobulinemia, or glomerulonephritis and lymphoma [1]. Other studies suggest that peripheral neuropathy can be the presenting feature of an otherwise isolated glandular disease with benign course [15, 17]. We believe that these discrepancies reflect the bias of the type of practice that reports the neuropathic symptoms. In our neurology practice, for example, small fiber sensory neuropathy and ataxic neuropathy are sometimes the presenting manifestations of Sjögren's syndrome. In contrast, sensorimotor polyneuropathies, cranial neuropathies, and autonomic neuropathies usually present in patients with established disease.

We have recently performed a retrospective study of the frequency of neuropathy in a large number of patients with bone fide Sjögren's syndrome diagnosed in our Department of Pathophysiology. We found that peripheral neuropathy is a rare manifestation of Sjögren's syndrome, occurring only in 1.8% of patients overall [18]. In the majority of our patients, peripheral neuropathy occurred late in the course of the disease, at a median time of 6 years after the diagnosis of Sjögren's syndrome. Most of our patients also had other prominent extraglandular features present (see below).

Table 21.2 Electrophysiologic findings in different neuropathy subtypes in Sjögren's syndrome

Axonal polyneuropathy	Reduced/absent nerve action potentials, normal conduction velocities
Demyelinating radiculoneuropathy	Reduced distal latencies, reduced conduction velocities, prolonged F-wave
Mononeuropathy/multiple mononeuropathy	Reduced/absent nerve action potentials, normal conduction velocities (corresponding to affected nerves), "pseudo-block" at sites of infarction
Small fiber neuropathy	Normal
Sensory neuronopathy	Absent sensory nerve action potentials, normal motor nerve action potentials, normal conduction velocities, normal F-wave, normal EMG

21.2 Sensory or Sensorimotor Axonal Polyneuropathy with Objective Clinical and Electrodiagnostic Findings

Axonaly polyneuropathies in Sjögren's syndrome typically have a slow onset and present as either a mixed sensorimotor polyneuropathy or a pure sensory neuropathy. Cases of pure motor neuropathy have rarely been reported [19]. In our small series of patients [18], polyneuropathy was found to be a feature of systemic Sjögren's syndrome. Sensorimotor polyneuropathy was associated with manifestations such as, palpable purpura, vasculitis, and cryoglobulinemia, which confer higher risk of lymphoma development [20]. On the other hand, sensory polyneuropathy, though often a feature of systemic Sjögren's syndrome, as well, was not associated with other specific disease manifestations.

Nerve conduction studies almost always reveal an axonal pattern of involvement (Table 21.2), with lower limbs being affected more often than upper limbs [15]. Patients usually present with distal paresthesias, including symmetric sensory deficits in a "glove-stocking" pattern. As the disease progresses, mild distal muscle weakness may be present. Tendon reflexes are diminished or absent in the affected limbs. Nerve biopsy usually yields nonspecific findings, typically loss of myelinated fibers, except if vasculitis is present. Although vasculitis is typically painful and asymmetric, when confluent multisegmental deficits have taken place, the neuropathy may present with a symmetric pattern. We recommend nerve biopsy to exclude inflammation and vasculitis based on critical review of the clinical and neurophysiological findings.

In patients with painful sensory paresthesias, tricyclic antidepressants, gabapentin, pregabalin, duloxetine, opioids, and topical local anesthetics can be effective [21] (Table 21.3).

21.3 Sensorimotor Demyelinating Polyneuropathy (CIDP)

These patients present with subacute onset of proximal and distal muscle weakness, sensory deficits, depressed reflexes, high CSF protein, and signs of demyelination on nerve conduction studies. This neuropathy, which is the most common form of acquired demyelinating neuropathy, can occur in patients with Sjögren's syndrome and should be always sought for and excluded because it is a treatable form of neuropathy responding to intravenous immunoglobulin (IVIg) and glucorticoids [22].

21.4   Multiple Mononeuropathy or Mononeuritis Multiplex

Mononeuropathy and multiple mononeuropathy are rare manifestations of Sjögren's syndrome. Patients present with acute or subacute onset of sensory and motor deficits in the distribution of single nerves. Deficits are almost invariably accompanied by pain over the same area. The symptoms are usually due to vasculitis of the vasa nervorum [15, 17]. Vessel wall inflammation, due to cellular infiltrates, results in endothelial damage, which in turn leads to vessel lumen occlusion and nerve infarction. Multiple deficits can give rise to an asymmetric, multifocal pattern. If the neurologic deficits become confluent, the resulting symmetric pattern may lead to the clinical impression of a generalized polyneuropathy [23]. Constitutional symptoms often accompany mononeuropathy or multiple mononeuropathy, reflecting the vasculitic involvement of other organs. Typical laboratory findings include an elevated erythrocyte sedimentation rate and C-reactive protein levels. Electrodiagnostic studies reveal an axonal pattern of nerve dysfunction with "pseudo-blocks" at the sites of nerve infarctions.

Nerve biopsy can be helpful in the diagnostically challenging cases [24]. Pathognomonic findings include damage of the vasa nervorum wall with fibrinoid necrosis and cellular infiltrates, mainly T cells and macrophages. We always recommend the combination of muscle and nerve biopsy if there is strong suspicion of vasculitis, because the focal nature of vasculitis often leads to false-negative nerve biopsies. The highly vascular nature of muscle tissues increases the yield of biopsy substantially. A number of studies have shown that dual biopsies of both muscle and nerve are associated with a sensitivity of up to 85% for vasculitis [25]. Necrotizing vasculitis usually responds well to immunosuppression, particularly if the diagnosis is made at an early stage [26].

Prompt recognition and treatment of this condition is needed in order to prevent the progression of neurological damage. Glucocorticoids and adjuvant immunosuppressive agents are the mainstay of treatment (Table 21.3). Cyclophosphamide plus glucocorticoids is presently the first-line therapy for remission induction in the setting of necrotizing vasculitis associated with Sjögren's syndrome [27]. After remission is achieved, safer agents such as azathioprine, methotrexate, or mycophenolate mofetil can be used as maintenance treatment [28, 29]. Rituximab is a highly promising approach to the treatment of this form of vasculitis, as B cell depletion has been proven to be as effective as cyclophosphamide for remission induction in forms of vasculitis associated with antineutrophil cytoplasmic antibodies (ANCA) [30]. Of interest are the results of another study, in which patients with Sjögren's syndrome and lymphoma were treated with rituximab and CHOP (cyclophosphamide, doxorubicin, vincristine, prednisone) [31]. Despite the use of vincristine, a potentially neurotoxic agent, complete remission of peripheral neuropathy was induced.

21.5   Sensory Ataxic Neuronopathy

Sensory ataxic neuropathy, also known by the names of ataxic neuropathy, sensory neuronopathy, or ganglionopathy, is a sensory neuropathy encountered in a number of different diseases, one of them being Sjögren's syndrome. The term "neuronopathy" is used to denote dysfunction of the sensory ganglionic neuronal cell body, located at the dorsal root. Because of the location of the lesion, a pure sensory neuropathy results. Muscle strength and motor electrodiagnostic studies are normal or nearly so, but sensory potentials are typically absent.

Sensory ataxic neuronopathy is the most disabling of all peripheral neuropathies encountered in Sjögren's syndrome. Its onset is usually subacute, although acute cases have also been described [32, 33]. Although all sensory modalities are affected, losses of position sense and vibration predominate because of involvement of large-size fibers [33]. Patients often present with paresthesias and unsteadiness of gait, due to deafferentiation [33]. Ataxic gait, Romberg sign, impaired proprioception and vibration sensation, as well as absent tendon reflexes are typical neurological findings [15, 17, 34].

An interesting and often misleading clinical finding in patients with sensory ataxic neuronopathy are pseudoathetoid movements of the hands. [33] This results from proprioceptive loss in the fingers. Neurological deficits are usually present bilaterally but involvement of the dorsal root ganglia can be asymmetric, affecting one side more than the other. Involvement of the upper limbs and trunk as well as the lower extremities is highly characteristic of sensory ataxic neuronopathies, in contrast to mononeuritis multiplex, for example. Patients usually progress to a wheel-chair confinement due to lack of proprioception, in spite of having normal strength [33]. Characteristic electrodiagnostic findings include absent sensory nerve action potentials, normal motor nerve action potentials, normal nerve conduction velocities, F-wave latencies, and a normal EMG (Table 21.2) [15, 17, 33, 34]. The F-wave latencies can be however prolonged when the roots are affected.

The main differential diagnostic entity of concern is paraneoplastic sensory ataxic neuropathy and the neuropathy associated with IgM monoclonal antimyelin-associated glycoprotein (MAG) antibodies [33]. Paraneoplastic neuronopathy most often accompanies or precedes small cell carcinoma of the lung, and rarely breast cancer or lymphoma [35]. Seropositivity for anti-Hu antibodies in these cases is a highly specific (99%) laboratory finding. The absence of anti-Hu antibodies, however, does not rule out a malignancy [36]. Immunofixation electrophoresis should be always performed to exclude an IgM monoclonal gammopathy. Other causes of sensory neuronopathy are listed in Table 21.3.

The pathogenesis of dorsal root ganglionopathy in Sjögren's syndrome is unclear. On the rare occasions when dorsal root ganglion tissue has been obtained through an open biopsy, neuronal degeneration and T cell infiltration of the dorsal root ganglia has been demonstrated [17, 34, 37]. However, the role of the other components of the immune system, namely B cells and autoantibodies, remains unknown.

Table 21.3 Sensory neuronopathy causes

Paraneoplastic (lung cancer, Hodgkin's lymphoma, neuroendocrine tumors, breast cancer, ovarian cancer, sarcoma)

Immune-mediated (Sjögren's syndrome, MGUS)[a]

Infectious (AIDS, HTLV-1)[b,c]

Iatrogenic (platin analogues, doxorubicin, bortezomib)

Vitamin related (pyridoxine intoxication, nicotinic acid deficiency, vitamin E deficiency, riboflavin deficiency)

Hereditary (Friedreich's ataxia)

Idiopathic

[a]MGUS: Monoclonal gammopathy of unknown significance
[b]AIDS: Acquired immune deficiency syndrome
[c]HTLV-1: Human T lymphotropic virus – 1

Treatment regimens including IVIg [38], plasmapheresis [39], D-penicillamine [40], infliximab [41], and interferon-α [42], have been employed, but none in a randomized clinical trial. The results are usually disappointing and the treatment of this neuronopathy remains challenging, particularly if treatment is not begun until an advanced stage. However, some cases with subacute onset appear to respond to immunotherapy. A case of IVIg-dependent sensory neuronopathy has been reported to respond to treatment with rituximab [43]. We recently treated five cases of autoimmune ataxic neuropathy with rituximab and, although there was not any dramatic change, minimal benefits were noted in four [44].

21.6   Small Fiber Painful Sensory Neuropathy

Small fiber neuropathy is the most common sensory neuropathy encountered in patients with Sjögren's syndrome. Small-diameter lightly myelinated Aδ and unmyelinated C fibers, which relay superficial sensation, are predominantly affected. Painful, burning dysesthesias, usually of the distal limbs is the presenting symptom. These patients are often labeled as having psychosomatic disorder, because they do not have any objective abnormal findings in the neurological examination. Reflexes, sensory examination, and nerve conduction studies are normal [45]. Two distinct patterns of small fiber neuropathy have been described in patients with Sjögren's syndrome [46, 47]. The first involves a distal, symmetric (length-dependent) pattern of neurologic involvement with centripetal progression, which is attributed to loss of small axons ("dying-back axonopathy"). The second involves an asymmetric, nonlength-dependent distribution of symptoms, which may reflect a neuronopathy affecting small sensory neurons located in the dorsal root ganglia, which give rise to small diameter nerve fibers [48]. Mixed, small and large fiber dysfunction has also been described, as well as progression from small fiber to large fiber dysfunction. The implication of this is that a patient with a nonlength-dependent small fiber neuropathy may later develop sensory ataxic neuropathy [46]. Sympathetic skin response, quantitative sensory testing, quantitative sudomotor axon reflex testing, and sensory evoked potentials are some of the methods used to assess small fiber function [49], but they are technically complex and not widely available. Skin biopsy, a simple outpatient procedure, is now used to assess epidermal nerve fiber density based on standardized methods of objective and reproducible quantification. Skin biopsy is the best and easiest method to diagnose small fiber neuropathy [24, 45]. We recommend it to establish the diagnosis and to exclude the possibility of psychosomatic complaints. Sural nerve biopsy, on the other hand, is not diagnostic and we do not recommend it [17, 46].

Treatment for small fiber neuropathy is mainly symptomatic, as described above. Of interest is a small uncontrolled study, which showed decrease of pain after IVIg [50]. However, the findings of this study need to be validated by further randomized controlled trials involving larger number of patients.

21.7   Restless Leg Syndrome

Restless legs syndrome is a constellation of symptoms [51], the most important being an unpleasant sensation of the legs, which is relieved by movement and exacerbated by limb immobilization. Symptoms typically follow a circadian pattern of fluctuation, being more intense when at rest or falling asleep during the night. The symptoms result in sleep loss, disruption of normal activities, and depression. Iron deficiency, end-stage renal disease, and pregnancy are common causes of restless leg syndrome that should be excluded before the condition is attributed to Sjögren's syndrome. The physical examination and laboratory evaluation are generally normal in this setting. Dopamine agonists, gabapentin, and the opiates methadone and oxycodone have been effective in the treatment of restless leg syndrome [52]. In a study focusing on sleep disorders, restless leg syndrome was more prevalent in patients with Sjögren's syndrome compared to rheumatoid arthritis or healthy controls [53]; however, this association requires confirmation. In our experience, restless leg syndrome is an overlooked symptom in Sjögren's syndrome patients and should be considered because the treatment is rewarding. Our experience suggests that dopamine agonists should be the treatment of choice.

References

1. Skopouli FN, Dafni U, Ioannidis JP, et al. Clinical evolution, and morbidity and mortality of primary Sjogren's syndrome. Semin Arthritis Rheum. 2000;29:296–304.
2. Harboe E, Tjensvoll AB, Maroni S, et al. Neuropsychiatric syndromes in patients with systemic lupus erythematosus and primary Sjogren syndrome: a comparative population-based study. Ann Rheum Dis. 2009;68:1541–6.
3. Goransson LG, Herigstad A, Tjensvoll AB, et al. Peripheral neuropathy in primary Sjogren syndrome: a population-based study. Arch Neurol. 2006;63:1612–5.

4. Govoni M, Bajocchi G, Rizzo N, et al. Neurological involvement in primary Sjogren's syndrome: clinical and instrumental evaluation in a cohort of Italian patients. Clin Rheumatol. 1999;18:299–303.
5. Ramos-Casals M, Solans R, Rosas J, et al. Primary Sjogren syndrome in Spain: clinical and immunologic expression in 1010 patients. Medicine (Baltimore). 2008;87:210–9.
6. Andonopoulos AP, Lagos G, Drosos AA, et al. The spectrum of neurological involvement in Sjogren's syndrome. Br J Rheumatol. 1990;29:21–3.
7. Vrethem M, Lindvall B, Holmgren H, et al. Neuropathy and myopathy in primary Sjogren's syndrome: neurophysiological, immunological and muscle biopsy results. Acta Neurol Scand. 1990;82:126–31.
8. Gemignani F, Marbini A, Pavesi G, et al. Peripheral neuropathy associated with primary Sjogren's syndrome. J Neurol Neurosurg Psychiatry. 1994;57:983–6.
9. Barendregt PJ, van den Bent MJ, van Raaij-van den Aarssen VJ, et al. Involvement of the peripheral nervous system in primary Sjogren's syndrome. Ann Rheum Dis. 2001;60:876–81.
10. Andonopoulos AP, Lagos G, Drosos AA, et al. Neurologic involvement in primary Sjogren's syndrome: a preliminary report. J Autoimmun. 1989;2:485–8.
11. Lopate G, Pestronk A, Al-Lozi M, et al. Peripheral neuropathy in an outpatient cohort of patients with Sjogren's syndrome. Muscle Nerve. 2006;33:672–6.
12. Lafitte C, Amoura Z, Cacoub P, et al. Neurological complications of primary Sjogren's syndrome. J Neurol. 2001;248:577–84.
13. Mauch E, Volk C, Kratzsch G, et al. Neurological and neuropsychiatric dysfunction in primary Sjogren's syndrome. Acta Neurol Scand. 1994;89:31–5.
14. Binder A, Snaith ML, Isenberg D. Sjogren's syndrome: a study of its neurological complications. Br J Rheumatol. 1988;27:275–80.
15. Grant IA, Hunder GG, Homburger HA, et al. Peripheral neuropathy associated with sicca complex. Neurology. 1997;48:855–62.
16. Delalande S, de Seze J, Fauchais AL, et al. Neurologic manifestations in primary Sjogren syndrome: a study of 82 patients. Medicine (Baltimore). 2004;83:280–91.
17. Mori K, Iijima M, Koike H, et al. The wide spectrum of clinical manifestations in Sjogren's syndrome-associated neuropathy. Brain. 2005;128:2518–34.
18. Pavlakis PP, Alexopoulos H, Kosmidis M, et al. Sjögren's syndrome associated polyneuropathy: clinical and immunological profiles. Neurology. 2010;74:491–2.
19. Mochizuki H, Kamakura K, Masaki T, et al. Motor dominant neuropathy in Sjogren's syndrome: report of two cases. Intern Med. 2002;41:142–6.
20. Ioannidis JP, Vassiliou VA, Moutsopoulos HM. Long-term risk of mortality and lymphoproliferative disease and predictive classification of primary Sjogren's syndrome. Arthritis Rheum. 2002;46:741–7.
21. Dworkin RH, O'Connor AB, Backonja M, et al. Pharmacologic management of neuropathic pain: evidence-based recommendations. Pain. 2007;132:237–51.
22. Hughes RA, Donofrio P, Bril V, et al. Intravenous immune globulin (10% caprylate-chromatography purified) for the treatment of chronic inflammatory demyelinating polyradiculoneuropathy (ICE study): a randomised placebo-controlled trial. Lancet Neurol. 2008;7:136–44.
23. Mellgren SI, Conn DL, Stevens JC, et al. Peripheral neuropathy in primary Sjogren's syndrome. Neurology. 1989;39:390–4.
24. England JD, Gronseth GS, Franklin G, et al. Evaluation of distal symmetric polyneuropathy: the role of autonomic testing, nerve biopsy, and skin biopsy (an evidence-based review). Muscle Nerve. 2009;39:106–15.
25. Collins MP, Mendell JR, Periquet MI, et al. Superficial peroneal nerve/peroneus brevis muscle biopsy in vasculitic neuropathy. Neurology. 2000;55:636–43.
26. Terrier B, Lacroix C, Guillevin L, et al. Diagnostic and prognostic relevance of neuromuscular biopsy in primary Sjogren's syndrome-related neuropathy. Arthritis Rheum. 2007;57:1520–9.
27. Schaublin GA, Michet Jr CJ, Dyck PJ, et al. An update on the classification and treatment of vasculitic neuropathy. Lancet Neurol. 2005;4:853–65.

28. Jayne D, Rasmussen N, Andrassy K, et al. A randomized trial of maintenance therapy for vasculitis associated with antineutrophil cytoplasmic autoantibodies. N Engl J Med. 2003;349: 36–44.
29. Pagnoux C, Mahr A, Hamidou MA, et al. Azathioprine or methotrexate maintenance for ANCA-associated vasculitis. N Engl J Med. 2008;359:2790–803.
30. Stone JH, Merkel PA, Spiera RF, et al. Rituximab compared with cyclophosphamide for remission induction in ANCA-associated vasculitis. N Engl J Med. 2010;15;363:221–32.
31. Voulgarelis M, Giannouli S, Tzioufas AG, et al. Long term remission of Sjogren's syndrome associated aggressive B cell non-Hodgkin's lymphomas following combined B cell depletion therapy and CHOP (cyclophosphamide, doxorubicin, vincristine, prednisone). Ann Rheum Dis. 2006;65:1033–7.
32. Souayah N, Chong PS, Cros D. Acute sensory neuronopathy as the presenting symptom of Sjogren's syndrome. J Clin Neurosci. 2006;13:862–5.
33. Dalakas MC. Chronic idiopathic ataxic neuropathy. Ann Neurol. 1986;19:545–54.
34. Griffin JW, Cornblath DR, Alexander E, et al. Ataxic sensory neuropathy and dorsal root ganglionitis associated with Sjogren's syndrome. Ann Neurol. 1990;27:304–15.
35. Sghirlanzoni A, Pareyson D, Lauria G. Sensory neuron diseases. Lancet Neurol. 2005;4:349–61.
36. Molinuevo JL, Graus F, Serrano C, et al. Utility of anti-Hu antibodies in the diagnosis of paraneoplastic sensory neuropathy. Ann Neurol. 1998;44:976–80.
37. Malinow K, Yannakakis GD, Glusman SM, et al. Subacute sensory neuronopathy secondary to dorsal root ganglionitis in primary Sjogren's syndrome. Ann Neurol. 1986;20:535–7.
38. Takahashi Y, Takata T, Hoshino M, et al. Benefit of IVIG for long-standing ataxic sensory neuronopathy with Sjogren's syndrome. IV immunoglobulin. Neurology. 2003;60:503–5.
39. Chen WH, Yeh JH, Chiu HC. Plasmapheresis in the treatment of ataxic sensory neuropathy associated with Sjogren's syndrome. Eur Neurol. 2001;45:270–4.
40. Asahina M, Kuwabara S, Nakajima M, et al. D-penicillamine treatment for chronic sensory ataxic neuropathy associated with Sjogren's syndrome. Neurology. 1998;51:1451–3.
41. Caroyer JM, Manto MU, Steinfeld SD. Severe sensory neuronopathy responsive to infliximab in primary Sjogren's syndrome. Neurology. 2002;59:1113–4.
42. Yamada S, Mori K, Matsuo K, et al. Interferon alfa treatment for Sjogren's syndrome associated neuropathy. J Neurol Neurosurg Psychiatry. 2005;76:576–8.
43. Gorson KC, Natarajan N, Ropper AH, et al. Rituximab treatment in patients with IVIg-dependent immune polyneuropathy: a prospective pilot trial. Muscle Nerve. 2007;35:66–9.
44. Kosmidis ML, Dalakas MC. Practical considerations on the use of rituximab in autoimmune neurological disorders. Ther Adv Neurol Disord. 2010;3:93–105.
45. Lacomis D. Small-fiber neuropathy. Muscle Nerve. 2002;26:173–88.
46. Mori K, Iijima M, Sugiura M, et al. Sjogren's syndrome associated painful sensory neuropathy without sensory ataxia. J Neurol Neurosurg Psychiatry. 2003;74:1320–2.
47. Chai J, Herrmann DN, Stanton M, et al. Painful small-fiber neuropathy in Sjogren syndrome. Neurology. 2005;65:925–7.
48. Gorson KC, Herrmann DN, Thiagarajan R, et al. Non-length dependent small fibre neuropathy/ganglionopathy. J Neurol Neurosurg Psychiatry. 2008;79:163–9.
49. Hoitsma E, Reulen JP, de Baets M, et al. Small fiber neuropathy: a common and important clinical disorder. J Neurol Sci. 2004;227:119–30.
50. Morozumi S, Kawagashira Y, Iijima M, et al. Intravenous immunoglobulin treatment for painful sensory neuropathy associated with Sjogren's syndrome. J Neurol Sci. 2009;279:57–61.
51. Kushida CA. Clinical presentation, diagnosis, and quality of life issues in restless legs syndrome. Am J Med. 2007;120:S4–12.
52. Jankovic J. Treatment of hyperkinetic movement disorders. Lancet Neurol. 2009;8:844–56.
53. Gudbjornsson B, Broman JE, Hetta J, et al. Sleep disturbances in patients with primary Sjogren's syndrome. Br J Rheumatol. 1993;32:1072–6.

Chapter 22
Autonomic Neuropathy

Thomas Mandl and Lennart Jacobsson

Contents

22.1 Introduction

Autonomic dysfunction (AD) is a feature of many different chronic diseases such as type I and II diabetes, rheumatoid arthritis, systemic lupus erythematosus, scleroderma, and inflammatory bowel disease. Patients with primary Sjögren's syndrome (pSS) may also show various symptoms of impaired autonomic nervous function such as orthostatic intolerance [1]. The use of autonomic reflex tests (ARTs) in pSS has demonstrated evidence of parasympathetic and sympathetic dysfunction [2–6]. In contrast, investigations of heart rate variability and baroreflex sensitivity in pSS have yielded contradictory results [6–9] (Table 22.1). A variety of AD symptoms have been reported in pSS patients [9, 15]. However, because the degree of exocrine

T. Mandl (✉) • L. Jacobsson
Department of Rheumatology, Skane University Hospital, Malmö, Sweden

M. Ramos-Casals et al. (eds.), *Sjögren's Syndrome*,
DOI 10.1007/978-0-85729-947-5_22, © Springer-Verlag London Limited 2012

Table 22.1 Studies on objective autonomic nervous function in patients with pSS

Year	Authors [Reference]	Inclusion criteria	Number of patients	Methods	Main findings in pSS patients
1997	Mandl et al. [10]	Cph/EC	19	ARTs	Parasympathetic dysfunction
1998	Andonopoulos et al. [3]	EC	32	ARTs	AD
1999	Barendregt et al. [4]	EC	41	ARTs Pupillography	Parasympathetic dysfunction
2000	Niemelä et al. [11]	EC	28	24 h HRV	No AD
2000	Tumiati et al. [8]	EC	16	HRV	Increased parasympathetic tone
2000	Kovacs et al. [12]	EC	22	CCh-induced vasodilatation in the skin	Impaired vasodilation to CCh
2001	Mandl et al. [13]	Cph/EC	30	ARTs	Parasympathetic dysfunction Sympathetic dysfunction
2002	Barendregt et al. [6]	EC	43	ARTs, BRS, HRV	Minor abnormalities
2003	Niemelä et al. [7]	AECC	30	ARTs, BRS, 24 h HRV	No AD
2004	Kovacs et al. [5]	AECC	51	ARTs, BRS, BPV, HRV	Abnormal ARTs Reduced HRV, BRS and BP variability
2007	Mandl et al. [2]	AECC	46	ARTs	Parasympathetic dysfunction Sympathetic dysfunction
2008	Cai et al. [9]	AECC	27	ARTs and HRV	Abnormal ARTs Reduced HRV, and BP variability
2010	Mandl et a l. [14]	AECC	27	ARTs	Parasympathetic dysfunction Sympathetic dysfunction

24hHRV 24-hour heart rate variability, *AD* autonomic dysfunction, *AECC* American-European Classification Criteria, *ARTs* autonomic reflex tests, *BP* blood pressure, *BPV* blood pressure variability, *BRS* baroreceptor sensitivity, *CCh* carbachol, *Cph* Copenhagen criteria, *EC* European community, *HRV* heart rate variability, *pSS* primary Sjögren's syndrome

gland destruction often correlates poorly with glandular function in pSS [16, 17], it is possible that the impaired exocrine gland function in this disorder relates in part to interference with nervous signals to the glands [18]. Exocrine secretion is modulated by the autonomic nervous system (ANS).

AD in pSS has been ascribed to various immunological factors, including anti-muscarinic 3 receptor (M3R) antibodies, inflammation of autonomic neural tissues, and cytokines interfering with neurotransmission [19–24]. Much interest has focused on anti-M3R antibodies, found in a subgroup of pSS patients [19–21].

These antibodies seem to block parasympathetic nervous signalling to exocrine glands, a signalling that is transmitted mainly via the parasympathetic M3R. Because the M3R is also found in other tissues, e.g., the bladder and the gastrointestinal system, these antibodies have also been proposed to cause symptoms such as irritable bladder and constipation [19]. However, anti-M3 antibodies do not account for all demonstrated disturbances of ANS function in pSS. Orthostatic hypotension, for example, often found in pSS patients, is usually considered a sign of sympathetic rather than parasympathetic dysfunction [25]. Orthostatic hypotension may be caused by inflammation of sympathetic ganglia or sympathetic nerves [22] or by cytokines that interfere with neurotransmission [24]. Thus, both subjective symptoms and objective signs of parasympathetic and sympathetic dysfunction have been described in pSS patients [1–5, 8, 9, 15].

The prevalence of AD in pSS is difficult to assess, for several reasons. First, the choice of methods, patients, and controls has varied between studies. Second, the standardization of autonomic test results and the definition of AD differ. Third, end-organ damage may obscure or mimic the effects of AD in some organ systems, e.g., in the exocrine glands. Fourth, cardiovascular autonomic nervous function, which is comparatively easy to assess, does not necessarily mirror ANS function in other parts of the body. Fifth, the proposed anti-M3R antibodies may mediate autonomic dysfunction in various organ systems but the effects of these antibodies are difficult to assess by the cardiovascular ANS tests that are used routinely. And finally, at this time no established, reproducible clinical test exists for the detection of these antibodies.

As a result of the limitations listed above, estimates of the prevalence of AD in pSS have varied widely. Taking all of the above limitations into account, objective signs of AD have been reported in 0–90% of pSS patients [3, 26] while approximately 50% have been reported to have an abnormal AD symptomatology using the Autonomic Symptom Profile questionnaire evaluating AD symptoms [26].

22.2 Pathogenesis of Autonomic Dysfunction in pSS

In pSS, AD has been ascribed to various immunological mechanisms, namely anti-M3R antibodies, cytokines interfering with neurotransmission, and inflammation of autonomic nerves, nerve vessels, and ganglia [19–24]. Although many chronic AD symptoms may be explained by the anti-M3R antibodies that interfere with parasympathetic nervous transduction in organs containing the M3R (e.g., secretomotor dysfunction, bladder symptoms, and gastroparesis), a more subacute occurrence of AD symptoms, e.g., orthostatic intolerance [1], would fit better with an autoimmune ganglionitis or a vasculitic process affecting autonomic nerves.

Adie's syndrome, a syndrome of parasympathetic nerve dysfunction involving the pupil, results in a dilated, tonic pupil that suffers from an impairment of the light reflex response. Adie's pupils, which affect some pSS patients [27], can be explained by inflammation affecting the ciliary ganglion, with or without a role for anti-M3-receptor antibodies.

AD is probably due to different mechanisms in different organs as well as different patients. The clinical manifestations and time course for the development of AD symptoms in pSS vary substantially across patients, with some symptoms developing over months/years and some symptoms occasionally developing over days/weeks. In contrast to what is found in patients with AD associated with diabetes, AD in pSS does not seem to be associated with excessive cardiovascular mortality [28], which suggests that there may be different types of ANS involvement in patients with diabetes and pSS. Because it has been shown that parasympathetic nerve signalling may have an attenuating effect on macrophage-induced inflammation and production of various cytokines [29], parasympathetic dysfunction may also affect the inflammatory process in pSS and possibly result in an exaggerated inflammatory response. The parasympathetic nervous system appears to exert its anti-inflammatory effects on macrophages mainly through ACh and the nicotine receptor [29]. Thus, the reduced focus scores and reduced prevalence of anti-SS-A antibodies reported in pSS patients who smoke could fit with an immunomodulatory effect of nicotine in addition to that of the parasympathetic nervous system [30]. Antimuscarinic antibodies may also increase the inflammatory response in pSS by increasing cycloxygenase-2 expression and prostaglandin E2 production [31].

The fact that pSS patients often have large amounts of acinar tissue in the exocrine glands that is morphologically intact but which functions at a subnormal level in vivo [22, 23] has heightened the interest in the mechanisms governing exocrine secretion and in possible mechanisms interfering with the normal signal transduction to and within acinar cells. The main parasympathetic receptor in exocrine glands is the M3R, which is also found elsewhere, e.g., in the gastrointestinal system and the bladder. In contrast, other muscarinic receptor subtypes, namely the M1- and M2-receptors, are more important in the brain and the heart, respectively. In healthy subjects, exocrine secretion starts when ACh stimulates the M3R. However, several factors could result in reduced stimulation of the M3R [18] with resulting exocrine dysfunction (Fig. 22.1), namely:

1. *Reduced innervation of the exocrine glands.* Although it is theoretically plausible that inflammation and neural degeneration could result in a reduced innervation of acinar, myoepithelial, and ductal cells in the exocrine glands, experimental data do not support this concept [18, 32].
2. *Reduced ACh release.* In vitro experiments using exocrine glands from MRL/lpr mice have indicated that certain cytokines (i.e., TNFα and IL-1β) may impair neuronal release of ACh [18, 33]. In addition, cytokines have also been proposed to affect the transcription and thus also the surface expression of neurotransmitter receptors, thereby interfering with signal transduction [34].
3. *Increased degradation of ACh by cholinesterases.* SS patients have been shown to have increased levels of cholinesterases, the enzymes that degrade ACh, in saliva. However, the implication of this finding is uncertain. Of note is that hydroxychloroquine, which is sometimes used as an immunomodulatory drug in pSS, is a cholinesterase inhibitor. This provides theoretical rationale for why treatment with this drug might affect ACh degradation in exocrine glands, thereby improving exocrine gland function [18, 35].

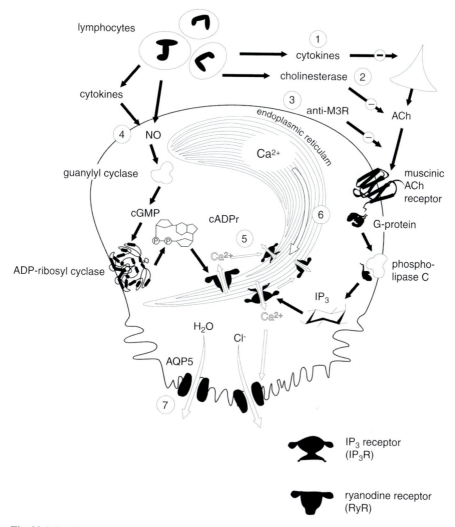

Fig. 22.1 Possible points of interaction between the immune system and the secretory process that could lead to glandular hypofunction. (*1*) Inhibition of neurotransmitter release by cytokines. (*2*) Enhanced breakdown of ACh by increased levels of cholinesterase. (*3*) Blockade of M3R by antimuscarinic autoantibodies. (*4*) Altered NO production. (*5*) Perturbation of Ca^{2+}- induced -Ca^{2+} release by altered levels of cADPr (possibly as a result of altered NO levels). (*6*) Altered Ca^{2+} tunneling. (*7*) Altered expression or distribution of AQP5 (By kind permission of Smith and Dawson [18])

4. *Antibodies directed against and blocking the M3R.* The presence of such antibodies in pSS patients has been reported by various authors using different techniques. These include:

   (a) Radioligand binding studies where sera from SS patients were found to bind non-competitively to the M3R of rat parotid and lacrimal gland membranes [36].

b) Various immunological techniques, e.g., a flow cytometric assay [37] and enzyme-linked immunosorbent assay (ELISA) [38]. However, neither technique has demonstrated sufficient reproducibility or specificity to date [18].

c) Bioassays in mouse colon or bladder strips demonstrating reductions of carbachol-induced contractility upon exposure to SS sera [19, 39].

d) Bioassays using human salivary gland cells where carbachol-induced, fluorometrically assessed intracellular increase in Ca^{2+} is blunted by antibodies in the IgG fraction of SS sera. Using this technique, the M3R was found to be blocked by the M3R-antibodies in a reversible manner [40].

Additional studies have shown that after a period of blockade of cholinergic transmission, these antibodies may induce a cholinergic hyperresponsiveness with upregulation of the M3R. This may explain the bladder irritability that is commonly encountered in pSS patients [41, 42]. These antibodies have also been suggested to cause gastrointestinal symptoms, e.g., gastroparesis [41], and microvascular responses to cholinergic stimulation [12]. Reports on abnormal distribution of aquaporins (AQP), protein water channels, in acinar cells [43] also show a disturbed intracellular signalling downstream of the M3R, a finding that is compatible with the presence of anti-M3R antibodies in patients with pSS. Furthermore, the physiologically measurable effects of the anti-M3R antibodies and the symptoms probably associated with them have also been reported to be diminished by anti-idiotypic antibodies/intravenous immunoglobulins [44].

In conclusion, there is substantial evidence that a serological factor exists in the IgG fraction of sera from patients with primary and secondary SS. This factor appears to interact with the response of the M3R to cholinergic stimuli. The exact target of these antibodies is still a matter of debate, but the second and third extracellular loops of the M3R have been implicated [45, 46] as well as cross-reactivity with the muscarinic-1 receptor [47]. Probably due to their low concentration and our lack of knowledge about their exact specificity, they are difficult to detect using conventional immunological methods such as ELISA. The best methods at present for their detection seem to be various bioassays studying their effects on murine colon and bladder contractility [18] or on increase in intracellular Ca^{2+} in human salivary gland cells as a result of cholinergic stimulation [18].

22.3 Diagnostic Tests

ANS functioning is assessed most commonly and easily in the cardiovascular system. Numerous cardiovascular tests can assess the effects of the parasympathetic and sympathetic nervous systems on the heart rate and blood pressure at rest and during various challenges. The cardiovascular tests are usually easy to perform, are reasonably standardized, and generally noninvasive. Autonomic reflex tests (ARTs) are used to measure various cardiovascular autonomic reflexes, which are modulated differently by the parasympathetic and sympathetic nervous systems. Examples of the ARTs are the *deep-breathing test*, which measures the degree of sinus arrhythmia to deep breathing (parasympathetic); the *orthostatic test* (Fig. 22.2),

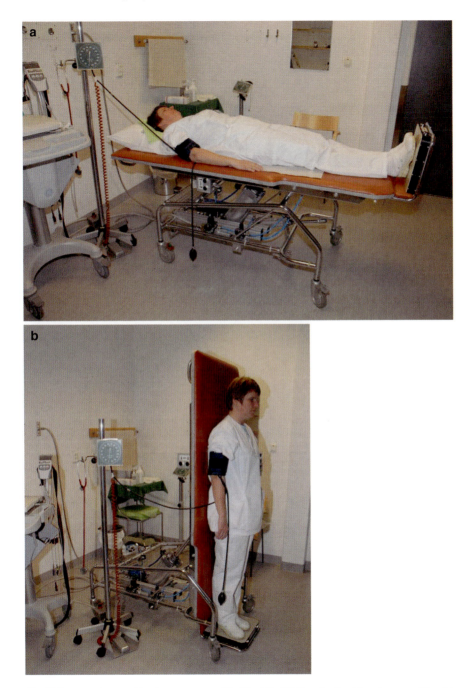

Fig. 22.2 The orthostatic blood pressure test – The Head Up Tilt Test. Supine (**a**) and erect position (**b**)

Fig. 22.3 The finger skin blood flow test is performed with the subject sitting in a semi-recumbent position (**a**) whilst the finger skin blood flow is monitored by a laser doppler imaging instrument (**b**) during rest and contralateral cooling

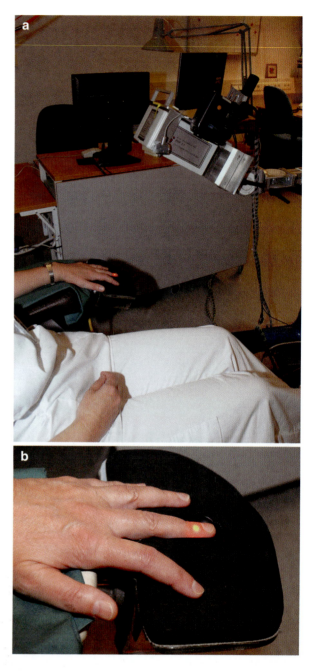

which measures the heart rate (mainly parasympathetic but partly also sympathetic) and blood pressure reaction (sympathetic) to orthostatic challenge; the *cold pressor test or finger skin blood flow test* (Fig. 22.3), which measures the vasoconstrictory response to cooling (sympathetic); the *Valsalva test*, which measures the heart rate reaction to the Valsalva manoeuvre (parasympathetic); and the *sustained hand grip test*, which measures the diastolic blood pressure reaction to sustained hand grip (sympathetic) [48].

More modern ways of assessing cardiovascular autonomic function include studies on heart rate variability (HRV), where fast HRV changes are considered to be mediated by the parasympathetic nervous system and slower changes by the sympathetic nervous system [48]. HRV can be studied in short-term electrocardiograms (ECGs) but it is better studied in 24-h ECGs. Baroreceptor sensitivity (BRS) involves the measurement of the sensitivity of the baroreflex by assessing the relationship between an increase in blood pressure and a decrease in heart rate, either by performing concomitant blood pressure and heart rate measurements during the day or during orthostatic challenge, but ideally during phenylephrine infusion [48].

ARTs are thought to measure ANS activity when the ANS is under stress while the HRV and BRS are thought to measure ANS function under basal conditions. The advantage of ARTs, in contrast to assessment of HRV and BRS, is their simplicity. However, ARTs depend upon the co-operation of the subject under study, a point that is less critical in the case of HRV. HRV and BRS investigations also have higher sensitivity and greater reproducibility compared to ARTs [49].

Because many factors affect the ART variables, it is of great importance that these be performed under standardized conditions, with uniform temperatures, during the same time of the day, without prior eating, drinking, or smoking and without medications that might affect ANS indices (e.g., various vasoactive drugs). Moreover, because autonomic function variables decline with advancing age and may demonstrate differences between the sexes, studies should include appropriate age- and sex-matched controls [50].

In addition to the cardiovascular ANS tests, additional assessments exist for the evaluation of other organs. Such tests include the quantitative sudomotor axon reflex test (QSART) and sympathetic skin response, which measure sudomotor function [51, 52]; pupillometry, which measures ophthalmologic ANS function [52]; urodynamic studies; gastric emptying scintigraphy [41]; and P-catecholamines, a surrogate marker of sympathetic nervous activity [52]. These tests are performed less frequently because of the need for specialized equipment, a lower degree of standardization of the methods, and greater invasiveness of the procedures. Because cardiovascular ANS tests do not necessarily mirror the function in other parts of the ANS and because AD is sometimes difficult to discriminate from the effects of end-organ damage (e.g., dryness can be both due to exocrine gland destruction and a parasympathetic dysfunction), it is ideal to combine different tests of autonomic function when evaluating the ANS [25].

In contrast to the numerous tests that exist to assess objective ANS function, few validated questionnaires exist for the documentation of subjective AD symptoms. One of the more commonly used is the Autonomic Symptom Profile (ASP) [53]. The ASP is the only questionnaire employed in pSS that addresses subjective AD symptoms. The questions in the ASP evaluate nine domains of autonomic symptoms: orthostatic intolerance, secretomotor dysfunction, male sexual dysfunction, urinary dysfunction, gastrointestinal dysfunction (divided into three subdomains, gastroparesis, diarrhoea, and constipation), pupillomotor dysfunction, vasomotor dysfunction, sleep disorder, and reflex syncope. The autonomic symptom domains of the ASP consist of questions that evaluate the presence, severity, distribution, frequency, and progression of various autonomic symptoms. The domain scores are weighted according to their clinical relevance and can be added to calculate a total ASP score that measures the total impact of AD symptoms.

Objective signs and subjective symptoms of AD correlate poorly in pSS patients [9, 15]. These discrepancies could be due to differences in mechanisms behind objective signs and subjective symptoms of AD. Furthermore, cardiovascular ARTs do not necessarily reflect autonomic nervous function in other parts of the ANS, and end-organ damage may obscure possible associations between objective and subjective AD. For these reasons, it seems reasonable to assess subjective AD symptoms as well as objective signs, as permitted by the ASP.

22.4 Parasympathetic and Sympathetic Disorders

In previous studies on cardiovascular AD, both the parasympathetic and the sympathetic nervous systems have been reported to be affected in pSS patients (Table 22.1). Since many symptoms of pSS mimic several AD symptoms [54], AD may not only be a feature of the disease but may also contribute to the various classical symptoms of the disease. For example, involvement of the parasympathetic nervous system and interference with the parasympathetic nervous transmission pathways may contribute to secretomotor dysfunction, bladder symptoms, and disturbed gastrointestinal motility in pSS. The sympathetic nervous system involvement may contribute to orthostatic intolerance, impaired sweating, and vasomotor dysfunction [52]. Fatigue in pSS may also relate to certain features of AD [9, 14, 54].

22.4.1 Secretomotor Disorder

Exocrine gland inflammation and dysfunction are hallmarks of pSS. In the past, the exocrine dysfunction of pSS has been ascribed principally to the presence of inflammation and its consequent destruction of the exocrine glands. As noted, however, the observed discrepancy between exocrine gland destruction and exocrine dysfunction requires other mechanisms to explain the exocrine insufficiency in pSS [16, 17]. The exocrine glands are innervated by both parasympathetic and sympathetic nerves. The liquid part of secretion appears to be modulated primarily by parasympathetic input, whereas protein secretion is principally under sympathetic control. However, the two parts of the ANS work synergistically in the exocrine glands.

Before secretion, the salivary gland blood flow is increased due to the release of nitric oxide and vasointestinal peptide from parasympathetic nerve endings. Otherwise, the main signal for secretion is acetylcholine (ACh), which is also released by parasympathetic nerve endings. ACh binds to the G-protein-coupled M3R on the acinar cells in the exocrine glands. The activated G protein stimulates phospholipase

C to generate inositol 1, 4, 5-trisphosphate (IP_3), which in its turn causes a release of Ca^{2+} ions from intracellular Ca^{2+} storages. The increment of intracellular Ca^{2+} activates apical membrane Cl- channels and basolateral K^+ channels, causing an efflux of Cl- and K^+ ions. The efflux of Cl- ions to the apical lumen also causes a similar movement of Na^+ ions in order to maintain electrochemical neutrality, resulting in an osmotic effect that brings water into the lumen, a process further facilitated by the presence of aquaporins in the acinar and myoepithelial cells.

Apart from the parasympathetic pathways, sympathetic pathways also affect the glandular cells. These act via noradrenaline and adrenaline, activating mainly the adenylate cyclase pathway, and also NPY. The sympathetic pathways play a role in modulating protein secretion in particular, but also liquid secretion to some extent. In addition to the secretory effects of autonomic nerve signals, there are also trophic effects as illustrated by the atrophy seen in a salivary gland deprived of parasympathetic signals. Following the production of primary saliva, its composition is modulated by the salivary ductal cells during its passage through the salivary gland ducts.

Various factors disturbing these signal transduction pathways may thus result in a decreased or altered exocrine gland secretion as well as dryness. Although AD thus may explain part of the secretomotor dysfunction seen in pSS, AD and exocrine dysfunction are generally poorly associated [2]. This could have several explanations. First, ANS function usually is evaluated by cardiovascular tests, which do not necessarily mirror exocrine ANS function. Second, anti-M3R antibodies may give rise to an exocrine AD that cannot be detected sufficiently by cardiovascular ANS function tests. And finally, end-organ damage may obscure possible associations, especially in late disease.

In analogy to what is seen in other exocrine glands, interference with nerve signalling to the sweat glands may result in a decreased and altered secretion from these and contribute to the xerosis of the skin. As is true for other exocrine glands, it is difficult to differentiate the effects of AD from end-organ damage in the sweat glands.

22.4.2   Urinary Disorder

The effects of AD on the bladder may explain the increased prevalence of urinary dysfunction symptoms, which appear to be overrepresented in pSS patients [9, 15]. Because M3R is found in the bladder and is important in eliciting bladder contraction, the putative anti-M3R antibodies have also been suggested as causatives of the pSS-related bladder symptoms. When studying objective signs of AD in the bladder, 56% of pSS patients were reported to show signs of decreased detrusor muscle tone and contractility [41]. An association with the anti-M3R antibodies has been proposed. Conversely, irritable bladder, which is also overrepresented in pSS patients, has also been suggested to be associated with anti-M3R antibodies [42, 55]. Although these results are contradictory, a hypothesis states that the anti-M3R antibodies, after a period of blockade of cholinergic transmission, may induce a cholinergic hyperresponsiveness with upregulation of the M3R, which in its turn may explain the bladder irritability seen in some pSS patients [42, 55].

22.4.3   Gastrointestinal Disorder

Dysphagia is a recognized feature in pSS and may be attributed both to lack of saliva, esophageal dysmotility, and esophageal webs. Because both exocrine secretion and esophageal motility are modulated by the ANS, dysphagia could partly be due to AD. Also constipation has been reported in pSS [16] and impaired gastric emptying has been found in 70% of pSS patients, studied by gastric emptying scintigraphy [41]. Such findings are all consistent with involvement of the enteric ANS or the putative anti-M3R antibodies, since the M3R are involved in gastrointestinal motility as well as secretion [41].

22.4.4   Pupillomotor Disorder

Adie's syndrome has been found in association with sensory neuropathy in pSS [27]. A ganglionitis affecting the ciliary and dorsal root ganglia was suggested to be the causative. Since the main parasympathetic receptor of the iris is again the M3R, it is possible that such symptoms could also be attributable to the anti-M3R antibodies.

22.4.5   Orthostatic Intolerance

Both objective signs of orthostatic blood pressure drops and subjective symptoms of orthostatic intolerance are encountered commonly in pSS [15, 26]. However, the objective signs of postural hypotension and subjective symptoms of lightheadedness usually correlate poorly with each other [15, 26]. Both orthostatic systolic and diastolic hypotension in pSS have been demonstrated in several studies [2, 13, 14]. Diastolic hypotension has been shown to progress during follow-up [14]. Orthostatic hypotension is generally considered a sign of sympathetic dysfunction [25]. The pathogenesis behind these finding thus seems to fit well with theories of inflammation that involves sympathetic ganglia or nerves [22] or cytokines that interfere with neurotransmission [24]. Because the anti-M3R antibodies can affect blood vessel tone and possibly blood pressure, an influence of these antibodies on the orthostatic blood pressure reaction cannot be excluded.

The subjective symptoms of orthostatic intolerance are very common in pSS patients [15], but their pathogenesis is complex and incompletely understood. Symptoms of orthostatic intolerance may be related to orthostatic hypotension, but the correlation of orthostatic intolerance is usually with an increased heart rate during orthostatic challenge rather than orthostatic hypotension. The pathogenesis of these symptoms is considered multifactorial and predisposing factors include: excessive venous pooling, impairment of renal sympathetic innervation, decreased plasma volume, sympathetic overactivity, beta-adrenergic hypersensitivity, and a reduced vagal cardioinhibitory reflex [52].

The relative importance of these factors in leading to symptoms of orthostatic intolerance in pSS remains to be determined. However, such symptoms have been reported to be associated with fatigue as well as symptoms of depression and anxiety in pSS patients, suggestive of a complex pathogenesis [14].

22.4.6 Vasomotor Disorder

Raynaud's phenomenon (RP) is one of the most common vascular disorders in pSS. Although our understanding of the underlying mechanisms of RP has increased over the last years, the pathogenesis is still not fully understood. The main mechanisms may be differentiated into vascular, neural, and intravascular factors [56]. The vascular abnormalities may be both structural with successive vessel occlusion as well as functional, with impaired vasodilation and increased vasoconstriction. The neural abnormalities include an imbalance between neural transmitters modulating muscular tone in the vessels, sympathetic hyperresponsiveness due to sensitization of alpha-2 receptors by cold exposure, and central nervous mechanisms. Intravascular factors, e.g., increased blood viscosity and platelet activation, and yet other factors such as smoking, hormonal, and genetic influences have also been suggested to contribute to RP pathogenesis [56]. Thus, in the absence of obvious morphological vascular changes, the pathogenesis of RP in pSS is likely multifactorial.

Beside RP, pSS patients have also been reported to show an impaired vasodilatory response to cholinergic stimulation [12]. M3R are found in blood vessels and it is conceivable that anti-M3R antibodies contribute to the pathophysiology of RP in pSS through interference with cholinergic nervous transmission [12]. However, this remains only a theoretical possibility.

22.5 Diagnostic Algorithm of pSS Patient with Autonomic Dysfunction

When assessing autonomic nervous function it is important to take into account that various parts of the ANS may be differently involved in different patients, even if having the same disease. Furthermore, autonomic nervous function in one part of the body cannot always be extrapolated from assessments of ANS function in other parts. Therefore, different ANS function tests, both evaluating parasympathetic and sympathetic nervous function, and ideally evaluating ANS function both in the cardiovascular and some other assessable system, should be combined to better evaluate the extent and severity of ANS involvement [25]. One proposed combination has been evaluation by: (1) parasympathetic cardiovascular tests, e.g., the deep breathing and Valsalva tests; (2) sympathetic cardiovascular tests, e.g., the orthostatic blood pressure test; and (3) a sudomotor function test, e.g., the QSART

Table 22.2 Proposed diagnostic algorithm for pSS-associated AD

(a) Evaluation of autonomic symptoms
   AD symptoms questionnaire (ASP)
(b) Diagnostic tests
   Cardiovascular parasympathetic function
   (i) Deep-breathing test
   (ii) Valsalva test
   Cardiovascular sympathetic function
   • Orthostatic blood pressure test
   Sudomotor function
   • QSART
(c) Laboratory tests
   Anti-M3R antibodies?

AD autonomic dysfunction, *QSART* quantitative sudomotor axon reflex test, *ASP* autonomic symptom profile, *M3R* muscarinic-3 receptor

(Table 22.2). By scoring the results semiquantitatively in each of these three domains, a Composite Autonomic Scoring Scale (CASS) score can be calculated that ranges from 0 to 10 and provides an overall estimate of objective autonomic nervous function [25].

Although the equipment for cardiovascular ARTs is available in many hospitals and these tests are easily performed, the equipment for assessing sudomotor function is less readily available. For that reason the sudomotor function tests are less commonly performed when assessing AD, although ideally they should be included in a comprehensive ANS evaluation. However, it is reasonable to think that there is a considerable risk of assessing end-organ damage as well as the effects of AD, when using the sudomotor function tests on patients with pSS, due to inflammation of the sweat glands in the disease.

In addition to the cardiovascular tests above, cardiovascular ANS function can also be assessed by measurement of HRV and BRS. These tests are usually considered more sensitive, more reproducible, and less dependent on co-operation of the subject under study in comparison with the ARTs. However, the advantage of the ARTs is the ease of performing these, in contrast with those involving HRV and BRS. Finally, when specifically evaluating objective ANS function in other organ systems, yet other methods must be employed, e.g., gastric emptying scintigraphy, urodynamic studies, and pupillometry.

22.6 Treatment

In case reports, severe autonomic neuropathy associated with pSS has been reported to respond to intravenous immunoglobulins [57, 58] and glucocorticoids [59]. The utility of rituximab as a therapeutic agent for severe autonomic neuropathy is unclear at this time [60]. Generally speaking, there is indeed a lack of larger studies on this topic. Moreover, since various pathogenetic mechanisms, e.g., vasculitis, ganglionitis, anti-M3R antibodies, and cytokines interfering with autonomic nervous transmission may underlie the various neurological complications of pSS, this also underscores the importance of individualization of treatment in different patients based on the clinical picture and the plausible pathophysiological mechanism in each case.

In patients with mild AD symptoms, symptomatic treatment may often be sufficient. For example, secretomotor dysfunction may be treated with pilocarpine or cevimeline. In addition, impaired gastrointestinal motility may be managed with metoclopramide, orthostatic hypotension with midodrine or etilefrine, and irritable bladder with tolterodine. Unfortunately, the use of some of these agents in pSS can be counterproductive. For example, tolterodine is an anticholinergic drug and its use can impair exocrine function, further exacerbating sicca symptoms. High-dose glucocorticoids can be tried when a vasculitic or a ganglionitic pathogenesis is suspected [59], and intravenous immune globulin has been used in refractory cases, with limited information on long-term clinical outcomes [57, 58].

References

1. Sakakibara R, Hirano S, Asahina M, et al. Primary Sjögren's syndrome presenting with generalized autonomic failure. Eur J Neurol. 2004;11:635–8.
2. Mandl T, Wollmer P, Manthorpe R, et al. Autonomic and orthostatic dysfunction in primary Sjögren's syndrome. J Rheumatol. 2007;34:1869–74.
3. Andonopoulos AP, Christodoulou J, Ballas C, et al. Autonomic cardiovascular neuropathy in Sjogren's syndrome. A controlled study. J Rheumatol. 1998;25:2385–8.
4. Barendregt PJ, van den Meiracker AH, Markusse HM, et al. Parasympathetic failure does not contribute to ocular dryness in primary Sjogren's syndrome. Ann Rheum Dis. 1999;58: 746–50.
5. Kovacs L, Paprika D, Takacs R, et al. Cardiovascular autonomic dysfunction in primary Sjogren's syndrome. Rheumatology. 2004;43:95–9.
6. Barendregt PJ, Tulen JH, van den Meiracker AH, et al. Spectral analysis of heart rate and blood pressure variability in primary Sjogren's syndrome. Ann Rheum Dis. 2002;61:232–6.
7. Niemela RK, Hakala M, Huikuri HV, et al. Comprehensive study of autonomic function in a population with primary Sjögren's syndrome. No evidence of autonomic involvement. J Rheumatol. 2003;30:74–9.
8. Tumiati B, Perazzoli F, Negro A, et al. Heart rate variability in patients with Sjogren's syndrome. Clin Rheumatol. 2000;19:477–80.
9. Cai FZ, Lester S, Lu T, et al. Mild autonomic dysfunction in primary Sjögren's syndrome: a controlled study. Arthritis Res Ther. 2008;10:R31.
10. Mandl T, Jacobsson L, Lilja B, Sundkvist G, Manthorpe R. Disturbances of autonomic nervous function in primary Sjögren's syndrome. Scand J Rheumatol. 1997;26:401–6.
11. Niemela RK, Pikkujamsa SM, Hakala M, Huikuri HV, Airaksinen KE. No signs of autonomic nervous system dysfunction in primary Sjorgen's syndrome evaluated by 24 hour heart rate variability. J Rheumatol. 2000;27:2605–10.
12. Kovacs L, Torok T, Bari F, et al. Impaired microvascular response to cholinergic stimuli in primary Sjogren's syndrome. Ann Rheum Dis. 2000;59:48–53.
13. Mandl T, Bornmyr SV, Castenfors J, Jacobsson LT, Manthorpe R, Wollmer P. Sympathetic dysfunction in patients with primary Sjögren's syndrome. J Rheumatol. 2001;28:296–301.

14. Mandl T, Hammar O, Theander E, Wollmer P, Ohlsson B. Autonomic nervous dysfunction development in patients with primary Sjögren's syndrome – a follow-up study. Rheumatology. 2010;49(6):1101–6.

15. Mandl T, Granberg V, Apelqvist J, et al. Autonomic nervous symptoms in primary Sjogren's syndrome. Rheumatology. 2008;47:914–9.

16. Humphreys-Beher MG, Brayer J, Yamachika S, et al. An alternative perspective to the immune response in autoimmune exocrinopathy: induction of functional quiescence rather than destructive autoaggression. Scand J Immunol. 1999;49:7–10.

17. Jonsson R, Kroneld U, Tarkowski A. Histological and functional features of salivary glands in rheumatic patients with oral sicca symptoms. Scand J Rheumatol. 1988;17:387–91.

18. Dawson LJ, Fox PC, Smith PM. Sjögren's syndrome – the non-apoptotic model of glandular hypofunction. Rheumatology. 2006;45:792–8.

19. Waterman SA, Gordon TP, Rischmueller M. Inhibitory effects of muscarinic receptor autoantibodies on parasympathetic neurotransmission in Sjogren's syndrome. Arthritis Rheum. 2000;43:1647–54.

20. Gordon TP, Bolstad AI, Rischmueller M, et al. Autoantibodies in primary Sjogren's syndrome: new insights into mechanisms of autoantibody diversification and disease pathogenesis. Autoimmunity. 2001;34:123–32.

21. Dawson L, Tobin A, Smith P, et al. Antimuscarinic antibodies in Sjogren's syndrome: where are we, and where are we going? Arthritis Rheum. 2005;52:2984–95.

22. Mori K, Iijima M, Koike H, et al. The wide spectrum of clinical manifestations in SS associated neuropathy. Brain. 2005;128:2518–34.

23. Fox RI, Stern M. Sjogren's syndrome: mechanisms of pathogenesis involve interaction of immune and neurosecretory systems. Scand J Rheumatol. 2002;116:3–13.

24. Zoukhri D, Hodges RR, Byon D, et al. Role of proinflammatory cytokines in the impaired lacrimation associated with autoimmune xerophthalmia. Invest Ophthalmol Vis Sci. 2002;43:1429–36.

25. Low PA. Composite autonomic scoring scale for laboratory quantification of generalized autonomic failure. Mayo Clin Proc. 1993;68:748–52.

26. Mandl T. Autonomic dysfunction in primary Sjögren's syndrome. Thesis. Lund University; 2008.

27. Waterschoot MP, Guerit JM, Lambert M, et al. Bilateral tonic pupils and polyneuropathy in Sjögren's syndrome: a common pathophysiological mechanism? Eur Neurol. 1991;31:114–6.

28. Theander E, Manthorpe R, Jacobsson LT. Mortality and causes of death in primary Sjogren's syndrome: a prospective cohort study. Arthritis Rheum. 2004;50:1262–9.

29. Borovikova LV, Ivanova S, Zhang M, et al. Vagus nerve stimulation attenuates the systemic inflammatory response to endotoxin. Nature. 2000;405:458–62.

30. Manthorpe R, Benoni C, Jacobsson L, et al. Lower frequency of focal lip sialadenitis (focus score) in smoking patients. Can tobacco diminish the salivary gland involvement as judged by histological examination and anti-SSA/Ro and anti-SSB/La antibodies in Sjogren's syndrome? Ann Rheum Dis. 2000;59:54–60.

31. Reina S, Orman B, Anaya JM, et al. Cholinoreceptor autoantibodies in Sjögren's syndrome. J Dent Res. 2007;86:832–6.

32. Konttinen YT, Sorsa T, Hukkanen M, et al. Topology of innervation of labial salivary glands by protein gene product 9.5 and synaptophysin immunoreactive nerves in patients with Sjögren's syndrome. J Rheumatol. 1992;19:30–7.

33. Zoukhri D, Kublin CL. Impaired neurotransmitter release from lacrimal and salivary gland nerves of a murine model of Sjögren's syndrome. Invest Ophthalmol Vis Sci. 2001;42:925–32.

34. Haddad EB, Rousell J, Lindsay MA, et al. Synergy between tumor necrosis factor alpha and interleukin 1 beta in inducing transcriptional down-regulation of muscarinic M2 receptor gene expression. Involvement of protein kinase A and ceramide pathways. J Biol Chem. 1996;271: 32586–92.

35. Dawson LJ, Caulfield VL, Stanbury JB, et al. Hydroxychloroquine therapy in patients with primary Sjögren's syndrome may improve salivary gland hypofunction by inhibition of glandular cholinesterase. Rheumatology. 2005;44:449–55.

36. Bacman S, Sterin-Borda L, Camusso JJ, et al. Circulating antibodies against rat parotid gland M3 muscarinic receptors in primary Sjogren's syndrome. Clin Exp Immunol. 1996;104:454–9.

37. Gao J, Cha S, Jonsson R, Opalko J, et al. Detection of anti-type 3 muscarinic acetylcholine receptor autoantibodies in the sera of Sjogren's syndrome patients by use of a transfected cell line assay. Arthritis Rheum. 2004;50:2615–21.
38. Kovacs L, Marczinovits I, Gyorgy A, et al. Clinical associations of autoantibodies to human muscarinic acetylcholine receptor 3(213–228) in primary Sjogren's syndrome. Rheumatology. 2005;44:1021–5.
39. Cavill D, Waterman SA, Gordon TP. Antiidiotypic antibodies neutralize autoantibodies that inhibit cholinergic neurotransmission. Arthritis Rheum. 2003;48:3597–602.
40. Dawson LJ, Stanbury J, Venn N, et al. Antimuscarinic antibodies in primary Sjogren's syndrome reversibly inhibit the mechanism of fluid secretion by human submandibular salivary acinar cells. Arthritis Rheum. 2006;54:1165–73.
41. Kovacs L, Papos M, Takacs R, et al. Autonomic nervous system dysfunction involving the gastrointestinal and the urinary tracts in primary Sjogren's syndrome. Clin Exp Rheumatol. 2003;21:697–703.
42. Wang F, Jackson MW, Maughan V, et al. Passive transfer of Sjogren's syndrome IgG produces the pathophysiology of overactive bladder. Arthritis Rheum. 2004;50:3637–45.
43. Beroukas D, Hiscock J, Gannon BJ, et al. Selective down-regulation of aquaporin-1 in salivary glands in primary Sjogren's syndrome. Lab Invest. 2002;82:1547–52.
44. Smith AJ, Jackson MW, Wang F, et al. Neutralization of muscarinic receptor autoantibodies by intravenous immunoglobulin in Sjogren syndrome. Hum Immunol. 2005;66:411–6.
45. Cavill D, Waterman SA, Gordon TP. Antibodies raised against the second extracellular loop of the human muscarinic M3 receptor mimic functional autoantibodies in Sjogren's syndrome. Scand J Immunol. 2004;59:261–6.
46. Koo NY, Li J, Hwang SM, et al. Functional epitope of muscarinic type 3 receptor which interacts with autoantibodies from Sjögren's syndrome patients. Rheumatology. 2008;47:828–33.
47. Schegg V, Vogel M, Didichenko S, et al. Evidence that anti-muscarinic antibodies in Sjögren's syndrome recognize both M3R and M1R. Biologicals. 2008;36:213–22.
48. Freeman R. Assessment of cardiovascular autonomic function. Clin Neurophysiol. 2006;117:716–30.
49. Huikuri HV, Kessler KM, Terracall E, et al. Reproducibility and circadian rhythm of heart rate variability in healthy subjects. Am J Cardiol. 1990;65:391–3.
50. Low PA, Denq J-C, Opfer-Gehrking TL, et al. Effect of age and gender on sudomotor and cardiovagal function and blood pressure response to tilt in normal subjects. Muscle Nerve. 1997;20:1561–8.
51. Riedel A, Braune S, Kerum G, et al. Quantitative sudomotor axon reflex test (QSART): a new approach for testing distal sites. Muscle Nerve. 1999;22:1257–64.
52. Robertson D, Biaggioni I, Burnstock G, Low PA, editors. Primer on the autonomic nervous system. 2nd ed. San Diego: Elsevier Academic press; 2004.
53. Suarez GA, Opfer-Gehrkring TL, Offord KP, et al. The autonomic symptom profile. A new instrument to assess autonomic symptoms. Neurology. 1999;52:523–8.
54. Nikolov NP, Illei GG. Pathogenesis of Sjögren's syndrome. Curr Opin Rheumatol. 2009;21:465–70.
55. Walker J, Gordon T, Lester S, et al. Increased severity of lower urinary tract symptoms and daytime somnolence in primary Sjogren's syndrome. J Rheumatol. 2003;30:2406–12.
56. Herrick AL. Pathogenesis of Raynaud's phenomenon. Rheumatology. 2005;44:587–96.
57. Kizawa M, Mori K, Iijima M, Koike H, Hattori N, Sobue G. Intravenous immunoglobulin treatment in painful sensory neuropathy without sensory ataxia associated with Sjögren's syndrome. J Neurol Neurosurg Psychiatry. 2006;77:967–9.
58. Dupond JL, Gil H, de Wazieres B. Five-year efficacy of intravenous gammaglobulin to treat dysautonomia in Sjogren's syndrome. Am J Med. 1999;106:125.
59. Sorajja P, Poirier MK, Bundrick JB, Matteson EL. Autonomic failure and proximal skeletal myopathy in a patient with primary Sjögren syndrome. Mayo Clin Proc. 1999;74:695–7.
60. Sève P, Gachon E, Petiot P, Stankovic K, Chahon A, Broussolle C. Successful treatment with rituximab in a patient with mental nerve neuropathy in primary Sjögren's syndrome. Rheumatol Int. 2007;28:175–7.

Chapter 23
Endocrine Involvement

Luis J. Jara, Gabriela Medina, Carmen Navarro, Olga Vera-Lastra,
and Miguel A. Saavedra

Contents

L.J. Jara (✉)
Direction of Education and Research, Hospital de Especialidades, Centro Médico La Raza,
IMSS, Universidad Nacional Autónoma de México, Mexico City, DF, Mexico

G. Medina
Clinical and Epidemiology Research Unit, Hospital de Especialidades Centro Médico La Raza,
IMSS, Mexico City, DF, Mexico

C. Navarro
Deputy Director of Clinical Research, Instituto Nacional de Enfermedades
Respiratorias, SSA, Mexico City, DF, Mexico

O. Vera-Lastra
Department of Internal Medicine, Hospital de Especialidades, Centro Médico Nacional La Raza,
IMSS, Universidad Nacional Autónoma de México, Mexico City, DF, Mexico

M.A. Saavedra
Department of Rheumatology, Hospital de Especialidades Centro Médico La Raza, Universidad
Nacional Autónoma de México, Mexico City, DF, Mexico

M. Ramos-Casals et al. (eds.), *Sjögren's Syndrome*,
DOI 10.1007/978-0-85729-947-5_23, © Springer-Verlag London Limited 2012

23.1   Introduction

Over the last decades much evidence of communication between the immune, nervous, and endocrine systems has accumulated. This communication has a solid molecular basis. The messengers are hormones, neuropeptides, neurotransmitters, cytokines, and their receptors. These messengers have endocrine action (at a distance), paracrine action (on the neighboring cells), and autocrine action (on the cells themselves). The integrated bidirectional communication of the three systems, now called the immune-neuroendocrine system, regulates the adaptive response to stress [1]. Stressful situations, such as the ones induced by an inflammatory or infectious process, the activation of autoimmunity, trauma, surgery, and emotional events, trigger a series of reactions that activate the immune-neuroendocrine system.

The immuno-neuroendocrine system includes the hypothalamic-pituitary-adrenal axis, the hypothalamic-pituitary-gonadal axis, the hypothalamic-pituitary-thyroid axis, prolactin,/and growth hormone. The autonomic nervous system, comprised of the sympathetic and parasympathetic nervous systems, also participates in the stress response through its sympathetic limb [2].

The interactions of the stress response systems support the concept that the immune-neuroendocrine system plays an important role in modulating host susceptibility and resistance to inflammatory disease. Recent studies have demonstrated that a disruption or an abnormal response of the immune-neuroendocrine communication may be associated with susceptibility to or severity of autoimmune diseases, including rheumatoid arthritis (RA), systemic lupus erythematosus (SLE), and Sjögren's syndrome (SS). The immune-neuroendocrine system may influence the activity of lymphoid organs and cells via endocrine and local autocrine/paracrine pathways or alter the function of different cell types in target organs involved in SS [3].

The aim of this chapter is to analyze the role of the immune-neuroendocrine system in the pathogenesis and clinical picture of SS and the hormonal treatment as a new perspective in this disease.

23.2   Immune-Neuroendocrine System in Sjögren Syndrome

During a stressful situation such as one involving inflammation, activated immune system cells release proinflammatory cytokines (IL-1-β, TNF-α, IL-6) that reach the liver via the blood stream. In the liver, these proinflammatory cytokines stimulate the production of acute phase reactants. The cytokines also traverse the blood–brain barrier and exert direct stimulation on the hypothalamus, leading to the production of corticotropin releasing hormone (CRH) and arginine-vasopressin. These hormones, in turn, activate anterior pituitary cells to release adrenocorticotrophin hormone (ACTH), β-endorphins, prolactin, and the melanocyte stimulation hormone. These anterior pituitary hormones then exert endocrine effects on distant organs. As an example, ACTH, produced under the direction of CRH, induces the production of corticosteroids by the adrenal glands. Stressful events also activate the autonomic nervous system, leading to the release of adrenaline and noradrenaline and resultant increases in blood glucose, heart rate, blood pressure, and the state of alertness; inhibition of the immune system; and decreases in reproductive function [2].

The impact of stress following major and minor life events before the onset of primary SS (pSS) has been investigated [4]. A disproportionate percentage of pSS patients report the occurrence of negative stressful life events within 1 year of disease onset, compared to patients with lymphoma and healthy controls. Coping strategies were defective and the overall social support was lower in patients with pSS. After SS is established, nearly half of the patients suffer from anxiety and 32% have depression [5]. Conversely, up to 52% of patients with chronic fatigue syndrome report mucosal dryness, and salivary gland biopsies demonstrate findings consistent with SS in 32% of cases [6].

23.3 Hypothalamus-Pituitary-Adrenal Axis

Several neuroendocrine functions appear to be impaired in SS. The HPA axis produces basal ACTH and cortisol levels that are significantly lower than those of healthy controls, and pSS patients have correspondingly diminished responses of the pituitary and adrenal glands in response to ovine CRH [3, 7]. The lack of response to CRH suggests an important defect in the hypothalamic influence over the anterior pituitary. However, another study on both the basal state and following stimulation with CRH, TRH, and LHRH demonstrated that women with pSS without glucocorticoid treatment have intact cortisol synthesis but decreased serum concentrations of dehydroepiandrosterone sulphate (DHEAS) and increased cortisol/DHEAS ratios compared with healthy controls. These findings suggest a constitutional or disease-mediated influence on adrenal steroid synthesis [8]. Other authors have found an increase of IL-6 in the serum and saliva of patients with pSS and a slight increase of tumor necrosis factor (TNF) levels. Stimulation of host IL-6 increases the protective host responses such as acute phase response and HPA axis. IL-6 stimulates CRH, ACTH, and cortisol synthesis [9]. According with these findings, patients with SS have not only HPA hypoactivity, but also varying patterns of dysfunction of other hormonal axes [10].

23.4 Hypothalamus-Pituitary-Gonadal Axis

The role of androgens and estrogens in SS has been of interest since the 1980s. The first demonstration of the role of sex hormones in SS was derived from experimental models. In 1984, a synthetic androgen, nandrolone decanoate that has strong immunosuppressive but only weak androgenic effects was used in B/W mice, an experimental model of SLE and SS. Three weekly injections of this androgen therapy reduced the development of mononuclear infiltrates in the submandibular gland, thereby preventing the destruction of glandular tissue [11].

In humans, the role of sex steroid hormones in SS syndrome was studied for the first time in five patients with hypogonadism and Klinefelter's syndrome, three of whom had SS and two had SLE. All patients had low serum testosterone but high LH levels, and reduced total T lymphocytes and suppressor/cytotoxic T lymphocytes. The erythrocyte sedimentation rate (ESR) was above normal in all patients, and all had high titers of antinuclear antibodies (ANA) and rheumatoid factor (RF). After 60 days of testosterone therapy, serum testosterone levels had increased and LH levels had decreased in comparison with placebo group. The numbers of total T lymphocytes and suppresor/cytotoxic T lymphocytes normalized, titers of ANA and RF decreased, and the ESR declined in all patients. After therapy, the patients' SS and SLE entered clinical remissions [12].

Dihydrotestosterone, estrogen, and testosterone were studied in the minor salivary glands of women with SS and normal controls, using the Peroxidase–Antiperoxidase method. In normal controls, estrogen was positive in the epithelial cells of duct, but testosterone and dihydrotesterone were negative. However, estrogen, testosterone, and dihydrotestosterone were positive in the labial minor salivary glands of the SS patients, suggesting an influence of sex hormones in SS [13].

The incidence of SS in women increases from menarche and is highest near the menopause. However, the prevalence of SS in men increases with older age (e.g., age >70 years). Previous studies have shown that androgens reduce the development of experimental SS. These observations suggest that androgens may play an immunosuppressive and "protective" role for SS in young men [14, 15].

Women with primary and secondary SS have low levels of testosterone. The function of the meibomian glands and the secretion of tears are regulated in part by androgens. Thus, androgen deficiency might be associated with eye dryness [16]. Meibomian gland tissue contains androgen receptor mRNA, androgen receptor protein within acinar epithelial cell nuclei, and types 1 and 2 5[alpha]-reductase mRNAs. Androgens deficiency may lead to meibomian gland dysfunction, altered lipid profiles in meibomian gland secretions, tear film instability, and evaporative dry eye [17].

Activation of the cysteine-rich secretory protein-3 (CRISP-3) gene has been identified in the minor salivary glands of women with SS. This gene is expressed under normal conditions in the testicles and salivary glands of men, and is regulated by androgens. The CRISP-3 gene is important in cellular growth, differentiation, proliferation, and apoptosis. The finding of CRISP-3 gene activation and expression by mononuclear cells infiltrating the labial minor salivary glands of SS women patients was unexpected, especially in light of the androgen deficiency that is characteristic of pSS. Activation of the CRISP-3 gene within the minor salivary glands of pSS patients is consistent with an immune-neuroendocrine molecular communication [18].

The serum concentration of androgens correlates with parameters of SS activity such as serum IgG concentrations, the ESR, and inflammatory infiltrates within minor salivary glands. In contrast, negative correlations exist between dihydrotestosterone and C-reactive protein concentrations. No correlation has been reported between estrogen concentrations and pSS disease activity, but higher levels of disease activity are associated with increasing testosterone concentrations [19].

These controversial results had led to other investigations. In fact, only DHEA and DHEAS but not testosterone are affected in SS. Low serum levels of DHEAS in pSS might be the common denominator and a shared pathogenetic factor contributing to salivary gland involvement in pSS or sSS. Thus, androgen levels, normally low in women at the time of menopause and adrenopause, are decreased in SS patients compared with age- and sex-matched healthy controls [8]. In support of this hypothesis, it has been demonstrated that the epithelial cells of the healthy human labial salivary glands house a well-organized intracrine machinery capable of converting the DHEAS prohormone to its most active sex steroid metabolites, dihydrotestosterone and 17β-estradiol. In contrast, the salivary glands of patients with SS demonstrate derangements of the intracrine enzymes and a deficiency of androgens. This dysfunction, together with low serum levels of DHEAS, may explain the local androgen deficiency observed in salivary glands of patients with SS [20]. In support to these findings, the expression of CRISP-3 within glandular tissue and salivary in pSS patients is weak, indicating that the expression level of DHEA-regulated CRISP-3 is pathologically low in association with low salivary levels of DHEA [21] (Fig. 23.1). Moreover, the upregulation of integrins by androgens in tubuloepithelial cells and in labial salivary glands in SS is defective, also contributing to defective outside-in signaling, acinar atrophy, and ductal cell hyperplasia [22]. Other studies confirm that women with SS are androgen-deficient [23].

Estrogens increase the inflammatory infiltrate in salivary glands of normal mice in a manner that is indistinguishable from human SS [24]. In contrast, in another murine model for SS, estrogen deficiency was associated with inflammation and destruction of salivary and lacrimal glands. These effects, which appeared to be mediated by functional alterations of T lymphocytes, disappeared with estrogen treatment. The dysfunction of regulatory T cells by estrogen deficiency may play a crucial role on acceleration of autoimmune lesions. A murine model of SS suggested that Fas-mediated apoptosis controls the action of estrogens on epithelial cells [25]. One model of estrogen deficiency in rodents is the aromatase-knockout (ArKO) mouse. These animals have an elevated B lymphopoiesis in bone marrow and develop a severe autoimmune exocrinopathy that resembles SS [26].

In humans, a possible role for estrogen in the induction or acceleration of SS has been described. Some patients who received estrogen therapy developed full-blown SS 3 years after starting the treatment [27]. It is of interest that normal salivary epithelium constitutively expresses the same functional estrogen receptors that appear to mediate immunomodulatory effects [28].

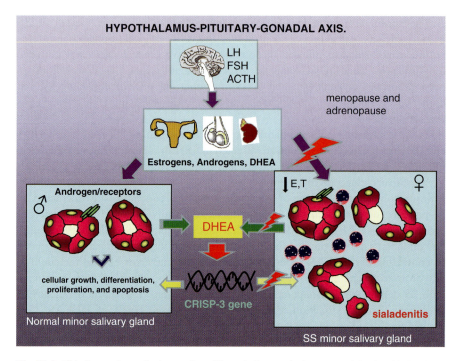

Fig. 23.1 This figure shows the interaction of hypothalamus-pituitary-gonadal axis with CRISP-3 gen in normal minor salivary gland and SS syndrome salivary gland. In SS salivary glands the architecture of the intracrine enzymes producing active A is deranged. This dysfunction, together with low serum levels of DHEAS, may explain the local A deficiency seen in salivary glands of patients with SS. In consequence, glandular and salivary CRISP-3 of SS patients was very weak, indicating that the expression level of DHEA-regulated CRISP-3 is pathologically low in association with low salivary levels of DHEA

23.5   Prolactin and Sjögren Syndrome

Hyperprolactinemia at serum concentrations between 20 and 40 ng/ml participates in the clinical expression of a variety of autoimmune rheumatic diseases, notably SLE. This hypothesis is based on several experimental studies that demonstrated prolactin's role as a neuroendocrine hormone with immunostimulatory properties. In addition, controversial reports suggest an association between hyperprolactinemia and lupus activity [29, 30].

Gutierrez et al. [31] studied basal serum levels of prolactin in 11 patients with pSS (9 women). Prolactin levels were significantly higher in patients with pSS compared with normal controls [31]. These preliminary data demonstrated hyperprolactinemia in a subset of patients with pSS, supporting the hypothesis of immune-neuroendocrine dysfunction characterized by an increase in prolactin and a decrease in cortisol in patients with pSS. Another study reported hyperprolactinemia in 21% of women between the ages of 51 and 81 who had anti-Ro and anti-La antibodies [32]. Some of those patients had clinical diagnoses of pSS, supporting an association between hyperprolactinemia and pSS [32].

Haga et al. [33] investigated the prevalence and clinical significance of hyperprolactinemia in 55 patients with pSS. Patients with pSS showed significantly higher prolactin levels than normal controls, and this difference was more striking in patients younger than age 45. Serum prolactin levels did not correlate with disease duration, serum immunoglobulin, autoantibodies, or focus score in biopsies from minor salivary glands, but did correlate with internal organ involvement. Two patients, both of whom had aggressive pSS with extraglandular manifestations, developed pSS 12 years after hyperprolactinemia was detected.

A recent study compares the level and relative ratio of estrogen, progesterone, and prolactin in postmenopausal (without hormone replacement therapy) patients with SS and healthy controls. A significantly higher level of prolactin in patients than controls was found with significantly higher prolactin/progesterone and estrogen/progesterone ratios [34]. Another study confirmed hyperprolactinemia in 16.3% of SS patients. Hyperprolactinemia was persistent after subgrouping the patients and the controls based on their menstrual history [35]. IgA-rheumatoid factor (RF), detected in the sera of 26% of the pSS patients and in 1% of the controls, correlated with serum prolactin levels [36]. As a whole, these studies suggest that hyperprolactinemia is prevalent in patients with pSS and that it correlates with internal organ involvement and the presence of autoantibodies. Primary SS may be preceded by hyperprolactinemia for many years.

Recently, Steinfeld et al. [37] investigated the role of prolactin in salivary glands of patients with pSS and normal controls. The investigators demonstrated prolactin receptors in the ductal epithelial cells of the salivary glands and increased synthesis of this hormone (prolactin of 16 and 60 kDa) by acinar cells among the patients with pSS. Furthermore, they found prolactin gene expression in the salivary glands and a positive correlation between the presence of prolactin in the acinar epithelial cells, extraglandular clinical manifestations, and positive anti-Ro and anti-La antibodies. Based on these findings and considering that diverse proteases are found in the minor salivary glands of patients with pSS, the same investigators studied the influence of prolactin on the expression of cathepsin B and D in the minor salivary glands of patients with pSS in comparison with normal controls. They found that under the direct influence of prolactin, patients had a significant increase of the proteases cathepsin B and D and their respective mRNAs [38].

The interaction between prolactin and cytokines is quite complex. IL-6 is a potent stimulator of both the synthesis and secretion of prolactin. The finding of elevated levels of IL-6 and prolactin in the cerebrospinal fluid of patients with SLE and CNS involvement supports the concept that these mediators may also participate in the pathophysiology of pSS [39].

Decreased serum levels of DHEA and DHEAS are perhaps the most important hormonal alterations observed in SS. DHEA and DHEAS (the major androgen products of the adrenal gland) inhibit IL-6 production and blunt the acute phase reaction. The mechanism of this effect is through the potentiation of an inhibitor of nuclear factor Kappa B [40].

23.6 Hypothalamus-Pituitary-Thyroid Axis

The thyroid, salivary, and lacrimal glands are susceptible to immunological damage, which can be expressed as thyroiditis or as SS. Indeed, the histopathology of both diseases characteristically shows focal or diffuse T and B lymphocyte infiltrates. These findings suggest that SS and autoimmune thyroid disease could share pathogenic mechanisms and antigens, which might explain the frequent co-occurrence of these conditions. The most common thyroid disorder found in SS is autoimmune thyroiditis and the most common hormonal pattern is subclinical hypothyroidism [41].

Tanaka et al. [42] performed serological and histopathological examination of the thyroid gland in 89 cases of SS. Thyroidal microsomal and thyroglobulin antibodies were detected in 34.5% and 21.4%, respectively. A direct correlation between thyroidal microsomal antibody and histopathology of the thyroid gland were found. Approximately 30% of SS had chronic thyroiditis as a complication.

Alpha-fodrin, an intracellular organ-specific cytoskeleton protein that is known to serve as an autoantigen, may be relevant to both SS and autoimmune thyroid disease [43–45].

23.7 Perspectives of Hormonal Treatment on Sjögren Syndrome

The main hormonal alterations in SS are hypofunction of the HPA axis and selective failure to produce DHEA-S. Based on these findings, several studies have proposed that pSS patients might benefit from DHEA supplementation. In a pilot study, 28 female pSS patients with severe fatigue and low serum DHEAS were treated with 200 mg of DHEA or placebo, (14 patients per group) during 24 weeks [46]. At the end of treatment, no significant differences were observed between both groups for dry eye symptoms, objective measures of ocular dryness, stimulated salivary flow, fatigue reduction, hypergammaglobulinemia, or ESR. Four DHEA and one placebo group patient dropped out because of adverse effects. However, a previous randomized, controlled trial had shown improvement of fatigue and well-being in the DHEA group [47].

Effects of 50 mg oral DHEA/day on changes in serum levels of DHEA and 12 of its metabolites, the relationships between steroid levels and disease characteristics; and the influence of DHEA on these parameters, were analyzed in a randomized, 9 month, controlled, double-blind crossover study. All metabolites increased during DHEA but not during placebo, with relief of symptoms as dry mouth during DHEA therapy [48].

Adiponectin is involved in the immune functions of several biologic systems. Its effect on the proliferation and apoptosis of salivary gland epithelial cells has been investigated. Adiponectin treatment resulted in a Dose-Dependent suppression of proliferation of salivary gland epithelial cells in pSS and protected the cells from spontaneous and interferon-gamma-induced apoptosis [49]. Additional studies of this immunoregulatory hormone are indicated in pSS.

23.8   Conclusions

1. Experimental and human studies suggest a dysfunction of immune-neuroendocrine system
2. The principal alterations in SS are hypofunction of the hypothalamus-pituitary-adrenal axis and the hyphothalamus-pituitary-gonadal axis
3. SS is characterized by androgen deficiency in salivary glands and defects in local processing of DHEA, with downregulation of CRISP-3 gene expression.
4. Prolactin and IL-6 may play a role in the pathogenesis of SS.
5. The treatment of SS with DHEA may be useful, but further investigations are required.

References

1. Wilder RL. Neuroendocrine-immune system interactions and autoimmunity. Annu Rev Immunol. 1995;13:307–38.
2. Jara LJ, Navarro C, Medina G, Vera-Lastra O, Blanco F. Immune-neuroendocrine interactions and autoimmune diseases. Clin Dev Immunol. 2006;13:109–23.
3. Tzioufas AG, Tsonis J, Moutsopoulos HM. Neuroendocrine dysfunction in Sjogren's syndrome. Neuroimmunomodulation. 2008;15:37–45.
4. Karaiskos D, Mavragani CP, Makaroni S, Zinzaras E, Voulgarelis M, Rabavilas A, et al. Stress, coping strategies and social support in patients with primary Sjögren's syndrome prior to disease onset: a retrospective case-control study. Ann Rheum Dis. 2009;68:40–6.
5. Valtýsdóttir ST, Gudbjörnsson B, Lindqvist U, Hällgren R, Hetta J. Anxiety and depression in patients with primary Sjögren's syndrome. J Rheumatol. 2000;27:165–9.
6. Sirois DA, Natelson B. Clinicopathological findings consistent with primary Sjögren's syndrome in a subset of patients diagnosed with chronic fatigue syndrome: preliminary observations. J Rheumatol. 2001;28:126–31.
7. Johnson EO, Vlachoyiannopoulos PG, Skopouli FN, Tzioufas AG, Moutsopoulos HM. Hypofunction of the stress axis in Sjögren's syndrome. J Rheumatol. 1998;25:1508–14.
8. Valtysdóttir ST, Wide L, Hällgren R. Low serum dehydroepiandrosterone sulfate in women with primary Sjögren's syndrome as an isolated sign of impaired HPA axis function. J Rheumatol. 2001;28:1259–65.
9. d'Elia HF, Bjurman C, Rehnberg E, Kvist G, Konttinen YT. Interleukin 6 and its soluble receptor in a central role at the neuroimmunoendocrine interface in Sjögren syndrome: an explanatory interventional study. Ann Rheum Dis. 2009;68:285–6.
10. Johnson EO, Kostandi M, Moutsopoulos HM. Hypothalamic-pituitary-adrenal axis function in Sjögren's syndrome: mechanisms of neuroendocrine and immune system homeostasis. Clin Rheumatol. 2001;20:44–8.

11. Schot LP, Verheul HA, Schuurs AH. Effect of nandrolone decanoate on Sjögren's syndrome like disorders in NZB/NZW mice. Clin Exp Immunol. 1984;57:571–4.
12. Bizzarro A, Valentini G, Di Martino G, DaPonte A, De Bellis A, Iacono G. Influence of testosterone therapy on clinical and immunological features of autoimmune diseases associated with Klinefelter's syndrome. J Clin Endocrinol Metab. 1987;64:32–6.
13. Kumagami H, Onitsuka T. Estradiol and testosterone in minor salivary glands of Sjögren's syndrome. Auris Nasus Larynx. 1993;20:137–43.
14. Anaya JM, Liu GT, D'Souza E, Ogawa N, Luan X, Talal N. Primary Sjögren's syndrome in men. Ann Rheum Dis. 1995;54:748–51.
15. García-Carrasco M, Cervera R, Rosas J, Ramos-Casals M, Morlà RM, Sisó A, et al. Primary Sjögren's syndrome in the elderly: clinical and immunological characteristics. Lupus. 1999;8:20–3.
16. Sullivan DA, Wickham LA, Rocha EM, Krenzer KL, Sullivan BD, Steagall R, et al. Androgens and dry eye in Sjögren's syndrome. Ann N Y Acad Sci. 1999;876:312–24.
17. Sullivan DA, Sullivan BD, Evans JE, Schirra F, Yamagami H, Liu M, et al. Androgen deficiency, Meibomian gland dysfunction, and evaporative dry eye. Ann N Y Acad Sci. 2002;966:211–22.
18. Tapinos NI, Polihronis M, Thyphronitis G, Moutsopoulos HM. Characterization of the cysteine-rich secretory protein 3 gene as an early-transcribed gene with a putative role in the pathophysiology of Sjögren's syndrome. Arthritis Rheum. 2002;46:215–22.
19. Brennan MT, Sankar V, Leakan RA, Grisius MM, Collins MT, Fox PC, et al. Sex steroid hormones in primary Sjögren's syndrome. J Rheumatol. 2003;30:1267–71.
20. Spaan M, Porola P, Laine M, Rozman B, Azuma M, Konttinen YT. Healthy human salivary glands contain a DHEA-sulphate processing intracrine machinery, which is deranged in primary Sjögren's syndrome. J Cell Mol Med. 2009;13:1261–70.
21. Laine M, Porola P, Udby L, Kjeldsen L, Cowland JB, Borregaard N, et al. Low salivary dehydroepiandrosterone and androgen-regulated cysteine-rich secretory protein 3 levels in Sjögren's syndrome. Arthritis Rheum. 2007;56:2575–84.
22. Porola P, Laine M, Virtanen I, Pöllänen R, Przybyla BD, Konttinen YT. Androgens and integrins in salivary glands in Sjogren's syndrome. J Rheumatol. 2010;37:1181–7.
23. Sullivan DA, Bélanger A, Cermak JM, Bérubé R, Papas AS, Sullivan RM, et al. Are women with Sjögren's syndrome androgen-deficient? J Rheumatol. 2003;30:2413–9.
24. Ahmed SA, Aufdemorte TB, Chen JR, Montoya AI, Olive D, Talal N. Estrogen induces the development of autoantibodies and promotes salivary gland lymphoid infiltrates in normal mice. J Autoimmun. 1989;2:543–52.
25. Ishimaru N, Saegusa K, Yanagi K, Haneji N, Saito I, Hayashi Y. Estrogen deficiency accelerates autoimmune exocrinopathy in murine Sjögren's syndrome through fas-mediated apoptosis. Am J Pathol. 1999;155:173–81.
26. Shim GJ, Warner M, Kim HJ, Andersson S, Liu L, Ekman J, et al. Aromatase-deficient mice spontaneously develop a lymphoproliferative autoimmune disease resembling Sjogren's syndrome. Proc Natl Acad Sci USA. 2004;101:12628–33.
27. Nagler RM, Pollack S. Sjögren's syndrome induced by estrogen therapy. Semin Arthritis Rheum. 2000;30:209–14.
28. Tsinti M, Kassi E, Korkolopoulou P, Kapsogeorgou E, Moutsatsou P, Patsouris E, et al. Functional estrogen receptors alpha and beta are expressed in normal human salivary gland epithelium and apparently mediate immunomodulatory effects. Eur J Oral Sci. 2009;117:498–505.
29. Walker SE, Jacobson JD. Roles of prolactin and gonadotropin-releasing hormone in rheumatic diseases. Rheum Dis Clin North Am. 2000;26:713–36.
30. Jara LJ, Vera-Lastra O, Miranda JM, Alcala M, Alvarez-Nemegyei J. Prolactin in human systemic lupus erythematosus. Lupus. 2001;10:748–56.
31. Gutiérrez MA, Anaya JM, Scopelitis E, Citera G, Silveira L, Espinoza LR. Hyperprolactinaemia in primary Sjögren's syndrome. Ann Rheum Dis. 1994;53:425.

32. Allen SH, Sharp GC, Wang G, Conley C, Takeda Y, Conroy SE, et al. Prolactin levels and antinuclear antibody profiles in women tested for connective tissue disease. Lupus. 1996;5:30–7.
33. Haga HJ, Rygh T. The prevalence of hyperprolactinemia in patients with primary Sjögren's syndrome. J Rheumatol. 1999;26:1291–5.
34. Taiym S, Haghighat N, Al-Hashimi I. A comparison of the hormone levels in patients with Sjogren's syndrome and healthy controls. Oral Surg Oral Med Oral Pathol Oral Radiol Endod. 2004;97:579–83.
35. El Miedany YM, Ahmed I, Moustafa H, El BM. Hyperprolactinemia in Sjogren's syndrome: a patient subset or a disease manifestation? Joint Bone Spine. 2004;71:203–8.
36. Peen E, Mellbye OJ, Haga HJ. IgA rheumatoid factor in primary Sjogren's syndrome. Scand J Rheumatol. 2009;38:46–9.
37. Steinfeld S, Rommes S, François C, Decaestecker C, Maho A, Appelboom T, et al. Big prolactin 60 kDa is overexpressed in salivary glandular epithelial cells from patients with Sjögren's syndrome. Lab Invest. 2000;80:239–47.
38. Steinfeld S, Maho A, Chaboteaux C, Daelemans P, Pochet R, Appelboom T, et al. Prolactin up-regulates cathepsin B and D expression in minor salivary glands of patients with Sjögren's syndrome. Lab Invest. 2000;80:1711–20.
39. Jara LJ, Irigoyen L, Ortiz MJ, Zazueta B, Bravo G, Espinoza LR. Prolactin and interleukin-6 in neuropsychiatric lupus erythematosus. Clin Rheumatol. 1998;17:110–4.
40. Kim SK, Shin MS, Jung BK, Shim JY, Won HS, Lee PR, et al. Effect of dehydroepiandrosterone on lipopolysaccharide-induced interleukin-6 production in DH82 cultured canine macrophage cells. J Reprod Immunol. 2006;70:71–81.
41. Jara LJ, Navarro C, Brito-Zerón Mdel P, García-Carrasco M, Escárcega RO, Ramos-Casals M. Thyroid disease in Sjögren's syndrome. Clin Rheumatol. 2007;26:16016.
42. Tanaka OA. A diagnosis and etiologic studies of Sjögren's syndrome – II: on the relationship between Sjögren's syndrome and chronic thyroiditis. Nippon Jibiinkoka Gakkai Kaiho. 1989;92:374–82.
43. Kahaly GJ, Bang H, Berg W, Dittmar M. Alpha-fodrin as a putative autoantigen in Graves' ophthalmopathy. Clin Exp Immunol. 2005;140:166–72.
44. Szanto A, Csipo I, Horvath I, Biro E, Szodoray P, Zeher M. Autoantibodies to alfa-fodrin in patients with Hashimoto thyroiditis and Sjögren's syndrome: possible markers for a common secretory disorder. Rheumatol Int. 2008;11:1169–72.
45. Nakamura H, Usa T, Motomura M, Ichikawa T, Nakao K, Kawasaki E, et al. Prevalence of interrelated autoantibodies in thyroid diseases and autoimmune disorders. J Endocrinol Invest. 2008;10:861–5.
46. Virkki LM, Porola P, Forsblad-d'Elia H, Valtysdottir S, Solovieva SA, Konttinen YT. Dehydroepiandrosterone (DHEA) substitution treatment for severe fatigue in DHEA-deficient patients with primary Sjögren's syndrome. Arthritis Care Res (Hoboken). 2010;62:118–24.
47. Hartkamp A, Geenen R, Godaert GL, Bootsma H, Kruize AA, Bijlsma JW, et al. Effect of dehydroepiandrosterone administration on fatigue, well-being, and functioning in women with primary Sjögren syndrome: a randomised controlled trial. Ann Rheum Dis. 2008;67:91–7.
48. d'Elia FH, Carlsten H, Labrie F, Konttinen YT, Ohlsson C. Low serum levels of sex steroids are associated with disease characteristics in primary Sjogren's syndrome; supplementation with dehydroepiandrosterone restores the concentrations. J Clin Endocrinol Metab. 2009;94: 2044–51.
49. Katsiougiannis S, Tenta R, Skopouli FN. Activation of AMP-activated protein kinase by adiponectin rescues salivary gland epithelial cells from spontaneous and interferon-gamma-induced apoptosis. Arthritis Rheum. 2010;62:414–9.

Chapter 24
Gynecological and Reproductive Complications in Primary Sjögren's Syndrome

Andreas V. Goules and Athanasios G. Tzioufas

Contents

24.1 Introduction

Primary Sjögren's syndrome (SS) almost exclusively afflicts women. The external genitalia are commonly affected and as a result, vaginal dryness and dypareunia may occur. Other less common gynecological problems have also been described.

The mean age at diagnosis for patients with SS occurs around menopause. Thus, the disease does not usually become clinically apparent until the fourth decade of life. Although a considerable number of patients are affected during reproductive age, SS does not appear to affect the fertility of patients. However, the presence of anti-Ro/SSA and/or anti-La/SSB autoantibodies posses a significant concern, because these autoantibodies can enter the embryonic circulation and lead in a subset of patients to the neonatal lupus syndrome (NLS).

A.V. Goules • A.G. Tzioufas (✉)

Department of Pathophysiology, School of Medicine, University of Athens, Athens, Greece

M. Ramos-Casals et al. (eds.), *Sjögren's Syndrome*,
DOI 10.1007/978-0-85729-947-5_24, © Springer-Verlag London Limited 2012

24.2   Gynecological Manifestations in Sjögren's Syndrome

Capriello et al. first described the common symptoms of dyspareunia and pruritus caused by vaginal dryness among women with SS [1]. In a systematic study that included 51 female SS patients (mean age 51 years) and 57 healthy, age-matched controls, Skopouli et al. described the disease effects on parity, fertility, and sexual activity [2]. Thirty-one (61%) of the 51 SS patients and 22 (39%) of the controls were postmenopausal. The reported age at the beginning of menopause was similar in the two groups. Sicca symptoms appeared in 34 (67%) of the SS patients before the menopause and in 17 (33%) after the menopause.

Fertility and parity rates, as well as the reproductive success rate were similar in both groups. Forty-eight of 51 patients with SS reported a total of 207 pregnancies and 50 of 57 healthy women had 187 pregnancies. The first sexual activity, frequency of intercourse, and libido were also similar in patients and controls. Twenty-five of 49 (51%) SS patients reported of dyspareunia, compared to only 3% of the controls. Eight of 20 (40%) SS patients were premenopausal and 17 of 29 (58.6%) were postmenopausal. Of the eight premenopausal patients, four had an obvious aetiology of dyspareunia (two had a perineal operation and two had vaginitis) and after appropriate treatment the dyspareunia disappeared. In the remaining four patients, the physical examination was normal and the cytological examination did not show signs of atrophy or inflammation. Vaginal biopsies from symptomatic patients disclosed nonkeratinised stratified squamous epithelia and a mild to moderate perivascular inflammatory lymphocytic infiltration in the underlying stroma.

Mulherin et al. assessed 11 patients with SS and also found that chronic dyspareunia could be the presenting symptom in these patients, preceding sicca symptoms in the eyes or mouth by many years [3]. These findings have been confirmed by other investigators despite the fact that their frequency did not always reach a statistically significant difference with an age-matched control population [4, 5]. Cirpan et al. evaluated 33 women with SS and 67 healthy controls who underwent cytology and colposcopic examination as well as DNA testing for the human papilloma virus [4]. No significant differences were observed between the two groups except for a higher prevalence of dyspareunia and vaginal dryness among patients with SS.

In a study of 58 patients with pSS and 157 controls, gynecological problems and relevant interventions were evaluated using a self-administered questionnaire [6]. Amenorrhea lasting for more than 3 months, menorrhagia/metrorrhagia (54.5% vs. 35.7%, $p = 0.012$), vaginal dryness (52.9% vs. 28.3%, $p = 0.005$), endometriosis (8.5% vs. 2.1%, $p = 0.03$), and surgical intervention for endometriosis (6.3% vs. 0.7%, $p = 0.009$) were found to occur more frequently in patients with SS compared to healthy individuals. In conclusion, women with SS have more gynecological problems compared to the general female population, with dyspareunia and vaginal dryness being the leading symptoms. Amenorrhoea, menorrhagia/metrorrhagia, and endometriosis are also reported to occur in younger patients with SS, but further research is needed in order to confirm these data and establish their underlying mechanisms. Table 24.1 shows the major gynecological problems affecting women with SS.

Table 24.1 Major gynecological problems in patients with pSS

Dyspareunia
Vaginal dryness
Menorrhagia
Metrorrhagia
Amenorrhoea
Endometriosis

pSS primary Sjögren's syndrome

24.3 Pregnancy Complications-Neonatal Lupus Syndrome

24.3.1 Epidemiology and Clinical Features of NLS and Congenital Heart Block (CHB)

NLS is a systemic disorder in which the skin, liver, blood cells, and heart can be involved. The syndrome, which affects newborns of anti-Ro/SSA and/or anti-La/SSB-positive mothers [7], results from the passive transfer of maternal autoantibodies through the placenta, leading to damage of the developing fetal tissues. CHB is the most serious extracutaneous manifestation of the syndrome, often requiring permanent cardiac pacing and sometimes resulting in intrauterine fetal demise.

In the context of NLS, CHB is defined as atrioventricular block diagnosed in utero, at birth, or within the neonatal period (0–27 days after birth) in an offspring of the anti-Ro/SSA and/or anti-La/SSB-positive woman [8, 9]. Anti-Ro/SSA and anti-La/SSB antibodies are detected in 60–90% and 30–60% of SS patients, respectively [10]. These autoantibodies are included in the diagnostic criteria of SS [11]. Because these autoantibodies can be associated with NLS and the development of CHB, it is important to provide prenatal counseling to women with anti-Ro/SSA and/or anti-La/SSB antibodies who wish to become pregnant.

The incidence of CHB varies between 1:17,000 and 1:20,000 live births [12, 13].

Approximately 50% of children affected by NLS have skin disease and approximately 50% have CHB [14]; 10% have both. NLS is characterized by specific skin lesions that resemble those of subacute cutaneous lupus erythematosus (SCLE) [7, 15]. The rash typically occurs within a few days after birth and affects sun-exposed areas such as the head and neck area, often following a malar distribution (Fig. 24.1). Erythematous, annular plaques with scaling are the most common lesions but discoid lesions can be also observed. The rash usually resolves after 6–8 months leaving residual hypopigmentation and skin atrophy. The histological features of the skin lesions include hyperkeratosis, vacuolar basal degeneration, interstitial edema, and perivascular lymphocytic infiltration. Immunofluorescence reveals immune deposits around the basal keratinocytes and along the dermal–epidermal junction [7, 16]. Other cutaneous manifestations of NLS include purpura (caused by thrombocytopenia rather than vasculitis) and jaundice due to hepatic involvement.

Fig. 24.1 The classic periorbital rash consistent with neonatal lupus (This figure was kindly provided by Dr. Jill Buyon)

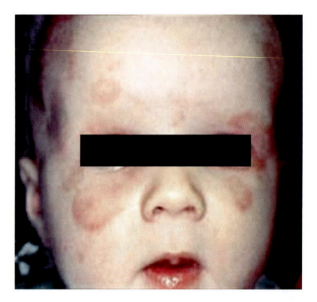

Because the neonatal rash is self-limited, no treatment is required, but topical steroids can be used with caution. In general, the long-term prognosis of children with skin disease is excellent.

The hematologic abnormalities reported in the literature include thrombocytopenia in 10–20% of patients [17] and neutropenia [18]. However, these abnormalities are transient and follow a benign course. Approximately 20–40% of the affected children present with hepatomegaly as a result of congestive heart failure [7, 19]. Asymptomatic elevation of liver enzymes has been observed in 26% [20]. Other rare extracutaneous manifestations reported in children with NLS include learning disabilities [21], anemia [7], and hydrocephalus [22].

Heart involvement is generally the most serious complication of NLS. Fetal clinical manifestations include heart block of various degrees, valve disease, myocarditis, and hydropic changes of the heart. CHB may have the form of first-, second-, or third-degree atrioventricular (AV) block. In complete CHB, the ventricular rate ranges from 30 to 110 beats/min [23]. Fetal heart rates less than 50 beats/min have been associated with fetal hydrops, heart failure, and neonatal death [23, 24]. Progression of CHB has been reported rarely to occur in the postpartum period, despite clearance of the maternal antibodies. This fact confirms that in utero injury to the fetal conduction system is the key pathophsyiological event. However, even if a partial heart block appears to regress after birth, the infant should be followed well into childhood to ensure that conduction disturbances do not emerge from subclinical damage (Fig. 24.2).

Approximately 6% of newborns with CHB may develop dilated cardiomyopathy and congestive heart failure [25, 26]. Most of these patients require cardiac transplantation. CHB has been also reported to be associated with endocardial fibroelastosis [27]. Unconfirmed cardiac manifestations possibly associated with NLS are sinus bradycardia and QT prolongation [28–31]. Rare complications of

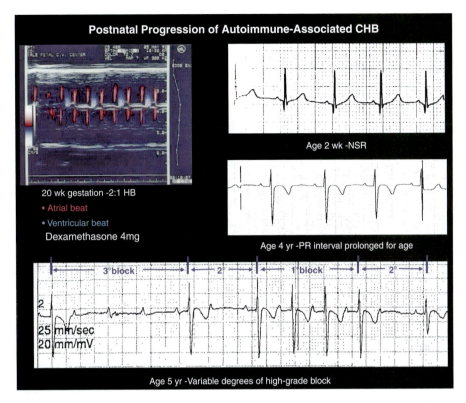

Fig. 24.2 Heart involvement in NLS. In the *upper left panel* is an in utero echocardiogram demonstrating second-degree block, 2:1. In red is the atrial beat and in blue the ventricular beat. The mother was treated with dexamethasone at 4 mg. At 2 weeks after birth the EKG showed normal sinus rhythm. However, over time the block progressed and at the age of 4 years a prolonged PR interval was noticed (*middle panel*). By the age of 5 years, the Holter showed variable degrees of high-grade block (*lower panel*) (This figure was kindly provided by Dr. Jill Buyon)

NLS included isolated endomyocardial elastosis with subsequent mitral and tricuspid avulsion, dysfunction of the sinus or sino-atrial nodes, conduction disturbances below the His bundle, and atrial flutter [32].

24.3.2   Maternal and Fetal Outcomes in NLS

Several studies assessed the clinical picture and long-term outcome of mothers who have given birth to children with NLS and/or CHB (Table 24.2). At least 50% of mothers whose offspring develop NLS or CHB are themselves entirely asymptomatic and have no idea that they possess antibodies to the Ro/SSA or La/SSB antigens. The true figure may be 80% [33–35]. The remaining 30–50% are known to have SLE, SS, or an undifferentiated autoimmune syndrome. Approximately half of women who are asymptomatic at the time of giving birth to a child with NLS will

Table 24.2 Evolution of the clinical picture of mothers giving birth to a child with NLS

Number of mothers	Follow-up (years)	Percent of asymptomatic mothers	Percent of progression and disease phenotype	References
57	3.7	50	48 (50% UAS, 30% SLE, 20% SS)	Waltuck and Buyon [33]
64	10.0	65	14 (50% UAS, 15% SLE)	Press et al. [34]
229	0.5	16	50 (55% UAS, 25% SS, 20% SLE)	Rivera et al. [35]

UAS undifferentiated autoimmune syndrome, *SS* Sjögren's syndrome, *SLE* systemic lupus erythematosus

eventually develop a systemic autoimmune disease, usually SLE or SS. The probabilities of developing full-blown SLE or SS during a 10 year period are approximately 19% and 28%, respectively [35]. However, the evolution of the underlying disease can be relatively slow for months: the median time to the development of any symptom related to a connective tissue disorder is more than 3 years.

The prognosis of children with NLS varies according to the clinical manifestations. The skin and hematologic manifestations subside after maturation of newborn's immune system, usually around the 6th month of life. In contrast, prognosis of children with CHB is poor. In fact, the mortality approaches 30%. Death usually occurs in utero or within the first 3 months of life [8]. However, children who will survive CHB and undergo pacemaker implantation may have normal lives. The probability that these children will develop an autoimmune disease in the future is low. Consequently, it is recommended that mothers at risk for carrying or delivering a child with CHB should have ultrasound evaluation every week between the 18th and 24th weeks of gestation.

Brucato et al. studied 16 newborns with CHB and found that 3 of them died either in utero or within 2 days of delivery [36]. An additional child died at the age of 6 years [36]. Among the 13 living children, whose mean age was 18.3 years (range 2–34 years), 8 required a cardiac pacemaker. However, none had developed an autoimmune disease despite lengthy follow-up.

A somewhat larger study of 49 children with a history of NLS yielded slightly different findings [37]. Six had been identified as having some form of autoimmune disease. The diagnoses included two with juvenile inflammatory arthritis and one each with Hashimoto's thyroiditis, psoriasis, type I diabetes mellitus and psoriasis, and congenital hypothyroidism and nephritic syndrome. Although autoimmune diseases can emerge in individuals as children, it is not clear that this risk is any higher than that conferred by being the offspring of a parent with primary SS or SLE.

24.3.3 Diagnosis

CHB is diagnosed in utero by prenatal ultrasound between the 18th and 24th weeks of gestation. Several methods have been used to detect conductive abnormalities, particularly first-degree AV block, since this may precede complete

CHB. One study employed gated, pulsed Doppler ultrasound to the mechanical PR interval in 98 pregnancies in 95 anti-Ro/SSA-positive mothers. The study detected three newborns with complete CHB, of whom none had a preceding prolonged PR interval [31].

In another study of 24 women with anti-Ro/SSA antibodies, the delay between atrial and ventricular depolarization was estimated by two Doppler echocardiographic methods [38]. Eight fetus in that study were found to have first-degree AV block, but only one progressed to complete CHB. Another fetus converted from second-degree heart block to first-degree heart block after treatment with betamethasone. In the remaining six babies, spontaneous normalization of the heart rhythm occurred.

Finally, fetal kinetocardiogram aiming to detect first-degree AV block was performed in 70 fetuses of 56 mothers with anti-Ro/SSA antibodies. Six fetuses had first-degree AV block, but all six recovered normal cardiac conduction features following treatment with dexamethasone [39].

In summary, several studies to date support the utility of a variety of echocardiographic methods in detecting fetal conduction defects. Further research is needed to establish their role to optimal approach this problem.

24.3.4 Risk Factors

The first clinical study addressing the risk of CHB in newborns of anti-Ro/SSA antibody-positive mothers was conducted by Brucato et al. [40]. In that study, 100 anti-Ro/SSA antibody-positive women with a history of an underlying connective tissue disease were followed before and after pregnancy. The risk of delivering an infant with complete CHB was found to be 2%. Since then, several other studies have confirmed that the risk of CHB in an anti-Ro/SSA pregnant woman ranges between 1% and 2.7% [20, 30, 31]. Other studies have reported even lower estimates [41, 42].

The presence of anti-La/SSB autoantibodies appears to increase the risk of CHB. In one study, the presence of anti-La/SSB autoantibodies increased the risk of CHB to 3.1%, compared to 0.9% for women without anti-La/SSB autoantibodies [43]. The likelihood of having a second child with CHB is at least two- to threefold higher in women with a previous pregnancy complicated by fetal CHB compared with the risk of who never had an affected child. The risk of recurrence may be as high as 15–20% (Table 24.3). Llanos et al. have shown that the recurrence rate of cardiac disease in 161 pregnancies of 129 anti-Ro/SSA-positive mothers was 17.4% (95% confidence intervals 11.1–23.6%) [44]. Another study estimated the risk of women CHB following the birth of an earlier child with cutaneous NLS to be 12.8% [45].

Hypothyroidism may also be a risk factor for CHB. Spence et al. showed that women with hypothyroidism and anti-Ro/SSA antibodies had a ninefold increased risk for delivering a child with complete CHB compared to women with antibodies but normal thyroid function [46].

Factor	Risk for CHB
Anti-Ro/SSA	1–2.7%
Anti-Ro/SSA and anti-La/SSB	3.1%
Anti-La/SSB negativity	0.9%
History of a previously affected child	15–20%
Initial birth of child with cutaneous NLS	12.8%
Hypothyroidism	~18% (9 fold higher)

Table 24.3 Factors affecting the risk of congenital heart block

CHB congenital heart block, *NLS* neonatal lupus syndrome

Finally, specific laboratory parameters may identify women and pregnancies at risk for NLS and CHB. Several studies have attempted to address the fine specificity of autoantibodies against Ro/SSA and La/SSB, by defining B-cell epitopes specific for NLS. Salomonsson et al. found that autoantibodies recognizing a specific epitope within the leucine zipper domain of Ro52, spanning the region 200–239aa (p200), correlated with the prolongation of fetal AV time and heart block. These autoantibodies were also found in women with unaffected children, but their levels were significantly higher in mothers of children with CHB [47, 48].

Regulation of autoantibody response and penetrance through placenta, via the idiotypic–anti-idiotypic network, appear to be also important. Indeed, the prevalence in maternal sera of anti-idiotypic antibodies targeting antibodies against the major B cell epitope of La/SSB, spanning the sequence 349–364aa, was higher in anti-Ro/SSA and/or anti-La/SSB-positive mothers carrying a healthy child and no history of a previous affected child (79%), compared to mothers carrying a child with NLS (24%) [49]. Furthermore, hidden antibodies against the major epitope of La/SSB were found in only 28% of mothers carrying a child with NLS compared to 89% of mothers carrying healthy children. This finding suggests that anti-idiotypic antibodies may exert a protective effect by neutralizing anti-La/SSB antibodies and decreasing the risk of NLS and CHB. Testing for anti-idiotypic responses by using this specific technique could be used to predict a decreased risk of NLS-related CHB.

24.3.5 Pathogenesis of Congenital Heart Block

The human cardiac conduction system is formed by the 12th week and undergoes further embryonic remodeling until the 20th week of gestation, during which time the transplacental transfer of maternal anti-Ro/SSA or anti-La/SSB autoantibodies occurs [8]. The proposed model of pathogenesis is based on the finding that apoptosis of cardiomyocytes during heart development may lead to translocation of the intracellular Ro/SSA and La/SSB autoantigens onto the cell surface [50]. Anti-Ro/SSA and anti-La/SSB antibodies then bound to apoptotic cells, which are subsequently phagocytosed by macrophages.

In vitro studies have shown that following ingestion of apoptotic cardiomyocytes, the macrophages become activated and secrete TNF-α [51] and TGF-β [52]. TGF-β is a pivotal cytokine involved in the fibrotic process, leading ultimately to injury of the conductive system. Exposure of cardiac fibroblasts to supernatants derived from macrophage cultures, after incubation with autoantibody-coated apoptotic cells, shifts their phenotype toward scar promotion. This process is mediated by TGF-β and inhibited specifically by anti-TGF-β monoclonal antibodies. Studying the role of clearance of apoptotic cells in the heart, Clancy et al. showed that the proliferating cardiomyocytes can eliminate the neighboring apoptotic cardiomyocytes. This process was inhibited by the presence of anti-Ro/SSA antibodies, suggesting that autoantibodies bound to apoptotic cells delay their clearance, leading eventually to their accumulation and contributing further to inflammation and fibrosis [53].

Genetics appear also to be involved in the pathogenesis of CHB. One study evaluated codons 10 and 25 of the TGF-β gene in 40 children with CHB, 17 children with NLS-related rash, 31 unaffected siblings, and 74 mothers who had at least one child with NLS [54]. The investigators found that the Leu^{10} TGF-β polymorphism was higher among CHB with CHB compared to both unaffected offspring and controls, implying that this specific polymorphism is associated with increased expression of TGF-β by macrophages [54]. Genome-wide association studies to address the genetic profile of these patients are pending.

24.3.6 Management of Pregnancy in Women with Anti-Ro/La Autoantibodies

The risk of an anti-Ro/SSA- or anti-La/SSB-antibody-positive mother with no history of a previous CHB delivery giving birth to a newborn with CHB does not exceed 3%. These pregnancies are viewed as low risk compared with those of a woman whose previous pregnancy was complicated by NLS or CHB, in whom the risk of having a child with CHB may be as high as 20%. These individuals comprise the high-risk group.

Low-risk patients require close monitoring to detect cardiac involvement as early as possible. Glucocorticoids are the cornerstone of therapy for CHB. Once CHB has become established, glucocorticoids cannot revert the disease but may improve the overall prognosis [55], probably through their effects on inflammation-related manifestations such as hydrops and pleural effusions [56, 57]. Because fluorinated glucocorticoids are not metabolized by the placenta, these preparations (e.g., betamethasone and dexamethasone) are the medications of choice in this setting. Glucocorticoid treatment has been reported in some studies to revert first- and second-degree AV block [38, 42, 56], but other studies have not confirmed these observations [58, 59]. Treatment complications observed in mothers treated with glucocorticoids include diabetes mellitus, infections, and osteoporosis. In fetuses, oligohydroamnios and intrauterine growth retardation may occur. A recent study on 13 children with CHB who were exposed to a high dose of dexamethasone demonstrated no adverse effects on neuropsycological development [60].

Table 24.4 Intrauterine and postnatal management of congenital heart block

Indication	Management
Incomplete or complete CHB less than 2 weeks	Betamethasone of 4–8 mg/daily and tapered after few weeks
Presence of myocarditis, heart failure, or hydrops	Betamethasone of 4–8 mg/daily and tapered after few weeks
Complete CHB more than 2 weeks	Serial echograms, no therapy
Increased heart rate	Selective beta 2 agonists (e.g., salbutamol)
Postnatal CHB	Pacemaker implantation

CHB congenital heart block

Brucato et al. suggested that betamethasone or dexamethasone of 4 mg daily should be administered to mothers if fetal heart block is incomplete or recent, or if heart block is complicated by myocarditis, heart failure, and hydropic changes [8]. The dexamethasone dose should be tapered and discontinued if no changes are evident within several weeks. In contrast, if the heart block is complete and known to be present for more than 2 weeks, a watchful waiting with serial echocardiography is recommended [8].

IVIG administration has been also proposed to prevent CHB in high-risk pregnancies [61, 62]. The possible mechanisms by which IVIG could prevent the development of CHB include elimination of maternal anti-Ro/SSA and La/SSB autoantibodies through anti-idiotypic antibodies, decreased transplacental transport of pathogenetic autoantibodies, and inhibition of macrophage activation. The value of IVIG at a dose of 400 mg/kg administered at 12, 15, 18, 21, and 24 weeks of high-risk pregnancies was recently addressed by two double-blind studies [63, 64]. Both failed to demonstrate a beneficial effect of IVIG, since CHB developed in 15% [66] of fetuses on one study and 20% of those in another, figures similar to those observed in the control groups. More specific immunotherapies, aimed at providing high-affinity blocking anti-idiotypic antibodies, are worthy of study in this disorder. In both studies the reasons of IVIG treatment failure could be attributed to: i) the chosen dose was low, ii) IVIG might not be effective in preventing transplacental passage of pathogenetic autoantibodies because it contains a small amount of specific anti-idiotypic antibodies with low affinity or iii) other, still undetermined, environmental factors are also involved.

Beta 2 adrenergic agonists such as salbutamol or ritodrine could also be administrated to the mothers in order to increase fetal heart rate and improve ventricular function [8, 65]. For newborns with CHB, the cornerstone of therapy is implantation of a permanent pacemaker [8]. Isopreterenol can be used to control bradycardia. In Table 24.4, the management of CHB proposed by Brucato et al. is shown. In regard to low-risk pregnancies, the administration of hydroxychloroquine is a therapeutic option, since exposure of SLE mothers with anti-Ro/SSA and/or anti-La/SSB antibodies to hydroxychloroquine has been found to decrease the risk of CHB [67].

References

1. Capriello P, Barale E, Cappelli N, Lupo S, Teti G. Sjogren's syndrome: clinical, cytological, histological and colposcopic aspects in women. Clin Exp Obstet Gynecol. 1988;15:9–12.
2. Skopouli FN, Papanikolaou S, Malamou-Mitsi V, Papanikolaou N, Moutsopoulos HM. Obstetric and gynaecological profile in patients with primary Sjogren's syndrome. Ann Rheum Dis. 1994;53:569–73.
3. Mulherin DM, Sheeran TP, Kumararatne DS, Speculand B, Luesley D, Situnayake RD. Sjogren's syndrome in women presenting with chronic dyspareunia. Br J Obstet Gynaecol. 1997;104:1019–23.
4. Cirpan T, Guliyeva A, Onder G, Terek MC, Ozsaran A, Kabasakal Y, et al. Comparison of human papillomavirus testing and cervical cytology with colposcopic examination and biopsy in cervical cancer screening in a cohort of patients with Sjogren's syndrome. Eur J Gynaecol Oncol. 2007;28:302–6.
5. Marchesoni D, Mozzanega B, De Sandre P, Romagnolo C, Gambari PF, Maggino T. Gynaecological aspects of primary Sjogren's syndrome. Eur J Obstet Gynecol Reprod Biol. 1995;63:49–53.
6. Haga HJ, Gjesdal CG, Irgens LM, Ostensen M. Reproduction and gynaecological manifestations in women with primary Sjogren's syndrome: a case-control study. Scand J Rheumatol. 2005;34:45–8.
7. Boh EE. Neonatal lupus erythematosus. Clin Dermatol. 2004;22:125–8.
8. Brucato A, Cimaz R, Caporali R, Ramoni V, Buyon J. Pregnancy outcomes in patients with autoimmune diseases and anti-Ro/SSA antibodies. Clin Rev Allergy Immunol. 2011;40(1): 27–41.
9. Buyon JP, Brucato A, Friedman DM. What's in a name? Ann Rheum Dis. 2008;67:732; discussion 732.
10. Routsias JG, Tzioufas AG. Sjogren's syndrome – study of autoantigens and autoantibodies. Clin Rev Allergy Immunol. 2007;32:238–51.
11. Vitali C, Bombardieri S, Jonsson R, Moutsopoulos HM, Alexander EL, Carsons SE, et al. Classification criteria for Sjogren's syndrome: a revised version of the European criteria proposed by the American-European Consensus Group. Ann Rheum Dis. 2002;61:554–8.
12. Siren MK, Julkunen H, Kaaja R. The increasing incidence of isolated congenital heart block in Finland. J Rheumatol. 1998;25:1862–4.
13. Michaelsson M, Engle MA. Congenital complete heart block: an international study of the natural history. Cardiovasc Clin. 1972;4:85–101.
14. Lee LA. Neonatal lupus erythematosus. J Invest Dermatol. 1993;100:9S–13S.
15. Sontheimer RD, Maddison PJ, Reichlin M, Jordon RE, Stastny P, Gilliam JN. Serologic and HLA associations in subacute cutaneous lupus erythematosus, a clinical subset of lupus erythematosus. Ann Intern Med. 1982;97:664–71.
16. Sontheimer RD, McCauliffe DP. Pathogenesis of anti-Ro/SS-A autoantibody-associated cutaneous lupus erythematosus. Dermatol Clin. 1990;8:751–8.
17. Watson R, Kang JE, May M, Hudak M, Kickler T, Provost TT. Thrombocytopenia in the neonatal lupus syndrome. Arch Dermatol. 1988;124:560–3.
18. Kanagasegar S, Cimaz R, Kurien BT, Brucato A, Scofield RH. Neonatal lupus manifests as isolated neutropenia and mildly abnormal liver functions. J Rheumatol. 2002;29:187–91.
19. Laxer RM, Roberts EA, Gross KR, Britton JR, Cutz E, Dimmick J, et al. Liver disease in neonatal lupus erythematosus. J Pediatr. 1990;116:238–42.
20. Cimaz R, Spence DL, Hornberger L, Silverman ED. Incidence and spectrum of neonatal lupus erythematosus: a prospective study of infants born to mothers with anti-Ro autoantibodies. J Pediatr. 2003;142:678–83.
21. Ross G, Sammaritano L, Nass R, Lockshin M. Effects of mothers' autoimmune disease during pregnancy on learning disabilities and hand preference in their children. Arch Pediatr Adolesc Med. 2003;157:397–402.

22. Boros CA, Spence D, Blaser S, Silverman ED. Hydrocephalus and macrocephaly: new manifestations of neonatal lupus erythematosus. Arthritis Rheum. 2007;57:261–6.
23. Schmidt KG, Ulmer HE, Silverman NH, Kleinman CS, Copel JA. Perinatal outcome of fetal complete atrioventricular block: a multicenter experience. J Am Coll Cardiol. 1991;17:1360–6.
24. Fesslova V, Vignati G, Brucato A, De Sanctis M, Butera G, Pisoni MP, et al. The impact of treatment of the fetus by maternal therapy on the fetal and postnatal outcomes for fetuses diagnosed with isolated complete atrioventricular block. Cardiol Young. 2009;19:282–90.
25. Moak JP, Barron KS, Hougen TJ, Wiles HB, Balaji S, Sreeram N, et al. Congenital heart block: development of late-onset cardiomyopathy, a previously underappreciated sequela. J Am Coll Cardiol. 2001;37:238–42.
26. Udink ten Cate FE, Breur JM, Cohen MI, Boramanand N, Kapusta L, Crosson JE, et al. Dilated cardiomyopathy in isolated congenital complete atrioventricular block: early and long-term risk in children. J Am Coll Cardiol. 2001;37:1129–34.
27. Nield LE, Silverman ED, Smallhorn JF, Taylor GP, Mullen JB, Benson LN, et al. Endocardial fibroelastosis associated with maternal anti-Ro and anti-La antibodies in the absence of atrioventricular block. J Am Coll Cardiol. 2002;40:796–802.
28. Brucato A, Cimaz R, Catelli L, Meroni P. Anti-Ro-associated sinus bradycardia in newborns. Circulation. 2000;102:E88–9.
29. Cimaz R, Stramba-Badiale M, Brucato A, Catelli L, Panzeri P, Meroni PL. QT interval prolongation in asymptomatic anti-SSA/Ro-positive infants without congenital heart block. Arthritis Rheum. 2000;43:1049–53.
30. Costedoat-Chalumeau N, Amoura Z, Lupoglazoff JM, Huong DL, Denjoy I, Vauthier D, et al. Outcome of pregnancies in patients with anti-SSA/Ro antibodies: a study of 165 pregnancies, with special focus on electrocardiographic variations in the children and comparison with a control group. Arthritis Rheum. 2004;50:3187–94.
31. Friedman DM, Kim MY, Copel JA, Davis C, Phoon CK, Glickstein JS, et al. Utility of cardiac monitoring in fetuses at risk for congenital heart block: the PR Interval and Dexamethasone Evaluation (PRIDE) prospective study. Circulation. 2008;117:485–93.
32. Cuneo BF, Strasburger JF, Niksch A, Ovadia M, Wakai RT. An expanded phenotype of maternal SSA/SSB antibody-associated fetal cardiac disease. J Matern Fetal Neonatal Med. 2009;22:233–8.
33. Waltuck J, Buyon JP. Autoantibody-associated congenital heart block: outcome in mothers and children. Ann Intern Med. 1994;120:544–51.
34. Press J, Uziel Y, Laxer RM, Luy L, Hamilton RM, Silverman ED. Long-term outcome of mothers of children with complete congenital heart block. Am J Med. 1996;100:328–32.
35. Rivera TL, Izmirly PM, Birnbaum BK, Byrne P, Brauth JB, Katholi M, et al. Disease progression in mothers of children enrolled in the Research Registry for Neonatal Lupus. Ann Rheum Dis. 2009;68:828–35.
36. Brucato A, Gasparini M, Vignati G, Riccobono S, De Juli E, Quinzanini M, et al. Isolated congenital complete heart block: longterm outcome of children and immunogenetic study. J Rheumatol. 1995;22:541–3.
37. Martin V, Lee LA, Askanase AD, Katholi M, Buyon JP. Long-term followup of children with neonatal lupus and their unaffected siblings. Arthritis Rheum. 2002;46:2377–83.
38. Sonesson SE, Salomonsson S, Jacobsson LA, Bremme K, Wahren-Herlenius M. Signs of first-degree heart block occur in one-third of fetuses of pregnant women with anti-SSA/Ro 52-kd antibodies. Arthritis Rheum. 2004;50:1253–61.
39. Rein AJ, Mevorach D, Perles Z, Gavri S, Nadjari M, Nir A, et al. Early diagnosis and treatment of atrioventricular block in the fetus exposed to maternal anti-SSA/Ro-SSB/La antibodies: a prospective, observational, fetal kinetocardiogram-based study. Circulation. 2009;119:1867–72.
40. Brucato A, Frassi M, Franceschini F, Cimaz R, Faden D, Pisoni MP, et al. Risk of congenital complete heart block in newborns of mothers with anti-Ro/SSA antibodies detected by counterimmunoelectrophoresis: a prospective study of 100 women. Arthritis Rheum. 2001;44:1832–5.

41. Gladman G, Silverman ED, Yuk L, Luy L, Boutin C, Laskin C, et al. Fetal echocardiographic screening of pregnancies of mothers with anti-Ro and/or anti-La antibodies. Am J Perinatol. 2002;19:73–80.

42. Gerosa M, Cimaz R, Stramba-Badiale M, Goulene K, Meregalli E, Trespidi L, et al. Electrocardiographic abnormalities in infants born from mothers with autoimmune diseases – a multicentre prospective study. Rheumatology (Oxford). 2007;46:1285–9.

43. Gordon P, Khamashta MA, Rosenthal E, Simpson JM, Sharland G, Brucato A, et al. Anti-52 kDa Ro, anti-60 kDa Ro, and anti-La antibody profiles in neonatal lupus. J Rheumatol. 2004;31:2480–7.

44. Salomonsson S, Sonesson SE, Ottosson L, Muhallab S, Olsson T, Sunnerhagen M, et al. Ro/SSA autoantibodies directly bind cardiomyocytes, disturb calcium homeostasis, and mediate congenital heart block. J Exp Med. 2005;201:11–7.

45. Izmirly PM, Llanos C, Lee LA, Askanase A, Kim MY, Buyon JP. Cutaneous manifestations of neonatal lupus and risk of subsequent congenital heart block. Arthritis Rheum. 2010;62: 1153–7.

46. Spence D, Hornberger L, Hamilton R, Silverman ED. Increased risk of complete congenital heart block in infants born to women with hypothyroidism and anti-Ro and/or anti-La antibodies. J Rheumatol. 2006;33:167–70.

47. Llanos C, Izmirly PM, Katholi M, Clancy RM, Friedman DM, Kim MY, et al. Recurrence rates of cardiac manifestations associated with neonatal lupus and maternal/fetal risk factors. Arthritis Rheum. 2009;60:3091–7.

48. Strandberg L, Winqvist O, Sonesson SE, Mohseni S, Salomonsson S, Bremme K, et al. Antibodies to amino acid 200–239 (p200) of Ro52 as serological markers for the risk of developing congenital heart block. Clin Exp Immunol. 2008;154:30–7.

49. Stea EA, Routsias JG, Clancy RM, Buyon JP, Moutsopoulos HM, Tzioufas AG. Anti-La/SSB antiidiotypic antibodies in maternal serum: a marker of low risk for neonatal lupus in an offspring. Arthritis Rheum. 2006;54:2228–34.

50. James TN. Normal and abnormal consequences of apoptosis in the human heart: from postnatal morphogenesis to paroxysmal arrhythmias. Circulation. 1994;90:556–73.

51. Miranda-Carus ME, Askanase AD, Clancy RM, Di Donato F, Chou TM, Libera MR, et al. Anti-SSA/Ro and anti-SSB/La autoantibodies bind the surface of apoptotic fetal cardiocytes and promote secretion of TNF-alpha by macrophages. J Immunol. 2000;165:5345–51.

52. Clancy RM, Buyon JP. Clearance of apoptotic cells: TGF-beta in the balance between inflammation and fibrosis. J Leukoc Biol. 2003;74:959–60.

53. Clancy RM, Neufing PJ, Zheng P, O'Mahony M, Nimmerjahn F, Gordon TP, et al. Impaired clearance of apoptotic cardiocytes is linked to anti-SSA/Ro and -SSB/La antibodies in the pathogenesis of congenital heart block. J Clin Invest. 2006;116:2413–22.

54. Clancy RM, Backer CB, Yin X, Kapur RP, Molad Y, Buyon JP. Cytokine polymorphisms and histologic expression in autopsy studies: contribution of TNF-alpha and TGF-beta 1 to the pathogenesis of autoimmune-associated congenital heart block. J Immunol. 2003;171:3253–61.

55. Jaeggi ET, Fouron JC, Silverman ED, Ryan G, Smallhorn J, Hornberger LK. Transplacental fetal treatment improves the outcome of prenatally diagnosed complete atrioventricular block without structural heart disease. Circulation. 2004;110:1542–8.

56. Theander E, Brucato A, Gudmundsson S, Salomonsson S, Wahren-Herlenius M, Manthorpe R. Primary Sjogren's syndrome – treatment of fetal incomplete atrioventricular block with dexamethasone. J Rheumatol. 2001;28:373–6.

57. Saleeb S, Copel J, Friedman D, Buyon JP. Comparison of treatment with fluorinated glucocorticoids to the natural history of autoantibody-associated congenital heart block: retrospective review of the research registry for neonatal lupus. Arthritis Rheum. 1999;42:2335–45.

58. Lopes LM, Tavares GM, Damiano AP, Lopes MA, Aiello VD, Schultz R, et al. Perinatal outcome of fetal atrioventricular block: one-hundred-sixteen cases from a single institution. Circulation. 2008;118:1268–75.

59. Breur JM, Visser GH, Kruize AA, Stoutenbeek P, Meijboom EJ. Treatment of fetal heart block with maternal steroid therapy: case report and review of the literature. Ultrasound Obstet Gynecol. 2004;24:467–72.
60. Brucato A, Astori MG, Cimaz R, Villa P, Li Destri M, Chimini L, et al. Normal neuropsychological development in children with congenital complete heart block who may or may not be exposed to high-dose dexamethasone in utero. Ann Rheum Dis. 2006;65:1422–6.
61. Kaaja R, Julkunen H. Prevention of recurrence of congenital heart block with intravenous immunoglobulin and corticosteroid therapy: comment on the editorial by Buyon et al. Arthritis Rheum. 2003;48:280–1; author reply 281–282.
62. Kaaja R, Julkunen H, Ammala P, Teppo AM, Kurki P. Congenital heart block: successful prophylactic treatment with intravenous gamma globulin and corticosteroid therapy. Am J Obstet Gynecol. 1991;165:1333–4.
63. Pisoni CN, Brucato A, Ruffatti A, Espinosa G, Cervera R, Belmonte-Serrano M, et al. Failure of intravenous immunoglobulin to prevent congenital heart block: findings of a multicenter, prospective, observational study. Arthritis Rheum. 2010;62:1147–52.
64. Friedman DM, Llanos C, Izmirly PM, Brock B, Byron J, Copel J, et al. Evaluation of fetuses in a study of intravenous immunoglobulin as preventive therapy for congenital heart block: results of a multicenter, prospective, open-label clinical trial. Arthritis Rheum. 2010;62: 1138–46.
65. Matsubara S, Morimatsu Y, Shiraishi H, Kuwata T, Ohkuchi A, Izumi A, et al. Fetus with heart failure due to congenital atrioventricular block treated by maternally administered ritodrine. Arch Gynecol Obstet. 2008;278:85–8.
66. Izmirly PM, Kim MY, Llanos C, Le PU, Guerra MM, Askanase AD, et al. Evaluation of the risk of anti-SSA/Ro-SSB/La antibody-associated cardiac manifestations of neonatal lupus in fetuses of mothers with systemic lupus erythematosus exposed to hydroxychloroquine. Ann Rheum Dis. 2010;69(10):1827–30.
67. Routsias JG, Kyriakidis NC, Friedman DM, Llanos C, Clancy R, Moutsopoulos HM, Buyon J, Tzioufas AG. Association of idiotypic/anti-idiotypic antibody ratio with therapeutic response of IVIG in the prevention of recurrent autoimmune associated congenital heart block. Arthritis Rheum. 2011 May 25. doi: 10.1002/art.30464. [Epub ahead of print]

Chapter 25
Laboratory Abnormalities in Primary Sjögren's Syndrome

Pilar Brito-Zerón, Roberto Pérez-Alvarez, Marta Pérez-de-Lis,
Carmen Hidalgo-Tenorio, and Manuel Ramos-Casals

Contents

P. Brito-Zerón • M. Ramos-Casals (✉)
Sjögren Syndrome Research Group (AGAUR), Laboratory of Autoimmune Diseases Josep Font,
Institut d'Investigacions Biomèdiques August Pi i Sunyer (IDIBAPS), Department of
Autoimmune Diseases, Hospital Clínic, Barcelona, Spain

R. Pérez-Alvarez • M. Pérez-de-Lis
Department of Internal Medicine, Hospital Meixoeiro, Vigo, Spain

C. Hidalgo-Tenorio
Department of Internal Medicine, Hospital Virgen de las Nieves, Granada, Spain

M. Ramos-Casals et al. (eds.), *Sjögren's Syndrome*,
DOI 10.1007/978-0-85729-947-5_25, © Springer-Verlag London Limited 2012

347

25.1 Introduction

Sjögren's syndrome (SS) is a systemic autoimmune disease that presents with sicca symptomatology of the main mucosa surfaces. The spectrum of the disease extends from sicca syndrome to systemic involvement (extraglandular manifestations) and may be complicated by the development of lymphoma. Patients with SS may present with a broad spectrum of autoantibodies and laboratory abnormalities. Most of the laboratory abnormalities have been described more frequently in patients with positive immunological markers. Some may be the first manifestation of primary SS, while others have no clinical significance. The most frequent cytopenias are normocytic anemia, leukopenia, and thrombocytopenia, which are all found more frequently in patients with positive immunological markers. Cytopenias are usually asymptomatic, but may be clinically overt in some cases. Erythrocyte sedimentation rates (ESRs) correlate closely with the percentage of circulating gammaglobulins (hypergammaglobulinemia) – frequently elevated in primary SS – but serum C-reactive protein concentrations are usually normal. Laboratory studies are a simple, useful, and noninvasive tool that can help identify subsets of patients with a high risk of developing of systemic manifestations and lymphoma.

25.2 Serum Proteins

25.2.1 Acute Phase Reactants

The erythrocyte sedimentation rate (ESR) is a common, nonspecific hematological test that indirectly measures systemic inflammation. In primary SS, nearly 25% of patients have an ESR >50 mm/h [1]. Patients with elevated ESRs have a high prevalence of extraglandular involvement [1] and other laboratory abnormalities such as anemia [1], anti-Ro/SS-A and –La/SS-B autoantibodies [1, 2], and rheumatoid factor (RF) [1]. A close relationship has also been found between ESR values and the percentage of serum gammaglobulins. ESR measurement is a useful hematologic marker in primary SS that seems to be related to B-cell polyclonal hyperactivity and the amount of circulating autoantibodies.

In contrast to the ESR, the C-reactive protein (CRP) has relatively little clinical significance in primary SS. Although 22% of patients with primary SS have minimal-to-moderate increases in CRP [3] levels, these patients do not differ clinically from those with normal CRP levels. In addition, no significant differences in CRP levels have been found in primary SS patients grouped according to the immunological profile (e.g., positivity or negativity for anti-Ro/SS-A and anti-La/SS-B autoantibodies) [2]. Higher CRP levels have been found in patients with associated SS [4]. Testing CRP levels in patients with primary SS may be most useful in the differential diagnosis between infection and systemic involvement.

Table 25.1 Prevalence of hypergammaglobulinemia in SS

Author	Year	Classification criteria for SS	Hypergammaglo-bulinemia definition	Patients (n)	Hypergammaglo-bulinemia n (%)
Bloch et al. [7]	1965	NS	>1.4 g/100 mL	62	62 (100)
Martínez et al. [8]	1979	Bloch	NS	30	29 (97)
Alexander et al. [9]	1983	NS	>4 g/L	75	27 (36)
Sutcliffe et al. [10]	1998	European, 1993	NS	72	26 (36)
Skopouli et al. [11]	2000	European, 1993	>2 g/L	261	109 (42)
Ramos-Casals et al. [1]	2002	European, 1993	>25% of total plasmatic proteins	252	56 (22)
			>35% of total plasmatic proteins	252	15 (6)
Baimpa et al. [12]	2009	American-European, 2002	>20 g/L (>22% of total serum proteins)	536	194 (36)[a]

NS not specified

[a] 141 patients at diagnosis and 53 during follow-up

25.2.2   Gammaglobulins

25.2.2.1   Polyclonal Hypergammaglobulinemia

Polyclonal hypergammaglobulinemia is one of the most characteristic laboratory abnormalities in primary SS. It reflects the polyclonal B-cell activation implicated in the pathogenesis of the disease and provides useful analytical data that may strengthen the diagnosis of primary SS in a patient with sicca syndrome [5]. Although it has been described in both the primary and secondary forms of SS, hypergammaglobulinemia is more typical of primary SS [6, 7].

The prevalence of hypergammaglobulinemia varies according to the classification criteria and the parameter used to define hypergammaglobulinemia (Table 25.1) [1, 7–12]. Studies from the 1960s and 1970s [7, 8] reported hypergammaglobulinemia in almost 100% of patients with SS, although subsequent studies have described a lower prevalence, ranging from 22% to 42% [1, 9–12].

Hypergammaglobulinemia is closely associated with the key immunological markers of SS (RF, anti-Ro/SS-A and anti-La/SS-B autoantibodies). In 1993, Markusse et al. [13] found a correlation between hypergammaglobulinemia and the presence of anti-Ro/SS-A and anti-La/SS-B antibodies. In 1999, Davidson et al. [2] found that the mean serum immunoglobulin G concentration was higher in anti-Ro/anti-La/SS-B positive patients than in those patients who were seronegative and in those who were either RF- or ANA-positive. Subsequent studies in larger series of patients [1] confirmed a correlation between hypergammaglobulinemia and the presence of the anti-Ro/SS-A antibody and RF. Baimpa et al. [12] reported a higher prevalence of hypergammaglobulinemia in patients with positivity for ANA, RF, anti-Ro/SS-A, and anti-La antibodies. In addition, a close

Table 25.2 Prevalence of hypogammaglobulinemia in primary SS

Author	Year	Hypogammaglo-bulinemia definition	Patients (n)	Hypogammaglobulinemia n (%)
Ramos-Casals et al. [1]	2002	<15% of total plasmatic proteins	252	37 (15)
Baimpa et al. [12]	2009	<8 g/L	536	31 (6)[a]

[a]16 patients at diagnosis and 15 during follow-up

relationship has been found between ESR values and the percentage of serum gammaglobulins, suggesting that raised ESR in patients with primary SS may be directly related to higher levels of circulating gammaglobulins [1].

25.2.2.2 Hypogammaglobulinemia and Immunoglobulin Deficiency

The prevalence and clinical significance of hypogammaglobulinemia in primary SS have been little studied. According to two large series of primary SS patients, the prevalence of hypogammaglobulinemia ranges between 6% and 15% (Table 25.2) [1, 12]. In 1965, Bloch et al. [7] described the development of reticulosarcoma in two SS patients with hypogammaglobulinemia. In 2002, Ramos-Casals et al. [1] reported that half of the SS patients who developed lymphoma had hypogammaglobulinemia. In this study, hypogammaglobulinemia was associated with a lower frequency of autoantibodies such as ANA, anti-Ro/SS-A, and anti-La. Baimpa et al. [12] have demonstrated that hypogammaglobulinemia is associated with palpable purpura, splenomegaly, and biopsy-proven vasculitis.

Humoral immunodeficiencies have rarely been reported in patients with primary SS. Ramos-Casals et al. [1] described three patients diagnosed with humoral immunodeficiencies in a series of 252 primary SS patients; two had common variable immunodeficiency and one had selective immunoglobulin A deficiency. Additional cases of selective immunoglobulin A deficiency and immunoglobulin G-subclass deficiency have been reported [1, 14–21]. In these patients, immunoglobulin deficiency was not associated with severe infections.

25.2.2.3 Circulating Monoclonal Immunoglobulins

Detection of circulating monoclonal immunoglobulins should be considered to be a marker of a potential underlying monoclonal B-cell population. Monoclonal immunoglobulins can be associated with multiple myeloma, lymphoma, or monoclonal gammopathy of undetermined significance (MGUS). Thirty years ago, studies identified free monoclonal bands within the serum and urine of SS patients [3, 22, 23]. Since then, additional studies have investigated the prevalence and clinical significance of monoclonal immunoglobulins in SS (Table 25.3). Although a preliminary study found a prevalence of 70%, subsequent studies in larger series of primary SS patients found lower figures, ranging from 8 to 25% (Table 25.3) [12, 24–26]. Monoclonal immunoglobulin G is the most frequent type of circulating monoclonal

Table 25.3 Prevalence of circulating monoclonal immunoglobulins in primary SS

Author	Year	Patients (n)	Monoclonal immunoglobulins (%)
Moutsopoulos et al. [3]	1983	21	14 (67)
Pariente et al. [24]	1992	62	5 (8)
Sibilia and Cohen-Solal [25]	1999	150	37 (25)
Brito-Zerón et al. [26]	2005	200	35 (17.5)
Baimpa et al. [12]	2009	536	41 (7.6)

immunoglobulin in primary SS (60%), followed by monoclonal immunoglobulin M (30%), and, less frequently, immunoglobulin A and free monoclonal bands. The most frequent type of light chain is "κ" (60%). Biclonal gammapathies are uncommon in primary SS, with a prevalence of less than 1% [26].

The clinical significance of circulating monoclonal immunoglobulins in primary SS has been little studied. The first studies suggested the association of free circulating monoclonal bands with extraglandular manifestations and lymphoma [3, 22, 23]. In 2005, an observational study in a large cohort of primary SS patients [26] showed that those with monoclonal immunoglobulins had a high prevalence of extraglandular manifestations, mainly lung involvement (interstitial lung disease). In that study, patients with monoclonal immunoglobulins also had a higher prevalence of laboratory abnormalities such as anemia, hypergammaglobulinemia, elevated ESR, and cryoglobulins compared to patients without monoclonal immunoglobulins, suggesting that SS patients with monoclonal spikes immunoglobulin have a more active pattern of disease expression. The association between circulating monoclonal immunoglobulins and hypergammaglobulinemia suggests that the appearance of a monoclonal B-cell population is more frequent in patients with greater B-cell hyperactivity.

The association between monoclonal free light chains in either serum or urine and lymphoproliferation was first suggested in the 1980s [3, 23]. Walters et al. [23] reported three SS patients in whom the detection of urinary monoclonal free light chains was followed by the development of lymphoma. In 1999, a study in 37 primary SS patients with monoclonal immunoglobulins found that 8% developed multiple myeloma [25], while a recent study [26] including 35 patients with primary SS and monoclonal immunoglobulins found that 6% of patients developed lymphoma. According to these studies and the cases reported in the literature, IgMκ is the most common type of monoclonal immunoglobulin associated with B-cell lymphoma and IgGκ the most common type of monoclonal immunoglobulin associated with multiple myeloma.

Since the emergence of a significant quantitatively monoclonal band may be the first biological manifestation of an underlying lymphoproliferative process, the development of monoclonal immunoglobulins in a patient with primary SS should be closely monitored, and should alert the clinician to the possible presence of cryoglobulinemia and/or lymphoproliferative disease [27].

Peripheral monoclonal expression differs substantially between patients with SS associated with chronic hepatitis C virus (HCV) infection and those with primary

SS [26]. HCV-SS patients have a prevalence of circulating monoclonal immuno-globulins of 43%, with IgMκ being the most common type. Monoclonal IgMκ is closely related to a higher frequency of mixed cryoglobulinemia. HCV-associated SS patients with circulating monoclonal immunoglobulins show a more restrictive monoclonal expression (limited to either monoclonal IgMκ or IgGλ) than do patients with primary SS, who can demonstrate all types of monoclonal heavy and light chains. This suggests that HCV may play an important role in the clonal selec-tion of specific B-cells, with a more restricted use of specific gene segments in assembling the immunoglobulin receptor variable regions [28].

25.2.3 β_2-Microglobulin

β_2-microglobulin is a low molecular weight protein (11,700 Da) secreted by nucleated cells. It forms the light chain of the human leukocyte antigen (HLA) and binds non-covalently to various transmembrane glycoproteins such as the HLA class I molecule. It is usually found in low concentrations in serum, bodily fluids, and secretions [29], and is of proven utility in evaluating various neoplastic, inflam-matory, and infectious conditions [30]. β_2-microglobulin is also used in renal disor-ders, particularly in kidney-transplant recipients, and in patients with suspected tubulointerstitial disease.

The role of β_2-microglobulin in primary SS was first analyzed in 1975 [29], when high levels were detected in the salivary glands of patients with primary SS in com-parison with patients with associated SS or sicca syndrome, suggesting a close asso-ciation with the degree of lymphocytic infiltration. Subsequent studies have also found higher salivary levels of β_2-microglobulin in primary SS patients in com-parison with sicca syndrome patients [31–33] and healthy individuals [31, 32, 34]. High levels of β_2-microglobulin have been also found in tears from primary SS patients [35].

Increased serum levels of β_2-microglobulin have also been found in patients with primary SS [29, 31, 32, 36, 37], systemic lupus erythematosus (SLE) [37], and healthy individuals [31, 37, 38]. An increase in serum β_2-microglobulin levels in patients with sicca syndrome has also been considered a predictor of progression to primary SS [39] and has been associated with the haplotype HLA DR3 [40]. With respect to immunological markers, β_2-microglobulin levels have been associated with positive anti-Ro/SS-A and anti-La/SS-B autoantibodies [2].

Some studies have suggested a close association between serum β_2-microglobulin levels and extraglandular involvement [41]. Lahdensuo et al. [42] found high serum β_2-microglobulin levels in patients with pulmonary emphysema and obstructive disease of the small airways, with β_2-microglobulin levels being inversely propor-tional to the forced vital capacity (FVC), forced expiratory volume (FEV1), and carbon monoxide diffusing capacity (DLCO) values [42]. High levels of this pro-tein have also been reported in primary SS patients with lymphocytic/neutrophilic alveolitis [43]. Some studies have also reported high levels of β_2-microglobulin in

Table 25.4 Prevalence of anemia in primary SS

Author	Year	Anemia definition	Patients (n)	Anemia n (%)
Bloch et al. [7]	1965	Htc <38%	62	15 (24)
Alexander et al. [9]	1983	Htc <35%	75	25 (33)
Ramakrishna et al. [47]	1992	Hb <13 g/dL	27	10 (37)
Skopouli et al. [11]	2000	Htc <35%	261	42 (16)
Ramos-Casals et al. [1]	2002	Hb <11 g/dL	380	76 (20)
Ramos-Casals et al. [48]	2008	Hb <11 g/dL	1,010	182 (18)
Baimpa et al. [12]	2009	Hb <12 g/dL in women	536	241 (45)[a]
		Hb <13.5 g/dL in men		

Hct hematocrit, *Hb* hemoglobin
[a]153 at diagnosis, 88 during follow-up

SS patients with renal disease. Pertovaara et al. [44] found distal tubular renal acidosis (dTRA) in 18 of 55 patients (33%) who showed elevated levels of serum β_2-microglobulin. The β_2-microglobulin levels correlated with hypertension and duration of dryness.

Finally, β_2-microglobulin has also been associated with lymphoma development in primary SS. In 1975, Michalski et al. [29] found increased levels of β_2-microglobulin in 77% of patients with SS and lymphoma or pseudolymphoma. In 2001, Pertovaara et al. [45], described β_2-microglobulin as an independent predictive factor for the development of lymphoma in patients with primary SS. β_2-microglobulin has also been postulated to be a predictive factor for the development of amyloidosis in primary SS [46].

25.3   Hematological Abnormalities

25.3.1   Normocytic Anemia

The prevalence of anemia in primary SS patients ranges between 16% and 45% (Table 25.4) [1, 7, 9, 11, 12, 47, 48]. The classification of a patient as "anemic" in this setting may be due to several factors, including the different parameters used to define anemia; the inclusion of patients with anemia secondary to causes other than SS; and the classification criteria used for SS. Only four studies have specified the causes of anemia in patients with primary SS (Table 25.5) [1, 7, 12, 47], and in these, the prevalence of anemia attributed to SS ranged from 11% to 34%. The most common type of anemia was mild, normocytic, normochromic anemia, similar to that seen in other chronic inflammatory diseases [1, 6, 8].

Recent studies have described an association between anemia and some extraglandular manifestations such as palpable purpura [12], lymphadenopathy [12], and peripheral neuropathy [1], and positive autoantibodies, mainly anti-Ro/SS-A and anti-La/SS-B antibodies [1, 9, 12], ANA [1, 12], and RF [12]. Some experimental

Table 25.5 Detailed causes of anemia in patients with primary SS

Author	Anemia definition	Patients (n)	Anemia n (%)	Anemia due to SS n (%)	Anemia associated to other causes than SS (n)
Bloch et al. [7]	Htc<38%	62	15 (24)	12 (19)	Iron deficiency (2), Felty syndrome (1)
Ramakrishna et al. [47]	Hb<13 g/dL	27	10 (37)	3 (11)	AHAI (3), MDS (2), PRCA (1), aplastic anemia (1)
Ramos-Casals et al. [1]	Hb<11 g/dL	380	76 (20)	55 (14)	GI bleeding (12), CAG (2), Lymphoproliferative disease (2), AHAI (1), MDS (1), aplastic anemia (1), other causes (2)
Baimpa et al. [12]	Hb<12 g/dL[a] Hb<13.5 g/dL[b]	536	241 (45)	183 (34)	B-thalassemia trait (16), iron deficiency (5), B12/folate deficiency (4), AHAI (6), renal failure (5), drug toxicity (18)

AHAI autoimmune hemolytic anemia, *MDS* myelodysplastic syndrome, *PRCA* pure red cell aplasia, *GI* gastrointestinal, *CAG* Chronic atrophic gastritis
[a]In women
[b]In men

studies [49, 50] have suggested that anti-Ro/SS-A and anti-La/SS-B antibodies directly mediate the development of these cytopenias. Cell membrane expression of Ro/SS-A and La/SS-B antigens, mainly located in the nucleus, can be induced by various stimuli. It is possible that some viruses with specific bone marrow tropism may affect the bone marrow of patients with SS, inducing cell membrane expression of Ro/SS-A and La/SS-B and leading to an autoantibody-induced lysis of blood cells [47]. Ramos-Casals et al. [51] found a higher prevalence of cytopenias in patients with primary SS and past parvovirus B19 infection. It has been reported that anti-Ro/SS-A antibodies can coexist with markers of B-cell hyperreactivity (hypergammaglobulinemia, RF) and other cytopenias, thus supporting an autoimmune pathogenesis of the anemia [52].

Other causes of anemia that have rarely been reported in patients with primary SS (Table 25.5) [1, 7, 12, 47] include drug-induced anemia due to gastrointestinal bleeding [6] or bone marrow hypoplasia and renal failure. Finally, hematological neoplasia may be another cause of anemia in SS patients [9, 11, 19, 47, 52–63].

25.3.2 Autoimmune Hemolytic Anemia

Although some studies consider a positive Coombs test a frequent hematological abnormality in SS (range from 22 to 47%), overt hemolysis is unusual [52]. Autoimmune hemolytic anemia (AIHA) has rarely been reported in patients with primary SS, with only 10 cases out of 327 (3%) primary SS patients reported with anemia (Table 25.5). The outcome of these patients was excellent, with improvement of hemoglobin values after receiving treatment with glucocorticoids, although immunosuppressive agents were added in some cases [18, 47, 52, 54, 55, 57].

AIHA may be the first clinical manifestation of underlying primary SS [52]. Thus, primary SS should be included in the differential diagnosis of AIHA.

The etiopathogenesis of AIHA in primary SS is unknown. Autoantibodies against red cells might play a role [54]. In addition, the abnormal expression of Ro/SS-A and La/SS-B antigens on the cell membrane may also contribute to the hemolysis [47]. This abnormal location of Ro/La antigens may be caused by external triggering factors, including cellular exposure to ultraviolet light or viral infections (such as adenovirus or viruses with specific bone marrow tropism), which might induce red blood cell lysis by autoantibodies. One case of AIHA has been reported in a newborn from a SS mother carrying anti-Ro/SS-A antibodies, suggesting a role for these autoantibodies in the etiopathogenesis of AIHA [47].

Due to the low prevalence of AIHA in patients with primary SS, hemolytic assays (haptoglobin, Coombs test) should only be performed in patients with clinical evidence of acute anemia or biological evidence of hemolysis such as the finding of spherocytosis on the peripheral blood smear and an elevation in the serum lactate dehydrogenase and bilirubin concentrations.

25.3.3   Aplastic Anemia

Although the first case of aplastic anemia in SS was reported in a patient with lymphoma [58], seven additional cases not associated with lymphoproliferative disorders have been reported [47, 58–60, 64–66]. Aplastic anemia has also been described in association with other systemic autoimmune diseases, particularly SLE. This clinical occurrence is associated most commonly with immunosuppressive therapy. In primary SS, aplastic anemia represents less than 1% of the total cases of anemia [1]. Translocation q24, p23 in the gene 14q 24 (where tumor necrosis factor, a hematopoietic suppressor lymphokine, is encoded) was identified in one patient with primary SS [60]. This translocation might lead to an abnormal gene expression of tumor necrosis factor and, therefore, hematopoietic suppression [60]. Studies in vitro have identified IgG antibodies that inhibit the proliferation of bone marrow in patients with SLE [47], but there are no similar studies in patients with SS.

25.3.4   Pure Red Cell Aplasia

Only eight cases of pure red cell aplasia (PRCA) have been described in primary SS [47, 67–72]. Two cases were associated with neoplasia (thymoma in one case and T-gamma large granular lymphocyte leukemia in the other) [71, 72]. PRCA was the first manifestation of primary SS in 2 patients [68, 69], and was associated with AIHA in another patient [70] who was refractory to treatment with glucocorticoids, intravenous immunoglobulins, and rituximab treatment [70].

Some in vitro studies have suggested that both serum erythropoietic-inhibitor IgG and cytotoxic lymphocytes may play a role in the etiopathogenesis of red cell aplasia [47, 67], affecting erythroid cells at different development stages. However, another study did not confirm this hypothesis [73]. Since patients with primary SS have an increased risk of lymphoma, and considering that PRCA may be the first manifestation of leukemia (lymphocytic or lymphoblastic) or lymphoma, these patients should be followed [67].

25.3.5 Myelodysplasia

Nine cases of myelodysplasia (MDS) have been reported in primary SS patients [1, 47, 74–76]. Some studies have analyzed the prevalence of systemic autoimmune diseases or rheumatic manifestations in patients with MDS [75, 77]. Castro et al. [77] found that 16 of 162 patients with MDS patients had rheumatic manifestations (mainly cutaneous vasculitis, but also primary SS in one patient). Roy-Peaud et al. [75] found systemic autoimmune diseases in 14 out of 97 patients with MDS, with primary SS being the most common diagnosis (4/14, 29%). A prospective study in 40 patients with MDS also found one patient with underdiagnosed primary SS [74].

25.3.6 Pernicious Anemia

Pernicious anemia is an uncommon cause of anemia in patients with primary SS [5, 7–63, 78–80]. Baimpa et al. [12] reported that pernicious anemia due to chronic atrophic gastritis represents less than 1% of all causes of anemia in primary SS, and a previous study found a similar figure (3%) [1]. However, chronic atrophic gastritis is not always associated with the development of pernicious anemia [63]. This may be explained by the patchy pattern of chronic atrophic gastritis and the existence of mucosa free of disease. Some studies have suggested that chronic atrophic gastritis might be caused by primary SS, because mononuclear infiltrates have been found in the gastric mucosa [63]. Anti-parietal cell autoantibodies have been associated with chronic atrophic gastritis and pernicious anemia, but the majority of patients with primary SS with anti-parietal cell autoantibodies do not have anemia (see chapter 28).

25.3.7 Leukopenia

Leukopenia is the second most frequently reported hematological abnormality in primary SS. The prevalence of leukopenia in primary SS ranges between 12% and 32% (Table 25.6) [1, 7, 9, 11, 12, 48]. Early studies found a close association between leukopenia and positive autoantibodies (mainly anti-Ro/SS-A and anti-La/SS-B antibodies) [9, 81]. This association was confirmed in subsequent studies

Table 25.6 Prevalence of leukopenia in primary SS

Author	Year	Leukopenia definition	Patients (n)	Leukopenia n (%)
Bloch et al. [7]	1965	<4,000/mm^3	62	20 (32)
Alexander et al. [9]	1983	<4,000/mm^3	75	17 (23)
Skopouli et al. [11]	2000	<4,000/mm^3	261	31 (12)
Ramos-Casals et al. [1]	2002	<4,000×10^9/L	380	59 (16)
Ramos-Casals et al. [48]	2008	<4,000×10^9/L	1,010	162 (16)
Baimpa et al. [12]	2009	<4,000/μL	536	139 (26)[a]

[a]75 patients had leukopenia at diagnosis, 64 during follow-up

Table 25.7 Prevalence of lymphopenia and neutropenia in primary SS

Author	Year	Patients (n)	Lymphopenia n (%)	Neutropenia n (%)
Ramos-Casals et al. [1]	2002	268	23 (9)[a]	19 (7)[b]
Brito-Zerón et al. [82]	2009	300	66 (22)[c]	90 (27)[d]
Baimpa et al. [12]	2009	536	49 (9)[e]	17 (3)[f]

[a]<1×10^9/L, [b]<1.5×10^9/L, [c]<0.9×10^9/L, [d]<2.5×10^9/L, [e]<1,000/μL, [f]<1500/μL

including large series of patients that described an association between leukopenia, anti-Ro/SS-A antibodies, and RF [1]. These findings underline the striking relationship between positive autoantibodies and cytopenias in primary SS. Some experimental studies [49, 50] have suggested a possible etiopathogenic mechanism played by anti-Ro/SS-A and anti-La/SS-B antibodies, as suggested in the etiopathogenesis of other cytopenias (AIHA, above).

The differential leukocyte count has been studied in large series of patients with primary SS. The most frequent abnormality was lymphopenia, closely followed by neutropenia (Table 25.7) [1, 12, 82]. Brito-Zerón et al. [82] reported a prevalence of neutropenia (<2.5×10^9/L) of 27%. However, when using a definition of neutrophil count <1.5×10^9/L, the prevalence fell to 14%. Neutrophil counts may oscillate between normal and low values in the majority of patients, with values between 1.5×10^9/L and 2.5×10^9/L in 60% of cases [1].

25.3.8 Lymphopenia

In primary SS, lymphopenia has been associated with other cytopenias [82] and a higher prevalence of autoantibodies [83]. The cause of lymphopenia in SS is unknown. Kirtava et al. [84] reported persistently reduced CD4$^+$ lymphocyte counts in 5% of patients with primary SS without HIV infection, a prevalence higher than that reported for any other non-HIV population group. The prevalence of CD4+ lymphopenia was higher in anti-Ro/SS-A antibody-positive SS patients, compared with seronegative and sicca patients [85]. These authors also identified anti-CD4 autoantibodies in 13% of 214 patients with primary SS, although no correlation was found between anti-CD4 antibodies and lymphopenia.

CD4 lymphocyte depletion in primary SS suggests an altered balance between CD4+ and CD8+ cells. Viral infections are typical causes of lymphopenia, and HIV infection is the prototype of viral-induced CD4+ T lymphopenia associated with lymphoma development. In 2006, Theander et al. [86] were the first to suggest that CD4+ T lymphopenia and a low CD4+/CD8+ T-cell ratio were predictor factors for the development of lymphoma in primary SS. Baimpa et al. [12] have identified lymphopenia as the only independent predictive variable for the development of any type of lymphoma other than marginal zone B-cell lymphoma (MZBCL).

Whatever the mechanism by which lymphopenia (especially at the expense of CD4+ T-lymphocytes) is induced in primary SS, it reflects a state of decreased immune surveillance. In this context, the probability of a progression from autoimmunity to a more aggressive type of lymphoma, such as diffuse large B-cell lymphoma (DLBCL), may be greater.

25.3.9 Neutropenia

Neutropenia is an uncommon, but well-established, analytical finding in primary SS. It may be secondary to neoplasia, adverse drug reactions, or immune mediated. According to a recent study that analyzed the causes of neutropenia in a large series of patients with primary SS [82], the most frequent cause (90%) was idiopathic or autoimmune neutropenia, followed by neutropenia associated with neoplasia or drugs in 3% of cases. SS patients with neutropenia often have other cytopenias [82, 87, 88]; in a large cross-sectional study [1], a close correlation between hemoglobin values and leukocyte and platelet counts was found. This suggests that there may be a specific subset of patients with primary SS, probably genetically predisposed, with a higher risk of developing cytopenias. Gottenberg et al. [89] described an association between haplotype DQB1*01 and neutropenia ($<1 \times 10^9$/L), while other studies have suggested a possible role of cytokine polymorphisms in the etiopathogenesis of idiopathic chronic adult neutropenia [90, 91]. The possible influence of the innate immune system has also been postulated [92].

Patients with neutropenia also have a high frequency of altered immunological markers including positive autoantibodies and low complement levels, especially those with lower neutrophil counts ($< 1.5 \times 10^9$/L), who had a twofold higher prevalence of RF and a threefold higher prevalence of anti-Ro/La antibodies in comparison with patients without neutropenia [82]. The association of neutropenia with positive anti-Ro/La antibodies has been previously described for other cytopenias such as leukopenia [2, 9, 81], lymphopenia [2, 81, 83], and thrombocytopenia [83]. It is known that some viruses, such as parvovirus B19 and HCV, are linked to both primary SS and severe cytopenias [51, 93]. Abnormal Ro/La antigen expression in blood cell membranes may induce the synthesis of autoantibodies against these cells and their lysis by an antibody-mediated complement-dependent mechanism [94]. The high frequency of hypocomplementemia in neutropenic patients supports the possible role of this mechanism in the etiopathogenesis of SS-related autoimmune neutropenia. Although a possible etiopathogenic role of antineutrophil antibodies has been suggested in the peripheral destruction of neutrophils in primary SS, the majority of studies have found no correlation between these antibodies and the neutrophil count.

In addition to the association between neutropenia and autoantibodies, an association with the development of lymphoma and infections has been recently postulated. Baimpa et al. [12] described neutropenia as a significant predictive factor for the development of lymphoma, especially MZBCL, while Brito-Zerón et al. found a higher rate of hospital admissions due to infection in patients with primary SS and neutropenia [82], especially in those with neutrophil counts less than $1 \times 10^9/L$. Therefore, these patients should be closely followed due to the high risk of infection.

According to a recent study [82], most SS patients with autoimmune neutropenia required no specific therapy, with standard antibiotic therapy often being sufficient to deal with infections. However, specific treatment with glucocorticoids, intravenous immunoglobulins, or granulocyte colony-stimulating factor (G-CSF) has been suggested in patients with severe infections or those requiring surgery [95, 96], although refractory neutropenia has also been described in primary SS despite G-CSF [97].

Severe immune granulocytopenia or agranulocytosis is uncommon in systemic autoimmune disease and particularly in primary SS, and few cases have been reported [82, 87, 88]. Agranulocytosis was found in 7/300 primary SS patients [82] and was mainly related to the development of neoplasia (5 patients); in the remaining 2 patients, the cause of agranulocytosis was not identified. The first patient presented a steady, low neutrophil count, while the other patient presented cyclic episodes of agranulocytosis, resembling cyclic neutropenia, a rare hematologic disorder not described in patients with primary SS. Two recent studies [87, 88] found a close association between agranulocytosis and positive autoantibodies and coexisting cytopenias.

Autoimmune neutropenia has also been associated with the development of large granular lymphoma (LGL), a T-cell leukemia closely associated with agranulocytosis. In fact, a recent study found that almost 25% of patients with LGL have an underlying primary SS, suggesting a closer relationship than previously suspected [98].

Treatment for agranulocytosis in primary SS is controversial, with variable results with corticosteroids, immunosuppressive treatment, or G-CSF [87, 88].

Although previous studies reported antineutrophil antibodies in patients with primary SS [99, 100], it was not until 1995 [101] that their presence was specifically analyzed in a series of 66 patients, and a prevalence of 45% reported. However, no correlation was found between the presence of antibodies and the number of neutrophils, suggesting that autoantibody production follows the release of FcRIIIb, which in turn, follows the activation of polymorphonuclear leukocytes (PMN). These authors found a significant correlation between neutropenia and the presence of non-erosive arthritis, Raynaud phenomenon, lung disease, and the presence of HLA-DR3. However, they found no correlation with serum IgG or serum PMN counts. Therefore, according to currently available data, it is not possible to establish a clear role for antineutrophil antibodies in primary SS.

Table 25.8 Prevalence of thrombocytopenia in primary SS

Author	Year	Thrombocytopenia definition	Patients (n)	Thrombocytopenia n (%)
Bloch et al. [7]	1965	<150,000/mm³	62	5 (8)
Alexander et al. [9]	1983	<150,000/mm³	75	8 (11)
Ramakrishna et al. [47]	1992	<150×10⁹/L	27	5 (15)
Ramos-Casals et al. [1]	2002	<150×10⁹/L	380	48 (13)
Ramos-Casals et al. [48]	2008	<150×10⁹/L	1,010	131 (13)
Baimpa et al. [12]	2009	<140,000/mm³	536	28 (5)

25.3.10 Eosinophilia

In studies in the 1960s, eosinophilia was reported in about one third of patients with SS (30%) [7]. However, a subsequent study that analyzed the prevalence of eosinophilia in a large cohort of primary SS patients [1] found a prevalence of 12%. Its clinical significance in primary SS is unclear.

25.3.11 Thrombocytopenia

The prevalence of thrombocytopenia in patients with primary SS ranges from 5% to 15% (Table 25.8) [1, 7, 9, 12, 47, 48]. Most studies defined thrombocytopenia as a count of <150,000 platelets; however, Baimpa et al. [12], who reported a prevalence of 5%, used a low cut-off level for platelet counts (<140,000), which may explain its lower prevalence (Table 25.8).

Thrombocytopenia is usually mild [1, 7, 9, 47, 83] and, like other hematologic abnormalities, may be the first sign of underlying SS [52, 102], either primary or associated. Thrombocytopenia in SS patients seems to be caused by peripheral platelet destruction, mediated by immune complexes or antiplatelet antibodies, with a pathogenic mechanism similar to that described in SLE patients [103]. Thrombocytopenia has been associated with anti-Ro/SS-A and anti-La/SS-B antibodies. Ramos-Casals et al. [48] reported a higher prevalence of anti-Ro/anti-La/SS-B in patients with thrombocytopenia, as described in previous studies [9, 83].

Severe thrombocytopenia (<50,000/mm³) is uncommon in primary SS [47, 52, 103]. A good response to corticosteroids was observed in the majority of patients, although some required immunosuppressive treatment [47]. Intravenous immunoglobulins have been shown to be successful for severe thrombocytopenia refractory to steroid treatment [104].

25.4 Conclusions

Laboratory abnormalities are frequent in primary SS. A raised erythrosedimentation rate and hypergammaglobulinemia are present in around 20% of patients and are more frequently found in patients with positive autoantibodies. Serum monoclonal immunoglobulins are also frequently detected (20%), with IgG being the most frequent type of monoclonal spike and κ the most frequent light chain. Monoclonal bands are associated with extraglandular involvement, cryoglobulinemia, and B-cell lymphoma. $β_2$-microglobulin may be useful in differentiating patients with sicca syndrome from those with primary SS, who often have higher serum levels, and has also been associated with extraglandular involvement and lymphoma.

Cytopenias are key laboratory abnormalities in primary SS. Although they have no clinical significance in most cases, they may be the first sign of underlying primary SS. Anemia and leukopenia are the most common hematological abnormalities reported. Anemia is usually mild, normocytic and normochromic, and is principally related to primary SS itself. Other infrequent causes of anemia described in primary SS include autoimmune hemolytic anemia, aplastic anemia, pure red cell aplasia, myelodysplastic syndrome, and pernicious anemia. Cytopenias are more frequently found in patients with positive autoantibodies and have been related to the presence of extraglandular manifestations. Recently, lymphopenia (at the expense of the CD4+ T-lymphocyte count) and neutropenia have been associated with the development of lymphoproliferative diseases. Although the spectrum of laboratory abnormalities in primary SS is wide, early detection may help the physician to identify subsets of patients who may be at risk of more severe disease.

References

1. Ramos-Casals M, Font J, Garcia-Carrasco M, Brito MP, Rosas J, Calvo-Alen J, et al. Primary Sjogren syndrome: hematologic patterns of disease expression. Medicine (Baltimore). 2002;81:281–92.
2. Davidson BKS, Kelly CA, Griffiths ID. Primary Sjogren's syndrome in the North East of England: a long-term follow-up study. Rheumatology. 1999;38:245–53.
3. Moutsopoulos HM, Steinberg AD, Fauci AS, Lane HC, Papadopoulos NM. High incidence of free monoclonal light chains in the sera of patients with Sjögren's syndrome. J Immunol. 1983;130:2263–5.
4. Youinou P, Fauquert P, Pennec YL, Bendaoud B, Katsikis P, Le Goff P. Raised C-reactive protein response in rheumatoid arthritis patients with secondary Sjogren's syndrome. Rheumatol Int. 1990;10:39–41.
5. Yazisiz V, Avci AB, Erbasan F, Kiris E, Terzioglu E. Diagnostic performance of minor salivary gland biopsy, serological and clinical data in Sjögren's syndrome: a retrospective analysis. Rheumatol Int. 2009;29:403–9.
6. Kahn MF, Peltier AP, Meyer O, Piette JC Les Maladies systemiques. Gougerot Sjogren's syndrome. Ed. Flammarion, Paris; 1991. pp. 517–8.
7. Bloch KJ, Buchanan WW, Wohl MJ, Bunim JJ. Sjogren's syndrome a clinical, pathological and serological study of 62 cases. Medicine (Baltimore). 1965;44:187–231.
8. Martínez-Lavin M, Vaughan J, Tan E. Autoantibodies and the spectrum of Sjogren's syndrome. Ann Intern Med. 1979;91:185–90.
9. Alexander EL, Arnett FC, Provost TT, Stevens MB. Sjogren's syndrome: association of anti-Ro(SS-A) antibodies with vasculitis, hematologic abnormalities, and serologic hyperactivity. Ann Intern Med. 1983;98:155–9.
10. Sutcliffe N, Inanc M, Speight P, Isenberg D. Predictors of lymphoma development in primary Sjogren's syndrome. Semin Arthritis Rheum. 1998;28:80–7.

11. Skopouli FN, Dafni U, Ioannidis JP, Moutsopoulos HM. Clinical evolution, and morbidity and mortality of primary Sjogren's syndrome. Semin Arthritis Rheum. 2000;29:296–304.
12. Baimpa E, Dahabreh IJ, Voulgarelis M, Moutsopoulos HM. Hematological manifestations and predictors of lymphoma development in primary Sjögren syndrome: clinical and pathophysiologic aspects. Medicine (Baltimore). 2009;88:284–93.
13. Markusse HM, Veldhoven CH, Swaak AJ, Smeenk RT. The clinical significance of the detection of anti-Ro/SS-A and anti-La/SS-B autoantibodies using purified recombinant proteins in primary Sjögren's syndrome. Rheumatol Int. 1993;13:147–50.
14. Amman AJ, Hong R. Selective immunoglobulinA deficiency: presentation of 30 cases and a review of the literature. Medicine (Baltimore). 1971;50:226–36.
15. Rodriguez-Cuartero A, Ceballos A, Gómez del Cerro A. Síndrome de Sjogren primario y deficiencia de immunoglobulinA. Rev Clin Esp. 1991;198:299–300.
16. Perez Pena F, Martinez Santos P, Sanchez Ramos A, Mateos Sanchez A, Lopez Alonso G. Deficiencia selectiva de immunoglobulinA. Rev Clin Esp. 1978;148:521–3.
17. Matter L, Wilhelm J, Angehrn W. Selective antibody deficiency and recurrent pneumococcal bacteremia in a patient with Sjogren's syndrome: hyperimmunoglobulinemia G, and deficiencies of immunoglobulinG2 and immunoglobulinG4. N Engl J Med. 1985;312:1039–42.
18. Montecucco C, Cherie-Ligniere EL, Rosso R, Longhi M, Riccardi A. Sjogren-like syndrome in kappa chain deficiency. Arthritis Rheum. 1986;29:1532–3.
19. Eriksson P, Almroth G, Denneberg T, Lindstrom FD. ImmunoglobulinG2 deficiency in primary Sjogren's syndrome and hypergammaglobulinemic purpura. Clin Immunol Immunopathol. 1994;70:60–5.
20. Steuer A, McCrea DJ, Colaco CB. Primary Sjogren's syndrome, ulcerative colitis and selective immunoglobulinA deficiency. Postgrad Med J. 1996;72:499–500.
21. Wanchu A, Bambery P, Sud A, Chawla Y, Vaiphei K, Deodhar SD. Autoimmune hepatitis in a patient with primary Sjogren's syndrome and selective immunoglobulinA deficiency. Trop Gastroenterol. 1998;19:62–3.
22. Sugai S, Shimizu S, Konda S. Lymphoproliferative disorders in Japanese patients with Sjogren's syndrome. Scand J Rheumatol Suppl. 1986;61:118–22.
23. Walters MT, Stevenson FK, Herbert A, Cawley MI, Smith JL. Lymphoma in Sjogren's syndrome: urinary monoclonal free light chains as a diagnostic aid and a means of tumour monitoring. Scand J Rheumatol Suppl. 1986;61:114–7.
24. Pariente D, Anaya JM, Combe B, Jorgensen C, Emberger JM, Rossi JF, et al. Non-Hodgkin lymphoma associated with primary Sjogren's syndrome. Eur J Med. 1992;1:337–42.
25. Sibilia J, Cohen-Solal J. Prevalence of monoclonal gammopathy and myeloma in a cohort of primary Sjögren' syndrome. Arthritis Rheum. 1999;42 Suppl 9:S140. abstract.
26. Brito-Zerón P, Ramos-Casals M, Nardi N, Cervera R, Yagüe J, Ingelmo M, et al. Circulating monoclonal immunoglobulins in Sjögren syndrome. Medicine (Baltimore). 2005;84:90–7.
27. Ramos-Casals M, Cervera R, Yagüe J, García-Carrasco M, Trejo O, Jiménez S, et al. Cryoglobulinemia in primary SS: prevalence and clinical characteristics in a series of 115 patients. Semin Arthritis Rheum. 1998;28:200–5.
28. De Re V, De Vita S, Gasparotto D, Marzotto A, Carbone A, Ferraccioli G, et al. Salivary gland B cell lymphoproliferative disorders in Sjogren's syndrome present a restricted use of antigen receptor gene segments similar to those used by hepatitis C virus-associated non Hodgkins's lymphomas. Eur J Immunol. 2002;32:903–10.
29. Michalski JP, Daniels TE, Talal N, Grey HM. b2 microglobulin and lymphocytic infiltration in Sjogren's syndrome. N Engl J Med. 1975;293:1228–31.
30. Bethea M, Forman DT. Beta 2-microglobulin: its significance and clinical usefulness. Ann Clin Lab Sci. 1990;20:163–8.
31. Bianucci G, Campana G, Bongi SM, Palermo C, D'Agata A. Salivary and serum beta 2-microglobulin in the diagnosis of primary Sjögren syndrome. Minerva Med. 1992;83:705–13.
32. Maddali Bongi S, Campana G, D'Agata A, Palermo C, Bianucci G. The diagnosis value of beta 2-microglobulin and immunoglobulins in primary Sjögren's syndrome. Clin Rheumatol. 1995;14:151–6.

33. Mogi M, Kage T, Chino T, Yoshitake K, Harada M. Increased beta 2-microglobulin in both parotid and submandibular/sublingual saliva from patients with Sjögren's syndrome. Arch Oral Biol. 1994;39:913–5.

34. Van der Geest SA, Markusse HM, Swaak AJ. Beta 2 microglobulin measurements in saliva of patients with primary Sjögren's syndrome: influence of flow. Ann Rheum Dis. 1993;52:461–3.

35. Markusse HM, Huysen JC, Nieuwenhuys EJ, Swaak AJ. Beta 2 microglobulin in tear fluid from patients with primary Sjögren's syndrome. Ann Rheum Dis. 1992;51:503–5.

36. Ström T, Evrin PE, Karlsson A. Serum beta 2-microglobulin in Sjögren's syndrome. Scand J Rheumatol. 1978;7:97–100.

37. Du D, Pu Y, Zhao Y. The value of salivary beta 2 microglobulin concentration for diagnosis of Sjögren's syndrome. Zhongguo Yi Xue Ke Xue Yuan Xue Bao. 1997;19:72–4.

38. Krejsek J, Slezák R, Kopecky O, Derner V, Andrys C. Elevation of serum soluble intercellular adhesion molecule-1 (sICAM-1) and beta 2-microglobulin in Sjögren's syndrome. Clin Rheumatol. 1997;16:149–53.

39. Pertovaara M, Korpela M, Uusitalo H, Pukander J, Miettinen A, Helin H, et al. Clinical follow up study of 87 patients with sicca symptoms (dryness of eyes or mouth, or both). Ann Rheum Dis. 1999;58:423–7.

40. Bianucci G, Campana G, Maddali-Bongi S, D'Agata A, Pradella F, Colafranceschi M, et al. Serum beta 2-microglobulin and HLA alloantigens in primary Gougerot-Sjogren syndrome: a possible relation with HLA-DR3 specificity. Rev Rhum Mal Osteoartic. 1991;58:339–42.

41. Gottenberg JE, Busson M, Cohen-Solal J, Lavie F, Abbed K, Kimberly RP, et al. Correlation of serum B lymphocyte stimulator and beta 2 microglobulin with autoantibody secretion and systemic involvement in primary Sjögren's syndrome. Ann Rheum Dis. 2005;64:1050–5.

42. Lahdensuo A, Korpela M. Pulmonary findings in patients with primary Sjogren's syndrome. Chest. 1995;102:316–9.

43. Hatron PY, Wallaert B, Gosset D, Tonnel AB, Gosselin B, Voisin C, et al. Subclinical lung inflammation in primary Sjögren's syndrome: relationship between bronchoalveolar lavage cellular analysis finding and characteristics of the disease. Arthritis Rheum. 1987;30:1226–31.

44. Pertovaara M, Korpela M, Kouri T, Pasternack A. The occurrence of renal involvement in primary Sjögren's syndrome: a study of 78 patients. Rheumatology. 1999;38:1113–20.

45. Pertovaara M, Pukkala E, Laippala P, Miettinen A, Pasternack A. A longitudinal cohort study of Finnish patients with primary Sjögren's syndrome: clinical, immunological and epidemiological aspects. Ann Rheum Dis. 2001;60:467–72.

46. Benucci M, Li Gobbi F, Del Gobbo A, Gambacorta G, Mannoni A. [Association between serum amyloid A (SAA) in salivary glands and high levels of circulating beta 2-microglobulin in patients with Sjögren syndrome]. Reumatismo. 2003;55:98–101.

47. Ramakrishna R, Chaudhuri K, Sturgess A, Manoharan A. Haematological manifestations of primary Sjögren's syndrome: a clinicopathological study. Q J Med. 1992;84:547–54.

48. Ramos-Casals M, Solans R, Rosas J, Camps MT, Gil A, del Pino-Montes J, et al. Primary Sjögren syndrome in Spain: clinical and immunological expression in 1010 patients. Medicine (Baltimore). 2008;87:210–9.

49. Baboonian C, Venables PJW, Booth J, Williams DG, Roffe LM, Maini RN. Virus infection induces redistribution and membrane localisation of the nuclear antigen La (SSB): a possible mechanism for autoimmunity. Clin Exp Immunol. 1989;78:454–9.

50. Le Feber WP, Norris DA, Ryan S, Huff DC, Lee LA, Kubo M, et al. Ultraviolet light induced expression of selected nuclear antigens on cultured human keratinocytes. J Clin Invest. 1984;74:1545–51.

51. Ramos-Casals M, Cervera R, García-Carrasco M, Vidal J, Trejo O, Jimenez S, et al. Cytopenia and past human parvovirus B19 infection in patients with primary Sjögren's syndrome. Semin Arthritis Rheum. 2000;29:373–8.

52. Schattner A, Friedman J, Klepfish A, Berrebi A. Immune cytopenias as the presenting finding in primary Sjogren's syndrome. Q J Med. 2000;93:825–9.

53. Chudwin DS, Daniels TE, Wara DW, Ammann AJ, Barrett DJ, Whitcher JP, et al. Spectrum of Sjogren's syndrome in children. J Pediatr. 1981;98:213–7.
54. Boling EP, Wen J, Reveille JD, Bias WB, Chused TM, Arnett FC. Primary Sjogren's syndrome and autoimmune hemolytic anemia in sisters. Am J Med. 1983;74:1066–71.
55. Schattner A, Shtalrid M, Berrebi A. Autoimmune hemolytic anemia preceding Sjogren's syndrome. J Rheumatol. 1983;10:482–4.
56. de la Montane Roque P, Arlet P, Chartier JP, Cornu JJ, Juchet H, Ollier S, et al. Autoimmune hemolytic anemia disclosing primary Gougerot-Sjogren syndrome. Rev Med Interne. 1993;14:133–4.
57. Usui K, Anzai C, Sano K. Primary Sjogren's syndrome with pulmonary hypertension. Nihon Koyuki Gakkai Zasshi. 1998;36:478–81.
58. Fye KH, Daniels TE, Zulman J, Michalski JP, Jaffe R, Talal N. Aplastic anemia and lymphoma in Sjogren's syndrome. Arthritis Rheum. 1980;23:1321–5.
59. Yoshida H, Wakashin M, Okuda K. Successful treatment of aplastic anemia associated with chronic thyroiditis and Sjogren's syndrome. J Rheumatol. 1986;13:1189–90.
60. Quiquandon I, Morel P, Lai JL, Bauters F, Dresch C, Gluckman E, et al. Primary Sjogren's syndrome and aplastic anaemia. Ann Rheum Dis. 1997;56:438–41.
61. Williamson J, Paterson RW, McGavin DD, Greig WR, Whaley K. Sjogren's syndrome in relation to pernicious anaemia and idiopathic Addison's disease. Br J Ophthalmol. 1970;54: 31–6.
62. Wegelious O, Fyhrquist F, Adner PL. Sjogren's syndrome associated with vitamin B12 deficiency. Acta Rheumatol Scand. 1970;16:184–90.
63. Pedro-Botet J, Coll J, Tomas S, Soriano JC, Gutierrez-Cebollada J. Primary Sjogren's syndrome associated with chronic atrophic gastritis and pernicious anemia. J Clin Gastroenterol. 1993;16:146–8.
64. Koramaz I, Sonmez M, Pulathan Z, Cobanoglu U, Karti SS. Successful coronary artery bypass grafting in a patient with aplastic anemia and Sjögren syndrome. Saudi Med J. 2006;27: 1251–2.
65. Matsumoto N, Kagawa H, Ichiyoshi H, Iguchi T, Yamanaka Y, Kishimoto Y, et al. Aplastic anemia complicating Sjögren's syndrome. Intern Med. 1997;36:371–4.
66. Satoh M, Yamagata H, Watanabe F, Matsushita Y, Nakayama S, Murakami M, et al. A case of Sjögren's syndrome complicating immune-mediated aplastic anemia. Clin Rheumatol. 1993;12:257–60.
67. Giordano N, Senesi M, Battisti E, DeRegis FM, Gennari C. Sjogren's syndrome and pure red cell aplasia. Clin Exp Rheumatol. 1996;14:344–5.
68. García-García C, Jaén-Aguila F, Hidalgo-Tenorio C. Jiménez-Alonso JF [Pure red cell aplasia as first manifestation of primary Sjögren syndrome]. Rev Clin Esp. 2009;209:203–4.
69. Cavazzana I, Ceribelli A, Franceschini F, Cattaneo R. Unusual association between pure red cell aplasia and primary Sjogren's syndrome: a case report. Clin Exp Rheumatol. 2007; 25: 309–11.
70. Assimakopoulos SF, Michalopoulou S, Melachrinou M, Giannakoulas N, Papakonstantinou C, Lekkou A, et al. Primary Sjögren syndrome complicated by autoimmune haemolytic anemia and pure red cell aplasia. Am J Med Sci. 2007;334:493–6.
71. Fujiu K, Kanno R, Shio Y, Ohsugi J, Nozawa Y, Gotoh M. Triad of thymoma, myasthenia gravis and pure red cell aplasia combined with Sjögren's syndrome. Jpn J Thorac Cardiovasc Surg. 2004;52:345–8.
72. Ergas D, Tsimanis A, Shtalrid M, Duskin C, Berrebi A. T-gamma large granular lymphocyte leukaemia associated with a megakaryocytic thrombocytopenic purpura, Sjögren's syndrome and polyglandular autoimmune syndrome type II, with subsequent development of pure red cell aplasia. Am J Hematol. 2002;69:132–4.
73. Ibkhatra S, Jacobson L, Manthorpe R. The association of pure red cell aplasia and primary Sjogren's syndrome. Clin Exp Rheumatol. 1997;15:119–20.

74. Bouali F, Berrah A, Si Ahmed-Bouali D, Harrieche F, Benhalima M, Hamladji RM, et al. [Immunological abnormalities in myelodysplastic syndromes. Prospective study (series of 40 patients)]. Rev Med Interne. 2005;26:777–83.

75. Roy-Peaud F, Paccalin M, Le Moal G, Landron C, Juhel L, Roblot P, et al. [Association of systemic disease and myelodysplastic syndromes: a retrospective study of 14 cases]. Presse Med. 2003;32:538–43.

76. DeCoteau WE, Katakkar SB, Skinnider L, Hayton RC, Somerville EA. Sjögren's syndrome terminating as a myeloproliferative disorder. J Rheumatol. 1975;2:331–5.

77. Castro M, Conn DL, Su WP, Garton JP. Rheumatic manifestations in myelodysplastic syndromes. J Rheumatol. 1991;18:721–7.

78. Rodriguez-Cuartero A, Pérez-Blanco FJ, Urbano-Jiménez F. Sjögren's syndrome and pernicious anaemia. Scand J Rheumatol. 1998;27:83–5.

79. James JM, Zittoun R, Simon F, Slama G, Facquet-Danis J, Bilski-Pasquier G. Pernicious anaemia associated with Hashimoto's thyroiditis, Sjögren's syndrome and chondrocalcinosis. Sem Hop. 1978;54:1041–4.

80. Zittoun R, Debain P, James JM, Bilski-Pasquier G. Hematological manifestations and complications in Sjögren's syndrome. Sem Hop. 1978;54:1011–20.

81. Harley JB, Alexander EL, Bias WB, Fox OF, Provost TT, Reichlin M, et al. Anti-Ro(SS-A) and anti-La(SS-B) in patients with Sjogren's syndrome. Arthritis Rheum. 1986;29:196–206.

82. Brito-Zerón P, Soria N, Muñoz S, Bové A, Akasbi M, Berenguer R, et al. Prevalence and clinical relevance of autoimmune neutropenia in patients with primary Sjögren's syndrome. Semin Arthritis Rheum. 2009;38:389–95.

83. Aoki A, Ohno S, Ueda A. Hematological abnormalities of primary Sjogren's syndrome. Nihon Rinsho Meneki Gakkai Kaishi. 2000;23:124–8.

84. Kirtava Z, Blomberg J, Bredberg A, Henriksson G, Jacobsson L, Manthorpe R. CD4+ T-lymphocytopenia without HIV infection: increased prevalence among patients with primary Sjögren's syndrome. Clin Exp Rheumatol. 1995;13:609–16.

85. Mandl T, Bredberg A, Jacobsson LT, Manthorpe R, Henriksson G. CD4+ T-lymphocytopenia – a frequent finding in anti-SSA antibody seropositive patients with primary Sjögren's syndrome. J Rheumatol. 2004;31:726–8.

86. Theander E, Henriksson G, Ljungberg O, Mandl T, Manthorpe R, Jacobsson LT. Lymphoma and other malignancies in primary Sjogren's syndrome: a cohort study on cancer incidence and lymphoma predictors. Ann Rheum Dis. 2006;65:796–803.

87. Coppo P, Sibilia J, Maloisel F, et al. Primary Sjögren's syndrome associated agranulocytosis: a benign disorder? Ann Rheum Dis. 2003;62:476–8.

88. Friedman J, Klepfish A, Miller EB, Ognenovski V, Ike RW, Schattner A. Agranulocytosis in Sjögren's syndrome: two case reports and analysis of 11 additional reported cases. Semin Arthritis Rheum. 2002;31:338–45.

89. Gottenberg JE, Busson M, Loiseau P, et al. In primary Sjögren's syndrome, HLA class II is associated exclusively with autoantibody production and spreading of the autoimmune response. Arthritis Rheum. 2003;48:2240–5.

90. Addas-Carvalho M, de Paula EV, Lima CS, Saad ST. Polymorphisms of interleukin-1 gene complex, IL6 and tumour necrosis factor genes in chronic idiopathic neutropenia of adults. Ann Hematol. 2005;84:709–14.

91. Gavrikova N, Zeidler C, Stanulla M, Germeshausen M, Schwinzer B, Welte K. TNF and lymphotoxin-alpha polymorphisms in patients with severe chronic neutropenia. Int J Hematol. 2001;74:477–8.

92. Neth OW, Bajaj-Elliott M, Turner MW, Klein NJ. Susceptibility to infection in patients with neutropenia: the role of the innate immune system. Br J Haematol. 2005;129:713–22.

93. Ramos-Casals M, Loustaud-Ratti V, De Vita S, SS-HCV Study Group, et al. Sjogren syndrome associated with hepatitis C virus: a multicenter analysis of 137 cases. Medicine (Baltimore). 2005;84:81–9.

94. Lamy T, Dauriac C, MoriceP LePrisePY. Agranulocytose et connectivites distincttes due syndrome de Felty: 4 observations, succes dans un cas de la ciclosporine. Rev Med Interne. 1990;11:325–8.
95. Shastri KA, Logue GL. Autoimmune neutropenia. Blood. 1993;81:1984–95.
96. Bux J, Behrens G, Jaeger G, Welte K. Diagnosis and clinical course of autoimmune neutropenia in infancy: analysis of 240 cases. Blood. 1998;91:181–6.
97. Vivancos J, Vila M, Serra A, Loscos J, Anguita A. Failure of G-CSF therapy in neutropenia associated with Sjogren's syndrome. Rheumatology (Oxford). 2002;41:471–3.
98. Friedman J, Schattner A, Shvidel L, Berrebi A. Characterization of T-cell large granular lymphocyte leukemia associated with Sjogren's syndrome-an important but under-recognized association. Semin Arthritis Rheum. 2006;35:306–11.
99. Boros P, Odin JA, Chen J, Unkeless JC. Specificity and class distribution of FcγR-specific autoantibodies in patients with autoimmune disease. J Immunol. 1994;152:302.
100. Yamato E, Fujioka Y, Masugi F, Nakamaru M, Tahara Y, Kurata Y, et al. Autoimmune neutropenia with anti-neutrophil autoantibody associated with Sjogren's syndrome. Am J Med Sci. 1990;300:102–3.
101. Lamour A, Le Corre R, Pennec YL, Cartron J, Youinou P. Heterogeneity of neutrophil antibodies in patients with primary Sjogren's syndrome. Blood. 1995;86:3553–9.
102. Berrebi A, Shtalrid M, Talmor M, Vorst E. Thrombocytopenia in Sjogren's syndrome. Arthritis Rheum. 1982;25:1510.
103. Sugai S, Shimizu S, Tachibana J, Sawada M, Hirose Y, Takiguchi T, et al. Monoclonal gammopathies in patients with Sjogren's syndrome. Jpn J Med. 1988;27:2–9.
104. Choung BS, Yoo WH. Successful treatment with intravenous immunoglobulin of severe thrombocytopenia complicated in primary Sjögren's syndrome. Rheumatol Int. 2010;(Epub ahead of print).

Part III
Diagnosis and Prognosis

Chapter 26
Diagnostic Procedures (I): Ocular and Oral Tests

Gabriela Hernández-Molina, Francisco Cárdenas-Velazquez,
Claudia Recillas-Gispert, and Jorge Sánchez-Guerrero

Contents

G. Hernández-Molina • J. Sánchez-Guerrero (✉)
Immunology and Rheumatology Department, Instituto Nacional de Ciencias Médicas y Nutrición
Salvador Zubirán, Mexico City, Mexico

F. Cárdenas-Velazquez • C. Recillas-Gispert
Ophthalmology Service, Instituto Nacional de Ciencias Médicas y Nutrición Salvador Zubirán,
Mexico City, Mexico

M. Ramos-Casals et al. (eds.), *Sjögren's Syndrome*,
DOI 10.1007/978-0-85729-947-5_26, © Springer-Verlag London Limited 2012

Table 26.1 Conditions associated with eye and mouth dryness

Eye
    Meibomian gland deficiency
    Local infection
    Neurologic defects: V or VII paralysis
    Eyelid defects: ectropion, hyperthyroidism, proptosis
    Contact lens use
    Deficient nourishment: hypovitaminosis, A-avitaminosis
    Conjunctival cicatrization: Stevens–Johnson syndrome, ocular pemphigoid, trachoma
Mouth
    Dehydration
Mouth breathing
    Hypoplasia or aplasia of salivary glands
Both
    Irradiation head and neck therapy
    Surgical glands excision
    Uncontrolled diabetes mellitus
    Liver diseases, graft-vs.-host disease, sarcoidosis, tuberculosis, HIV or hepatitis C infection,
      amyloidosis
Medications
    Antihistamines: pseudoephedrine, chlorpheniramine, diphenhydramine
    Blood pressure drugs: β-blockers, α-blockers, diuretics
    Antidepressants: amitriptyline, nortriptyline, imipramine, and others
Muscle relaxants: cyclobenzaprine, methocarbamol
    Urologic drugs: oxybutynin, bethanechol
    Parkinson drugs: carbidopa, levodopa, biperiden
    Anti-arrhythmic: disopyramide, mexiletine
Neuroleptics
Sedatives and hypnotics
Anticholinergics: atropine

Primary Sjögren's syndrome (SS) is a clinical disease characterized by keratoconjunctivitis sicca (KCS) and xerostomia due to an autoimmune background. Although the presence of one or both components is important for the diagnosis, these clinical features are not exclusively present in this syndrome.

For instance, in the general population, the prevalence of xerostomia varies between 6% and 29% [1] and of dry eye between 16% and 50% [2]. Among patients attending a rheumatologic clinic, the prevalence of dry eye and dry mouth symptoms has been reported as 45% and 43%, respectively [3]. In contrast, in primary SS patients, the prevalence of xerostomia and xerophthalmia is as high as 96% [4]. Patients with sicca syndrome usually describe a burning or foreign body sensation, itching, inability to tear, photophobia, intermittent mild visual disturbances, oral dryness, increased need of drinking water, difficulties chewing dry food, speech difficulties, and other symptoms [5]. Because there are multiple other causes of dry mouth and dry eye – particularly medications (Table 26.1) – clinicians must be certain to consider other etiologies, as well [6].

Table 26.2 Symptoms evaluation according to the American-European Consensus Group

I. Ocular symptoms: a positive response to at least one of the following questions:
1. Have you had daily, persistent, troublesome dry eyes for more than 3 months?
2. Do you have a recurrent sensation of sand or gravel in the eyes?
3. Do you use tear substitutes more than three times a day?
II. Oral symptoms: a positive response to at least one of the following questions:
1. Have you had a daily feeling of dry mouth for more than 3 months?
2. Have you had recurrently or persistently swollen salivary glands as an adult?
3. Do you frequently drink liquids to aid in swallowing dry food?

26.1   Definitions

KCS is defined as a tear deficiency or an excessive tear evaporation that causes damage to the cornea and/or conjunctiva. It may be associated with ocular discomfort secondary to dryness. SS is the prototype of an aqueous deficient dry eye [7]. Symptomatic xerostomia is the subjective feeling of oral dryness [8]. Xerostomia is defined as flow rates ≤ 0.1 mL/min.

26.2   Questionnaires

Some questionnaires are available to evaluate the presence dry eye. However, most of these questionnaires do not assess symptomatology with sufficient thoroughness [9]. In contrast, the Dry Eye Questionnaire (DEQ) characterizes the frequency of ocular surface symptoms and their diurnal intensity. The DEQ has been validated for the study of KCS [10, 11].

Two questions regarding oral and ocular symptoms are customarily included as items of the current primary SS classification criteria [12] (Table 26.2). These questions yield a sensitivity of 81.4% and 84.9%, respectively, with a specificity higher than 80% [13]. Moreover, the retest reliability of these questions 1 year later are 96.4% and 98.2%, respectively [14]. Nevertheless, the correlation between sicca symptoms and objective signs of glandular dysfunction is only moderate [1, 15]. A precise measure of symptoms, therefore, is an important aspect of making the diagnosis of either dry eyes or dry mouth. With regard to xerostomia, careful inspection of the mouth looking for angular cheilitis, saliva in the mouth's floor, deep tongue fissures, candidiasis, and atypical caries is useful [5].

26.3   Ocular Tests

The tests used most frequently to assess the integrity of the corneal surface and the volume and quality of tear film are the Schirmer-I test (Schirmer test), Rose Bengal staining, fluorescein or lissamine green staining, and the tear break-up time (Table 26.3) [16].

Table 26.3 Methods for evaluating dry eye

Test	Basis and method	Abnormal test	Reference
SchirmSchirmer-I and -II tests	Measure of tear secretion See text for details	≤5 mm Sensitivity 76% Specificity 72%	[13, 26]
Break-up time	Index of tear film stability See text for details	≤10 s Sensitivity 77% Specificity 38%	[16]
Vital stains	Stain the ocular surface to discover abnormalities	Grading Bijsterveld score ≥4	[29, 31, 32]
Rose Bengal Lissamine green Fluorescein	See text for details	Sensitivity 78% Specificity 67%	
Tear meniscus	Measure of basal tear volume with a video meniscometer	Normal value 0.3 ± 0.1 mm	[16, 19]
Tear osmolarity	Osmolarity is increased as a result of cytokines' liberation. It is measured with an osmometer	Normal value 304 ± 1.4 mOsm/L A value ≥312 mOsm/L identifies dry eyes (sensitivity 94%, specificity 97%)	[19]
Tear proteins: lysozyme, lactoferrin	Decrease in these proteins is a reflex of glandular dysfunction. Measured by immunonephelometry, agars gels, ELISA, spectrophotometry	Normal value for lysozyme 1–3 mg/mL and for lactoferrin 2 ± 1.1 mg/mL Lysozyme specificity 96%, sensitivity 25% Lactoferrin specificity 67–90%, sensitivity 78–28%	[17–19]
Ferning test	An index of tear film stability. A freshly produced tear is dropped on light micros-copy slides, after evaporation at room temperature. Crystallization is observed without staining	Uniform and abundant arborization (Ferning phenomenon) is absent	[20]
Brush cytology	Analysis of conjunctival morphology. Type and grade of inflammation	Only conjunctival epithelial cells should be found. It is pathological when mononuclear cells or neutrophils are present	[19]
Imprint cytology	Evaluation of squamous metaplasia. It is performed under local anesthesia using cellulose filters. Score 0 (normal epithe-lium) to 5 (advanced keratinization)	Score ≥2 has a specificity or 93% and sensitivity 30%	[19]

Rose Bengal staining, once a standard test in this disease, is now used less frequently because the application of the ocular stain is intensely uncomfortable to patients with KCS.

Because gradual destruction of the lacrimal gland in SS leads to diminished levels of tear proteins (lysozyme, lactoferrin, tear-specific prealbumin), some authors have proposed to measure these proteins to identify patients with dry eyes [17, 18]. Other tests, such as the tear film osmolarity, tear evaporation, tear meniscus, and ocular surface impression cytology, and crystallization, have also been studied (Table 26.3) [19, 20]. Although all of these methods provide different qualitative information, they have not achieved general clinical acceptance because of their lack of broad accessibility and general applicability.

26.3.1 Schirmer Test

The Schirmer test, a practical, semiquantitative method, is a commonly used initial screening procedure for SS [13]. Some studies have reported a good correlation between in vivo fluorometric measurement of basal tear turnover and tear flow [21], as well as with the rose Bengal test [22]. Other studies, however, have not [23–25].

The Schirmer test may be performed with or without topical anesthetic. In order to assess the maximal tear production, a cotton-tipped swab can be introduced gently into the nose to stimulate the nasolacrimal gland reflex (via the trigeminal nerve) while performing the Schirmer test [26]. This is known as a Schirmer-II test. For some authors, the Schirmer-II test has a better correlation with staining tests [24].

During the Schirmer test, a standardized tear test strip is placed between the eye and the lateral part of the inferior eyelid. The patient is then inclined forward in a resting position at 45°, with eyes closed. After 5 min, the length of the wetted strip area is measured (Fig. 26.1). Humidification of ≤5 mm at least in one eye is required for a test result to be positive. The sensitivity and specificity of the test are 76.9% and 72.4%, respectively, when this cutoff value is used [13]. When the first test is positive in both eyes, the test-retest reliability at 1 year is 77.4% for one eye and 84.2% for both [14].

One of the factors that influences the results of the Schirmer test is the tear clearance rate. Consequently, a tear function index (TFI) has been proposed as a better tear measurement. The TFI is derived from dividing the Schirmer's test value by the tear clearance rate, which is calculated by instilling 10 μL of fluorescein into the conjunctival fornix [27, 28]. Although the TFI is theoretically useful, it is not as simple to perform as the Schirmer's test and is not widely used in clinical practice.

Fig. 26.1 Schirmer-I test. Patient with absence of tear flow strip humidification after a time interval of 5 min. The lack of tear meniscus is also evident

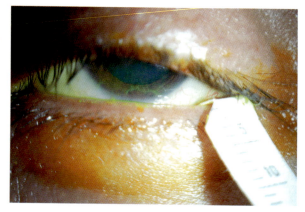

26.3.2 Vital Dyes

Vital dyes are any colored substance that contain auxochromes and are therefore capable of staining tissues. Vital dyes used in the field of ophthalmology have acceptable physiological and toxicological profiles. These dyes are used to detect abnormalities on the ocular surface. Positive staining is usually a relatively late manifestation of tear film disturbances or abnormalities of the ocular surface.

26.3.3 Rose Bengal

The Rose Bengal method stains degenerated dead cells and cells that have a tendency to keratinization. Van Bijsterveld created a grading scale that divides the ocular surface into three zones: the nasal bulbar conjunctiva, cornea, and the temporal bulbar conjunctiva [29]. After instillation of the 1% Rose Bengal solution into the conjunctiva and asking the patient to blink one or two times, the intensity of staining of each area is scored. Each section is scored 1 (sparsely scattered), 2 (densely scattered), or 3 (confluent staining), such that a maximum score of 9 can be obtained.

KCS diagnosed when a grading Bijsterveld score ≥4 in at least one eye is present (Fig. 26.2) [29]. The evaluation of the conjunctiva and cornea can be determined with an ophthalmoscope, although a more accurate evaluation with a slit lamp outfitted with a cobalt filter is preferred. Solutions of rose Bengal should not be left in the patient's eye for a prolonged period, as this stain may be irritating and uncomfortable. In addition, it is important to remember that the specificity of the test is poor: Patients with infectious conjunctivitis or chronic, irritative conjunctivitis may also show an increased score [30]. The method has a sensitivity of 64.3% and a specificity of 81.7% [13].

Fig. 26.2 Rose Bengal staining. Staining is mainly present at the medial bulbar conjunctiva and cornea

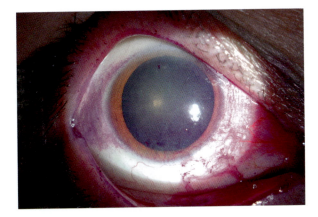

26.3.4 Fluorescein

Fluorescein stains denuded areas of the epithelium (Fig. 26.3). This method is an alternative for Rose Bengal. The same grading Bijsterveld score ≥4 is considered positive for the presence of KCS [31].

26.3.5 Lissamine Green

Like fluorescein, lissamine green stains corneal and collagenous stroma and can demonstrate epithelial defects within the corneal and conjunctivae (Fig. 26.4). Its capacity to stain membrane-damaged epithelial cells, combined with its ability to stain denuded corneal stroma, makes this dye a useful alternative to Rose Bengal and fluorescein. Lissamine green also causes less irritation than these other two dyes, but requires a slit lamp examination for adequate quantification of the staining [32].

26.3.6 Tear Break-Up Time

The tear break-up time measures the stability of the tear film and is useful in the evaluation of an evaporative dry eye. The tear break-up time is defined as the interval between a complete blink and the appearance of the first randomly distributed dry spots. In order to perform the test, a 1% fluorescein solution is instilled in the inferior fornix of both eyes. After blinking, the interval in seconds between the last and first bead in the tear film is measured. A tear film break-up time of less than 10 s is considered positive [33].

The break-up time depends on variables such as the concentration of fluorescein, age, and the number of blinks [30]. The method has a sensitivity of 77.8% and a

Fig. 26.3 Fluorescein staining. Severe keratoconjunctivitis sicca visualized with fluorescein staining (**a**), mucine filaments are also evident when using a blue cobalt filter (**b**)

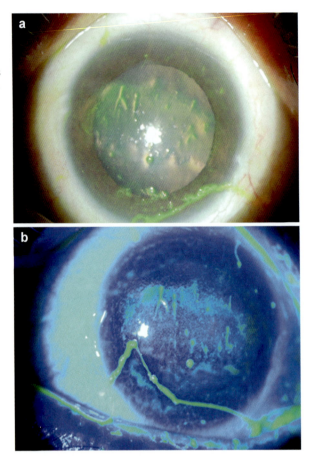

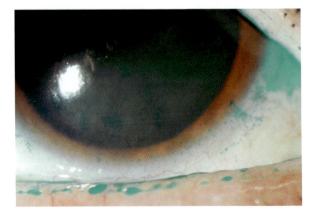

Fig. 26.4 Green lissamine staining. The staining shows areas of denuded corneal stroma

specificity of 38.9% [13, 34]. The use of this test is generally limited to ophthalmo-logical practice because the need for a slit lamp to assess the results.

26.3.7   Tear Osmolarity

Reduction of aqueous secretion and increased evaporation in patients with SS can combine to produce a tear film with an increased osmolarity. This has been shown to damage the ocular surface in and of itself. The normal tear osmolarity value varies around 304 ± 1.4 mOsm/L. Values greater than 320 mOsm/L have a sensitivity of 94% and a specificity of 97% in the detection of dry eye [19].

26.3.8   Tear Meniscus

Most of the tear film is located at the lacrimal meniscus area that is found between the ocular surface and the lower lid margin. This zone has been used as a measure-ment of the basal lacrimal basal volume. Its normal height is approximately 0.3 ± 0.1 mm. The ideal means of measuring the tear meniscus is through the use of a video meniscometer, but subjective assessments (visible, poor, absent) have also been employed [16, 19].

26.3.9   Tear Proteins

Diminished lactoferrin or lysozyme content usually signals impaired lacrimal gland function. The most frequent cause of decreases in the lactoferrin or lysozyme con-centrations is related to aging. The normal concentrations of lysozyme and lactofer-rin are 1–3 mg/mL and 2.05 ± 1.2 mg/mL in normal subjects respectively [17–19].

26.3.10   Ferning Test

Saliva crystallizes in the form of ferns when it is dried at room temperature and observed by polarized light microscopy. This is known as the "ferning phenome-non." Patterns of crystallization can then be identified based on the uniformity, integrity, and spreading of the ferning phenomenon. Grade I ferning (uniform arborization, without spaces among the ferns) is normal. Grades II (shorter and thicker ferns), III (smaller ferns and incompletely formed), and IV (absence of fern-ing phenomenon) are abnormal patterns seen in patients with SS [20].

Table 26.4 Methods for evaluating dry mouth

Test	Basis and method	Abnormal test	Reference
Whole saliva flow collection Stimulated Non-stimulated	Saliva collection may be performed with or without stimulus during a 5- or 15-min period	For the non-stimulated collection, an abnormal value is ≤1.5 mL/15 min	[36]
Wafer test	The main outcome is the time of dissolution of the wafer in the oral cavity	The test is positive if the time of dissolution is >4 min	[40]
Saxon test	Saliva production is quantified by weighing a gauze before and after chewing it for 2 min	Normal production of saliva in 2 min is ≥2.75 g	[41]
Imprint cytology of buccal mucosa	Cellulose acetate paper is applied in the internal surface or the inferior lip and stained with hematoxylin and PAS	As the normal epithelium is nonkeratinized, the presence of keratinized epithelium is abnormal	[37]
Iodine-starch reaction	A test tape 1 × 1 cm containing iodine and starch is set on labial mucosa anterior to the labial frenulum for 30 s. The number of blue spots corresponds to the number of salivary gland ostia	Controls 9.4 ± 2.5 spots Oral dryness 4.5 ± 3.1 spots Sjögren 2.1 ± 1.3 spots	[38]

26.3.11   Ocular Cytology

Ocular cytology is an approach to analyzing the conjunctival surface. Cells are collected by imprint (using cellulose filters in the bulbar superior conjunctiva) or by brush cytology. The specimen is then evaluated for the presence of squamous metaplasia (Grade 0 = absent; Grade 5 = advanced keratinization), cell morphology (small and homogenous is the normal pattern), and presence of inflammatory cells (mononuclear, neutrophils). All of these features are abnormal in dry eye patients [19].

26.4   Oral Tests

Methods for determining salivary gland function include salivary flow rate measurements (sialometry) and analysis of salivary composition (sialochemistry) [35, 36]. Other methods such as impression cytology of the buccal mucosa [37] and the use of iodine-starch reaction to know the number of lip salivary gland ostia have been described (Table 26.4) [38].

Sialometry is easy to perform and provides an objective measure, although normal values decrease with aging [39]. Some of the methods to quantify saliva production are the wafer test [40], the Saxon test [41], and the whole saliva collection (Table 26.4) [36]. On the other hand, sialochemistry is hampered by the lack of salivary reference values and the need for specialized equipment. Thus, their use is not common.

26.4.1 Wafer Test

The wafer test is a semiquantitative assessment that is useful for screening patients with early salivary gland dysfunction and xerostomia. The results of the wafer test correlate with the flow of non-stimulated whole saliva. The main outcome of the test is the time of dissolution of the wafer. The patient is asked to sit in a relaxed and upright position and not to speak during the test. After swallowing any residual saliva, the wafer is put on the center of the subject's tongue. Then the patient is asked to close the mouth and keep the wafer in the mouth without chewing or swallowing it. The swallowing of saliva is allowed. The test is considered as positive if the time to the dissolution of the wafer is more than 4 min [40].

26.4.2 Whole Saliva Flow Collection

This is the most straightforward test in the determination of salivary flow. Flow rates ≥0.3 mL/min are considered normal [42]. The collection may be performed with or without stimulus. Stimulated parotid flow may not correlate with the symptoms and may be normal even if basal secretion is reduced. In addition, it is difficult to obtain in patients who do not tolerate the cannula or the stimulus. Moreover, because a variety of stimulants (e.g., citric acid, gum, and others) have been used, there is a lack of agreement for normal values. Conversely, the non-stimulated whole saliva flow (NSWSF) reflects the basal flow from all glands taking place during most of the day. It is easy to measure and reproducible. The NSWSF is measured by the spitting method. Subjects are instructed to rest for 5 min before the test, to minimize orofacial movements, and not to speak. Before starting the procedure, the patient must swallow any residual saliva and allow all saliva to accumulate on the floor of the mouth and to spit it into a graduated test tube every minute. Saliva is collected for a period of 15 min and the measured volume expressed in mL/min [43]. A shortened version of the previously described technique more suitable for use in community surveys measures the volume in a 5 min period and is also available [1].

For the current SS criteria, an abnormal value is ≤1.5 mL/15 min [12]. The method has a sensitivity of 56.1%–64% and a specificity of 80.7% for SS [13, 44]. Salivary flow measurements are influenced by the time of day (maximal in the afternoon), degree of hydration, body position, smoking, exposure to light, and multiple different medications [45]. Thus, standardized procedures before the collection procedure are important. For example, patients should fast for at least 1 h before the procedure and refrain from brushing their teeth or smoking during this time.

26.4.3 Saxon Test

A sterile 10×10 gauze sponge is weighted. After swallowing to remove any preexisting oral fluid, saliva is collected by vigorously chewing for 2 min. The amount of saliva produced is determined by subtracting the original weight from the weight obtained after chewing. Normal production of saliva in 2 min is ≥2.75 g [41].

26.4.4 Iodine-Starch Reaction

A test tape (1 × 1 cm) containing iodine and starch is set in the mucosal area anterior to the labial frenulum for 30 s. The number of blue spots appearing on the strip corresponds to the number of ostia of the salivary gland on the lower lip. The average number of spots in patients with oral dryness is 4.5 ± 3.1 and in normal controls of 9.4 ± 2.5. SS patients have fewer spots than controls (2.1 ± 1.3) [38].

26.4.5 Impression Cytology

Cellulose acetate paper is applied in the internal surface of the inferior lip and stained with hematoxylin and PAS. The normal lip epithelium is a stratified, nonkeratinized with absence of goblet cells. An abnormal cytology consists of poorly cohesive normal epithelial cells or isolated keratinized cells [37].

26.5 Conclusion

Multiple different techniques exist to measure the production of tears or saliva either quantitatively or qualitatively. Some tests are most appropriate as screening assessments. Others are useful in the evaluation of gland function in subjects in whom suspicion of dysfunction has already been raised [46]. No single test of oral or ocular involvement is sufficiently sensitive and specific. The use of a combination of several tests is often recommended.

Currently, the European Study Group on Diagnostic criteria for SS recognizes as diagnostic ocular tests the use of the Schirmer test and the Rose Bengal staining test [12]. Non-stimulated whole saliva flow is the preferred oral test. Among all of the tests discussed in the present chapter, several have not been validated sufficiently for diagnostic purposes. However, we consider that they may be useful for screening patients with dry eyes/mouth or replace any of the validated tests in centers with enough experience with them.

References

1. Hay E, Thomas E, Pal B, et al. Weak association between subjective symptoms of and objective testing for dry eyes and dry mouth: results from a population based study. Ann Rheum Dis. 1998;57:20–4.

2. Nichols K, Nichols J, Zadnik K. Frequency of dry eye diagnostic test procedures used in various models of opthtalmic practice. Cornea. 2000;19:477–82.

3. Sánchez-Guerrero J, Pérez-Dorsal M, Cárdenas-Velázquez F, et al. Prevalence of Sjögren's syndrome in ambulatory patients according to the American-European Consensus Group criteria. Rheumatology. 2005;44:235–40.

4. Ramos-Casals M, Solans R, Rosas J, et al. Primary Sjögren syndrome in Spain. Medicine. 2008;87:210–9.

5. Manthorpe R, Axéll T. Xerostomia. Clin Exp Rheumatol. 1990;8 Suppl 5:7–12.

6. Konsen J. Xerostomia. Scand J Rheumatol Suppl. 1986;61:185–9.

7. Lemp M. Report of the National Eye Institute/Industry workshop on clinical trials in dry eyes. CLAO J.1995;21(4):221–32.

8. Speight PM, Kaul A, Melsom R. Measurement of whole unstimulated saliva flow in the diagnosis of Sjögren's syndrome. Ann Rheum Dis. 1992;51:499–502.

9. Hochberg M, Tielsch J, Muñoz B, et al. Prevalence of symptoms of dry mouth and their relationship to saliva production in community dwelling elderly: the SEE Project. J Rheumatol. 1998;25:486–91.

10. Begley C, Chalmer R, Mitchell G, et al. Characterization of ocular surface symptoms from optometric practices in North America. Cornea. 2001;20:610–8.

11. Begley C, Caffery B, Chalmers R, et al. Use of the dry eye questionnaire to measure symptoms of ocular irritation in patients with aqueous tear deficit dry eye. Cornea. 2002;21(7):664–70.

12. Vitali C, Bombardieri S, Jonsson R, et al. Classification criteria for Sjögren's Syndrome: a revised version of the European criteria proposed by the American-European Consensus group. Ann Rheum Dis. 2002;61:554–8.

13. Vitali C, Moutsopoulos H, Bombardieri S, et al. The European Community Study Group on diagnostic criteria for Sjögren's syndrome. Sensitivity and specificity of tests for ocular and oral involvement in Sjögren's syndrome. Ann Rheum Dis. 1994;53:637–47.

14. Haga H, Hulten B, Bolstad A, et al. Reliability and sensitivity of diagnostic tests for primary Sjögren's syndrome. J Rheumatol. 1999;26:604–8.

15. Begley C, Chalmers R, Abetz L, et al. The relationship between habitual patients reported symptoms and clinical signs among patients with dry eye of varying severity. Invest Ophtalmol Vis Sci. 2003;44:4753–61.

16. Goren M, Goren S. Diagnostic tests in patients with symptoms of keratoconjunctivitis sicca. Am J Ophthalmol. 1988;106:570–4.

17. Holly F. Dry eye and the Sjögren's syndrome. Scand J Rheumatol Suppl. 1986;61:201–5.

18. Mackie I, Seal D. Confirmatory tests for the dry eye of Sjögren's syndrome. Scand J Rheumatol Suppl. 1986;61:220–3.

19. Labbé A, Brignole-Baudouin F, Baudouin C. Méthodes d'évaluation de la surface oculaire dans les syndromes secs. J Fr Ophtalmol. 2007;30:76–97.

20. Maragou M, Vaikousis E, Ntre A, et al. Tear and saliva ferning test in Sjögren's syndrome. Clin Rheumatol. 1996;15:125–32.

21. Afonso A, Monroy D, Stern M, et al. Correlation of tear fluorescein clearance and Schirmer test scores with ocular irritation symptoms. Ophthalmology. 1999;106:803–10.

22. Coll J, Porta M, Rubiés-Prat J, et al. Sjögren's syndrome: a stepwise approach to the use of diagnostic test. An inverse correlation was noted between symptoms severity and Schirmer I test score. Ann Rheum Dis. 1992;51:607–10.

23. Versura P, Frigato M, Mulé R, et al. A proposal of new ocular items in Sjögren's syndrome classification criteria. Clin Exp Rheumatol. 2006;24:567–72.

24. Tsubota K, Kaido M, Yagi Y, et al. Diseases associated with ocular surface abnormalities: the importance of reflex tearing. Br J Ophthalmol. 1999;83:89–91.

25. Versura P, Frigato M, Cellini M, et al. Diagnostic performance of tear function test in Sjögren's syndrome patients. Eye. 2007;21:229–37.

26. Workshop participants. Manual of methods procedures. Clin Exp Rheumatol. 1989;7:213–18.

27. Xu KP, Yagi Y, Toda I. Tear function index. Arch Ophthalmol. 1995;113:84–8.

28. Kaye S, Sims G, Willoughby C, et al. Modification of the tear function index and its use in the diagnosis of Sjögren's syndrome. Br J Opthalmol. 2001;85:193–9.

29. Van Bijsterveld O. Diagnostic test in the sicca syndrome. Arch Ophtalmol. 1969;82:10–4.
30. Van Bijsterveld O. Diagnosis and differential diagnosis of keratoconjunctivitis sicca associated with tear gland degeneration. Clin Exp Rheumatol. 1990;8 Suppl 5:3–6.
31. Norn M. Vital staining of the cornea and conjunctiva. Am J Ophthalmol. 1967;64:1078–80.
32. Chodosh J, Dix R, Howell C, et al. Staining characteristics and antiviral activity of sulphorodamine B and lissamine green B. Invest Ophthalmol Vis Sci. 1994;35:1046–58.
33. Norn M. Tear secretion in diseased eyes. Acta Ophthalmol. 1966;44:25–32.
34. Kalk W, Mansour K, Vissink A, et al. Oral and ocular manifestations in Sjögren's syndrome. J Rheumatol. 2002;29:924–30.
35. Kalk W, Vissink A, Stegenga B, et al. Sialometry and sialochemistry: a non-invasive approach for diagnosing Sjögren's syndrome. Ann Rheum Dis. 2002;61:137–44.
36. Kalk W, Vissink A, Spijkervet F, et al. Sialometry and sialochemistry diagnostic tools for Sjögren's syndrome. Ann Rheum Dis. 2001;60(12):1110–6.
37. Aguilar A, Fonseca L, Craxatto O. Sjogren's syndrome: a comparative study of impression cytology of the conjunctiva and buccal mucosa, and salivary gland biopsy. Cornea. 1991;10:203–6.
38. Inamura T, Ino C, Katoh M, et al. A simple method to estimate the secretion of saliva from minor salivary glands using iodine-starch reaction. Laryngoscope. 2001;111:272–7.
39. Dawes C. Physiological factors affecting salivary flow rate, oral sugar clearance and the sensation of dry mouth in men. J Dent Res. 1987;66:648–53.
40. Sánchez-Guerrero J, Aguirre-Garcia E, Pérez-Dosal M, et al. The wafer test: a semi-quantitative test to screen for xerostomia. Rheumatology. 2002;41:381–9.
41. Kohler P, Winter M. A quantitative test for xerostomia. The Saxon test, an oral equivalent of the Schirmer test. Arthritis Rheum. 1985;28:1128–32.
42. Speight P, Kaul A, Melson R. Measurement of whole unstimulated saliva flow in the diagnosis of Sjögren's syndrome. Ann Rheum Dis. 1992;51:499–502.
43. Navazesh M. Methods of collecting saliva. Ann N Y Acad Sci. 1993;694:72–7.
44. Pennec Y, Letoux G, Leroy J, et al. Reappraisal of tests for xerostomia. Clin Exp Rheumatol. 1993;11:523–8.
45. Flink H, Tegelberg A, Lagerlöf F. Influence of the time of measurement of unstimulated whole salivary flow on the diagnosis of hyposalivation. Arch Oral Biol. 2005;50:553–9.
46. Sánchez-Guerrero J, Pérez-Dosal M, Celis-Aguilar E, et al. Validity of screening test for Sjögren's syndrome in ambulatory patients with chronic diseases. J Rheumatol. 2006;33:907–11.

Chapter 27
Diagnostic Procedures (II): Parotid Scintigraphy, Parotid Ultrasound, Magnetic Resonance, Salivary Gland Biopsy

Gabriela Hernández-Molina, Eric Kimura-Hayama, María del Carmen Ávila-Casado, and Jorge Sánchez-Guerrero

Contents

Salivary gland involvement is a hallmark of Sjögren's syndrome (SS). Besides the assessment of salivary gland function with objective tests such as sialometric methods, the analysis of gland specimens as well as some image methods are useful in the evaluation of these patients. For instance, the current American-European Consensus Group (AECG) criteria for SS [1] consider the performance of a labial salivary gland biopsy, salivary gland scintigraphy, and a sialography as tests to evaluate these patients. However, a standard algorithm for the evaluation of SS has not been established.

G. Hernández-Molina • J. Sánchez-Guerrero (✉)
Immunology and Rheumatology Department, Instituto Nacional de Ciencias Médicas y Nutrición Salvador Zubirán, Mexico City, Mexico

E. Kimura-Hayama
Tomography Department, Instituto Nacional de Cardiología Ignacio, Chávez, Mexico City, Mexico

M.C. Ávila-Casado
Department of Pathology, Instituto Nacional de Cardiología Ignacio, Chávez, Mexico City, Mexico

M. Ramos-Casals et al. (eds.), *Sjögren's Syndrome*,
DOI 10.1007/978-0-85729-947-5_27, © Springer-Verlag London Limited 2012

383

Herein, we describe these tests as well as other imaging methods that are used frequently in the evaluation of patients with possible SS.

27.1   Salivary Scintigraphy

The salivary gland scintigraphy is a simple, noninvasive method that provides a functional evaluation of saliva production. It measures the amount and speed of uptake and excretion of the four major salivary glands following an intravenous injection of $^{99}Tc^m$ pertechnetate [2]. Both the resting and the stimulated states are assessed. After the injection, the uptake and distribution in the salivary glands is evaluated during a variable time interval of 20–45 min (resting state). During the excretion phase, the tracer elimination 10–15 min following citrus stimulation is registered. Among patients with SS, the quantity of isotope recorded over the glands is generally reduced by at least 50%. Once the images have been obtained, visual inspection is performed to assess the pattern of salivary glands uptake and excretion (Fig. 27.1).

Patients can be classified according to a four category grading system proposed by Schall that varies from normal to very severe dysfunction (Table 27.1) [3]. Some readers score the highest value of both parotids and both submandibular glands together [4]. Others count only the maximum glandular value. Salivary gland scintigraphy has an overall sensitivity for SS of 71–87%, and a specificity of 78.9% [5, 6]. The submandibular glands are most commonly abnormal when assessed by scintigraphy [7–9]. Impaired excretion is usually present before a defect in tracer accumulation is evident.

Other qualitative measures such as time–activity curves [7], semiquantitative assessments [8], and quantitative indices have been developed in order to improve the study of SS patients. Quantitative indexes may identify mild degrees of glandular dysfunction. Some of these approaches include computer-assisted time–activity curves [10], the percent uptake of counts injected, gland-to-background ratio, uptake slope, time elapsed to peak counts, maximum-to initial count ratio, and gland-to-thyroid count ratio [2]. Despite the number of different approaches employed, there remains no consensus about their utility.

The classification 2002 AECG criteria for SS defines a positive salivary scintigraphy result as the presence of delayed uptake and reduced concentration and/or delayed excretion of tracer, without reference to any specific classification score [1]. One weakness of this definition is that scintigraphies in which the concentration of tracer within the gland and glandular excretion are practically absent are not considered strictly positive (Class 4 Schall grading system).

An ideal noninvasive measure of salivary gland function correlates with histopathologic findings. Some studies have demonstrated that the qualitative and quantitative characteristics of scintigraphic abnormalities progress in tandem with histopathologic grades of glandular damage [11–13]. One study found that patients with SS who presented with severe scintigraphic involvement (Class 4) had higher

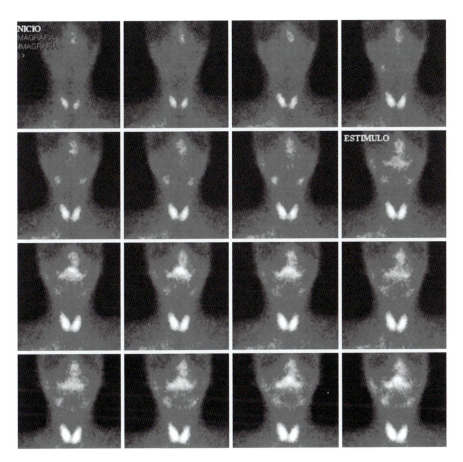

Fig. 27.1 Scintigraphy in a patient with Sjögren's syndrome. Impaired uptake of the nuclear tracer mainly in parotids glands. Absence of tracer elimination after gland stimulation

Table 27.1 Scintigraphy Schall´s grading system

Scale	Description
Normal	Rapid uptake, progressive increase in concentration in the first 10 min and prompt excretion within 20–30 min
Mild/moderate	Delayed uptake or oral excretion or both. At the end of the study, the oral activity is approximately equal to the tracer concentration in the gland
Severe	Tracer uptake is reduced and delayed, the oral activity is not always evident at the end of the study
Very severe	Concentration of tracer into the gland and excretion is practically absent

frequency of positivity for SS antibodies, extraglandular manifestations, lymphoma, and a lower survival rate [14]. That study also evaluated the results of a second parotid scintigraphy after a mean of 5 years in 40 patients with SS. The investigators reported that two-thirds of the patients had stabilized or improved, and one-third had worsened.

Scintigraphic abnormalities are not specific for SS. Patients with chronic sialad-enitis, drug-induced xerostomia, metabolic disorders, and radiation damage can also show evidence of impaired salivary function by scintigraphy. Some studies have attempted to find scintigraphic features that are specific for SS. A pilot study of SS patients and patients with isolated sicca symptoms found that a reversed parotid/submandibular uptake ratio, prolonged tracer uptake, and a reduced tracer secretion of the parotid glands characterized the SS patients and distinguished between the study groups [10]. Conversely, another study that compared patients with chronic sialadenitis and SS patients reported that even though SS patients are more likely to have multi-glandular involvement, biphasic kinetics defects, and more severe dysfunction, SS and chronic sialadenitis shared a number of features including a predilection for submandibular involvement [15].

In conclusion, salivary gland scintigraphy is a simple, noninvasive test that helps in the evaluation of salivary gland function in SS. Even though standard-ized quantitative indices have been proposed, however, the interpretation of scintigraphy results continues to be qualitative and observer-dependent. In addi-tion, most scintigraphic abnormalities are not specific for SS but rather can be seen in a variety of conditions with associated with salivary gland dysfunction.

27.2   Sialography

Digital subtraction sialography delineates the ductal system and traditionally has been considered the most reliable method of evaluating obstructive salivary disease and salivary gland involvement in SS. Positive sialographic findings correlate well with pathologic changes [16] and are included in a proposal for revised SS diagnostic criteria [1].

Sialographic staging of SS is based on the criteria of Rubin and Holt [17] obtained from lateral views. This criteria set divides findings into five categories: normal, punctate, globular, destructive, and cavitary (Table 27.2). The destructive and cavi-tary stages are considered to represent advanced disease. Sialographic findings cor-respond to the collection of contrast material within ductal and acinar dilatations [17]. The invasive nature of the method limits its widespread use and contraindi-cates its use in the presence of infection [16]. Moreover, duct cannulation is opera-tor dependent and stenosis of the ductal orifice may preclude the cannulation. The major advantage of sialography is that it facilitates minimally invasive interventions to remove calculi and repair ductal stenoses.

27.3   Ultrasound

Ultrasound is potentially an important tool for both diagnosis and longitudinal fol-low-up of salivary gland involvement in SS. The technique is inexpensive, swift to perform, widely available, and noninvasive. Moreover, it does not employ ionizing radiation. It also facilitates real-time image guidance for fine-needle aspiration cytology [16]. However, there are two substantial drawbacks to ultrasound. First,

Table 27.2 Sialographic findings in Sjögren's syndrome

Sialographic category	Stage of disease	Findings
1. Punctate	Earliest stage	Diffusely distributed, <1 mm in size, spherical collections within the gland. Main duct is normal in diameter
2. Globular	Intermediate stage	Larger collections (1–2 mm in size) with diffuse involvement of the gland due to acinar atrophy. Main duct still normal but intraglandular ducts are no longer seen
3. Destructive	Advanced stage	Coalescence of collections irregular in size and less in number. Main duct is deformed and dilated
4. Cavitary	Most advanced stage	Contrast material dissects into the subcapsular spaces. There is no recognizable branching pattern

the technique is highly operator dependent. Few ultrasonographers develop sufficient skill in examining patients with SS to deploy the technique effectively. Second, ultrasound is most effective for the parotid gland and is less helpful in evaluations of the submandibular and sublingual glands. In addition, ultrasonographers are sometimes unable to visualize the entire parotid gland because the gland is positioned behind the acoustic shadow of the mandible [18].

When imaging the parotid gland, usually a 5–12 MHz wide-band linear transducer is selected (median frequency of 7–7.5 MHz) with multiple focal zones. The gland is assessed in orthogonal planes both parallel and perpendicular relative to the Frankfurt horizontal plane of the parotid gland [18, 19]. For deeply located parotid lesions, an oral approach with an endocavitary probe or a fingertip transducer may be used. Normal gland parenchyma has a fine and homogeneous echogenicity, similar to the normal thyroid gland and hypoechoic compared to the surrounding soft tissue and muscles, but higher echogenicity can be observed in glands that are infiltrated by fat. The normal volume ranges from 13 to 15±4–5 mL or 20±3 mm in width. A normal, non-dilated Stenson's duct is usually not visible by ultrasound. Submandibular glands are smaller, with an average volume of 4.5±1.6 mL or 13±2 mm in width [18, 20]. Fine short bands might be seen representing the ductal and vessel wall and the normal fibrous septum; these lines run parallel to each other with a minimal distance of 1.4–2 mm between them [19]. The tissue within these lines is the normal lobules which are generally uniform in size.

The ultrasonographic findings most suggestive of SS are a non-homogenous salivary gland (corresponding to an early stage of disease); a coarse salivary gland with multiple hypoechoic areas (intermediate stage of disease); and the presence of echogenic lines that give the gland a reticular pattern (late stage of disease) [16, 21]. The hypoechoic zones, typically 2–5 mm in diameter, represent enlarged lobules caused by lymphocyte infiltration. The echogenic lines represent fibrosis and the accumulation of fat within the gland [19].

The sensitivities of hypoechoic zones and echogenic lines are quite low: 56% (95% CI 0.51–0.58) and 43% (95% CI 0.37–0.45), respectively [19]. The overall sensitivity of ultrasound in the diagnosis of SS ranges from 40% to 90% (average of

Table 27.3 Ultrasonographic grading of Sjögren's syndrome

Ultrasound category	Findings
Grade 0	Normal gland (see text for further description)
Grade 1	Normal or increased gland volume with regular contours and regular small hypoechoic areas, and ill-defined posterior gland border. No echogenic bands noticed
Grade 2	Grade 1 plus increased in number hypoechoic areas of variable size (<2 mm)
Grade 3	Irregular contour, multiple large circumscribed or confluent hypoechoic areas (2–6 mm) and/or multiple cysts, echogenic bands, normal or decreased gland volume, and non-visible posterior bland border
Grade 4	Grade 3 but hypoechoic areas are larger (>6 mm) and multiple calcifications might be seen

A 0–16 point scale is obtained by summing up the single scores (0–4) for each parotid and submandibular gland

63%) [20–23]. Parenchymal inhomogenicity identified by ultrasound correlates with the presence of serological markers of SS, including antinuclear antibodies and anti-Ro and/or anti-La antibody positivity in 97% of the cases. IgM RF positivity and hypergammaglobulinemia have been reported in 89% and 69% of patients with parenchymal inhomogenicity, respectively [20].

Many studies have proven the semiquantitative analysis of the parenchymal inhomogeneity by ultrasound scores to be a good method to evaluate the state of the parotid gland (Table 27.3) (Fig. 27.2) when compared to histologic analysis [24]. However, an ultrasound classification by grade is highly dependent upon the experience of the observer. Quantitative analysis studies on the texture of the gland have been reported to correlate well with sialographic findings [19, 22].

The submandibular glands have been noted by ultrasound to decrease in size by as much as 30% as SS progresses to advanced stages [20]. In contrast, correlations between parotid size and the diagnosis of SS appear to be poor. These findings are consistent with the knowledge that functional impairment of the submandibular glands in SS tends to be more severe than in the parotid glands.

Other uncommon ultrasonographic findings include dilatation of the main duct, increased parenchymal blood flow as seen by color/power Doppler, pseudo masses, ill-defined irregular cystic masses that might represent areas of previously formed abscesses, and intraparotid lymph node enlargement disease [18, 25]. Moreover, because SS is associated with an increased risk of neoplasic lymphoproliferative disease, ultrasound monitoring may be useful for the detection of lesions that exceed 2 cm or appear to be fast-growing on serial examinations [18]. There is diffuse hypervascularization in the acute setting; however, there is impairment of the salivary production in the chronic stage due to fibrosis with decreased arterial blood flow. The differential diagnosis by ultrasound of diffuse parotid swelling and hypoechoic focal areas includes chronic sialadenitis, sclerosing sialadenitis (Küttner tumor), abscesses, sialolithiasis, sarcoidosis, and other granulomatous sialadenitis, lymphoma, and parotitis (i.e., benign lymphoepithelial lesions) associated with the acquired immunodeficiency syndrome [18].

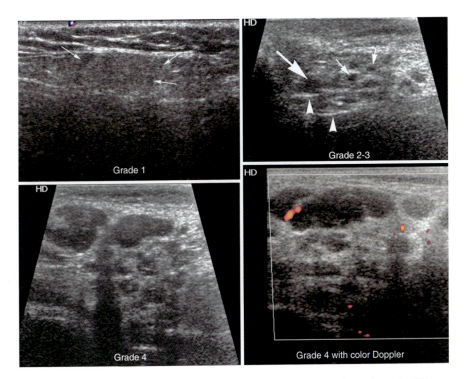

Fig. 27.2 Ultrasonographic images from different patients with Sjögren's syndrome in different grades of disease. In grade 1, a barely seen heterogeneous parenchyma is noted due to ill-defined and small hypoechoic areas (*arrows*). Conversely, in grade 2–3, these areas are larger [*small arrows* representing lesions <2 mm, and the *large arrow* a larger hypoechoic area (>6 mm)] and echogenic bands (*arrowheads*) representing fibrotic changes are seen. Finally, in grade 4, multiple large and irregular but with well-defined hypoechoic cystic cavities are easily demonstrated. There is no increase in vascularity with color Doppler

27.4 Tomography

Non-enhanced computed tomography (CT) scans can be employed when sialo-lithiasis is suspected (Fig. 27.3). CT examinations are helpful in distinguishing a single large stone from a cluster of stones [16]. Contrast-enhanced scans are indicated when complications such as abscess cannot be defined by ultrasound.

27.5 Magnetic Resonance

Magnetic resonance imaging (MRI) has emerged as a reliable, noninvasive modality that can demonstrate glandular changes. The main advantages of the method include its multiplanar capability, the use of non-ionizing radiation, and the high-contrast

Fig. 27.3 Fifty-six-year-old female with Sjögren's syndrome and an indurated palpable mass in the right parotid. The axial CT image demonstrates fatty infiltration of the left parotid with multiple tiny calcifications (sialolithiasis) (*arrows*) in the parenchyma. Conversely, notice the enlarged right parotid gland (*) with mildly heterogeneous density. When compared to MR Imaging (Fig. 27.4), CT has low tissue contrast resolution

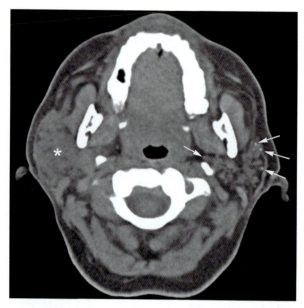

tissue resolution. MRI sialography has now largely replaced conventional sialography for evaluations of the duct system [26, 27].

MRI findings that are characteristic of SS include inhomogeneous internal pattern on both T1 and T2 sequences. This pattern, described as a "salt and pepper" or "honeycomb" appearance, represents areas of increased fat and decreases in intact lobules. Such a pattern is characterized by multiple hypo- and hyper-intense nodules of different sizes [26, 27] (Fig. 27.4). An MRI classification scheme for grading the structure of the parotid gland has been proposed (Table 27.4) [26]. Comparison studies between MRI and ultrasound have demonstrated good agreement (85%) in patients with primary SS, other patients with sicca symptoms without SS, and healthy controls [28, 29].

One investigation that validated MRI findings by comparison to histological analysis reported a sensitivity of 71% and a specificity of 100% for SS [30]. In another study that considered all MRI abnormalities (Grades 1–3) to be positive, the sensitivity of MRI was 100% and its specificity only 40%. The application of stricter criteria for a positive MRI study – grades 2 and 3 only – decreased the sensitivity to 88% but increased the specificity dramatically, to 100%. This discrepancy is explained by the fact that grade 1 MRI findings might be detected in normal subjects and patients with *sicca* symptoms who do not fulfill the criteria for SS [28].

Other MR modalities used in the evaluation of SS patients include MR sialography, functional MR sialography, and dynamic contrast-enhanced MRI. Dynamic, contrast-enhanced studies enable quantification of the microvascular characteristics of the gland [27].

In summary of the imaging section, there now exist many noninvasive imaging modalities for use in the assessment of salivary gland involvement in SS.

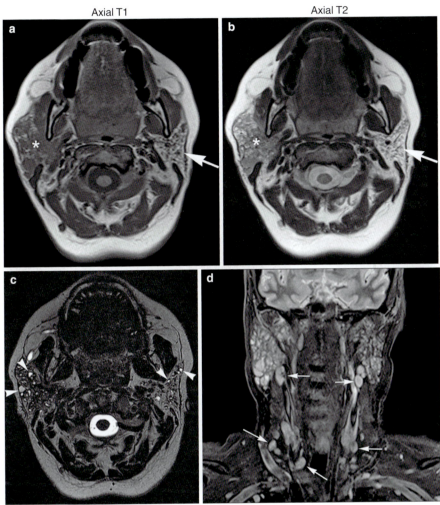

Fig. 27.4 Same patient as shown in Fig. 27.3. Axial T1w (**a**), T2w (**b**), T2w gradient echo (**c**), and coronal T2w (**d**) images showing heterogeneous intensity of parotid parenchyma, best seen in the right side (*** in **a** and **b**) with fatty infiltration of the left gland (*arrows* in **a** and **b**). There are multiple cystic lesions in both sides (*arrowheads* in **c**) and nonspecific lymph nodes in multiple levels of the head and neck (*arrows* in **d**)

Ultrasonography is a useful tool in the hands of an experienced operator. MRI can be used in lieu of ultrasound if there is not sufficient expertise with ultrasound. MRI is also useful when ultrasonographic studies have been negative, and when broader evaluation (e.g., for lymphadenopathy) is required in the setting of a tumor (Fig. 27.5). CT is mainly reserved for study of suspected sialolithiasis. It is likely that both ultrasound and MRI will find greater applications in the evaluation and care of patients with SS in the future.

Table 27.4 MRI classification
of Sjögren's syndrome
parenchymal abnormalities

MRI category	Findings
Grade 0	Normal gland with homogeneous parenchyma (intermediate signal intensity on both T1-weighted and T2-weighted, higher than the masseter muscle and lower than tissue)
Grade 1	Fine reticular or small nodular
Grade 2	Medium nodular
Grade 3	Coarsely nodular

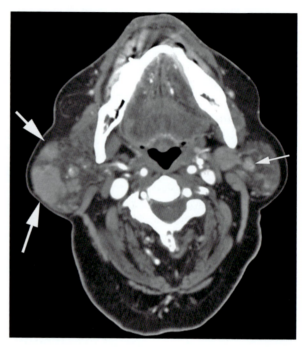

Fig. 27.5 Forty-five-year-old female with Sjögren's syndrome and a fast-growing mass in the right parotid that was originally followed up with ultrasound. Further evaluation with CT was requested. The contrast-enhanced axial CT image demonstrates at least two large (>2 cm) enhancing lesions (*large arrows*) in the right parotid. Notice the small intraparotid lymph node in the left side (*small arrow*). Histopathologic analysis revealed a non-malignant lymphoepithelial lesion

27.6 Salivary Gland Biopsy

Salivary biopsy is a common procedure in the assessment of SS. Histopathologic examination of the salivary glands offers the advantage of directly examining the affected organ. In addition, salivary gland biopsy is often essential to exclude SS mimickers such as sarcoidosis, amyloidosis, and chronic sclerosing sialadenitis (IgG4-related sialadenitis) [31].

27.6.1 Labial Gland Biopsy

Labial salivary gland biopsy is the hallmark of the diagnosis of SS. In order to obtain the specimens, various techniques have been described. Each has advantages and disadvantages.

27.6.2 Daniels' Technique

The biopsy specimen is obtained through mucosa that appears normal and should contain at least five labial salivary glands. Following local anesthesia with 2% xylocaine, a horizontal incision (1.5–2 cm) is made on the inner surface of the lower lip between the midline and the commissure. Incisions in the midline of the lip should be avoided because there are fewer labial salivary glands in that zone. Blunt dissection is performed and salivary glands are removed. Closure of the incision is performed with suture material [32].

Variations on this technique have been described. For instance: (a) palpation of the lower lip to locate the lip salivary glands (submucosal nodules) instead of simply performing a blind incision in a conventional location [33]; (b) leaving the incision open and allowing spontaneous healing [33, 34]; and (c) holding an ice-pack on the lip for 20 min after the procedure to achieve better hemostasis.

27.6.3 Punch Biopsy

This technique is also performed through normal-appearing mucosa of the lower lip. The lip is everted, anesthesia injected, and a 4-mm punch incision is made. The vermilion border of the lip should be avoided. The lip specimen is removed with an insulin needle. Patient is instructed to rinse her/his mouth. No suturing is required [35].

Short-term adverse events of the lip biopsy are local swelling (10%), local infection (4%), short-term local pain (25%), and long-term local numbness (1.7%). Among a cohort of 502 procedures, transient adverse events were reported in 13% of cases [36]. No permanent morbidity resulted from the procedure. Thus, minor salivary gland biopsy is simple, safe, reliable tool for the diagnosis of SS. However, under normal conditions, only two lower lip biopsies can be performed on an individual, therefore its use in clinical drug trials is limited [37].

27.6.4 Major Salivary Gland Biopsy

Parotid gland tissue can be harvested easily and repeated biopsies may be performed [38]. In addition, some authors have reported a better yield from parotid biopsies compared to minor labial salivary gland biopsies. However, parotid biopsy is usually not recommended because it may be associated with fistula formation, injuries to the facial nerve, and scarring.

In contrast to labial salivary glands, lymphoepithelial islands and well-formed lymphoid follicles or germinal centers are found easily in the major salivary glands. One study reported that lip biopsy identified 58% of patients with SS, compared with 100% of such patients confirmed by parotid gland biopsy [39]. On the other hand, another study of 15 SS patients with SS indicated similar sensitivities and specificities. Many patients experienced transient (6 months) hypoanesthesia of the preauricular region after parotid biopsy, but no sialoceles or fistulas were reported [38].

27.6.5 Lacrimal Gland Biopsy

The lacrimal glands are another major target organ of SS. However, complications of biopsies that might affect lacrimation or lead to hemorrhage or fistula formation have prevented the routine use of this biopsy. One study evaluated 32 subjects with SS with both labial and lacrimal gland biopsies. The authors found that epimyoepithelial islands and severe lymphocyte infiltration with germinal centers were observed only in lacrimal specimens. In addition, 19% of the cases failed to show early changes in labial salivary glands biopsies, indicating that lymphocytic infiltration in lacrimal glands may occur earlier and more extensively than in the labial gland [40].

27.6.6 Focus Score

The characteristic histopathologic feature of the labial salivary gland in SS is the presence of focal lymphocytic sialadenitis (Fig. 27.6) at most of the glands in the specimen. Thus, once the lip biopsy is obtained, the specimen is evaluated with a semiquantitative technique to assess sialadenitis, originally described by Chisholm and Manson in 1968. These authors reviewed lip biopsy specimens from 40 patients with rheumatologic diseases as well as 60 postmortem controls. They observed that the presence of more than one focus of lymphocytes per 4 mm^2 gland section was found only in patients with SS.

A focus is defined as a dense aggregate (round cell infiltrate) of 50 or more lymphocytes/plasma cells and macrophages in perivascular or periductal location [41]. In 1984, Daniels evaluating 362 lower lip biopsies concluded that a focus score >1 per 4 mm^2 tissue sample was indicative of SS [32]. The focus score correlates directly with the presence of keratoconjunctivitis sicca and inversely with the parotid flow rate [31].

For Daniels and colleagues, the finding of a focus score of exactly one may represent an early or mild form of the salivary component of SS [31]. Other grading systems (Table 27.5) besides the Chisholm–Manson scale (class I normal salivary gland with few lymphocytes to class IV [>1 lymphocyte foci]) [41] have been proposed. Greenspan et al. modified this system by recording the actual focus score. On the modified scale, which ranges from 0 (normal) to 12 (confluent infiltrates), a focus score of ≥2 is indicative of SS [42]. In the grading system of Tarpley, biopsies are classified as normal (Grade 0), with 1–2 focus (Grade 1), >2 focus (Grade 2), diffuse infiltrate + partial acinar destruction (Grade 3), and diffuse infiltrate + total acinar destruction with or without fibrosis (Grade 4). On that scale, classes 2, 3, and 4 are considered to be diagnostic of SS [43].

In 1993, a group of investigators of the European Community proposed preliminary criteria set for the classification of SS, where a focus ≥1 is considered a positive item [44]. They found a good balance between sensitivity (83.5%) and specificity (81.8%) when the presence of at least 1 focus was considered as indicative or SS. Conversely, when the cut-off value was raised to two or more foci, the sensitivity fell to 65% with only a slight increase of specificity (92.4%) [6].

Fig. 27.6 Nodular
lymphocytic infiltration in a
patient with Sjögren's
syndrome

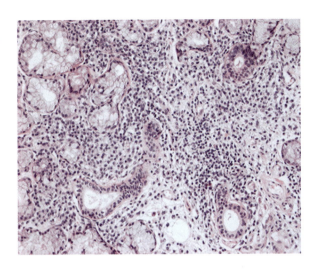

Table 27.5 Histopathologic
classification of minor
salivary gland biopsies

Chisholm and Manson classification	Greenspan classification	Tarpley classification
Grade 0 No infiltrate	Focus score 0	Class 0
Grade 1 Slight infiltrate	Focus score 0	Class 1
Grade 2 Moderate infiltrate but <1 focus	Focus score 0	Class 1
Grade 3 One focus	Focus score 1	Class 1
Grade 4	Focus score 2 (so on until 11 focus)	Class 2
>1 focus	Focus score 12 (confluent infiltrate)	>2 focus Class 3 Partial acinar destruction Class 4 Total acinar destruction

In a subsequent multicentre study, these investigators demonstrated that a focus score > 1 had a specificity similar to that obtained using a combination of four of the six items of the 1993 criteria set (96% vs. 93%) [45]. The sensitivity of labial salivary gland biopsy, however, was lower (68% vs. 97%). Thus, the current AECG criteria consider a focus score ≥1 as a major parameter for the diagnosis [1]; however patients should achieve other positive items (clinical or serologic) of the criteria, as well.

Several attempts to standardize the focus score methodology have been made, but demonstration of reproducibility has been challenging. A variety of factors may contribute to variability across pathologic evaluations of the same specimen, including non-homogenous distribution of the inflammatory infiltrates and the small size of some biopsy specimens. Small specimens (less than 5 glands) or those in which the glands remain embedded in a connective tissue block may lead to unreliable focus score values [32]. For instance, in a study that reevaluated lip biopsy specimens several years after the first assessment, the grading system had been applied incorrectly during the initial interpretation in 45% of specimens. This resulted in misdiagnoses in 10% of the cases and non-diagnoses in 34% [46]. Other studies have demonstrated that the grade of infiltration varied within the same biopsy depending on the depth of tissue examined. The lack of reproducibility and standardization with regard to the interpretation of labial salivary gland biopsies has hampered progress in SS [47].

A variety of strategies have been proposed to improve the reliability of salivary gland biopsies. Multiple tissue levels should be evaluated in order to maximize the number of foci, the glandular area, and the technical quality of the material. One expert group suggested that within a single 4 mm^2 biopsy, a minimum of three tissue levels separated by a minimum of 200 nm should be evaluated, thereby insuring the detection of independent foci on each section [48]. Another group suggested that the histopathological evaluation should be performed with multilevel sectioning as well as with the assessment of a cumulative focus score (cFS). Thus, for each patient, the total number of foci at all three levels and the total surface area measured at all levels are used to calculate this cFS. This approach in a study of 120 SS patients altered the baseline classification in 6% of the patients and increased the specificity of the AECG criteria from 84.5% to 94.4% [49].

Cigarette smoking has been linked with a reduced glandular focus score in lower lip biopsies of patients primary SS [50]. It has also been proposed that cigarette smoking reduces the production of anti-Ro and anti-La antibodies by lowering the accumulation of lymphocytes within salivary glands [50].

Finally, it must be remembered that focal sialadenitis can occur in conditions other than SS. Focal or diffuse inflammatory infiltration has been reported in cases of sialolithiasis cases [51], other connective tissue diseases, in the elderly, in chronic hepatitis C virus infections, and in sarcoidosis. Moreover, focus score >1 has been found in 15% of healthy asymptomatic volunteers without correlation with age, smoking, serologic findings, or salivary flow [52]. This type of infiltrate has also been reported in postmortem series of submandibular glands from subjects who had no clinical evidence of SS during life [53].

27.7   Is There an Alternative to Labial Salivary Gland Biopsy?

Some studies have sought to identify adequate surrogates of minor salivary gland biopsy in order to spare patients this invasive procedure. Subjects with both sicca symptoms and positive serology (elevated anti-SSA or anti-SSB) have been reported more likely to have strongly positive lip biopsies [54, 55]. Similarly, more widespread glandular inflammatory changes have been observed in the presence of multiple systemic extraglandular manifestations and disease-specific autoantibodies

[56, 57]. Two studies of patients with sicca symptoms reported that high serum levels of IgG were associated with biopsy results [58, 59]. Although the specificity and positive predictive values of elevated serum IgG were both 97%, the sensitivity was only 40%. Conversely, another study found that neither the symptoms nor the serology could predict the result of the biopsy [46].

In conclusion, biopsy of the minor salivary gland is valuable in the diagnosis of SS. However, the diagnosis requires additional findings, such as abnormal immunologic essays, the presence of keratoconjunctivitis sicca, and demonstration of salivary gland hypofunction. For some authors, patients who have typical presentations of SS, including positive assays for anti-Ro or –La antibodies, do not derive additional benefit from a lip biopsy. In contrast, labial salivary gland biopsy may contribute importantly to the evaluation of patients with equivocal symptoms and/or negative serological testing [54].

References

1. Vitali C, Bombardieri S, Jonsson R, et al. Classification criteria for Sjögren's Syndrome: a revised version of the European criteria proposed by the American-European Consensus group. Ann Rheum Dis. 2002;61:554–8.
2. Vivino F, Hermann G. Role of nuclear scintigraphy in the characterization and management of the salivary component of Sjögren's syndrome. Rheum Dis Clin North Am. 2008;34:973–86.
3. Shall G, Anderson L, Wolf R, et al. Xerostomia in Sjögren's syndrome: evaluation by sequential scintigraphy. JAMA. 1971;216:2109–16.
4. Vinagre F, Santos M, Prata A, et al. Assessment of salivary gland function in Sjögren's syndrome: the role of salivary gland scintigraphy. Autoimmun Rev 2009;8(8):672–6.
5. Pennec Y, Letoux G, Leroy J, et al. Reappraisal of tests of xerostomia. Clin Exp Rheumatol. 1993;11:523–8.
6. Vitali C, Moutsopoulos H, Bombardieri S, The European Study Group on Diagnostic Criteria for Sjögren's syndrome. The European Community Study Group on diagnostic criteria for Sjögren's syndrome. Sensitivity and specificity of tests for ocular and oral involvement in Sjögren's syndrome. Ann Rheum Dis. 1994;53:637–47.
7. Sugihara T, Yoshimura Y. Scintigraphic evaluation of the salivary glands in patients with Sjögren's syndrome. Int J Oral Maxillofac Surg. 1988;17:71–5.
8. Loutfi I, Nair M, Ebrahim A. Salivary gland scintigraphy: the use of semiquantitative analysis for uptake and clearance. J Nucl Med Technol. 2003;31:81–5.
9. Tensing E, Nordström D, Solovieva S, et al. Salivary gland scintigraphy in Sjögren's syndrome and patients with sicca symptoms but without Sjögren's syndrome the psychological profiles and predictors for salivary gland dysfunction. Ann Rheum Dis. 2003;62:964–8.
10. Henriksen A, Nossent H. Quantitative salivary gland scintigraphy can distinguish patients with primary Sjögren's syndrome during the evaluation of sicca symptoms. Clin Rheumatol. 2007;26:1837–41.
11. Daniels T, Powell M, Sylvester R, et al. An evaluation of salivary scintigraphy in Sjögren's syndrome. Arthritis Rheum. 1979;22:809–14.
12. Saito T, Fakuda H, Horikawa M, et al. Salivary gland scintigraphy with 99mTC-pertechnetate in Sjögren's syndrome: relationship to clinicopathologic features of salivary and lacrimal glands. J Oral Pathol Med. 1997;26:46–50.
13. Nishiyama S, Miyawaki S, Yoshinaga Y. A study to standardize quantitative evaluation of parotid gland scintigraphy in patients with Sjögren's syndrome. J Rheumatol. 2006;33:2470–4.
14. Ramos-Casals M, Brito-Zeron P, Perez-De-Lis M, et al. Clinical and prognostic significance of parotid scintigraphy in 405 patients with primary Sjögren's syndrome. J Rheumatol. 2010;37:585–90.

15. Hermann G, Vivino F, Goin J. Scintigraphic features of chronic sialadenitis and Sjögren's syndrome: a comparison. Nucl Med Commun. 1999;20:1123–32.
16. Madani G, Beale T. Inflammatory conditions of the salivary glands. Semin Ultrasound CT MR. 2006;27:440–51.
17. Rubin H, Holt M. Secretory sialography in diseases of the major salivary glands. AJR Am J Roentgenol. 1957;77:575–98.
18. Bialek EW, Jakubowski W, Zajkowski P, Szopinski KT, Osmolski A. US of the major salivary glands: anatomy and spatial relationships, pathologic conditions, and pitfalls. Radiographics. 2006;26:745–63.
19. Chikui T, Shimizu M, Kawazu T, Okamura K, Shiraishi T, Yoshiura K. A quantitative analysis of sonographic images of the salivary gland: a comparison between sonographic and sialographic findings. Ultrasound Med Biol. 2009;35:1254–64.
20. Wernicke D, Hess H, Gromnica-Ihle E, Krause A, Schmidt WA. Ultrasonography of salivary glands – a highly specific imaging procedure for diagnosis of Sjögren's syndrome. J Rheumatol. 2008;35:285–93.
21. Makula E, Pokorny G, Rajtar M, et al. Parotid gland ultrasonography as a diagnostic tool in primary Sjögren's syndrome. Br J Rheumatol. 1996;35:972–7.
22. Ariji Y, Ohki M, Eguchi K, et al. Texture analysis of sonographic features of the parotid gland in Sjögren's syndrome. AJR Am J Roentgenol. 1996;166:935–41.
23. Donets K, Takagi Y, Sumi M, Nakamura T. Sonography as a replacement for sialography for the diagnosis of salivary glands affected by Sjögren's syndrome (letter). Ann Rheum Dis. 2002;61:276–7.
24. Salaffi F, Argalia G, Carotti M, et al. Salivary gland ultrasonography in the evaluation of primary Sjögren's syndrome. Comparison with minor salivary gland biopsy. J Rheumatol. 2000;27:1229–36.
25. Martinoli C, Derchi LE, Solbiati L, Rizzatto G, Silvestri E, Giannoni M. Color Doppler sonography of the salivary glands. AJR Am J Roentgenol. 1994;163:933–41.
26. Spät M, Kruger K, Dresel S, et al. Magnetic resonance imaging of the parotid gland in patients with Sjögren's syndrome. J Rheumatol. 1991;18:1372–8.
27. Niemelä RA, Takalo R, Pääkkö E, et al. Ultrasonography in primary Sjögren's syndrome. A comparison with magnetic resonance imaging and magnetic resonance sialography of parotid glands. Rheumatology. 2004;43:875–9.
28. Makula E, Pokorny G, Kiss M, et al. The place of magnetic resonance and ultrasonographic examinations of the parotid gland in the diagnosis and follow-up of primary Sjögren's syndrome. Rheumatology. 2000;39:97–104.
29. El Miedany YM, Ahmed I, Mourad HG, et al. Quantitative ultrasonography and magnetic resonance imaging of the parotid gland: can they replace the histopathologic studies in patients with Sjögren's syndrome? Joint Bone Spine. 2004;71:29–38.
30. Valesini G, Gualdi GF, Priori R, et al. Magnetic resonance imaging of the parotid gland and the lip biopsy in the evaluation of xerostomy in Sjögren's syndrome. Scand J Rheumatol. 1994;23:103–6.
31. Daniels T, Whitcher J. Association of patterns of labial salivary gland inflammation with keratoconjunctivitis sicca. Arthritis Rheum. 1994;37:869–77.
32. Daniels T. Labial salivary gland biopsy in Sjögren's syndrome. Assessment as a diagnostic criterion in 362 suspected cases. Arthritis Rheum. 1984;27:147–8.
33. Friedman J, Miller E, Huszar M. A simple technique for minor salivary gland biopsy appropriate for use by rheumatologists in an outpatient setting. Clin Rheumatol. 2002;21:349–50.
34. Amigo M, Vidal M, Martinez-Lavin M. Minimally-invasive salivary gland biopsy technique. J Clin Rheumatol. 2007;8:236.
35. Guevara-Gutierrez W, Tlacuilo-Parra A, Minjares-Padilla L. Minor salivary gland punch biopsy for evaluation of Sjögren's syndrome. J Clin Rheumatol. 2001;7:401–2.
36. Caporali R, Bonacci E, Epis O, et al. Safety and usefulness of minor salivary gland biopsy: retrospective analysis of 502 procedures performed at a single center. Arthritis Rheum. 2008;59:714–20.

37. Manthorpe R. How should we interpret the lower lip biopsy finding in patients investigated for Sjögren's syndrome? Arthritis Rheum. 2002;47:114–5.
38. Pijpe J, Kalk W, van der Wal J, et al. Parotid gland biopsy compared with labial biopsy in the diagnosis of patients with primary Sjögren's syndrome. Rheumatology. 2007;46:335–41.
39. Segerber-Konttinen M. A postmortem study of focal adenitis in salivary and lachrymal glands. J Autoimmun. 1989;2:553–8.
40. Xu K, Katagiri S, Takeuchi T, Tsubota K. Biopsy of labial salivary glands and lachrymal glands in the diagnosis of Sjögren's syndrome. J Rheumatol. 1996;23:76–82.
41. Chisholm D, Manson D. Labial salivary gland biopsy in Sjögren's disease. J Clin Pathol. 1968;21:656.
42. Greenspan J, Daniels T, Talal N, et al. The histopathology of Sjögren's syndrome in labial salivary gland biopsies. Oral Surg Oral Med Oral Pathol. 1974;37:21–9.
43. Tarpley T, Anderson L, White C. Minor salivary gland involvement in Sjögren's syndrome. Oral Surg Oral Med Oral Pathol. 1974;37:64–73.
44. Vitali C, Bombardieri S, Moutsopoulos H, et al. Preliminary criteria for the classification of Sjögren's syndrome. Results of an EEC prospective concerted action. Arthritis Rheum. 1993;36:340–7.
45. Vitali C, Bombardieri S, Moutsopoulos M, et al. Assessment of the European classification criteria for Sjögren's syndrome in a series of clinically defined cases: results of a prospective multicentre study. Ann Rheum Dis. 1996;55:116–21.
46. Langerman A, Blair E, Sweiss N, et al. Utility of lip biopsy in the diagnosis and treatment of Sjögren's syndrome. Laryngoscope. 2007;117:1004–8.
47. Al-Hashimi I, Wright J, Cooley C, et al. Reproducibility of biopsy grade in Sjögren's syndrome. J Oral Pathol Med. 2001;30:408–12.
48. Scardina G, Spano G, Carini F, et al. Diagnostic evaluation of serial sections of labial salivary gland biopsies in Sjögren's syndrome. Med Oral Patol Oral Cir Bucal. 2007;12:E565–8.
49. Morbini P, Manzo A, Caporali R, et al. Multilevel examination of minor salivary gland biopsy for Sjögren's syndrome significantly improves diagnostic performance of AECG classification criteria. Arthritis Res Ther. 2005;7:R343–8.
50. Manthorpe R, Benoni C, Jacobsson L, et al. Lower frequency of focal lip sialadenitis (focus score) in smoking patients. Can tobacco diminish the salivary gland involvement as judged by histological examination and anti-SSA/Ro and anti-SSB/La antibodies in Sjögren's syndrome? Ann Rheum Dis. 2000;59:54–60.
51. Segerberg-Konttinen M. Focus score in sialolithiasis. Scand J Rheumatol. 1988;17:87–9.
52. Radfar L, Kleiner D, Fox P, et al. Prevalence and clinical significance of lymphocytic foci in minor salivary glands of healthy volunteers. Arthritis Rheum. 2002;47:520–4.
53. Segerber-Konttinen M, Konttinen Y, Bergroth V. Focus score in the diagnosis of Sjögren's syndrome. Scand J Rheumatol Suppl. 1986;61:47–51.
54. Bamba R, Sweiss N, Langerman A, et al. The minor salivary gland biopsy as a diagnostic tool for Sjögren's syndrome. Laryngoscope. 2009;119:1922–6.
55. Lee M, Rutka J, Slomovic A, et al. Establishing guidelines for the role of minor salivary gland biopsy in clinical practice for Sjögren's syndrome. J Rheumatol. 1998;25:247–53.
56. Gerli R, Muscat C, Giansanti M, et al. Quantitative assessment of salivary gland inflammatory infiltration in primary Sjögren's syndrome: its relationship to different demographic, clinical and serological features of the disorder. Br J Rheumatol. 1997;36:969–75.
57. Wise C, Woodruff R. Minor salivary gland biopsies in patients investigated for primary Sjögren's syndrome. A review of 187 patients. J Rheumatol. 1993;20:151–8.
58. Brennan M, Sankar V, Leakan R, et al. Risk factors for positive minor salivary gland biopsy findings in Sjögren's syndrome and dry mouth patients. Arthritis Rheum. 2002;4:189–95.
59. Govoni M, Trotta F, Cavazzini L. Risk factors for positive minor salivary gland biopsy findings in Sjögren's syndrome and dry mouth patients: something new? Arthritis Rheum. 2003;15(49):145–6.

Chapter 28
Immunological Tests in Primary Sjögren Syndrome

Soledad Retamozo, Pilar Brito-Zerón, Myriam Gandía, Lucio Pallarés, and Manuel Ramos-Casals

Contents

S. Retamozo • P. Brito-Zerón • M. Ramos-Casals (✉)
Spanish Group of Autoimmune Diseases (GEAS), Spanish Society of Internal Medicine (SEMI),
Sjögren Syndrome Research Group (AGAUR), Laboratory of Autoimmune Diseases Josep Font,
Institut d'Investigacions Biomèdiques August Pi i Sunyer (IDIBAPS),
Department of Autoimmune Diseases, ICMD Hospital Clínic, Barcelona, Spain

M. Gandía
Sjögren Syndrome Research Group (AGAUR), Laboratory of Autoimmune Diseases
Josep Font, Institut d'Investigacions Biomèdiques August Pi i Sunyer (IDIBAPS),
Department of Autoimmune Diseases, ICMD Hospital Clínic, Barcelona, Spain

Rheumatology Department, Hospital Puerta del Mar, Cadiz, Spain

L. Pallarés
Autoimmune Diseases Unit, Hospital Son Espases, Palma de Mallorca, Spain

M. Ramos-Casals et al. (eds.), *Sjögren's Syndrome*,
DOI 10.1007/978-0-85729-947-5_28, © Springer-Verlag London Limited 2012

Table 28.1 The immunological evaluation in Sjögren's syndrome

Test	Typical result
ANA	Positive in more than 80%
Rheumatoid factor	Positive in 40–50% of patients, often leading to diagnostic confusion with rheumatoid arthritis
Anti-ENA antibodies	Positive anti-SSA/Ro (30–60%) and anti-SSB/La (15–40%)
C3, C4, CH50	Complement levels are decreased in 10–20% of patients
Cryoglobulins	Present in 10–20% of patients
Other autoantibodies	Antimitochondrial antibodies (associated PBC)
	Antithyroid antibodies (associated thyroiditis)
	Anti-dsDNA (associated SLE)
	Anti-centromere (associated limited form of systemic sclerosis)
	Anti-CCP antibodies (associated RA)
	Antiphospholipid antibodies (associated APS in 10% of cases)

ANA antinuclear antibody, *ENA* extractable nuclear antigens, *PBC* primary biliary cirrhosis, *RA* rheumatoid arthritis, *SLE* systemic lupus erythematosus, *APS* antiphospholipid syndrome

Patients with primary Sjögren syndrome (SS) produce a wide variety of autoantibodies directed at specific nuclear or cytoplasmic antigens. In some cases, the target antigen is present within specific tissues (Table 28.1). B-lymphocyte hyperactivation, the most typical etiopathogenic abnormality of primary SS, accounts for these autoantibodies. Autoantibodies have traditionally been central to classification criteria for SS. The 1993 European Criteria [1] included the presence of one or more of the following four antibodies: antinuclear antibodies (ANA), rheumatoid factor, anti-SSA/Ro, and anti-SSB/La. However, in the 2002 Criteria [2], only anti-SSA/Ro and anti-SSB/La antibodies were included. Together with a positive salivary gland biopsy, the presence of these autoantibodies became mandatory criteria for the classification of primary SS.

Even so, the clinical significance of other autoantibodies against nuclear and nonnuclear antigens remains understudied in primary SS [3]. In addition, patients with primary SS sometimes demonstrate autoantibodies considered characteristic of other systemic autoimmune diseases. In most such cases, the clinical significance of this immunological overlap (if any) has not been established. Some studies have attributed the presence of certain autoantibodies merely to the B-cell hyperactivity that is characteristic of primary SS [4, 5]. In contrast, other studies have implied that the presence of such autoantibodies signals a predictive role and a greater likelihood for the emergence of an additional systemic autoimmune disease [6, 7].

28.1 Antinuclear Antibodies

ANA were found in more than 80% of our patients with primary SS, with nearly half having high titers (≥ 1/320). ANA, discovered during investigations of the LE cell phenomenon [8], have become a key immunological test for the diagnosis of systemic autoimmune diseases [1, 9]. Low titers are less significant than high titers [10]. Although positive ANA assays were not included in the 2002 Classification Criteria for SS, their role in the diagnosis of patients with suspected SS should be reconsidered for various reasons. First, ANA are the most frequently detected antibodies in primary SS, and their determination play a central role in differentiating SS from causes of sicca syndrome that do not relate to autoimmunity. Second, ANA were associated with various extraglandular and serological features of SS [11–13], including hypergammaglobulinemia, elevations in the erythrocyte sedimentation rate, and autoantibodies directed against extractable nuclear antigens (ENAs) [14]. Third, ANA titers ≥ 1/80 have an excellent positive predictive value (91%) for the classification of patients with primary SS according to the 2002 Criteria. Thus, a patient with xerostomia, xerophthalmia, positive ocular tests, positive parotid scintigraphy, and an ANA titer ≥ 1/80 should be classified as having primary SS, even in the absence of anti-SSA/Ro and anti-SSB/La antibodies, assuming the absence of a coexisting systemic autoimmune disease.

28.2 Anti-SSA/Ro and Anti-SSB/La Antibodies

ENAs are a heterogeneous group of ribonucleoproteins and nonhistone proteins that mediate different functions in nuclear metabolism. Anti-SSA/Ro, -SSB/La, -RNP, and -Sm autoantibodies are directed against small ribonucleoproteins, which are small constituents of cellular RNA [15].

Four molecular forms of the autoantigen Ro complex have been described: a Ro-lymphocyte peptide of 60 kDa, a Ro-erythrocyte peptide of 60 kDa peptide, a Ro-lymphocyte peptide of 52 kDa peptide, and a Ro-erythrocyte peptide of 54 kDa. The Ro complex is found in most tissues and cells (erythrocytes, platelets), with differences in structure and quantity across tissues, species, and embryonic development stages. The great majority of patients with primary SS have antibodies against the SSA/Ro or SSB/La antigens [16], and there is a close correlation between these autoantibodies and certain clinical features, including parotidomegaly [17, 18], lymphadenopathy [17], cutaneous vasculitis [18–21], neurologic disease [18–20], a focus score higher than 1 in salivary gland biopsy [12, 22], and serologic hallmarks such as the presence of hypergammaglobulinemia [17, 18, 21, 23], rheumatoid factor [18], and cryoglobulins [18]. Locht et al. [24] reported that the presence of anti-SSA/Ro and anti-SSB/La antibodies was a stronger predictor of internal organ involvement than was the presence of anti-SSA/Ro antibodies alone.

Although antibodies to the SSA/Ro and SSB/La antigens are characteristic of the most clinically and immunologically "active" subset of patients with primary SS, their use as mandatory criteria for primary SS would lead to the exclusion of some subsets of patients who are usually Ro/La negative (e.g., males, the elderly, and patients without extraglandular features) [16].

28.3   Antibodies Against Nonnuclear Antigens

In contrast to ANA, the clinical significance of antibodies directed against nonnuclear antigens has been little studied in primary SS. Nonnuclear antigens that are potentially relevant to systemic autoimmune conditions include antimitochondrial antibodies and anti-parietal cell antibodies, but an extensive list of other antibodies have also been investigated.

In 2006, the prevalence and clinical significance of these autoantibodies was studied in a large cohort of patients [25]. A variety of important observations were made. First, these antibodies are detected in primary SS at very different frequencies. As examples, anti-smooth muscle antibodies were detected most frequently. Anti-parietal cell antibodies were detected as often as were anti-SSB/La antibodies, but anti-LKM-1 antibody assays were negative in all patients. Despite the frequency of anti-parietal cell antibodies in SS, chronic atrophic gastritis and pernicious anemia are rare in this condition, being reported in only 2 of 380 patient in one study [26] and in less than a handful of other reports in the literature [27–29].

Second, the clinical significance of these autoantibodies directed against nonnuclear antigens differs from that of antibodies whose targets are nuclear antigens. In contrast to ANA, which are closely associated with extraglandular and laboratory features of SS, antibodies directed against nonnuclear antigens are mainly associated with organ-specific autoimmune diseases, particularly those associated with liver and thyroid autoimmune disease. However, it is important to note that many SS patients whose sera have autoantibodies "specific" for autoimmune liver or thyroid disease have no clinical evidence of dysfunction in these organs.

Third, there is a small subset of patients with primary SS and positive antimitochondrial antibodies (AMA) (8%), an immunological marker closely related to primary biliary cirrhosis (PBC) [30]. However, only 50% of our SS patients who had AMA demonstrated clinical or laboratory test evidence of liver disease. This suggests the existence of an incipient or incomplete PBC in some patients with primary SS.

28.4   Anti-DNA Antibodies

Few studies have analyzed the clinical significance of anti-DNA antibodies in patients with primary SS. Satoh et al. [7] described an elderly woman with primary SS who presented anti-Sm and anti-DNA antibodies prior to the development of systemic lupus erythematosus (SLE). Zufferey et al. [6] described the occurrence of SLE in two out of four primary SS patients in whom anti-DNA antibodies were detected between 2 and 11 years after the diagnosis of primary SS. In a study of 26 patients with primary SS who had anti-DNA autoantibodies [31], features of SLE included ANA positivity in all cases, leukopenia in 14 (54%), and articular involvement in 9 (35%). Other SLE features such as skin, renal, and central nervous disease were uncommon. After a median follow-up of nearly 6 years, 8 (31%) of the 26 SS patients with anti-dsDNA antibodies at baseline fulfilled 4 or more of the classification criteria for SLE and 10 (38%) fulfilled 3 criteria.

Manoussakis et al. [32] described the clinical characteristics of 26 patients with coexistence of SS and SLE. In comparison to patients with SLE, the SS-SLE patients were older and had a higher frequency of certain features (Raynaud's phenomenon, rheumatoid factor, and anti-SSA-Ro/SSB-La antibodies) but a lower frequency of others (glomerulonephritis and thrombocytopenia). Autoantibodies were not useful in distinguishing between SLE and SS-SLE patients. The clinical presentations of the two patient groups were similar. The substantial overlap in the clinical and serologic features of primary SS and SLE, and the consequent difficulties in using classification criteria to distinguish between them have been emphasized [33]. Thus, there seems to be a fine line separating primary SS and SS-SLE in patients older than 50 years [33, 34], since the main SLE-related features found in SS-SLE patients (ANA, articular involvement, and cytopenias) are also frequently found in primary SS [17, 27, 35–37]. Because some SS-DNA patients develop overlapping SLE over time, we suggest including anti-DNA antibodies in the immunological follow-up of patients with primary SS, especially in those with articular involvement or leukopenia.

28.5 Anti-Sm Antibodies

Anti-Sm antibodies are rarely found in patients with primary SS. To date, only nine cases are reported in the literature [6, 7, 31]. After a mean follow-up of nearly 5 years, the previously reported three SS-Sm patients developed SLE, while five out of our six SS-Sm+patients [31] presented an SLE-like disease with the fulfillment of three criteria (four presented cytopenia and one arthritis in addition to the two immunological criteria, ANA and anti-Sm). All nine SS-Sm patients had negative anti-DNA antibodies. These studies suggest that anti-Sm antibodies are an infrequent immunological event, and thus we do not recommend including anti-Sm antibodies in the routine immunological follow-up of patients with primary SS. However, we recommend a close follow-up of patients with primary SS with positive Sm antibodies, in order to detect clinical and/or analytical data suggesting the development of an additional systemic autoimmune disease, and thus, an evolution from a single autoimmune disease (primary SS) to an overlap syndrome (SS associated with SLE).

28.6 Anti-RNP Antibodies

A small number of patients with primary SS have anti-RNP antibodies (<2% of patients). In one study of eight anti-RNP antibody-positive patients who had primary SS, none fulfilled the classification criteria for mixed connective tissue disease (MCTD) [31]. However, some patients demonstrated various components of these criteria, such as Raynaud's phenomenon or synovitis. Several studies have analyzed anti-RNP antibodies in small series including patients with primary and associated SS and found a prevalence ranging between 8% and 28% [38–42]. In contrast, a recent study analyzed 55 patients with MCTD and found sicca symptoms in 23 (42%) patients and positive anti-SSA/Ro in 18 (33%) [43]. Thus, overlap syndromes between SS and MCTD occur in some patients.

28.7 Antiphospholipid Antibodies

Antiphospholipid antibodies (aPL) are the most frequently detected atypical autoantibodies in primary SS (Table 28.2). One study reported a total of 134 patients with aPL [31]. In spite of the frequency with which aPL are detected, the fully expressed antiphospholipid syndrome (APS) occurs in only a minority of primary SS patients. Only 13 (10%) SS-aPL patients presented thrombotic events, 12 (9%) had thrombocytopenia, 8 (6%) had histories of fetal loss, 2 (1.5%) had livedo reticularis, and 1 (1%) had hemolytic anemia. Only 12 (9%) of the 134 SS-aPL patients fulfilled the 1999 APS classification criteria [44].

Most experts regard aPL as nonspecific immunological markers in patients with primary SS, analysis of the clinical and immunological features of these 134 patients shows potentially greater clinical relevance than previously supposed. First, these patients presented with aPL profiles that differ from those of patients with fully expressed APS, with very infrequent detection of IgM anticardiolipin antibodies [45–47]. Second, in one-quarter of these SS-aPL patients, a heterogeneous spectrum of APS-related manifestations was observed, including patients with a prothrombotic history but only one isolated positive aPL determination; patients with hematological features (mainly thrombocytopenia and, more infrequently, hemolytic anemia); and patients with aPL but with obstetric complications not included in the current classification criteria (e.g., fewer than three fetal losses).

Although only 3% of patients with primary SS have associated APS, aPL are detected in nearly 25%. In contrast, aPL are detected in 43% of SLE patients [48] and while 15% of SLE patients fulfill the APS classification criteria [48, 49].

Table 28.2 Prevalence of atypical immunological markers in patients with primary SS [31]

Atypical antibodies	Patients (positive/tested)	Prevalence
Antiphospholipid antibodies	120/589	20.4%
ANCA	43/357	12%
ACA	11/137	8%
Anti-CCP	11/166	6.6%
Anti-DNA	34/718	4.7%
Anti-RNP	34/782	4.3%
Anti-Scl70	2/92	2.2%
Anti-Sm	8/457	1.7%

Haga et al. [50] found an incidence of 1.44 thromboembolic events per 100 patients-years in SS patients, which was lower than that reported for SLE patients [51]. Fauchais et al. [4] found that positive aPL was closely related to the presence of hypergammaglobulinemia and that SS-aPL patients had a high frequency of organ-specific autoimmune diseases associated with SS (thyroid disease, primary biliary cirrhosis, autoimmune thrombocytopenic purpura). The presence of cerebral white matter lesions in MRI did not correlate with positive aPL.

In summary, the coexistence of primary SS and APS should be considered an infrequent (but not exceptional) event that occurs in approximately 10% of primary SS patients who have aPL. We do not recommend routine aPL determination in patients with primary SS except in those with specific clinical (thrombosis or repeated miscarriages) or laboratory (thrombocytopenia, hemolytic anemia) features consistent with APS.

28.8 Anti-Scl70 Antibodies

We have described two patients with primary SS and anti-Scl70 or anti-topoisomerase I antibodies [31]. No previous studies have analyzed the prevalence and clinical significance of these autoantibodies in patients with primary SS, with only two isolated cases being reported in patients with coexisting SS and SLE [52]. None of these four patients presented clinical features suggestive of SSc. However, clinicians should be aware of the possibility of the development of scleroderma features in patients who have these autoantibodies.

28.9 Anticentromere Antibodies

In contrast to anti-Slc70 antibodies, anticentromere antibodies (ACA) seem to have a higher prevalence and greater clinical significance in patients with primary SS, with a total of 48 cases being reported [31, 53–57]. A combined analysis of these 48 patients suggests the frequent expression of a specific clinical phenotype. An analysis of the 38 well-described SS-ACA patients showed Raynaud's phenomenon and telangiectasias, observed in 61% of the patients, to be the predominant clinical features. The principal immunological findings were comprised of high titers of ANA but a relatively low prevalence of rheumatoid factor (28%) and anti-SSA/Ro antibodies (7%). During the follow-up, limited SSc emerged in 7 (25%) of the 28 patients, with the appearance of typical cutaneous signs and sclerodactylia.

Salliot et al. [58] reported a prevalence of anticentromere antibodies of 4.7% in patients with primary SS. In general, these patients did not fulfill the classification criteria for SSc but had a higher prevalence of Raynaud's phenomenon, peripheral neuropathy, and other autoantibodies or autoimmune diseases – especially primary biliary cirrhosis – compared to patients without anticentromere antibodies.

We recommend routine testing for ACA in patients with primary SS who have Raynaud's phenomenon, especially in patients with high titers of ANA and negative anti-Ro/La antibodies. A substantial portion of such patients are at risk for the development of coexistent limited SSc. Close inspection on physical examination for incipient cutaneous changes that suggest limited SSc, particularly a nailfold capillaroscopic analysis, is essential. In addition, SS-ACA patients should be monitored closely for the development of gastrointestinal or pulmonary manifestations that commonly complicate SSc.

28.10 Anti-neutrophil Cytoplasmic Antibodies (ANCA)

A total of 59 patients with primary SS and positive ANCA have been reported [31]. The potential clinical significance of these autoantibodies in patients with primary SS are defined by three points: the prevalence of the different immunofluorescence patterns and enzyme immunoassay specificities; the association of these autoantibodies with specific extraglandular features of SS; and the overlap with systemic vasculitis.

ANCA were detected in 36 (19%) of 194 primary SS patients included in 4 previous studies [59–62] but only 6% in another study [31]. Eighty percent of the patients with positive immunofluorescence assays for ANCA demonstrated a perinuclear (p-ANCA) pattern. An additional 19% of the patients showed atypical patterns of immunofluorescence, and only one patient (<1%) had cytoplasmic (c-ANCA) patterns [63]. The ANCA specificities, analyzed in 20 patients by enzyme immunoassay, were reported to be myeloperoxidase in 15 cases [59, 64–67], lactoferrin in 4 cases [59], and proteinase-3 in 1 case [63].

The clinical characteristics of SS-ANCA patients, in 19 of the 59 cases, included a high prevalence of such extraglandular features as Raynaud's phenomenon and pulmonary disease, necrotizing crescentic glomerulonephritis, peripheral neuropathy, or cutaneous vasculitis in 20–30% of patients. SS-ANCA patients had a high prevalence of other autoantibodies: 71% had high titers of ANA, anti-SSA/Ro and –SSB/La antibodies, and/or rheumatoid factor.

Coexistent systemic vasculitis develops in only a small number of patients. One of our patients developed an associated microscopic polyangiitis [31]; two similar cases have been previously reported [63, 68]. Radaeli et al. described the coexistence of primary SS and microscopic polyangiitis in a 72-year-old woman with ulcerative jejunitis [68]. Young et al. [63] described a patient with primary SS, cavitary lung disease, and ANCA directed against proteinase 3 and causing a c-ANCA pattern of immunofluorescence, all highly consistent with Wegener's granulomatosis.

The clinical significance of ANCA in patients with primary SS can be summarized by an overwhelming prevalence of the p-ANCA pattern. However, antibodies directed against myeloperoxidase are found in less than 20% of cases. There is a high frequency of extraglandular and immunological features among these patients, but true ANCA-associated vasculitis emergences in only a minority of the cases. Thus, there appears to be little utility to the routine determination of ANCA in patients with primary SS, and ANCA testing should be reserved for those in whom a high index of suspicion for a true "pauci-immune" form of systemic vasculitis exists.

28.11 Anti-citrullinated Antibodies

Antibodies to cyclic citrullinated peptides (CCP) are highly specific for the diagnosis of rheumatoid arthritis (RA) (95%) and have a sensitivity for RA that is on the order of 65% [69, 70]. Recent studies suggest that anti-CCP and anti-keratin antibodies are useful in discriminating SS patients with coexisting RA from those with primary SS. Goeb et al. found anti-CCP autoantibodies in only 4% of 137 women and 16% of 11 men with SS [71]. In a study of 134 patients with primary SS, Gottenberg et al. [72] found anti-CCP antibodies in 7.5% and anti-keratin antibodies in 5.2%. Other studies have confirmed that anti-CCP and anti-keratin antibodies occur in a minority of patients with primary SS, with or without evidence of erosive arthritis [73–76]. The presence of erosive arthritis and either anti-CCP or anti-keratin antibodies in a patient with primary SS likely signals the co-occurrence of two diseases, primary SS and rheumatoid arthritis.

28.12 Rheumatoid Factor and Cryoglobulins

Rheumatoid factor is the second most frequently detected antibody in patients with primary SS after ANA (40–60%). Patients with rheumatoid factor positivity show a higher frequency of extraglandular and immunological features including articular involvement, cutaneous vasculitis, ANA, and anti-SSA/Ro. The results in larger studies support a key role of rheumatoid factor in the diagnosis of primary SS because this immunological marker has an independent association with most of the main clinical and immunological features of the disease [22, 77–79]. Thus, rheumatoid factor is a useful immunological test for the diagnosis of some subsets of patients with primary SS, such as those with extraglandular manifestations or with circulating cryoglobulins.

The clinical significance of cryoglobulinemia in primary SS is threefold. First, cryoglobulins are associated with a higher prevalence of extraglandular disease [79–82]. Second, patients with cryoglobulinemia are at a higher risk of B-cell lymphoma than are those who do not have cryoglobulins [79]. Third, there is a close association between cryoglobulinemia and life-threatening vasculitis. In one study, all of the primary SS patients with small-vessel vasculitis who died presented with cryoglobulinemic vasculitis [76]. Thus, the finding of cryoglobulinemia in a patient with primary SS is a marker for enhanced risks of lymphoproliferative disease, vasculitis, and early mortality.

28.13 Complement

The complement system, a group of individual proteins that act sequentially to form enzyme cascades, is activated by three pathways: the classical, alternative, and mannose-binding protein pathways. Complement activation is usually assessed by determinations of levels of individual complement components, e.g., C3 and C4, and by the quantification of the CH50 activity, which reflects the sequential interaction of all the components of the classical and alternative pathways. The routine measurement of the serum complement profile (C3, C4, and CH50) is an important clinical tool in the management of some systemic autoimmune diseases. The best example is SLE, a disease in which hypocomplementemia correlates closely with disease activity in some patients [83]. However, the clinical significance of hypocomplementemia in systemic autoimmune diseases other than SLE has been little studied. In patients with primary SS, there is growing interest in the clinical significance of low complement levels due to recent studies that have associated low C4 levels with lymphoma development [36] and mortality [37, 84].

In patients with primary SS, hypocomplementemia is found in 10–25% of patients [36, 37, 84, 85], although the prevalence of low C3 or C4 levels varied according to the study. Skopouli et al. [36] detected low C3 levels in 4 (2%) and low C4 levels in 44 (17%) out of 261 Greek patients, while Ioannidis et al. [84] found low C3 in 17 (3%) and low C4 in 122 (20%) out of 601 Greek patients from a multicenter study. Recently, Theander et al. [37] described low C3 levels in 98 (25%) and low C4 levels in 105 (27%) out of 386 Swedish patients. These differences may be related to the different classification criteria used, the cut-off levels of the complement assays, or other differences in the study design.

The role of hypocomplementemia in the clinical expression of primary SS has not been analyzed thoroughly. Previous studies have described an association between hypocomplementemia and either neurological [86] or renal [87] involvement. We found a significant association between low complement levels and systemic SS features, including both extraglandular disease (fever, articular involvement, cutaneous vasculitis, and peripheral neuropathy) and immunological markers (cryoglobulinemia, rheumatoid factor) [88]. These features are typical of the clinical and immunological expression of cryoglobulinemic vasculitis, suggesting an important role for cryoglobulinemia in the systemic expression of SS in patients with hypocomplementemia. Cryoglobulinemia and hypocomplementemia are closely related immunological markers that suggest systemic involvement in patients with primary SS.

Hypocomplementemia is also closely associated with the two main adverse outcomes of primary SS (lymphoma development and death). We found that lymphoma was associated with low C3, C4, and CH50 levels in a univariate analysis, although only low C4 levels were an independent risk factor for these outcomes in the multivariate analysis [88]. This close association was also described in a recent multicenter study by Ioannidis et al. [84], who found a higher risk of lymphoproliferative disease among prevalent cases of primary SS than among incident cases, and also reported that low C4 levels were an independent predictor of lymphoproliferative disease in multivariate modeling.

Theander et al. found that patients with low C4 levels had an increased cause-specific standardized mortality ratio for lymphoproliferative disease and an increased hazard ratio for death compared with patients with normal C4 levels [37]. This close association between hypocomplementemia and lymphoma might be related directly to the presence of cryoglobulinemia. Tzioufas et al. were the first to demonstrate that mixed cryoglobulinemia was a predictive laboratory factor for lymphoma development in SS [79]. However, the studies by Theander and Ioannidis on mortality in primary SS patients did not analyze cryoglobulinemia at protocol entry [37, 84]. Prospective studies including both markers are needed to define their joint or independent value as predictive factors for lymphoma development in patients with primary SS. In addition, we found that low complement levels are prospectively associated with a higher risk of mortality in patients with primary SS [88]. This confirms the results of Ioannidis et al. [84] who showed that low C4 levels were an independent predictor of mortality, and Theander et al. [37] who described a similar association with low C3 and C4 levels.

Persistent, repeated, unquantifiable complement levels were infrequently observed in patients with primary SS, suggesting that acquired hypocomplementemia (rather than heritable complement deficiencies) are the main cause of low complement values in most patients. In one study of 336 patients, two (0.6%) were reported to have possible homozygous C4 deficiencies [88]. Both patients had serum C4 levels that were persistently below 0.07 g/L. The existence of possible inherited complement deficiencies in primary SS has been very little studied [89], with isolated cases also being reported [90, 91].

28.14 Conclusion

In conclusion, a great heterogeneity in the immunological presentation of primary SS is often observed, including the presence of multiple autoantibodies against both nuclear and nonnuclear antigens. ANA play a central role in the immunological expression of primary SS because of their frequency, their association with clinical SS features, and their close association with autoantibodies directed against ENA. Anti-SSA/Ro and Anti-SSB/La antibodies are related closely to the extraglandular expression of primary SS and identify the most clinically and immunologically "active" subset of primary SS patients. The presence of some antibodies directed against nonnuclear antigens, e.g., antimitochondrial antibodies, suggests an association between primary SS and other organ-specific autoimmune diseases, specifically primary biliary cirrhosis. For other antibodies directed against nonnuclear antigens, e.g., parietal cell antibodies and smooth muscle antibodies, the associations are less clear or even believed to be of little or no clinical significance.

Testing for atypical autoantibodies may be helpful in diagnosing a possible overlap between primary SS and other systemic autoimmune disease. Although patients with atypical autoantibodies are often classified initially as having primary SS (most of them also fulfilling the more restrictive 2002 classification criteria), 20% fulfilled classification criteria for an additional systemic autoimmune disease during follow-up. The risk of developing an additional systemic autoimmune disease differed according to the atypical autoantibody present at the diagnosis of "primary" SS. Patients having anti-DNA or anti-centromere antibodies are at higher risk of developing an additional disease and require closer follow-up in order to detect clinical and/or analytical data suggestive of coexisting SLE or SSc.

References

1. Vitali C, Bombardieri S, Moutsopoulos HM, Balestrieri G, Bencivelli W, Bernstein RM, et al. Preliminary criteria for the classification of Sjogren's syndrome. Arthritis Rheum. 1993;36: 340–7.
2. Vitali C, Bombardieri S, Jonsson R, Moutsopoulos HM, Alexander EL, Carsons SE, et al. Classification criteria for Sjogren's syndrome: a revised version of the European criteria proposed by the American-European Consensus Group. Ann Rheum Dis. 2002;61:554–8.
3. García-Carrasco M, Ramos-Casals M, Font J, Vives J. Interpretación de las pruebas inmunológicas en el síndrome de Sjögren. In: Ramos-Casals M, García-Carrasco M, Anaya JM, Coll J, Cervera R, Font J, Ingelmo M, editors. Síndrome de Sjögren. Barcelona: Masson; 2003. p. 445–66.
4. Fauchais AL, Lambert M, Launay D, Michon-Pasturel U, Queyrel V, Nguyen N, et al. Antiphospholipid antibodies in primary Sjogren's syndrome: prevalence and clinical significance in a series of 74 patients. Lupus. 2004;13:245–8.
5. Cervera R, Garcia-Carrasco M, Font J, Ramos M, Reverter JC, Munoz FJ, et al. Antiphospholipid antibodies in primary Sjogren's syndrome: prevalence and clinical significance in a series of 80 patients. Clin Exp Rheumatol. 1997;15:361–5.
6. Zufferey P, Meyer OC, Bourgeois P, Vayssairat M, Kahn MF. Primary Sjögren syndrome preceding systemic lupus erythematosus: a retrospective study of 4 cases in a cohort of 55 SS patients. Lupus. 1995;4:23–7.
7. Satoh M, Yamagata H, Watanabe F, Nakayama S, Ogasawara T, Tojo T, et al. Development of anti-Sm and anti-DNA antibodies followed by clinical manifestation of systemic lupus erythematosus in an elderly woman with long-standing Sjogren's syndrome. Lupus. 1995;4:63–5.
8. Hollingsworth PN, Pummer SC, Dawkins RL. Antinuclear antibodies. In: Peter JB, Shoenfeld Y, editors. Antibodies. Amsterdam: Elsevier; 1996. p. 74–90.
9. Hochberg MC. Updating the American College of Rheumatology revised criteria for the classification of systemic lupus erythematosus. Arthritis Rheum. 1997;40:1725.
10. Adams BB, Mutasim DF. The diagnostic value of anti-nuclear antibody testing. Int J Dermatol. 2000;39:887–91.
11. Asmussen K, Andersen V, Bendixen G, et al. A new model for classification of disease manifestations in primary Sjögren's syndrome. J Intern Med. 1996;239:475–82.
12. Wise CM, Woodruff RD. Minor salivary gland biopsies in patients investigated for primary Sjögren's syndrome. A review of 187 patients. J Rheumatol. 1993;20:1515–8.
13. Shah F, Rapini RP, Arnett FC, Warner NB, Smith CA. Association of labial salivary gland histopathology with clinical and serologic features of connective tissue diseases. Arthritis Rheum. 1990;33:1682–7.
14. Ramos-Casals M, Brito-Zerón P, Font J. The overlap of Sjögren's syndrome with other systemic autoimmune diseases. Semin Arthritis Rheum. 2007;36(4):246–55.

15. Wenzel J, Gerdsen R, Uerlich M, Bauer R, Bieber T, Boehm I. Antibodies targeting extractable nuclear antigens: historical development and current knowledge. Br J Dermatol. 2001;145: w859–67.
16. Garcia-Carrasco M, Ramos-Casals M, Rosas J, Pallares L, Calvo-Alen J, Cervera R, et al. Primary Sjogren syndrome: clinical and immunologic disease patterns in a cohort of 400 patients. Medicine (Baltimore). 2002;81:270–80.
17. Davidson BKS, Kelly CA, Griffiths ID. Primary Sjogren's syndrome in the North East of England: a long-term follow-up study. Rheumatology (Oxford). 1999;38:245–53.
18. Moutsopoulos HM, Zerva LV. Anti-Ro (SS-A)/La (SS-B) antibodies and Sjogren's syndrome. Clin Rheumatol. 1990;9 Suppl 1:123–30.
19. Alexander EL, Arnett FC, Provost TT, Stevens MB. Sjogren's syndrome: association of anti-Ro (SS-A) antibodies with vasculitis, hematologic abnormalities and serologic hyperreactivity. Ann Intern Med. 1983;98:155–9.
20. Alexander EL, Provost TT, Stevens MB, Alexander GE. Neurologic complications of primary Sjogren's syndrome. Medicine (Baltimore). 1982;61:247–57.
21. Harley JB, Alexander EL, Bias WB, et al. Anti-Ro(SS-A) and anti-La(SS-B) in patients with Sjogren's syndrome. Arthritis Rheum. 1986;29:196–206.
22. Manoussakis MN, Tzioufas AG, Pange PJ, Moutsopoulos HM. Serological profiles in subgroups of patients with Sjogren's syndrome. Scand J Rheumatol. 1986;61:89–92.
23. Markusse HM, Veldhoven CH, Swaak AJ, Smeenk RT. The clinical significance of the detection of anti-Ro/SS-A and anti-La/SS-B autoantibodies using purified recombinant proteins in primary Sjogren's syndrome. Rheumatol Int. 1993;13:147–50.
24. Locht H, Pelck R, Manthorpe R. Clinical manifestations correlated to the prevalence of autoantibodies in a large (n = 321) cohort of patients with primary Sjögren's syndrome: a comparison of patients initially diagnosed according to the Copenhagen classification criteria with the American-European consensus criteria. Autoimmun Rev. 2005;4:276–81.
25. Nardi N, Brito-Zerón P, Ramos-Casals M, et al. Circulating auto-antibodies against nuclear and non-nuclear antigens in primary Sjögren's syndrome: prevalence and clinical significance in 335 patients. Clin Rheumatol. 2006;25:341–6.
26. Ramos-Casals M, Font J, Garcia-Carrasco M, et al. Primary Sjogren syndrome: hematologic patterns of disease expression. Medicine (Baltimore). 2002;81:281–92.
27. Wegelious O, Fyhrquist F, Adner PL. Sjogren's syndrome associated with vitamin B12 deficiency. Acta Rheumatol Scand. 1970;16:184–90.
28. Williamson J, Paterson RW, McGavin DD, Greig WR, Whaley K. Sjogren's syndrome in relation to pernicious anaemia and idiopathic Addison's disease. Br J Ophthalmol. 1970;54:31–6.
29. Pedro-Botet J, Coll J, Tomás S, Soriano JC, Gutiérrez Cebollado J. Primary Sjogren's syndrome associated with chronic atrophic gastritis and pernicious anemia. J Clin Gastroenterol. 1993;16:146–8.
30. Talwalkar JA, Lindor KD. Primary biliary cirrhosis. Lancet. 2003;362(9377):53–61.
31. Ramos-Casals M, Nardi N, Brito-Zeron P, et al. Atypical autoantibodies in patients with primary Sjogren syndrome: clinical characteristics and follow-up of 82 cases. Semin Arthritis Rheum. 2006;35:312–21.
32. Manoussakis MN, Georgopoulou C, Zintzaras E, et al. Sjogren's syndrome associated with systemic lupus erythematosus: clinical and laboratory profiles and comparison with primary Sjogren's syndrome. Arthritis Rheum. 2004;50:882–91.
33. Isenberg DA. Systemic lupus erythematosus and Sjogren's syndrome: historical perspective and ongoing concerns. Arthritis Rheum. 2004;50:681–3.
34. Bell DA. SLE in the elderly – is it really SLE or systemic Sjogren's syndrome? J Rheumatol. 1988;15:723–4.
35. Ramos-Casals M, Anaya JM, Garcia-Carrasco M, et al. Cutaneous vasculitis in primary Sjogren syndrome: classification and clinical significance of 52 patients. Medicine (Baltimore). 2004;83:96–106.
36. Skopouli FN, Dafni U, Ioannidis JP, Moutsopoulos HM. Clinical evolution, and morbidity and mortality of primary Sjogren's syndrome. Semin Arthritis Rheum. 2000;29:296–304.

37. Theander E, Manthorpe R, Jacobsson LT. Mortality and causes of death in primary Sjogren's syndrome: a prospective cohort study. Arthritis Rheum. 2004;50:1262–9.
38. Juby A, Johnston C, Davis P. Specificity, sensitivity and diagnostic predictive value of selected laboratory generated autoantibody profiles in patients with connective tissue diseases. J Rheumatol. 1991;18:354–8.
39. Habets WJ, de Rooij DJ, Salden MH, Verhagen AP, van Eekelen CA, van de Putte LB, et al. Antibodies against distinct nuclear matrix proteins are characteristic for mixed connective tissue disease. Clin Exp Immunol. 1983;54:265–76.
40. Kurata N, Tan EM. Identification of antibodies to nuclear acidic antigens by counterimmunoelectrophoresis. Arthritis Rheum. 1976;19:574–80.
41. Tsuzaka K, Ogasawara T, Tojo T, et al. Relationship between autoantibodies and clinical parameters in Sjögren's syndrome. Scand J Rheumatol. 1993;22:1–9.
42. Fujii T, Mimori T, Hama N, et al. Characterization of autoantibodies that recognize U4/U6 small ribonucleoprotein particles in serum from a patient with primary Sjögren's syndrome. J Biol Chem. 1992;267:1641–6.
43. Setty YN, Pittman CB, Mahale AS, Greidinger EL, Hoffman RW. Sicca symptoms and anti-SSA/Ro antibodies are common in mixed connective tissue disease. J Rheumatol. 2002;29: 487–9.
44. Wilson WA, Gharavi AE, Koike T, et al. International consensus statement on preliminary classification criteria for definite antiphospholipid syndrome: report of an international workshop. Arthritis Rheum. 1999;42:1309–11.
45. Manoussakis MN, Gharavi AE, Drosos AA, Kitridou RC, Moutsopoulos HM. Anticardiolipin antibodies in unselected autoimmune rheumatic disease patients. Clin Immunol Immunopathol. 1987;44:297–307.
46. Asherson RA, Fei HM, Staub HL, Khamashta MA, Hughes GR, Fox RI. Antiphospholipid antibodies and HLA associations in primary Sjogren's syndrome. Ann Rheum Dis. 1992;51:495–8.
47. Jedryka-Goral A, Jagiello P, D'Cruz DP, et al. Isotype profile and clinical relevance of anticardiolipin antibodies in Sjogren's syndrome. Ann Rheum Dis. 1992;51:889–91.
48. Ruiz-Irastorza G, Egurbide MV, Ugalde J, Aguirre C. High impact of antiphospholipid syndrome on irreversible organ damage and survival of patients with systemic lupus erythematosus. Arch Intern Med. 2004;164:77–82.
49. Perez-Vazquez ME, Villa AR, Drenkard C, Cabiedes J, Alarcon-Segovia D. Influence of disease duration, continued follow-up and further antiphospholipid testing on the frequency and classification category of antiphospholipid syndrome in a cohort of patients with systemic lupus erythematosus. J Rheumatol. 1993;20:437–42.
50. Haga HJ, Jacobsen EM, Peen E. Incidence of thromboembolic events in patients with primary Sjögren's syndrome. Scand J Rheumatol. 2008;37:127–9.
51. Cervera R, Khamashta MA, Font J, et al. Morbidity and mortality in systemic lupus erythematosus during a 5 year period. A multicenter prospective study of 1000 patients. Medicine (Baltimore). 1999;78:167–75.
52. Al Attia HM, D'Souza MS. Antitopoisomerase I antibody in patients with systemic lupus erythematosus/sicca syndrome without a concomitant scleroderma: two case reports. Clin Rheumatol. 2003;22:70–2.
53. Tubach F, Hayem G, Elias A, Nicaise P, Haim T, Kahn MF, et al. Anticentromere antibodies in rheumatologic practice are not consistently associated with scleroderma. Rev Rhum Engl Ed. 1997;64:362–7.
54. Tektonidou M, Kaskani E, Skopouli FN, Moutsopoulos HM. Microvascular abnormalities in Sjogren's syndrome: nailfold capillaroscopy. Rheumatology (Oxford). 1999;38:826–30.
55. Caramaschi P, Biasi D, Carletto A, et al. Sjögren's syndrome with anticentromere antibodies. Rev Rhum Engl Ed. 1997;64:785–8.
56. Chan HL, Lee YS, Hong HS, Kuo TT. Anticentromere antibodies (ACA): clinical distribution and disease specificity. Clin Exp Dermatol. 1994;19:298–302.

57. Katano K, Kawano M, Koni I, Sugai S, Muro Y. Clinical and laboratory features of anticentromere antibody positive primary Sjogren's syndrome. J Rheumatol. 2001;28:2238–44.
58. Salliot C, Gottenberg JE, Bengoufa D, Desmoulins F, Miceli-Richard C, Mariette X. Anticentromere antibodies identify patients with Sjögren's syndrome and autoimmune overlap syndrome. J Rheumatol. 2007;34(11):2253–8.
59. Nishiya K, Chikazawa H, Hashimoto K, Miyawaki S. Antineutrophil cytoplasmic antibody in patients with primary Sjogren's syndrome. Clin Rheumatol. 1999;18:268–71.
60. Font J, Ramos-Casals M, Cervera R, et al. Antineutrophil cytoplasmic antibodies in primary Sjögren's syndrome: prevalence and clinical significance. Br J Rheumatol. 1998;37:1287–91.
61. Gross WL, Schmitt WH, Csernok E. Antineutrophil cytoplasmic autoantibody-associated diseases: a rheumatologist's perspective. Am J Kidney Dis. 1991;18:175–9.
62. Fukase S, Ohta N, Inamura K, Kimura Y, Aoyagi M, Koike Y. Diagnostic specificity of antineutrophil cytoplasmic antibodies (ANCA) in otorhinolaryngological diseases. Acta Otolaryngol Suppl. 1994;511:204–7.
63. Young C, Hunt S, Watkinson A, Beynon H. Sjogren's syndrome, cavitating lung disease and high sustained levels of antibodies to serine proteinase 3. Scand J Rheumatol. 2000;29:267–9.
64. Hiromura K, Kitahara T, Kuroiwa T, et al. Clinical analysis of 14 patients with anti-myeloperoxidase antibody positive rapid progressive glomerulonephritic syndrome. Nippon Jinzo Gakkai Shi. 1995;37:573–9.
65. Hernandez JL, Rodrigo E, De Francisco AL, Val F, Gonzalez-Macias J, Riancho JA. ANCA-associated pauci-immune crescentic glomerulonephritis complicating Sjogren's syndrome. Nephrol Dial Transplant. 1996;11:2313–5.
66. Tatsumi H, Tateno S, Hiki Y, Kobayashi Y. Crescentic glomerulonephritis and primary Sjogren's syndrome. Nephron. 2000;86:505–6.
67. Akposso K, Martinant de Preneuf H, Larousserie F, Sraer JD, Rondeau E. Rapidly progressive acute renal failure. A rare complication of primary Sjogren syndrome. Presse Med. 2000;29:1647–9.
68. Radaelli F, Meucci G, Spinzi G, et al. Acute self-limiting jejunitis as the first manifestation of microscopic polyangiitis associated with Sjogren's disease: report of one case and review of the literature. Eur J Gastroenterol Hepatol. 1999;11:931–4.
69. Schellekens GA, de Jong BA, van den Hoogen FH, van de Putte LB, van Venrooij WJ. Citrulline is an essential constituent of antigenic determinants recognized by rheumatoid arthritis-specific autoantibodies. J Clin Invest. 1998;101(1):273–81.
70. Van Gaalen FA, Linn-Rasker SP, van Venrooij WJ, et al. Autoantibodies to cyclic citrullinated peptides predict progression to rheumatoid arthritis in patients with undifferentiated arthritis: a prospective cohort study. Arthritis Rheum. 2004;50:709–15.
71. Goëb V, Salle V, Duhaut P, et al. Clinical significance of autoantibodies recognizing Sjögren's syndrome A (SSA), SSB, calpastatin and alpha-fodrin in primary Sjögren's syndrome. Clin Exp Immunol. 2007;148:281–7.
72. Gottenberg JE, Mignot S, Nicaise-Rolland P, et al. Prevalence of anti-cyclic citrullinated peptide and anti-keratin antibodies in patients with primary Sjögren's syndrome. Ann Rheum Dis. 2005;64:114–7.
73. Kamali S, Polat NG, Kasapoglu E, et al. Anti-CCP and antikeratin antibodies in rheumatoid arthritis, primary Sjögren's syndrome, and Wegener's granulomatosis. Clin Rheumatol. 2005;24:673–6.
74. Atzeni F, Sarzi-Puttini P, Lama N, et al. Anti-cyclic citrullinated peptide antibodies in primary Sjögren syndrome may be associated with non-erosive synovitis. Arthritis Res Ther. 2008;10:R51.
75. Iwamoto N, Kawakami A, Tamai M, et al. Determination of the subset of Sjögren's syndrome with articular manifestations by anticyclic citrullinated peptide antibodies. J Rheumatol. 2009;36:113–5.
76. Mohammed K, Pope J, Le Riche N, et al. Association of severe inflammatory polyarthritis in primary Sjögren's syndrome: clinical, serologic, and HLA analysis. J Rheumatol. 2009;36: 1937–42.

77. Müller K, Manthorpe R, Permin H, Høier-Madsen M, Oxholm P. Circulating IgM rheumatoid factors in patients with primary Sjögren's syndrome. Scand J Rheumatol Suppl. 1988;75:265–8.

78. Müller K, Oxholm P, Mier-Madsen M, Wiik A. Circulating IgA- and IgM-rheumatoid factors in patients with primary Sjögren syndrome. Correlation to extraglandular manifestations. Scand J Rheumatol. 1989;18(1):29–31.

79. Ohara T, Itoh Y, Itoh K. Reevaluation of laboratory parameters in relation to histological findings in primary and secondary Sjogren's syndrome. Nippon Naika Gakkai Zasshi. 2000;89: 1337–42.

80. Tzioufas AG, Boumba DS, Skopouli FN, Moutsopoulos HM. Mixed monoclonal cryoglobulinemia and monoclonal rheumatoid factor cross-reactive idiotypes as predictive factors for the development of lymphoma in primary Sjögren's syndrome. Arthritis Rheum. 1996;39:767–72.

81. Tzioufas AG, Manoussakis MN, Costello R, Silis M, Papadopoulos NM, Moutsopoulos HM. Cryoglobulinemia in autoimmune rheumatic diseases. Evidence of circulating monoclonal cryoglobulins in patients with primary Sjögren's syndrome. Arthritis Rheum. 1986;29:1098–104.

82. Ramos-Casals M, Cervera R, Yague J, et al. Cryoglobulinemia in primary Sjögren's syndrome: prevalence and clinical characteristics in a series of 115 patients. Semin Arthritis Rheum. 1998;28:200–5.

83. Cervera R, Khamashta MA, Font J, et al. Systemic lupus erythematosus: clinical and immunologic patterns of disease expression in a cohort of 1,000 patients. The European Working Party on Systemic Lupus Erythematosus. Medicine (Baltimore). 1993;72:113–24.

84. Ioannidis JP, Vassiliou VA, Moutsopoulos HM. Long-term risk of mortality and lymphoproliferative disease and predictive classification of primary Sjögren's syndrome. Arthritis Rheum. 2002;46:741–7.

85. Lindgren S, Hansen B, Sjoholm AG, Manthorpe R. Complement activation in patients with primary Sjögren's syndrome: an indicator of systemic disease. Autoimmunity. 1993;16: 297–300.

86. Alexander EL, Provost TT, Sanders ME, Frank MM, Joiner KA. Serum complement activation in central nervous system disease in Sjögren's syndrome. Am J Med. 1988;85:513–8.

87. Goules A, Masouridi S, Tzioufas AG, Ioannidis JP, Skopouli FN, Moutsopoulos HM. Clinically significant and biopsy-documented renal involvement in primary Sjogren syndrome. Medicine (Baltimore). 2000;79:241–9.

88. Ramos-Casals M, Brito-Zerón P, Yagüe J, et al. Hypocomplementaemia as an immunological marker of morbidity and mortality in patients with primary Sjögren's syndrome. Rheumatology (Oxford). 2005;44:89–94.

89. Moriuchi J, Ichikawa Y, Takaya M, et al. Association of the complement allele C4AQ0 with primary Sjögren's syndrome in Japanese patients. Arthritis Rheum. 1991;34:224–7.

90. Suzuki Y, Hinoshita F, Yokoyama K, Katori H, Ubara Y, Hara S, et al. Association of Sjogren's syndrome with hereditary angioneurotic edema: report of a case. Clin Immunol Immunopathol. 1997;84:95–7.

91. Schoonbrood TH, Hannema A, Fijen CA, Markusse HM, Swaak AJ. C5 deficiency in a patient with primary Sjögren's syndrome. J Rheumatol. 1995;22:1389.

Chapter 29
Classification Criteria

Chiara Baldini, Rosaria Talarico, and Stefano Bombardieri

Contents

29.1   Introduction

SS is a chronic, systemic inflammatory disorder that mainly affects the salivary and lacrimal glands with focal lymphocytic infiltration of the exocrine glands, leading to sicca symptoms [1]. Although xerostomia and keratoconjunctivitis sicca are the hallmarks of SS, over the course of disease progression any organ or mucosal surface may be involved. The disease also has an important association with non-Hodgkin's lymphoma [2, 3]. Thus, pSS is a heterogeneous autoimmune entity that possesses both organ-specific and systemic features and encompasses a wide spectrum of clinical manifestations, serological abnormalities, and short- and long-term complications. The complexity of SS clinical presentation is increased by the fact that SS can occur alone as pSS or in association with other connective tissue diseases, including rheumatoid arthritis (RA), systemic lupus erythematosus (SLE), and systemic sclerosis (SSc), in which case the disorder is considered to be a secondary SS (sSS) variant [4].

Disease heterogeneity is probably the most important reason why multiple classification criteria sets have cropped up through the years, all proposed by leading

C. Baldini • R. Talarico • S. Bombardieri (✉)
Rheumatology Unit, Department of Internal Medicine, University of Pisa, Pisa, Italy

M. Ramos-Casals et al. (eds.), *Sjögren's Syndrome*,
DOI 10.1007/978-0-85729-947-5_29, © Springer-Verlag London Limited 2012

experts in the field, yet none has been widely accepted until 2002 [5]. The key question the different sets of classification criteria have had to address was whether the term "Sjögren's syndrome" can only be applied to a rather restricted group of individuals whose exocrinopathy is linked to a systemic, autoimmune basis, to the larger group of patients who share the similar sicca complex symptoms [6, 7]. In 2002, the American-European Consensus Group (AECG) proposed a criteria set that is now considered by most experts in the field to provide a sufficient basis for the diagnoses of pSS and sSS [5]. Nevertheless, classification criteria for SS remain a subject of ongoing debate.

29.2   Historical Overview and Sets of Criteria

Four different criteria sets for the definition of SS were presented at the First International Seminar on SS in 1986. The four different sets were known as the Copenhagen [8], Japanese [9], Greek [10], and San Diego criteria [11], respectively. Eleven years earlier, yet another set – the San Francisco criteria for SS – had been proposed USA [12]. Table 29.1 summarizes their similarities and dissimilarities. All these criteria sets had been presented by leading experts in the field and were routinely used in the leading expert's own countries but had not been validated by multicenter studies or by means of standard statistical approaches. The sets focused primarily on assessing the glandular signs and symptoms of the disease, utilizing different procedures with variable levels of sensitivity, specificity and reliability (in many cases still not assessed). The criteria sets appeared to be more or less restrictive depending on their requirements for histological or serologic abnormalities in addition to features of dry eye and dry mouth.

All of the candidate criteria sets except Copenhagen employed the terms "probable" and "definite" SS. The Copenhagen, Greek, and San Francisco criteria used the terms "pSS" and "sSS" [8, 10, 12]. The concept of probable and definite was introduced in the 1958 classification criteria for rheumatoid arthritis but was viewed as problematic because of issues relating to giving a patient a diagnosis of a "probable" disorder [13]. The distinction between pSS and sSS, on the other hand, was justified by the fact that patients with sSS had different genetic, serological, and clinical profiles with respect to pSS patients.

Some of the proposed criteria sets included both subjective symptoms (e.g., sicca symptoms) and objective findings (e.g., positive lip biopsies). In contrast, others relied exclusively on objective findings, considering the subjective symptoms to be non-specific. The Copenhagen Criteria and San Francisco Criteria were the most restrictive criteria from this point of view, whereas the Greek criteria and the Japanese were more liberal. The San Diego criteria offered an intermediate view, focusing on objective evidence of sicca symptoms and signs but also including symptomatic xerostomia, provided that it was also proven on clinical examination and confirmed by decreases in the basal and stimulated salivary flow rates.

The choice of diagnostic tests and their ranges has been another topic of debate. For example, the Greek criteria required only one abnormal test for the diagnosis of

Table 29.1 Similarities and dissimilarities of the historical criteria sets for SS: Copenhagen, Japanese, Greek, San Diego and San Francisco criteria

	Copenhagen (1976)	Japanese (1977)	Greek (1979)	San Diego (1986)	San Francisco (1975, 1984)
Definition of probable/definite SS	–	+	+	+	+
Definition of pSS/sSS	+	–	+	–	+
Subjective xerophthalmia	–	+	+	–	–
Subjective xerostomia	–	+	+	+	–
Objective tests exclusively (no subjective symptoms)	+	–	–	–	+
Parotid gland swelling (history)	–	+	+	–	–
Ocular tests:					
Schirmer-I test	+ (≤ 10 mm/5′)	+ (≤ 10 mm/5′)	+ (≤ 10 mm/5′)	+ (< 9 mm/5′)	+ (≤ 10 mm/5′)
Break-up time	+ (≤ 10 s)	–	–	–	+
Rose bengal (van Bijesterveld score)	+ (≥4)	+(≥2)	+ (≥4)	+(≥4)	+(≥4)
Fluorescein test	–	+	–	+	–
At least two abnormal tests as evidence of KCS	+	+	–	+	+
Oral tests:					
Unstimulated whole saliva	+	–	–	+	–
Stimulated parotid flow rate	–	–	+	+	–
Scintigraphy	+	–	–	–	–
Sialography	–	+	–	–	–
Minor salivary obligatory criterion	No	no	yes	yes	yes
Focus score (minor salivary glands biopsy)	>1	>1	≥2	≥2	>1
Serological findings					
Antinuclear antibodies	–	–	–	+	–
Anti-SS-A/Ro	–	–	–	+	–
Anti-SS-B/La	–	–	–	+	–
IgM-rheumatoid factor	–	–	–	+	–

keratoconjunctivitis sicca (KCS). In contrast, the Copenhagen, Japanese, and San Diego criteria required at least two simultaneous tests of ocular dryness (see Table 29.1). The tests most commonly used to diagnose KCS were the Schirmer-I test, the tear break-up time, the slit lamp examination after rose Bengal staining, and the fluorescein test.

For the assessment of xerostomia, nearly all the four criteria sets mentioned salivary flow rate estimation. However, sialometry was performed by using different modalities, all of which essentially evaluated the unstimulated and stimulated flow rate. Only the Japanese criteria used abnormal sialography as a criterion for the diagnosis of SS. In contrast, the Copenhagen criteria employed salivary gland scintigraphy to provide a functional (albeit expensive) evaluation of all salivary glands.

In 1975, Daniels et al. [14] outlined the value of the minor gland biopsy as a basis for the salivary components of SS. Daniels differentiated focal sialoadenitis from chronic non-specific sialoadenitis, defining a focus as a cluster of at least 50 mononuclear cells. The Daniels group concluded that an average focus score per 4 mononuclear cells/mm^2 (based on the evaluation of at least four glands) should be required for diagnosis. Moreover, according to Daniels, the biopsy sample had to be obtained through clinically normal mucosa and lobules characterized by non-specific infiltrates had to be excluded from the evaluation. This criterion served as a substitute for symptoms or signs of salivary hypofunction in the San Francisco Criteria [12].

The importance of focal sialoadenitis was remarked upon by subsequent studies, which confirmed that the histological criterion was highly associated with parotid flow rate, diagnosis of KCS, and the presence of antinuclear or anti-Ro antibodies [15–18]. The minor salivary gland biopsy became an obligatory criterion for the San Francisco (focus score >1), for the Greek (focus score ≥2), and for the San Diego criteria (focus score ≥2). The inclusion of minor salivary gland biopsy as a criterion increased the homogeneity of patients classified as having pSS for the purpose of studies, but also conferred a degree of invasiveness to the diagnostic algorithm. The different criteria sets dealt with this issue in a variety of ways. The San Diego criteria required a minor salivary gland biopsy only for definite SS, whereas the category of "probable" SS could be fulfilled in the absence of a biopsy. On the other hand, the Copenhagen and Japanese criteria permitted the diagnosis of SS without an abnormal salivary gland biopsy. The latter also considered that a biopsy from tear glands might replace biopsy of the minor salivary glands.

The California (San Diego and San Francisco) criteria were the only sets to utilize the presence of autoantibodies (antinuclear antibodies, anti-SSA/Ro, anti-SSB/La and IgM-rheumatoid factor), underscoring the systemic autoimmune background of the disease.

During the First International Seminar on SS in 1986, comparisons among all of the criteria drew appropriate attention to the lack of diagnostic homogeneity in SS and the resulting potential discrepancies in clinical studies and epidemiological surveys [19]. Awareness of these shortcomings created the foundation for the subsequent development of a set of international criteria for SS.

29.3 Preliminary European Criteria

In 1988, 2 years after the First International Seminar on SS held in Copenhagen, a workshop sponsored by the Epidemiology Committee of the Commission of the European Communities (EEC-COMAC) was held in Pisa. The workshop was attended by 29 experts from 11 European countries and Israel. The aim of this collaboration was to define and validate simple standardized diagnostic tools for SS and to design a multicenter study to define classification criteria for SS [20]. The novelty was represented by the fact that previously proposed classification criteria had generally been formulated by experts on the basis of clinical experience or derived from data coming from single centers. The preliminary European classification criteria, in contrast, represented the first attempt to create criteria for pSS using the same methodology and statistics that have been used by the American College of Rheumatology for RA: a multicenter study using a generally agreed upon protocol, standardized methodologies, and the collection of data from real patients [13, 20].

The panel of experts included rheumatologists, ophthalmologists, oral pathologists, and epidemiologists and the study protocol was articulated in two parts. The preliminary groundwork was represented by the proposal of a panel of candidate tools for the diagnosis of glandular and extraglandular aspects of the disease. Clear guidelines for their application and interpretation were defined and collected in a manual of methods and procedures. Furthermore, the panel of experts decided that for subjective symptoms, a specific questionnaire should be validated on a separate protocol. A simple questionnaire (20 questions: 13 regarding ocular involvement and 7 regarding oral involvement) for dry eyes and dry mouth was therefore validated. Each expert was asked to complete these questionnaires in 15 patients who, in their judgment, had well-defined pSS, and also in 15 healthy age- and sex-matched controls.

Data on 480 patients (240 SS and 240 controls) were gathered. Monovariate and multivariate analyses and stepwise multiple regression were used to select those questions and combinations of questions that performed best in classifying patients and controls correctly. A simplified questionnaire consisting of three questions each for dry eyes and dry mouth emerged from this section of the study [20].

For part II, each center recruited 40 patients: ten each with pSS, sSS, other connective tissue disorders (CTDs) without SS, and ten controls. In these study subjects, a limited set of proposed diagnostic tests were validated. These included the Schirmer-I test, rose bengal test, tear break-up time, tear fluid lactoferrin level, stimulated and unstimulated saliva flow, biopsy of the minor salivary glands, parotid sialography, and salivary gland scintigraphy. The procedures for each test were described in the protocol. The data from part II were subjected to the same analysis as were those from part I, with the addition of a classification tree to assist in determining the optimal classification strategy. From the analysis, the consensus group established a set of four objective criteria for the diagnosis of SS [21]. These four criteria and the two subjective criteria are presented in Table 29.2. The preliminary European criteria were based on any four out of six items, including ocular and oral symptoms (oral and ocular dryness), ocular and oral signs (positive Schirmer-I test, Rose Bengal score, parotid sialography, scintigraphy and unstimulated salivary flow), immunological parameters, and focal sialoadenitis. For primary SS, the presence of four out of six items had good sensitivity (93.5%) and specificity (94%) [21]. Some exclusion criteria were also added to this classification set for SS following the recommendations made by Fox et al. [11], namely preexisting lymphoma, acquired immunodefi-

Table 29.2 European preliminary criteria for Sjögren's syndrome

I. Ocular symptoms: a positive response to at least one of the following questions:
    1. Have you had daily, persistent, troublesome dry eyes for more than 3 months?
    2. Do you have a recurrent sensation of sand or gravel in the eyes?
    3. Do you use tear substitutes more than 3 times a day

II. Oral symptoms: a positive response to at least one of the following questions:
    1. Have you had a daily feeling of dry mouth for more than 3 months?
    2. Have you had recurrently or persistently swollen salivary glands as an adult?
    3. Do you frequently drink liquids to aid in swallowing dry food?

III. Ocular signs – that is, objective evidence of ocular involvement defined as a positive result for at least one of the following two tests:
    1. Schirmer's I test ($\leq$5 mm in 5 min)
    2. Rose bengal score or other ocular dye score ($\geq$4 according to van Bijsterveld's scoring system)

IV. Histopathology: Focus score $\geq$1 on minor salivary gland biopsy (focus defined as an aggregation of at least 50 mononuclear cells; focus score defined as the number of foci per 4 mm^2 of glandular tissue)

V. Salivary gland involvement: objective evidence of salivary gland involvement defined by a positive result for at least one of the following diagnostic tests:
    1. Unstimulated whole salivary flow (<1.5 mL in 15 min)
    2. Parotid sialography showing the presence of diffuse sialectasias (punctate, cavitary or destructive pattern), without evidence of obstruction in the major ducts
    3. Salivary scintigraphy showing delayed uptake, reduced concentration and/or delayed excretion of tracer

VI. Autoantibodies: presence in the serum of the following autoantibodies:
    1. Antibodies to Ro(SSA) or La(SSB) antigens, or both
    2. Antinuclear antibodies
    3. Rheumatoid factor

Exclusion criteria:
    Pre-existing lymphoma
    Acquired immunodeficiency disease (AIDS)
    Sarcoidosis
    Graft versus host disease

ciency syndrome, sarcoidosis, and graft-versus-host disease. For the diagnosis of sSS, the criterion for any positive serological test was excluded and a consensus emerged from the group that three of five items were sufficient for diagnosis [21].

In 1996, the criteria set was validated on a total of 278 cases (157 SS patients and 121 non-SS controls) collected from 16 centers in ten countries. The criteria were confirmed to have a sensitivity of 97.5% and a specificity of 94.2% [22].

After these validation exercises, the European classification criteria have been widely received by the scientific community because of their excellent combination of sensitivity and specificity. In fact, when previously proposed criteria [8–12] had been used to classify patients with pSS and controls enrolled in the European study, they all demonstrated high specificities (range 97.9–100%) but low sensitivities (range 22.9–72.2%) [21]. Other advantageous characteristics of the European criteria were that they distinguished between pSS and sSS but avoided the concept of definite/possible SS. Furthermore, they relied upon unstimulated or basal tests [21, 22] and did not require an invasive procedure such as the minor salivary gland biopsy for diagnosis.

Despite their strong points, the European criteria for the classification of SS continue to generate extensive discussion. One key point of ongoing debate is that these criteria can be fulfilled in the absence of either the classic autoantibodies (i.e., antibodies directed against the SSA/Ro or SSB/La antigens) or positive findings on labial salivary gland biopsy. Further, the criteria can also be fulfilled by patients who have sicca symptoms caused by entities other than primary SS. Finally, in a criteria set in which two out of the six items are devoted to subjective complaints, it is difficult to classify asymptomatic patients precisely even if the abundance of objective data suggest that a diagnosis of pSS is likely [15, 23].

29.4 American-European Criteria: Strengths, Limitations, and Future Proposals

The European Preliminary Criteria represented the first attempt to validate a set of international criteria for pSS [21]. Because of the appropriate criticisms voiced against the European Preliminary Criteria, the SS Foundation proposed that a joint effort be undertaken by the European Study Group on Classification Criteria for SS and a group of American experts. The Foundation has organized meetings between the two groups since 1998. A detailed analysis of the European database of the patients and controls collected during the validation phase of the European Criteria was undertaken. A receiver operating characteristic (ROC) curve of the revised criteria was constructed, based on the analysis of 180 cases provided by 16 centers from ten European countries. The patient and control populations included 76 patients affected by pSS, 41 patients with a diagnosis of CTD without SS, and 63 healthy control subjects. The curve was obtained by plotting sensitivity and specificity values for each different combination of positive tests.

Based on these ROC curve analyses, the condition "positivity of any four out of the six items" and the condition "positivity of four out of six items with the exclusion of the cases in which both serology and histopathology were negative" showed the same accuracy, 92.7%. However, the second condition had a lower sensitivity (89.5% vs. 97.4%) but a higher specificity (95.2% vs. 89.4%). The presence of any three of the four objective criteria items performed as well a slightly lower accuracy (90.5%) but a specificity of 95.2% and a sensitivity of 84.2%. This combination was, therefore, judged to be reliable, as well. Thus, the American-European Consensus Group introduced the obligatory rule that for a definite diagnosis of SS either the minor salivary gland biopsy or serology had to be positive (see Table 29.3) [5]. Other proposed modifications were suggested to make with item definitions within the European criteria more precise. In particular, it was specified that Schirmer's I test should be performed with standardized paper strips in unanesthetized and closed eyes, following the European and the Japanese approaches. Moreover, as rose

Table 29.3 American-European Consensus Group Criteria. Revised international classification criteria for Sjögren's syndrome

I.   Ocular symptoms: a positive response to at least one of the following questions:
  1. Have you had daily, persistent, troublesome dry eyes for more than 3 months?
  2. Do you have a recurrent sensation of sand or gravel in the eyes?
  3. Do you use tear substitutes more than 3 times a day

II. Oral symptoms: a positive response to at least one of the following questions:
  1. Have you had a daily feeling of dry mouth for more than 3 months?
  2. Have you had recurrently or persistently swollen salivary glands as an adult?
  3. Do you frequently drink liquids to aid in swallowing dry food?

III. Ocular signs – that is, objective evidence of ocular involvement defined as a positive result for at least one of the following two tests:
  1. Schirmer's I test, performed without anesthesia (<5 mm in 5 min)
  2. Rose bengal score or other ocular dye score (>4 according to van Bijsterveld's scoring system)

IV. Histopathology: In minor salivary glands (obtained through normal-appearing mucosa) focal lymphocytic sialoadenitis, evaluated by an expert histopathologist, with a focus score >1, defined as a number of lymphocytic foci (which are adjacent to normal-appearing mucous acini and contain more than 50 lymphocytes) per 4 mm^2 of glandular tissue

V.   Salivary gland involvement: objective evidence of salivary gland involvement defined by a positive result for at least one of the following diagnostic tests:
  1. Unstimulated whole salivary flow (<1.5 mL in 15 min)
  2. Parotid sialography showing the presence of diffuse sialectasias (punctate, cavitary or destructive pattern), without evidence of obstruction in the major ducts
  3. Salivary scintigraphy showing delayed uptake, reduced concentration and/or delayed excretion of tracer

VI. Autoantibodies: presence in the serum of the following autoantibodies:
  1. Antibodies to Ro(SSA) or La(SSB) antigens, or both

Revised rules for classification

For primary SS

In patients without any potentially associated disease, primary SS may be defined as follows:
  (a) The presence of any 4 of the 6 items is indicative of primary SS, as long as either item IV (Histopathology) or VI (Serology) is positive
  (b) The presence of any 3 of the 4 objective criteria items (i.e., items III, IV, V, VI)
  (c) The classification tree procedure represents a valid alternative method for classification, although it should be more properly used in clinical-epidemiological survey

For secondary SS

  In patients with a potentially associated disease (for instance, another well-defined connective tissue disease), the presence of item I or item II plus any 2 from among items III, IV, and V may be considered as indicative of secondary SS

Exclusion criteria:

  Past head and neck radiation treatment
  Hepatitis C infection
  Acquired immunodeficiency disease (AIDS)
  Pre-existing lymphoma
  Sarcoidosis
  Graft versus host disease
  Use of anticholinergic drugs (since a time shorter than fourfold the half-life of the drug)

Bengal is not available in many countries, other ocular dye scores (i.e., fluorescein and lissamine green stains) were suggested.

The joint European and American experts defined a positive minor salivary gland biopsy as one or more foci of lymphocytes per 4 mm^2 glandular tissue, specifying that the foci had to be adjacent to normal-appearing mucous acini. Finally, a consensus on the list of exclusion criteria was also reached. In comparison to the exclusion criteria adopted by the European preliminary criteria, the category "anticholinergic" drugs was introduced, replacing "antidepressant, antihypertensive, parasympatholytic, parasympatholytic drugs and neuroleptic agents". In addition, the term sialoadenosis was deleted and the definition "past head and neck radiation treatment" was added. Finally, hepatitis C virus (HCV) infection was added as an exclusion criterion [24].

For sSS it was established that, in patients with a potentially associated disease, the presence of item I or II plus any two from among items III, IV and V had to be considered as indicative of the disorder [5].

The American–European Revised Classification Criteria preserved many aspects of the European Preliminary Criteria but appear to be more stringent [5, 25, 26]. In one study of the Copenhagen, San Diego, European, and AECG criteria sets conducted on 222 consecutive patients with possible SS, 90 patients (41%) fulfilled at least one classification criteria set. The highest number of patients fulfilled the European criteria (36%), followed by the Copenhagen criteria (28%), the AECG criteria (26%) and the San Diego criteria (9%) sets. The AECG criteria resulted therefore to be highly specific and quite restrictive [25].

The AECG criteria are the most widely accepted tool presently available for the classification of patients with pSS and sSS. The AECG criteria have been applied in a number of epidemiologic studies aimed at determining the prevalence of SS (Table 29.4 summarizes the data) [27–39]. According to these studies, the prevalence of pSS assessed by using the AECG criteria varies from 0.09% to 0.6% [28–30, 33–35], while the incidence of the diseases was estimated to be 5.3 per 10^5 (4.5–6.1) [33]. Prevalence of pSS estimated according to the Copenhagen Criteria and to the Preliminary European criteria varied from 0.2 to 2.7 and 0.35 to 3.59, respectively [28–32, 36–39]. When studies that have assessed the prevalence of pSS prevalence by different criteria sets are analyzed, the prevalence of pSS estimated by European Preliminary Criteria resulted estimates 1.67–2.5 higher than estimates made by the AECG [29].

In our series, 381 out of all the 506 (75%) patients screened for SS, fulfilled both the AECG and the 1993-EU criteria, whereas the other 125/506 (25%) fulfilled only the latter. Among the patients who only fulfilled European Preliminary Criteria, those with positive RF but negative Ro/SSA and/or La/SSB were clinically indistinguishable from AECG patients, over prolonged follow-up term, for both glandular and extraglandular disease manifestations.

These data suggest that excessive stringency may be the major drawback to the AECG when these criteria are employed in epidemiologic studies. The mandatory alternative items "positive minor salivary gland biopsy" or "positivity of Ro/SSA

Table 29.4 Prevalence of primary Sjögren's syndrome

	Study	Criteria sets	Prevalence
Intra-study comparisons	2009 Turkey [28]	European	0.35 (0.17–0.65)
		AECG	0.21 (0.08–0.46)
	2008 Norway [29]	European	0.44 (0.34–0.57)
		AECG	0.22 (0.15–0.32)
	2006 Turkey [30]	European	1.5 (0.85–2.5)
		AECG	0.6 (0.24–1.39)
	1997 Denmark [31]	European	0.6–2.1
		Copenhagen	0.2–0.8
	1995 China [32]	Copenhagen	0.77 (0.44–1.25)
		San Diego	0.34 (0.44–1.25)
Single observations	2006 Greece [33]	AECG	0.092 (0.08–0.10)
	2005 Greece [34]	AECG	0.15 (0.09–0.21)
	2004 UK [35]	AECG	0.45 (0.04–1.32)
	1999 Slovenia [36]	European	0.6 (0.07–2.16)
	1998 UK [37]	European	2.1 (1.13–2.58)
	1997 Greece [38]	European	0.6 (0.19–1.39)
	1989 Sweden [39]	Copenhagen	2.7 (1–4.5)

and La/SSB antibodies" tend to restrict the diagnosis, excluding those with sicca symptoms, positive ocular and oral tests, and serological profiles characterized by the ANA and RF positivity. For similar reasons, the AECG criteria may be too restrictive for use in daily clinical practice, particularly in early disease [40, 41]. The prevalence of Ro/SSA and La/SSB autoantibodies has been estimated to be respectively around 60% and 45% in pSS, these autoantibodies are particularly common in younger patients [42, 43]. Heavy reliance upon the minor salivary gland biopsy also creates potential problems, as the degree of lymphocytic infiltration may be strongly influenced by the age or smoking and the reproducibility of the test is imperfect [44].

In conclusion, although the AECG criteria have been now widely adopted by the scientific community, it is a common belief that some aspects of these criteria should be re-visited. Classification criteria for SS remain a work in progress. The NIH-sponsored longitudinal observational study known as the Sjögren's International Collaborative Clinical Alliance (SICCA) is likely to provide critical information on SS and future efforts on criteria development [45, 46].

Acknowledgments We thank Miss Wendy Doherty and Miss Luisa Marconcini for their valuable contribution in reviewing the text.

References

1. Nikolov NP, Illei GG. Pathogenesis of Sjögren's syndrome. Curr Opin Rheumatol. 2009;21(5): 465–70.
2. Fietta P, Delsante G, Quaini F. Hematologic manifestations of connective autoimmune diseases. Clin Exp Rheumatol. 2009;27(1):140–54.

3. Voulgarelis M, Tzioufas AG, Moutsopoulos HM. Mortality in Sjögren's syndrome. Clin Exp Rheumatol. 2008;26(5 Suppl 51):S66–71.

4. Theander E, Jacobsson LT. Relationship of Sjögren's syndrome to other connective tissue and autoimmune disorders. Rheum Dis Clin North Am. 2008;34(4):935–47, viii–ix.

5. Vitali C, Bombardieri S, Jonsson R, Moutsopoulos HM, Alexander EL, Carson SE, et al. Classification criteria for Sjögren's syndrome: a revised version of the European criteria proposed by the American-European Consensus Group. Ann Rheum Dis. 2002;61:554–8.

6. Iorgulescu G. Saliva between normal and pathological. Important factors in determining systemic and oral health. J Med Life. 2009;2(3):303–7.

7. Kikuchi M, Inagaki T, Ogawa K, Banno S, Matsumoto Y, Ueda R, et al. Histopathological investigation of salivary glands in the asymptomatic elderly. Arch Gerontol Geriatr. 2004;38(2):131–8.

8. Manthorpe R, Oxholm P, Prause JU, Schiodt M. The Copenhagen criteria for Sjögren's syndrome. Scand J Rheumatol. 1986;61:19–21.

9. Homma M, Tojo T, Akizuki M, Yamagata H. Criteria for Sjögren's syndrome in Japan. Scand J Rheumatol. 1986;61:26–7.

10. Skopouli FN, Drosos AA, Papaioannou T, Moutsopoulos HM. Preliminary diagnostic criteria for Sjögren's syndrome. Scand J Rheumatol. 1986;61:22–5.

11. Fox RI, Robinson CA, Curd JG, Kozin F, Howell FV. Sjögren's syndrome. Proposed criteria for classification. Arthritis Rheum. 1986;29(5):577–85.

12. Daniels TE, Silverman S, Michalski JP, Greenspan JS, Sylvester RA, Talal N. The oral component of Sjögren's syndrome. Oral Surg Oral Med Oral Pathol. 1975;39:875–85.

13. Arnett FC, Edworthy SM, Bloch DA, McShane DJ, Fries JF, Cooper NS, et al. The 1987 revised American association criteria for classification of rheumatoid arthritis. Arthritis Rheum. 1988;31:315–24.

14. Daniels TE. Labial salivary gland biopsy in Sjögren's syndrome: assessment as a diagnostic criterion in 362 suspected cases. Arthritis Rheum. 1984;27:147–56.

15. Fox RI, Saito I. Criteria for diagnosis of Sjögren's syndrome. Rheumatol Dis North Am. 1994;20(2):391–407.

16. Shah F, Rapini RP, Arnett FC, Warner NB, Smith CA. Association of labial salivary gland histopathology with clinical and serologic features of connective tissue diseases. Arthritis Rheum. 1990;33:1682–7.

17. Atkinson JC, Travis WD, Slocum L, Ebbs WL, Fox PC. Serum anti-SS-B/La and IgA rheumatoid factor are markers of salivary gland disease activity in primary Sjögren's syndrome. Arthritis Rheum. 1992;35:1368–72.

18. Daniels TE, Witcher JP. Association of patterns of labial salivary gland inflammation with keratoconjunctivitis sicca. Analysis of 618 patients with suspected Sjögren's syndrome. Arthritis Rheum. 1994;6:869–77.

19. Prause JU, Manthorpe R, Oxholm P, Schiødt M. Definition and criteria for Sjögren's syndrome used by the contributors to the First International Seminar on Sjögren's syndrome – 1986. Scand J Rheumatol Suppl. 1986;61:17–8.

20. Workshop on diagnostic criteria for Sjögren's syndrome: I. Questionnaires for dry eye and dry mouth. II Manual of methods and procedures. Clin Exp Rheumatol. 1989;7:212–19.

21. Vitali C, Bombardieri S, Moutsopoulos HM, Balestrieri G, Bencivelli W, Bernstein RM, et al. Preliminary criteria for the classification of Sjögren's syndrome. Results of a prospective concerted action supported by the European Community. Arthritis Rheum. 1993;36(3):340–7.

22. Vitali C, Bombardieri S, Moutsopoulos HM, Coll J, Gerli R, Hatron PY, et al. Assessment of the European classification criteria for Sjögren's syndrome in a series of clinically defined cases: results of a prospective multicentre study. The European Study Group on Diagnostic Criteria for Sjögren's Syndrome. Ann Rheum Dis. 1996;55(2):116–21.

23. Fox RI. Fifth international symposium on Sjögren's syndrome. Arthritis Rheum. 1996;39(2):195–6.

24. Ramos-Casals M, Garcia Carrasco M, Cervera R, Rosas J, Trejo O, de la Red G, et al. Hepatitis C virus infection mimicking primary Sjögren's syndrome. A clinical and immunologic description of 35 cases. Medicine (Baltimore). 2001;80:1–8.

25. Novljan MP, Rozman B, Jerse M, Rotar Z, Kveder T, Tomsic M. Comparison of the different classification criteria sets for primary Sjögren's syndrome. Scand J Rheumatol. 2006;35:463–7.

26. Langegger C, Wenger M, Duftner C, Dejaco C, Baldissera I, Moncayo R, et al. Use of the European preliminary criteria, the Breiman classification tree and the American–European criteria for diagnosis of primary Sjögren's Syndrome in daily practice: a retrospective analysis. Rheumatol Int. 2007;27(8):699–702.

27. Binard A, Devauchelle-Pensec V, Fautrel B, Jousse S, Youinou P, Saraux A. Epidemiology of Sjögren's syndrome: where are we now? Clin Exp Rheumatol. 2007;25(1):1–4.

28. Birlik M, Akar S, Gurler O, Sari I, Birlik B, Sarioglu S, et al. Prevalence of primary Sjögren's syndrome in Turkey: a population-based epidemiological study. Int J Clin Pract. 2009;63(6): 954–61.

29. Haugen AJ, Peen E, Hultén B, Johannessen AC, Brun JG, Halse AK, et al. Estimation of the prevalence of primary Sjögren's syndrome in two age-different community-based populations using two sets of classification criteria: the Hordaland Health Study. Scand J Rheumatol. 2008;37(1):30–4.

30. Kabasakal Y, Kitapcioglu G, Turk T, Oder G, Durusoy R, Mete N, et al. The prevalence of Sjögren's syndrome in adult women. Scand J Rheumatol. 2006;35(5):379–83.

31. Bjerrum KB. Keratoconjunctivitis sicca and primary Sjögren's syndrome in a Danish population aged 30–60 years. Acta Ophthalmol Scand. 1997;75:281–6.

32. Zhang NZ, Shi CS, Yao QP, Pan GX, Wang LL, Wen ZX, et al. Prevalence of primary Sjögren's syndrome in China. J Rheumatol. 1995;22(4):659–61.

33. Alamanos Y, Tsifetaki N, Voulgari PV, Venetsanopoulo AI, Siozos C, Drosos AA. Epidemiology of primary Sjögren's syndrome in north-west Greece, 1982–2003. Rheumatology. 2006;45:187–91.

34. Trontzas PI, Andrianakos AA. Sjögren's syndrome: a population-based study of prevalence in Greece: The ESORDIG study. Ann Rheum Dis. 2005;64:1240–1.

35. Bowman SJ, Ibrahim GH, Holmes G, Hamburger J, Ainsworth JR. Estimating the prevalence among Caucasian women of primary Sjögren's syndrome in two general practices in Birmingham, UK. Scand J Rheumatol. 2004;33:39–43.

36. Tomsic M, Logar D, Grmek M, Perkovic T, Kveder T. Prevalence of Sjögren's syndrome in Slovenia. Rheumatology. 1999;38:164–70.

37. Thomas E, Hay EM, Hajeer A, Silman AJ. Sjögren's syndrome: a community-based study of prevalence and impact. Br J Rheumatol. 1998;37:1069–76.

38. Dafni UG, Tzioufas AG, Staikos P, Skopouli FN, Moutsopoulos MH. Prevalence of primary Sjögren's syndrome in a closed rural community. Ann Rheum Dis. 1997;56:521–5.

39. Jacobsson LT, Axell TE, Hansen BU, Henricsson VJ, Larsson A, Lieberkind K, et al. Dry eyes or mouth – an epidemiological study in Swedish adults, with special reference to primary Sjögren's syndrome. J Autoimmun. 1989;2(4):521–7.

40. Brun JG, Madland TM, Gjesdal CB, Bertelsen LT. Sjögren's syndrome in an out-patient clinic: classification of patients according to the preliminary European criteria and the proposed modified European criteria. Rheumatology. 2002;41(3):301–4.

41. Sánchez-Guerrero J, Pérez-Dosal MR, Cárdenas-Velázquez F, Pérez-Reguera A, Celis-Aguilar E, Soto-Rojas AE, et al. Prevalence of Sjögren's syndrome in ambulatory patients according to the American-European Consensus Group criteria. Rheumatology. 2005;44(2):235–40.

42. Kassan SS, Mutsopoulos HM. Clinical manifestations and early diagnosis of Sjögren syndrome. Arch Intern Med. 2004;164:1275–84.

43. Ramos Casals M, Tzioufas AG, Font J. Primary Sjögren's syndrome: new clinical and therapeutic concepts. Ann Rheum Dis. 2005;64:347–54.

44. Morbini P, Manzo A, Caporali R, Epis O, Villa C, Tinelli C, et al. Multilevel examination of minor salivary gland biopsy for Sjögren's syndrome significantly improves diagnostic performance of AECG classification criteria. Arthritis Res Ther. 2005;7(2):R343–8.

45. Whitcher JP, Shiboski CH, Shiboski SC, Heidenreich AM, Kitagawa K, Zhang S, et al. A simplified quantitative method for assessing keratoconjunctivitis sicca from the Sjögren's Syndrome International Registry. Am J Ophthalmol. 2010;149(3):405–15.

46. Daniels TE, Criswell LA, Shiboski C, Shiboski S, Lanfranchi H, Dong Y, et al. An early view of the international Sjögren's syndrome registry. Arthritis Rheum. 2009;61(5):711–4.

Chapter 30
Measurement of Chronicity and Activity in Sjögren's Syndrome

Claudio Vitali

Contents

30.1   Introduction

Systemic autoimmune conditions such as Sjögren's syndrome (SS) are commonly characterized by prolonged episodes of activity, sustained by the underlying immunologic and inflammatory processes [1, 2]. The activity flares are clinically marked by the new appearance or worsening of signs and symptoms that are typical for each one of the different diseases. In some diseases, elevation of acute phase reactants or abnormalities of immunologic markers accompany active periods. If the active phase of the disease does not remit spontaneously or if remission is not achieved by treatment, a chronic phase of the disease may begin and irreversible damage can be produced in the involved organs and systems [1, 2].

Although the concepts of disease activity and damage are easy to formulate in theory, functional definitions have not been established for most autoimmune

C. Vitali
Department of Internal Medicine and Section of Rheumatology,
'Villamarina' Hospital, Piombino, Italy

M. Ramos-Casals et al. (eds.), *Sjögren's Syndrome*,
DOI 10.1007/978-0-85729-947-5_30, © Springer-Verlag London Limited 2012

conditions [3]. Generally speaking, activity can be defined as a reversible entity, because the related inflammatory process may have a fluctuating course and may respond to treatment. In contrast, damage, defined as a permanent loss of function, represents a chronic, irreversible component of the disease process. The concept of damage suggests histological or radiological evidence of structural derangement in tissues.

Disease severity may also influence the clinical perception of disease-related features. A clinical manifestation, either as a consequence of an activity flare or related to a permanent damage, is commonly judged more severe when it can cause the patient's death or important disability, or its treatment appears particularly difficult.

30.2 Clinical and Serological Peculiarities of Sjögren's Syndrome

Primary SS is a systemic autoimmune disease that mainly affects the exocrine glands. Thus, persistent dryness of the mouth and eyes caused by functional impairment and structural derangement of the salivary and lacrimal glands are the hallmarks of the disease. However, other epithelial organs, including the liver, lung, and kidney, can also be involved. The typical histological finding of SS is a focal lymphocytic infiltration of the involved tissues (exocrine and non exocrine epithelia). This infiltrate is comprised primarily by activated T cells in early lesions, but B cells become predominant in later phases of the disease. Indeed, chronic B cell activation and proliferation are considered to be chief disease characteristics [4].

B cell hyperactivity is usually characterized, from the serological point of view, by the production of autoantibodies, the presence of circulating immune complexes, hypergammaglobulinemia, and cryoglobulinemia, and the clinical correlates of cutaneous vasculitis, glomerulonephritis, and peripheral or central nervous system disease [5]. Benign B cell proliferation sometimes evolves to the development of different forms of B cell lymphoma. The presence of low complement level, type II cryoglobulins, cutaneous vasculitis, and persistent parotid gland swelling are risk factors for progression to lymphoma [6].

The clinical course of SS is slowly progressive in most of patients, in whom sicca symptoms, fatigue, and articular and muscular pain are the most common symptoms. The involvement of other epithelial tissues, e.g., those of the upper airways, renal tubules, and gastrointestinal tract, justifies the term "autoimmune epithelitis" that has been applied to the disease [4]. In contrast, in 20–30% of patients, the clinical course is marked by extra-epithelial systemic features of variable severity, including Raynaud's phenomenon, arthritis, palpable purpura, autoimmune cytopenias, peripheral neuropathy, glomerulonephritis, and higher risk of lymphoma development [6].

The different variants of SS proceed at different rates. The epithelitis is typically slowly progressive, whereas patients with extra-epithelial disease often have disease courses punctuated by highly evident disease flares. Some data from B cell depletion trials in SS suggest that clinical manifestations related to both the autoimmune epithelitis and systemic involvement are at least partially reversible [7–11]. However, the conduct and interpretation of clinical trials in SS poses a number of challenges. First, careful definition of the inclusion criteria is required for any given trial, such that a trial focuses upon a particular subset of patients. Excessive heterogeneity in clinical trials subjects leads to substantial difficulties in interpreting results. Second, the selection of patients must be guided by knowledge of the specific targeted approach and its intended effects. Finally, clinical trials require predefined endpoints that can be measured with reliable and validated outcome measures.

30.3 Assessment of Disease Activity or Damage in Systemic Autoimmune Diseases

Criteria for the assessment of disease activity and cumulative damage have been developed for a variety of systemic autoimmune conditions [2, 12]. These tools are essential in the conduct of clinical trials, but their use has also been extended to clinical practice. Fulfillment of the basic psychometric properties of face validity, construct validity, and content validity is crucial to any index of disease activity or damage [3, 13].

Face validity can be defined simply as the fact that an instrument seems to measure what it is designed to measure. To have construct validity means that the instrument has been demonstrated to correlate closely with an independent measure of same variable. When this independent parameter does not exist, as happens in the case of autoimmune systemic diseases, the physician's global assessment is commonly used as the gold standard. Although the physician's global assessment is often considered as the most effective and simplest index for the measurement of disease status domains, in some settings the physician's global assessment has poor accuracy and inter-rater reliability [14]. Content validity implies that the clinical scale built for a disease status may cover all of the relevant disease manifestations.

Sensitivity to change, i.e., the ability of a disease status index to detect significant clinical alterations in patients' status, is crucial to assess disease activity [14, 15]. The minimal significant change in any activity index should be defined. During the last decades, a number of activity criteria have been developed for most of the systemic autoimmune diseases [12]. A plethora of activity criteria have been proposed for systemic lupus erythematosus [13], although a more restricted number has been validated and recommended for the use in therapeutic trials and in daily practice [16].

Instruments aimed at measuring the disease activity in rheumatoid arthritis have also been designed and validated, and are currently in use as steady state and transition indices both in therapeutic trials and in clinical practice [12, 15]. Activity criteria for systemic sclerosis have been developed and validated by a European consensus study group [17].

A limited number of tools are available to measure the cumulated disease damage. An ad hoc committee of the American College of Rheumatology has defined a scoring system to measure chronicity and irreversible damage in lupus [18]. Standardized methods for radiographic evaluation are commonly applied to assess the articular damage in rheumatoid arthritis [19].

30.4 Methodological Procedures to Develop Disease Status Criteria

To quantify a global clinical assessment in a clinical scoring system is a simplification of a complex intellectual process that an expert clinician is able to do by elaborating all of the patient's physical, biological and imaging-related findings, by selecting only the relevant data, and eliciting those related to concomitant psychological status or different diseases. The selection of items to be included in a clinical scale can be done by using statistical procedures or on the basis of an expert consensus (Delphi method). In this latter case, an expert committee preliminarily chooses the variables that may predict a disease status. Construct validity, content validity, and sensitivity to change of the proposed scale are then verified in a sufficient number of true or simulated patients, with the physician's global assessment generally considered to be the external criterion (gold standard). Conversely, the variables to be included in the scale can be selected and stratified for severity by analyzing a sufficiently large series of real patients and building a multivariate model in which the physician's global assessment represents the dependent variable. Validation of this preliminary index should then be performed by using it on a different series of patients.

30.5 Development of Disease Status Indices for Sjögren's Syndrome

30.5.1 The Italian Approach

The first study aimed at defining activity and damage criteria for SS was conducted out by an Italian group [20]. A methodology similar to that used to develop ECLAM (European Consensus Lupus Activity Measurement) was employed [21]. Two multivariate models based on data collected from a rather large of patients recruited in a number of Italian centers were built in order to select the variables predictive of disease activity and damage, respectively. The physician's global scores, given by the observers in assessing both activity and damage, were used as dependent variables of the two multivariate linear models. The variables that significantly contributed to the definition of the two models were taken into account in the formulation of the two disease status scales: the SS Disease Damage Index (SSDDI) and SS Disease Activity Index (SSDAI). The weight of any variable in each scale was extrapolated by the correlation coefficient of the same variable in the corresponding model. The correlation between the scores for damage and activity obtained by applying SSDDI and SSDAI, respectively, and the scores assigned by the observers for the corresponding clinical status entities, was used to measure the construct validity of both indices. The ability of SSDAI to detect the variation of activity over time (sensitivity to change) was tested by applying SSDAI scale in two different observation times characterized by different levels of perceived activity.

Table 30.1 SSDDI (SS disease damage index)

Item	Definition	Score
Oral/salivary damage		
Salivary flow impairment	Unstimulated whole saliva collection <1.5 ml/15 min, by standard method	1
Loss of teeth	Complete or almost complete	1
Ocular damage		
Tear flow impairment	Schirmer I test <5 mm in 5 min, by standard method	1
Structural abnormalities	Corneal ulcers, cataracts, chronic blepharitis	1
Neurologic damage		
CNS involvement	Long-lasting stable CNS involvement	2
Peripheral neuropathy	Long-lasting stable peripheral or autonomic system impairment	1
Pleuropulmonary damage (any of the following)		2
Pleural fibrosis	Confirmed by imaging	
Interstitial fibrosis	Confirmed by imaging	
Significant irreversible functional damage	Confirmed by spirometry	
Renal impairment (any of the following)		2
Increased serum creatinine level or reduced GFR	Long-lasting stable abnormalities	
Tubular acidosis	Urinary pH>6 and serum bicarbonate <15 mmoles/l in two consecutive tests	
Nephrocalcinosis	Confirmed by imaging	
Lymphoproliferative disease (any of the following)		5
B cell lymphoma	Clinically and histologically confirmed	
Multiple myeloma	Clinically and histologically confirmed	
Waldenström's macroglobulinemia	Clinically and histologically confirmed	

Modified from Vitali et al. [21] with permission of John Wiley & Sons, Inc

The fact that SSDDI and SSDAI were built starting from a rather limited series of patients recruited in a single country may raise some doubts about their content validity. Therefore, the validity and reliability of these indices need to be verified in larger studies performed in different cohorts of patients collected on a multinational basis.

The SSDDI and SSDAI scoring systems are reported in Tables 30.1 and 30.2, respectively.

Table 30.2 SS disease activity index (SSDAI)

SSDAI		
Constitutional symptoms		
Fever	38°C, not due to infections	1
Fatigue	Sufficiently severe to affect normal activities	1
Change in fatigue	New appearance or worsening of fatigue	1
Change in salivary gland swelling	New appearance or increasing swelling of major salivary glands, not due to infection or stones	3
Articular symptoms (any of the following)		2
Arthritis	Inflammatory pain in ≥ 1 joint	
Evolving arthralgias	New appearance or worsening of joint pain without signs of articular inflammation	
Hematologic features		
Leukopenia/lymphopenia	$<3,500$ mm^3/$<1,000$ mm^3	1
Lymph node/spleen enlargement	Clinically palpable lymph node/spleen	2
Pleuropulmonary symptoms (any of the following)		4
Pleurisy	Confirmed by imaging, not due to infection	
Pneumonia (segmental or interstitial)	Ground-glass appearance on computed tomography scan, not due to infection	
Change in vasculitis	New appearance or worsening or recurrent flares of palpable purpura	3
Active renal involvement (any of the following)		2
New or worsening proteinuria	>0.5 gm/day	
Increasing serum creatinine level	Above the normal limits	
New or worsening nephritis	Glomerular or interstitial, histologically defined	
Peripheral neuropathy	Recent onset (<6 months), confirmed by nerve conduction studies	1

30.5.2 *The British Approach*

At the same time as the Italian group, a British Group performed a similar study aimed at developing and validating an activity index for SS [22]. The proposed scale was based on a modified version of the BILAG (British Island Lupus Activity Group) index for systemic lupus [23]. The BILAG scoring system is a multidimensional nominal scale, in which eight domains are separately considered and scored for activity according to changes since the previous observation. Stratification of each domain of the index for severity is done according the observer's intention to treat. An additional domain dedicated to specific features of SS was included in this BILAG-derived Sjögren's Syndrome Clinical Activity Index (SCAI). Because the analysis of the correlation matrix showed that a number of variables were interrelated, this instrument was reduced to a six-factor model. A correlation between the physician's global assessment and the SCAI derived score was used to test construct validity of the index. Furthermore, sensitivity to change was tested by comparing SCAI-derived and physician-defined disease flares, even based on the intention to treat analysis. Content validity of SCAI, similar to what has been argued for SSDAI, may have some limitations, because this index was derived from the analysis of a limited cohort of patients recruited in a single country.

A modified version of Systemic Lupus International Collaborating Clinics/American College of Rheumatology Damage Index (SLICC/ACR-DI) [18], adapted for the clinical peculiarities of SS, has been applied to lupus patients with secondary SS and patients with primary SS. This scale was shown to be a valid instrument for the measurement of some domains of disease damage related to sicca complaints [24]. Another version of SLICC/ACR-DI, with modifications included for specific use in SS, has been developed by a multidisciplinary British group. Specialists in rheumatology, ophthalmology, and oral medicine were part of the group. Ocular and oral domains and eight systemic domains represented the components of this new SS Damage Index (SSDI) [25]. A longitudinal study aimed at verifying the validity of this index in assessing cumulated damage of patients with SS is in an advanced phase.

30.5.3 The EULAR Initiative

Because studies conducted solely on a national scale suffer from inherent potential limitations with regard to content validity and amplitude of data collection, a multinational initiative sponsored by EULAR (European League Against Rheumatism) has recently started. This is aimed at defining and validating a EULAR activity index for SS. A promoting committee that includes leading investigators from Europe and overseas. The conceptual framework of the project stemmed from idea that the spectrum of SS varies between two poles: (a) a stable or slowly progressive disorder limited to epithelial regions (principally exocrine glands), characterized clinically by sicca complaints and constitutional symptoms such as fatigue and musculoskeletal pain; and (b) a more aggressive and systemic disorder, accompanied by extra-epithelial features and serological signs of autoimmune activation.

With this statement in mind, the task force of the project decided that two indices are needed to correctly define activity in SS. The first index, termed the EULAR SS Patient Reported Index (ESSPRI), is devoted to the assessment of sicca complaints and subjective symptoms such as dryness, fatigue and pain from the perspective of the patient. The second index, known as the EULAR SS Disease Activity Index (ESSDAI), addresses global activity related to the systemic features of the disease.

The Delphi methodology was followed initially in the design of ESSDAI. On the basis of their clinical experience and of the present knowledge from the literature review, the Steering Committee members first selected the organ- or system-specific domains they considered relevant to disease activity, and, in each domain, defined and ranked for severity all the possible related items. This proposal was submitted to the expert panel, who were asked to suggest and approve possible changes.

The final derived scale was preliminarily validated using a cohort of 702 simulated cases constructed, by means of a computer-assisted program, from a series of

96 real patient vignettes initially provided by members of the Steering Committee. Using the whole cohort of true and simulated cases, a multivariate model was built in which the ESSDAI domains represented the independent variables and the physician's global assessment, given by each expert to real and computer-derived clinical vignettes, was considered the dependent variable (gold standard). All of the domains listed in the ESSDAI were significantly associated with the physician's disease activity perception in the multivariate model. Finally, construct validity was assessed by correlation between the ESSDAI and physician's global scores [26].

Since the data on three consecutive visits (time 0, and after 3 and 6 months) for the 96 real patient profiles were available, it was possible to score these clinical vignettes in each observation time by applying both the ESSDAI and the previously described indices for activity (SSDAI and SCAI). Experts from the study group scored the same clinical vignettes in each observation time by simply judging whether disease activity had improved, worsened, or remained stable at visits 2 and 3 with respect to previous observation time. This procedure allowed testing sensitivity to change of the ESSDAI, SSDAI and SCAI and compare their performance in appreciating over time the variations of activity level. Analysis of performance characteristic curves, which Fig. 30.1 reports for the transition from visit 1 to visit 2,

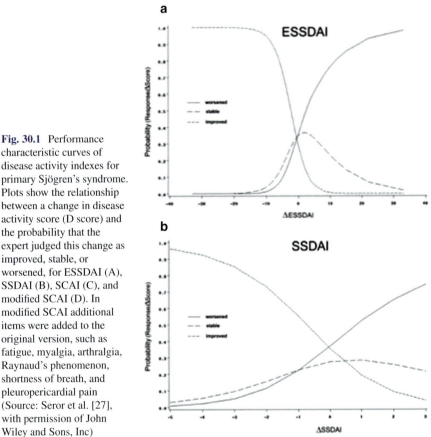

Fig. 30.1 Performance characteristic curves of disease activity indexes for primary Sjögren's syndrome. Plots show the relationship between a change in disease activity score (D score) and the probability that the expert judged this change as improved, stable, or worsened, for ESSDAI (A), SSDAI (B), SCAI (C), and modified SCAI (D). In modified SCAI additional items were added to the original version, such as fatigue, myalgia, arthralgia, Raynaud's phenomenon, shortness of breath, and pleuropericardial pain (Source: Seror et al. [27], with permission of John Wiley and Sons, Inc)

Fig. 30.1 (continued)

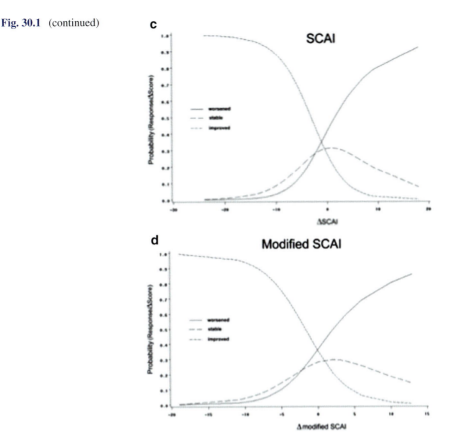

This kind of analysis showed that all scores discriminate improved and worsened disease activity effectively. However, the ESSDAI detected changes in activity and disease stability more accurately than the other indices [27].

The framework for ESSPRI development was consistently conditioned by the evidence that dryness, pain, and fatigue (somatic and mental) represent the key symptoms of patients with primary SS [28, 29]. These studies also indicated that a single numerical (or visual) scale for each domain is sufficient to assess these features. On the basis of this conceptual background, the preliminary ESSPRI was composed by specific questionnaires exploring these key symptoms of the disease. These questionnaires were applied in a large number of patients coming from different countries. A multiple regression model in which the patient's global assessment was considered the dependent variable (gold standard) was analyzed to select the most relevant domains in the patient perception and estimate their weights. In this multivariate model, dryness, limb pain, and physical fatigue were significantly associated with patient's global assessment, and weights derived from the regression were identical for these three domains. Thus, ESSPRI was redefined as a simple tool composed by three scales assessing the main symptoms, i.e., dryness, limb pain, and fatigue [30].

Final validation studies of both the ESSDAI and ESSPRI in a large series of real patients are under way. When this ongoing phase of the project is finished, valid and reliable instruments to assess activity in SS will finally be available for clinical trials and practice.

References

1. Symmonds DPM. Disease assessment indices: activity, damage and severity. Baillieres Clin Rheumatol. 1995;9:267–85.
2. Fries JF, Hochberg MC, Medsger TA. Criteria for rheumatic diseases: different types and different functions. Arthritis Rheum. 1994;37:454–62.
3. Liang MH. Translating outcomes measurement in experimental therapeutics of systemic rheumatic disease to patient care. Rheum Dis Clin North Am. 2006;32:1–8.
4. Mitsias DI, Kapsogeorgou EK, Moutsopoulos HM. Sjögren's syndrome: why autoimmune epithelitis? Oral Dis. 2006;12:523–32.
5. Garcia-Carrasco M, Ramos Casals M, Rasas J, et al. Primary Sjögren's syndrome: clinical and immunologic disease patterns in a cohort of 400 patients. Medicine (Baltimore). 2002;81:270–80.
6. Ioannidis JP, Vassiliou VA, Moutsopoulos HM. Long term risk of mortality and lymphoproliferative diseases and predictive classification of primary Sjögren's syndrome. Arthritis Rheum. 2002;46:741–7.
7. Ramos-Casals M, Brito-Zeron P. Emerging biological therapies in primary Sjögren's syndrome. Rheumatology (Oxford). 2007;46:1389–96.
8. Looney RJ. Will targeting B cells be the answer for Sjögren's syndrome. Arthritis Rheum. 2007;56:1371–7.
9. Seror R, Sordet C, Guillevin L, et al. Tolerance and efficacy of rituximab and changes in serum B cell biomarkers in patients with systemic complications of primary Sjögren's syndrome. Ann Rheum Dis. 2007;66:351–7.
10. Szororay P, Jonnson R. The BAFF/APRIL system in systemic autoimmune diseases with special emphasis on Sjögren's syndrome. Scand J Immunol. 2005;62:421–8.
11. Meijer JM, Meiners PM, Vissink A, et al. Effectiveness of rituximab treatment in primary Sjögren's syndrome: a randomized, double-blind, placebo-controlled trial. Arthritis Rheum. 2010;62:960–8.
12. Pincus T, Sokka T. Complexities in the quantitative assessment of patients with rheumatic diseases in clinical trials and clinical care. Clin Exp Rheumatol. 2005;23 Suppl 39:S1–9.
13. Liang MH, Socher SA, Neal Roberts W, et al. Measurement of systemic lupus erythematosus activity in clinical research. Arthritis Rheum. 1988;31(7):817–25.
14. American College of Rheumatology Ad Hoc Committee on Systemic Lupus Erythematosus Response Criteria. The American College of Rheumatology response criteria for systemic lupus erythematosus clinical trials: measures of overall disease activity. Arthritis Rheum. 2004;50:3418–26.
15. Pincus T, Sokka T. Quantitative measures for assessing rheumatoid arthritis in clinical trials and clinical care. Best Pract Res Clin Rheumatol. 2003;17:753–81.
16. Strand V, Gladman D, Isenberg D, et al. Outcome measures to be used in clinical trials in systemic lupus erythematosus. J Rheumatol. 1999;26:490–7.
17. Valentini G, Della Rossa A, Bombardieri S, et al. European multicentre study to define disease activity criteria for systemic sclerosis. II. Identification of disease activity variables and development of preliminary activity indexes. Ann Rheum Dis. 2001;60:592–8.
18. Gladman D, Ginzler E, Goldsmith C, et al. The development and initial validation of the Systemic Lupus International Collaborating Clinics/American College of Rheumatology damage index for systemic lupus erythematosus. Arthritis Rheum. 1996;39:363–9.

19. van der Heijde D. How to read radiographs according to the Sharp/van der Heijde method. J Rheumatol. 2000;27:261–3.
20. Vitali C, Palombi G, Baldini C, et al. Sjögren's syndrome disease damage index and disease activity index. Scoring systems for the assessment of disease damage and disease activity in Sjögren's syndrome, derived from an analysis of a cohort of Italian patients. Arthritis Rheum. 2007;56:2223–31.
21. Vitali C, Bencivelli W, Isenberg DA, et al. Disease activity in systemic lupus erythematosus: report of the Consensus Study Group of the European Workshop for Rheumatology Research. II Identification of the variables indicative of disease activity and their use in the development of an activity score. Clin Exp Rheumatol. 1992;10:541–7.
22. Bowman SJ, Sutcliffe N, Isenberg DA, et al. Sjögren's Syndrome Clinical Activity Index (SCAI) – a systemic disease activity measure for use in clinical trials in primary Sjögren's syndrome. Rheumatology (Oxford). 2007;46:1845–51.
23. Hay EM, Bacon PA, Gordon C, et al. The BILAG index: a reliable and valid instrument for measuring clinical disease activity in systemic lupus erythematosus. Q J Med. 1993;86: 447–58.
24. Sutcliffe N, Stoll T, Pyke S, et al. Functional disability and end organ damage in patients with systemic lupus erythematosus (SLE), SLE and Sjögren's syndrome (SS), and primary SS. J Rheumatol. 1998;25:63–8.
25. Barry RJ, Sutcliffe N, Isenberg DA, et al. The Sjögren's syndrome Damage Index (SSDI) – a damage index for use in clinical trials and observational studies in primary Sjögren's syndrome. Rheumatology (Oxford). 2008;47:1193–8.
26. Seror R, Ravaud P, Bowman SJ, et al. EULAR Sjogren's syndrome disease activity index: development of a consensus systemic disease activity index for primary Sjogren's syndrome. Ann Rheum Dis. 2010;69:1103–9.
27. Seror R, Mariette X, Bowman S, et al. Accurate detection of changes in disease activity in primary Sjogren's syndrome by the European League Against Rheumatism Sjogren's Syndrome Disease Activity Index. Arthritis Care Res. 2010;62:551–8.
28. Bowman SJ, Booth DA, Platts RG. Measurement of fatigue and discomfort in primary Sjögren's syndrome using a new questionnaire tool. Rheumatology (Oxford). 2004;43: 758–64.
29. Bowman SJ, Booth DA, Platts RG, et al. Validation of the Sicca Symptoms Inventory for clinical studies of Sjogren's syndrome. J Rheumatol. 2003;30:1259–66.
30. Seror R, Ravaud P, Mariette X, et al. EULAR Sjögren's Syndrome Patient Reported Index (ESSPRI). Development of a consensus patient index for primary Sjögren's syndrome. Ann Rheum Dis. 2011;70(6):968–72.

Chapter 31
Measurement of Quality of Life in Primary Sjögren's Syndrome

Simon J. Bowman and Wan-Fai Ng

Contents

31.1   Introduction

Primary Sjögren's syndrome (PSS) is an immune-mediated rheumatic disease in which inflammation of secretory (exocrine) glands leads to dry eyes and dry mouth [1]. Dryness of other surfaces such as the skin, vagina, airways, and gastrointestinal tract also occurs. The secretory glands are infiltrated by collections (focal aggregations) of lymphocytes. In the salivary glands, these focal lymphocyte aggregations are typically clustered around the salivary ducts. Patients typically also complain of reduced well-being, fatigue, and arthralgia. Approximately three-quarters of patients have autoantibodies in their blood – anti-Ro and/or anti-La antibodies – and a majority also have elevated total immunoglobulin levels (hypergammaglobulinaemia). A proportion of patients have other systemic organ involvement including neuropathies,

S.J. Bowman (✉)
Rheumatology Department, University Hospital Birmingham (Selly Oak), Birmingham, UK

W.-Fai Ng
Musculoskeletal Research Group, Institute of Cellular Medicine, Newcastle University,
Newcastle Upon Tyne, UK

M. Ramos-Casals et al. (eds.), *Sjögren's Syndrome*,
DOI 10.1007/978-0-85729-947-5_31, © Springer-Verlag London Limited 2012

skin rashes (purpura, vasculitis), interstitial lung disease, renal tubular acidosis, and hematological abnormalities. Finally, patients with PSS are at substantially increased risk for the occurrence of lymphomas, particularly mucosa-associated lymphoid tissue (MALT) B-cell lymphomas. In this chapter, we assess the issue of health-related quality of life (QoL) in PSS.

"Quality of life" is a broad concept that attempts to describe the general well-being of individuals and societies [2]. QoL studies often focus particularly on economic well-being. As an example, in terms of QoL within countries, the Economist's 2005 QoL Index (http://www.economist.com/media/pdf/QUALITY_OF_LIFE.pdf) scores a country's QoL according to scores on nine domains: health (life expectancy at birth), family life (divorce rate), community life (e.g., church attendance, trade union membership), material well-being (gross domestic product), political stability and security, climate and geography (latitude), job security (unemployment rate), political freedom, and gender equality (ratio of average male:female earnings). The World Health Organization (WHO) defines QoL as "individuals' perceptions of their position in life in the context of the culture and value systems in which they live and in relation to their goals, expectations, standards and concerns" (http://www.who.int/mental_health/media/68.pdf). Domains include a person's physical health, psychological state, level of independence, social relationships, personal beliefs and their relationship to salient features of their environment. The WHOQOL Group has developed questionnaires to measure generic QoL: the initial (WHOQOL-100) [3] and the shorter (26 item) WHOQOL-BREF [4]. The principal domains of the WHOQOL are of physical health, psychological well-being, social relationships, and environmental factors. The questionnaires also include questions pertaining to an individual's global QoL – "how would you rate your quality of life?" – and also introduce the generic concept of "health-related quality of life (HRQoL)"; for example: "how satisfied are you with your health?". The WHOQOL questionnaires were designed and piloted in centers around the world and in individuals with various states of health and illness. They are intended to measure QoL independently of cultural constraints.

The line between the concepts of "QoL" and "HRQoL" is often blurred. For example, HRQoL typically focuses on aspects of physical and psychological well-being and the consequences of ill-health on social relationships. The environment may have a major impact on individuals and populations quality of life but only indirectly on health status. In the context of evaluating a disease state such as PSS, the term HRQoL is more widely used in most papers but in some the terms HRQoL and QoL are used interchangeably. To some extent, a convention has developed whereby questionnaires such as the WHOQoL measure QoL and other questionnaires (discussed below) measure HRQoL.

QoL/HRQoL measures fall within the broader concept of "patient-reported outcome measures" (PROMs). These are patient-completed questionnaires that encompass symptom questionnaires as well as QoL measures. Some are generic and hence widely applicable, but others are specific to particular conditions or patient groups. They can be used in a number of situations, including clinical trials, economic evaluations, and routine clinical care. Their value is that they complement more

Study	Number of patients	SF-36 domains impaired
Table 31.1 Studies using the SF-36 in patients with PSS.		
Thomas et al. [6]	13	All except mental health
Strömbeck et al. [7]	42	All
Tensing et al. [8]	90	All
Rostron et al. [9]	43	All
Bowman et al. [10]	137	All
Belenguer et al. [11]	110	All
Champey et al. [12]	109	All
Stewart et al. [13]	39	All
López-Jornet et al. [14]	33	All
Meijer et al. [15]	155	All except bodily pain and mental health
Segal et al. [16]	277	All
Baturone et al. [17]	30	All

"traditional" measures of physician-focused disease assessment. To give an example from PSS: an improvement in salivary flow without a corresponding improvement in the patient's perception of oral dryness may only be of limited clinical value.

31.2   Measurement of Generic HRQoL in PSS: The SF-36 Questionnaire

The Medical Outcomes Study SF-36 questionnaire [5] was developed from work done by the RAND Corporation in the 1980s and 1990s. As its name suggests it comprises 36 questions forming eight domains: vitality, physical functioning, bodily pain, general health perceptions, physical role functioning, emotional role functioning, social role functioning and mental health. The raw scores are converted through a weighted algorithm into 0–100 scores for each domain where 100=perfect health and 0=poor HRQoL for that domain; i.e., the higher the score the better the level of HRQoL. Composite "physical health" and "mental health" scores can also be calculated and the scores can be used in health economics to generate estimates of quality adjusted life years. However, the SF-36 does not generate a single number for "total HRQoL". Population data, against which patient group scores can be compared, are available from many countries. The SF-36 and its more recent derivative, the SF-36 V2, have been used in thousands of research studies across the globe, making it the most successful HRQoL measure in current use.

The SF-36 has been used in many studies of PSS [6–17] (Table 31.1). Although there are some differences between the studies, the simple summary is that patients with PSS generally have reduced HRQoL across a range of domains. The HRQoL scores of PSS patients are comparable to those of patients with other rheumatic diseases, e.g., rheumatoid arthritis and systemic lupus erythematosus, as well as to

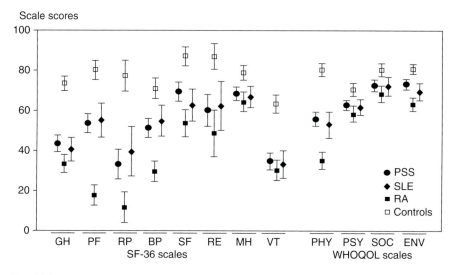

Fig. 31.1 Measurement of quality of life in patients with primary SS, SLE, RA and controls (SF-36 and WHOQOL scales).

non-inflammatory conditions such as fibromyalgia. Data in PSS using a shortened form of the SF-36, the SF-20, have also been reported [18].

31.3 Other Generic QoL/HRQoL Measures

Patients with PSS have been shown to have reduced QoL across all four domains of the WHOQoL-BREF compared with a community control comparator group [10]. The pattern was similar to a comparator group of patients with systemic lupus erythematosus. The main difference compared to a further control group of patients with rheumatoid arthritis was that the rheumatoid arthritis group had significantly lower scores on the physical domain scale (Fig. 31.1). The WHOQOL-BREF physical scale scores correlated with SF-36 vitality and physical domain scores.

Another HRQoL questionnaire that is increasingly likely to be used over the next few years is the EuroQoL 5-domain (EQ-5D) questionnaire [19]. The EuroQoL group, founded in 1987, includes researchers from the UK, Finland, the Netherlands, Norway, Sweden and other countries in Europe, North America, and Japan. Their goal was to develop a generic HRQoL measure for use across Europe and elsewhere. The EQ-5D comprises five domains: mobility, self-care, usual activities, pain/discomfort and anxiety/depression as well as a global health status "thermometer" (100 mm visual analogue scale). The EQ-5D is similar to the WHOQoL in that it generates a single global HRQoL score as well as individual domain scores. Rajagopalan et al. have reported on the EQ-5D in 32 patients with PSS and shown comparable reductions in HRQoL with the EQ-5D and SF-36 [20]. Two much larger studies are currently collecting EQ-5D data in PSS – the European League Against

Rheumatism (EULAR) Sjögren's working group [21] and the UK Primary Sjögren's Syndrome Registry (UKPSSR) [22].

Other HRQoL measures that have been widely used (although not in PSS) include the Nottingham Health Profile (NHP) [23], the Sickness Impact Profile (SIP) [24], and many others, e.g.: http://phi.uhce.ox.ac.uk/home.php and http://www.health-measurement.org/Measures.html. A Swedish group reported on reduced QoL in PSS using the Gothenburg Quality of Life Instrument (GQOL) [25].

31.4   "Disease-Specific" HRQoL Measures

A number of oral and ocular dryness symptom questionnaires can be applied in PSS [26]. The Sicca Symptoms Inventory measures both oral and ocular dryness as well as other sicca symptoms [27]. Some of these questionnaires, such as the Oral Health Impact Profile [28], have been proposed to be "disease-specific" HRQoL measures, on the basis that they do not only measure oral symptoms but also the social impact of oral disorders. The OHIP comprises 49 questions in seven domains: functional limitations (Q1–9), physical pain (Q10–18), psychological discomfort (Q19–23), physical disability (Q24–32), psychological disability (Q33–38), social disability (Q39–43) and handicap (Q44–49). The items range from simple symptoms (e.g., Q1: "Have you had difficulty chewing any foods because of problems with your teeth, mouth or dentures?") to more complex effects on social functioning (e.g., Q39: "Have you avoided going out because of problems with your teeth, mouth or dentures?"), and general health perception (e.g., Q44: "Have you felt that your general health has worsened because of problems with your teeth, mouth or dentures?"). In a study that compared different groups of patients lacking teeth to those with teeth, Allen et al. [29] demonstrated that the OHIP discriminated between groups whereas the SF-36 did not. Moreover, the OHIP was sensitive to change following the provision of dentures or dental implants [30].

In patients with PSS, OHIP-49 scores are reduced compared to controls and where the SF-36 was also used the scores parallel those of the latter [31–34]. In another study the OHIP-14 (a shortened version of the OHIP-49) total score correlated significantly with five of the eight SF-36 domain scores, particularly with the domains of social functioning ($p < 0.01$) and general health ($p < 0.01$) [13]. One important point to emphasize is that since the OHIP includes question items on both social functioning and general health (see above), one might predict correlations between the generic and "disease-specific" HRQoL measures. It is useful to see this borne out in a formal evaluation in this study. Other reported oral health HRQoL measures include the Oral Health-related QoL measure [35], the Geriatric Oral Health Assessment Index [36], and the Xerostomia-related QoL questionnaire [37].

With regard to ocular features, a comparison of the widely used Ocular Surface Disease Index (OSDI) (predominantly a dryness symptom questionnaire) and the National Eye Institute Visual Function Questionnaire (NEI-VFQ) (which includes a broad range of visual symptom questions but also some vision-related HRQoL domains such as vision-specific social functioning, mental health, role functioning and dependency) in 109 patients with dry eye showed significant correlations between the measures [38]. Similar correlations between the OSDI and the symptom components of the NEI-VFQ-25 were observed in a study of 42 patients with PSS [39]. The "HRQoL" components of the NEI-VFQ have been shown to correlate with relevant domains of the SF-36 in a study of patients with a variety of ocular disorders [40].

31.5 Predictors of HRQoL (SF-36) in PSS

We have described a variety of studies above that demonstrate reduced SF-36 scores in patients with PSS. What are the potential reasons for reduced HRQoL in this disorder? Belenguer et al. studied 110 patients with PSS [11]. Age correlated with SF-36 physical functioning and bodily pain domain scores. Patients with extraglandular features had lower scores for the vitality, social functioning, bodily pain and general health, whereas sicca features were not significantly associated with SF-36 domain scores. Champey et al. studied 111 patients with PSS and 65 patients with sicca symptoms without autoimmune features [12]. In both groups, fatigue and pain correlated with physical composite scores of the SF-36. In addition, psychological distress, measured by the symptom checklist 90 revised (SCL-90-R) questionnaire, correlated with SF-36 physical and mental domain composite scores. However, sicca symptoms did not.

In a study by Meijer et al. that included 185 patients with PSS and 50 with secondary SS, fatigue was correlated strongly with physical and mental composite scores in the combined population [15]. Multivariate regression analysis also identified that "tendomyalgia", comorbidity, male sex, and disability compensation correlated with SF-36 physical composite scores. Articular involvement, the use of anti-depressants, and comorbidity were associated with reduced SF-36 mental composite scores. However, the data interpretation was complicated by the fact that both PSS and secondary SS were included in the study. Another study of 277 patients with PSS demonstrated that somatic fatigue was the unique predictor of the general health domain scores of SF-36, pain, severity and depression of emotional well-being [16]. Depression accounted for 25% of the variance of emotional well-being. Age, pain severity, and somatic fatigue predicted the overall level of physical functioning [16].

A recent study of 30 patients with PSS examined the correlations between SF-36 scores and serum cytokine levels [17]. This study identified an inverse relationship between serum IL-6 levels and SF-36 bodily pain, physical functioning, and the physical composite score [17]. D'Elia and colleagues have also shown that baseline serum soluble IL-6 receptor (sIL6R) correlates inversely with fatigue as measured by MFI and VAS and positively with vitality and mental component scores of the SF-36 [41]. Data from other studies, however, report different findings. Hartkamp et al. [42] compared serum cytokine levels including of IL-6 in PSS patients and controls and found no correlation between the levels of fatigue (assessed using MFI) and the levels of these cytokines.

Table 31.2 Summary of published data on the clinical and biological predictors of HRQoL (SF-36 Domain Scores) in PSS [11, 12, 15–17, 41, 44, 45]

Predictors[a]	SF-36 domain scores
	Physical health
Age [11, 16], pain severity [16], somatic fatigue [16], total SSDI score [45], serum IL6 [17]	Physical functioning (PF)
	Role-physical (RP)
Age [11], extraglandular features [11], serum IL6 [17]	Bodily pain (BP)
Extraglandular features [11], somatic fatigue [16]	General health (GH)
	Mental health
Extraglandular features [11], SCAI fatigue [44], serum sIL6R [41]	Vitality (VT)
Extraglandular features [11]	Social functioning (SF)
Pain severity [16], depression [16]	Role-emotional (RE)
Serum sIL6R [41]	Mental health (MH)
	Composite scores
Fatigue [12, 15], pain [12], psychological distress [12], tendomyalgia [15], male [15], disability compensation [15], co-morbidity [15], SCAI arthritis [44], serum IL6 [17]	Physical composite
Psychological distress [12], fatigue [15], co-morbidity [15], articular involvement [15], anti-depressant use [15]	Mental composite

[a]Sicca was not a predictor for any of the SF-36 domains listed [11, 12]

Fatigue is identified as a predictor of SF-36 domain scores in a variety of studies. In an investigation of 94 patients with PSS, pain, helplessness, and depression were predictors of physical and mental fatigue [43]. Table 31.2 indicates some of the predictors of reduced HRQoL identified in studies of PSS.

31.6 Predictors of QoL and HRQoL (WHOQoL) in PSS

In validation studies of instruments for the assessment of systemic disease activity and accumulated damage in patients with PSS, we evaluated 104 patients at baseline and at 12 months. For the Sjögren's systemic Clinical Activity Index (SCAI), the SF-36 vitality domain correlated with the SCAI fatigue domain and the SF-36 physical summary score correlated with the SCAI arthritis domain score [44]. A 29-item damage score that incorporated ocular, oral, and systemic domains was also agreed upon. Total damage score correlated with disease activity and duration at study entry and also with physical function as measured by the SF-36 [45].

We can also examine this same data looking for correlations between the WHO "global" QoL question "how do you rate your QoL?", the WHO "global" HRQoL question "how satisfied are you with your health?" and multiple other symptomatic and "objective" measures (Table 31.3). One observation from these data is that age, disease duration and objective measures of disease activity SCAI (Sjögren's Clinical

Table 31.3 Correlation analysis of variables with WHOQoL 'global' QoL and HRQoL questions [3, 4]

	How do you rate your QoL?		How satisfied are you with your health? (HRQoL)	
	r value	p value	r value	p value
WHO HRQoL	0.445	<0.001		
Age	−0.203	0.042	0.084	0.402
Disease duration	−0.064	0.523	0.029	0.776
Modified Beck depression inventory score [44]	−0.454	<0.001	−0.490	<0.001
Profile of fatigue and discomfort				
Somatic fatigue	−0.441	<0.001	−0.426	<0.001
Mental fatigue	−0.440	<0.001	−0.273	<0.001
Arthralgia	−0.403	<0.001	−0.365	<0.001
Profile of fatigue [10]	−0.476	<0.001	−0.386	<0.001
PROFAD [10]	−0.541	<0.001	−0.416	<0.001
Occ dryness	−0.383	<0.001	−0.370	<0.001
Oral dryness	−0.310	0.002	−0.312	0.002
Sicca symptoms inventory total score [27]	−0.357	<0.001	−0.365	<0.001
SF-36				
Physical function	0.404	<0.001	0.344	<0.001
Role physical	0.352	<0.001	0.377	<0.001
Bodily pain	0.379	<0.001	0.525	<0.001
General health	0.414	<0.001	0.66	<0.001
Vitality	0.426	<0.001	0.439	<0.001
Social functioning	0.516	<0.001	0.571	<0.001
Role emotional	0.367	<0.001	0.341	<0.001
Mental health	0.439	<0.001	0.391	<0.001
Physical summary score	0.344	<0.001	0.444	<0.001
Mental summary score	0.567	<0.001	0.552	<0.001
Sjögren's clinical activity index				
SCAI total [44]	−0.228	0.022	−0.29	0.003
SCAI objective total [45]	−0.109	0.28	−0.154	0.125
Schirmers average	−0.259	0.01	−0.104	0.305
Unstimulated salivary flow	0.132	0.199	−0.029	0.777

Source: Data is derived from PSS patients recruited in Bowman et al. [44] and Barry et al. [45]
IgG, IgA, anti-Ro and anti-La antibody titers*, SSDI [45] ocular*, oral*, systemic and total* damage: r between −0.146 and 0.206 p = not significant at 0.05. Patient n between 98 and 104 for all analyses above except for * where n is between 84 and 87

Activity Index) scores, Sjögren's Syndrome Damage Index (SSDI) scores, tear production (Schirmer's I test), the unstimulated salivary flow rate, and biological markers such as immunoglobulin and autoantibody titers correlate poorly with global WHOQoL item ratings. The symptomatic measures: a measure of depression (a modified short 10-item version of the Beck Depression Inventory (BDI)), components of the Profile of Fatigue and Discomfort (PROFAD), Sicca Symptoms Inventory (SSI), and the SF-36 all correlate highly with each other, such that it is impossible to ascribe a percentage variance to these in a combined multivariate regression analysis. If one performs single regression analyses for each variable (BDI, PROFAD, SSI, SF-36 physical summary score (PCS) and SF-36 mental summary score (MCS)) against the WHO HRQoL global item the individual R^2 are: 23.3%, 16.5%, 12.4%, 18.9% and 29.7% respectively (Minitab version 12). The corresponding figures for the same variables analyzed against the WHOQoL global items are 19.8%, 28.6%, 11.8%, 10.9% and 31.5%, respectively. In stepwise regression analysis, the best-fit model for the HRQoL global item includes the BDI and SF-36 PCS and MCS scores and for the QoL global item the PROFAD and SF-36 MCS. These data demonstrate the importance of psychological factors, fatigue/discomfort, and to a significant but lesser extent, dryness symptoms in determining patients' assessment of their QoL/HRQoL. In contrast, in PSS, biological factors and objective measures of dryness play little part.

31.7   Therapeutic Interventions

Studies in the 1990s, whether of cyclosporine ophthalmic emulsion for ocular dryness [46], pilocarpine for oral dryness [47], or hydroxychloroquine for systemic features [48], did not always incorporate generic HRQoL assessment as a component of outcome assessment. More recent studies of PSS have included such measures routinely. In the study by Mariette et al. [49] in 103 patients with PSS who received either infliximab or placebo there was no difference in the SF-36 physical or mental summary scores at week 10 compared with baseline in either group [49]. However, that clinical trial was a negative study in that the symptomatic responses (pain, fatigue, dryness visual analogue scales) did not differ between the groups, either.

More recently, initial studies using rituximab have been more positive. Pijpe et al. [50] reported an open-label study of eight patients with early PSS treated with 375 mg/m^2 of rituximab plus 25 mg intravenous prednisolone on four occasions. At week 12, improvement was seen in oral symptoms, stimulated salivary flow rate, multidimensional fatigue inventory domains (except for the mental fatigue domain) and SF-36 physical functioning and vitality domains. Meijer et al. [51] updated progress after five of these patients had been retreated and followed for up to 48 weeks with similar improvement in SF-36 scores. In another open-label study using 375 mg/m^2 of rituximab but given on only two occasions, significant improvement at 36 weeks was seen for both symptomatic (fatigue, dryness, joint pain visual analogue scales) and SF-36 physical and mental summary scores [52].

In our double blind, placebo-controlled, randomized pilot study of the efficacy of rituximab in 17 patients with pSS who were randomized to receive either two infusions of rituximab 1 g or placebo, there was significant improvement from baseline in fatigue VAS in the rituximab group ($p<0.001$) in contrast to the placebo group ($p=0.147$). There was a significant difference between the groups at 6 months in the social functioning score of SF-36 ($p=0.01$) and a trend to significant difference in the mental health domain score of SF-36 ($p=0.06$) [53]. A double-blind randomized controlled study of 120 patients with PSS receiving either rituximab or placebo is currently ongoing in France (http://clinicaltrials.gov/ct2/show/NCT00740948) and a similar study is planned to start in the UK. These should address clearly whether rituximab can improve HRQoL in patients with PSS.

There are a number of randomized controlled studies of other therapies in PSS, which have included some data on SF-36 scores. Androgen deficiency has been proposed to be a contributory factor in developing PSS and in a double-blind, randomized placebo-controlled trial of 60 PSS patients, Hartkamp et al. [54] demonstrated that both dehydroepiandrosterone and placebo significantly reduced the levels of fatigue as assessed by MFI and mental summary score of the SF-36, whereas there was no change in the SF-36 physical summary score in either group. Leflunomide 20 mg daily has also been studied in a phase II open-labeled study in 15 patients with pSS. At 24 weeks, there was a statistically significant reduction of the general fatigue domain score (from 17 to 11) and an increase in the physical dimension score (from 39.8 to 43.8) of the SF-36 [55].

Non-pharmacologic approaches have also been studied. Strombeck and colleagues investigated the effect of moderate to high intensity exercise programme on the aerobic capacity and fatigue in patients with PSS [56]. Eleven PSS patients were given a medium to high intensity aerobic exercise programme and ten were given low-intensity home exercises. The level of fatigue was assessed before and after the 12-week study period. Patients allocated to the medium to high intensity programme reported a significant improvement of fatigue visual analogue scale and aerobic capacity compared to the home exercise group. There were reductions in the total, somatic and mental components of the Profile of Fatigue score in both interventional groups. No changes, however, were seen in SF-36 domain scores in either group after intervention compared with baseline.

31.8   Conclusions and Summary

A series of studies over the past decade have demonstrated consistently that HRQoL as measured by the SF-36 is reduced in patients with PSS [6–17]. Studies examining what factors might be contributing to this have identified fatigue as a major factor and indicated that psychological factors also play a part [12, 15, 16]. In contrast, dryness symptoms appear to contribute relatively little to SF-36 scores. The difficulty inherent in this conclusion about sicca symptoms, however, is that the content of the SF-36 favors physical and mental difficulties and does not incorporate question items to which dryness symptoms would necessarily correlate. To this end, assessment of HRQoL though the "global" component of WHOQoL [4] or EQ-5D [19] may be more useful in this type of analysis. Data should be available for the EQ-5D over the next few years from two currently active collaborative studies (The EULAR study [21] and the UK Primary Sjögren's syndrome Registry [22]). An alternative approach, which has been adopted by oral and ocular specialists interested in PSS, is to use a measure such as the OHIP [28] or NEI-VFQ [39] which combine some symptomatic assessment items as well as "disease-specific" HRQoL items such as the effect of their oral/ocular symptoms on social functioning and other QoL components.

A number of interventional studies including anti-B-cell therapy [49–53] and non-pharmacological approaches [56] suggest that there is scope to intervene to improve HRQoL in patients with PSS. Two studies of rituximab, one in France (actively recruiting) and one due to start in the UK should address clearly whether anti-B-cell therapy has a role to play in improving HRQoL and other features in PSS. What is important to note, however, in all of these studies, is that HRQoL has become an integral part of global patient assessment in PSS as it has increasingly become a part of patient assessment across the health spectrum.

Acknowledgements and Conflicts of Interest WFN has received salary support from the Arthritis Research Campaign and grant support from the Medical Research Council, Arthritis Research Campaign, British Sjögren's Syndrome Association and the JGW Patterson Foundation. The UK Primary Sjögren's Syndrome Registry is funded by the Medical Research Council. SJB has consulted for Roche, Genentech, UCB, Glaxo-Smith-Kline and Astra-Zeneca and has received grant support from the Arthritis Research Campaign, University Hospital Birmingham Charities and the British Sjögren's Syndrome Association.

References

1. Jonsson R, Bowman SJ, Gordon TP. Sjögren's Syndrome. In: Koopman WJ, Moreland LW, editors. Arthritis and allied conditions, Chapter 78. 15th ed. Philadelphia: Lippincott Williams & Wilkins; 2005. p. 1681–705.
2. Carr AJ, Thompson PW, Kirwan JR. Quality of life measures. Br J Rheumatol. 1996;35: 275–81.
3. WHOQOL Group. Development of the WHOQOL: rationale and current status. Int J Ment Health. 1994;23:24–56.
4. WHOQOL Group. Development of the World Health Organization WHOQOL-BREF Quality of Life Assessment. Psychol Med. 1998;28:551–8.
5. Ware JE, Snow KK, Kosinski M, Gandek B. SF-36 Health Survey. Manual and interpretation guide. Boston: The Health Institute, New England Medical Centre; 1993.
6. Thomas E, Hay EM, Hajeer A, Silman AJ. Sjogren's syndrome: a community based study of prevalence and impact. Br J Rheumatol. 1998;37:1069–76.
7. Strömbeck B, Ekdahl C, Manthorpe R, et al. Health-related quality of life in primary Sjogren's syndrome, rheumatoid arthritis and fibromyalgia compared to normal population data using SF-36. Scand J Rheumatol. 2000;29:20–8.
8. Tensing EK, Soloviyeva SA, Tervahartiala T, et al. Fatigue and health profile in sicca syndrome of Sjogren's and non-Sjogren's syndrome origin. Clin Exp Rheumatol. 2001;19:313–6.
9. Rostron J, Rogers S, Longman L, et al. Health-related quality of life in patients with primary Sjogren's syndrome and xerostomia: a comparative study. Gerodontology. 2002;19:53–9.
10. Bowman SJ, Booth DA, Platts RG, UK Sjögren's Interest Group. Measurement of fatigue and discomfort in primary Sjogren's syndrome using a new questionnaire tool. Rheumatology (Oxford). 2004;43:758–64.
11. Belenguer R, Ramos-Casals M, Brito-Zerón P, et al. Influence of clinical and immunological parameters on the health-related quality of life in patients with primary Sjogren's syndrome. Clin Exp Rheumatol. 2005;23:351–6.

12. Champey J, Corruble E, Gottenberg JE, et al. Quality of life and psychological status in patients with primary Sjogren's syndrome and sicca symptoms without autoimmune features. Arthritis Rheum. 2006;55:451–7.
13. Stewart CM, Berg KM, Cha S, Reeves WH. Salivary dysfunction and quality of life in Sjogren's syndrome: a critical oral-systemic connection. J Am Dent Assoc. 2008;139:291–9.
14. López-Jornet P, Camacho-Alonso F. Quality of life in patients with Sjogren's syndrome and sicca complex. J Oral Rehabil. 2008;35:875–81.
15. Meijer JM, Meiners PM, Huddleston Slater JJ, et al. Health-related quality of life, employment and disability in patients with Sjogren's syndrome. Rheumatology (Oxford). 2009;48:1077–82.
16. Segal B, Bowman SJ, Fox PC, et al. Primary Sjogren's syndrome: health experiences and predictors of health quality among patients in the United States. Health Qual Life Outcomes. 2009;27:7–46.
17. Baturone R, Soto M, Marquez M, et al. Health-related quality of life in patients with primary Sjogren's syndrome: relationship with serum levels of proinflammatory cytokines. Scand J Rheumatol. 2009;2:1–4.
18. Sutcliffe N, Stoll T, Pyke S, Isenberg D. Functional disability and end-organ damage in patients with systemic lupus erythematosus (SLE), SLE and Sjögren's syndrome (SS), and primary SS. J Rheumatol. 1998;25:63–8.
19. Group EuroQoL. EuroQoL – a new facility for the measurement of health-related quality of life. Health Policy. 1990;16:199–208.
20. Rajagopalan K, Abetz L, Mertzanis P, et al. Comparing the discriminative validity of two generic and one disease-specific health-related quality of life measures in a sample of patients with dry eye. Value Health. 2005;8:168–74.
21. Seror R, Ravaud P, Bowman S, et al. EULAR Sjogren's Syndrome Disease Activity Index (ESSDAI): development of a consensus systemic disease activity index in primary Sjogren's syndrome. Ann Rheum Dis. 2009;69:1103–9.
22. Ng WF, Griffiths B, Griffiths ID, Bowman SJ. United Kingdom primary Sjogren's syndrome registry (UKPSSR). London: Medical Research Council; 2008.
23. Hunt SM, McEwan J. The development of a subjective health indicator. Sociol Health Illn. 1980;2:231–46.
24. Gilson BS, Gilson JS, Bergner M, et al. The sickness impact profile. Development of an outcome measure of health care. Am J Public Health. 1975;65:1304–10.
25. Valtysdottir ST, Gudbjornsson B, Lindqvist U, et al. Anxiety and depression in patients with primary Sjogren's syndrome. J Rheumatol. 2000;27:165–9.
26. Bowman SJ. Patient-reported outcomes including fatigue in primary Sjogren's syndrome. Rheum Dis Clin North Am. 2008;34:949–62.
27. Bowman SJ, Booth DA, Platts RG, et al. Validation of the sicca symptoms inventory for clinical studies of Sjogren's syndrome. J Rheumatol. 2003;30:1259–66.
28. Slade GD, Spencer AJ. Development and evaluation of the Oral Health Impact Profile. Community Dent Health. 1994;11:3–11.
29. Allen PF, McMillan AS, Walshaw D, Locker D. A comparison of the validity of generic and disease-specific measures in the assessment of oral health-related quality of life. Community Dent Oral Epidemiol. 1999;27:344–52.
30. Allen PF, McMillan AS, Locker D. An assessment of sensitivity to change of the Oral Health Impact Profile in a clinical trial. Community Dent Oral Epidemiol. 2001;29:175–82.
31. Lopez-Jornet P, Camacho-Alonso F. Quality of life in patients with Sjogren's syndrome and sicca complex. J Oral Rehabil. 2008;35:875–81.
32. McMillan AS, Leung KC, Leung WK, et al. Impact of Sjogren's syndrome on oral health-related quality of life in southern Chinese. J Oral Rehabil. 2004;31:653–9.
33. Larsson P, List T, Lundström I, et al. Reliability and validity of a Swedish version of the Oral Health Impact Profile (OHIP-S). Acta Odontol Scand. 2004;62:147–52.
34. Barcelos F, Patto JV, Parente M, et al. Applicability of sialometry and other instruments to evaluate xerostomia and xerophthalmia in a Sjogren's syndrome outpatient clinic. Acta Reumatol Port. 2009;34:212–8.

35. McGrath C, Bedi R, Bowling A. Evaluation of OHQoL-UK(c): a measure of oral health related quality of life. J Dent Res. 1999;78:1051.
36. Locker D, Matear D, Stephens M, et al. Comparison of the GOHAI and OHIP-14 as measures of the oral health-related quality of life of the elderly. Community Dent Oral Epidemiol. 2001;29:373–81.
37. Henson BS, Inglehart MR, Eisbruch A, Ship JA. Preserved salivary output and xerostomia-related quality of life in head and neck cancer patients receiving parotid-sparing radiotherapy. Oral Oncol. 2001;37:84–93.
38. Schiffman RM, Christianson MD, Jacobsen G, et al. Reliability and validity of the Ocular Surface Disease Index. Arch Ophthalmol. 2000;118:615–21.
39. Vitale S, Goodman LA, Reed GF, Smith JA. Comparison of the NEI-VFQ and OSDI questionnaires in patients with Sjogren's syndrome-related dry eye. Health Qual Life Outcomes. 2004;2:44.
40. Mangione CM, Lee PP, Pitts J, et al. Psychometric properties of the National Eye Institute Visual Function Questionnaire (NEI-VFQ). Arch Ophthalmol. 1998;116:1496–504.
41. d'Elia HF, Bjurman C, Rehnberg E, et al. Interleukin 6 and its soluble receptor in a central role at the neuroendocrine interface in Sjogren's syndrome: an exploratory interventional study. Ann Rheum Dis. 2009;68:285–6.
42. Hartkamp A, Geenen R, Bijl M, et al. Serum cytokine levels related to multiple dimensions of fatigue in patients with primary Sjogren's syndrome. Ann Rheum Dis. 2004;63:1335–7.
43. Segal B, Thomas W, Rogers T, et al. Prevalence, severity and predictors of fatigue in subjects with primary Sjogren's syndrome. Arthritis Rheum. 2008;59:1780–7.
44. Bowman SJ, Sutcliffe N, Isenberg DA, et al. Sjogren's systemic clinical activity index (SCAI): a systemic disease activity measure for use in clinical trials in primary Sjogren's syndrome. Rheumatology (Oxford). 2007;46:1845–51.
45. Barry RJ, Sutcliffe N, Isenberg DA, et al. The Sjogren's Syndrome Damage Index: a damage index for use in clinical trials and observational studies in primary Sjogren's syndrome. Rheumatology (Oxford). 2008;47:1193–8.
46. Sall K, Stevenson OD, Mundorf TK, et al. Two multicenter, randomised studies of the efficacy and safety of cyclosporine ophthalmic emulsion in moderate to severe dry eye disease. Ophthalmology. 2000;107:631–9.
47. Vivino FB, Al-Hashimi I, Khan Z, et al. Pilocarpine tablets for the treatment of dry mouth and dry eye symptoms in patients with Sjogren's syndrome. Arch Intern Med. 1999;159:174–81.
48. Kruize AA, Hené RJ, Kallenberg CG, et al. Hydroxychloroquine treatment for primary Sjogren's syndrome: a two year double blind crossover trial. Ann Rheum Dis. 1993;52:360–4.
49. Mariette X, Ravaud P, Steinfeld S, et al. Inefficacy of infliximab in primary Sjogren's syndrome. Results of the randomised, controlled trial of Remicade in primary Sjogren's syndrome (TRIPSS). Arthritis Rheum. 2004;50:1270–6.
50. Pijpe J, van Imhoff GW, Spijkervet FK, et al. Rituximab treatment in patients with primary Sjogren's syndrome: an open-label phase II study. Arthritis Rheum. 2005;52:2740–50.
51. Meijer JM, Pijpe J, Vissink A, et al. Treatment of primary Sjogren's syndrome with rituximab: extended follow-up, safety and efficacy of treatment. Ann Rheum Dis. 2009;68:284–5.
52. Devauchelle-Pensec V, Pennec Y, Morvan J, et al. Improvement of Sjogren's syndrome after two infusions of rituximab (anti CD20). Arthritis Rheum. 2007;57:310–7.
53. Dass S, Bowman SJ, Vital EM, et al. Reduction of fatigue in Sjogren's syndrome with rituximab: results of a randomised, double-blind, placebo-controlled pilot study. Ann Rheum Dis. 2008;67:1541–4.
54. Hartkamp A, Geenen R, Godaert GL, et al. Effect of dehydroepiandrosterone administration on fatigue, well-being, and functioning in women with primary Sjogren's syndrome: a randomised controlled trial. Ann Rheum Dis. 2008;67:91–7.
55. van Woerkom JM, Kruize AA, Geenen R, et al. Safety and efficacy of leflunomide in primary Sjogren's syndrome: a phase II pilot study. Ann Rheum Dis. 2007;66:1026–32.
56. Strombeck BE, Theander E, Jacobsson LT. Effects of exercise on aerobic capacity and fatigue in women with primary Sjogren's syndrome. Rheumatology (Oxford). 2007;46:868–71.

Chapter 32
Sjögren's Syndrome and Associations with Other Autoimmune and Rheumatic Diseases

James E. Peters and David A. Isenberg

Contents

32.1 Introduction

Sjögren's syndrome (SS) is an autoimmune exocrinopathy that manifests itself most commonly as dryness of the mucosal surfaces. Systemic or extraglandular features can also occur. Both primary and secondary forms of SS are recognized to exist. In the latter, the syndrome develops in a patient with another systemic

J.E. Peters • D.A. Isenberg (✉)
Department of Rheumatology, University College London Hospital,
London, UK

M. Ramos-Casals et al. (eds.), *Sjögren's Syndrome*,
DOI 10.1007/978-0-85729-947-5_32, © Springer-Verlag London Limited 2012

autoimmune disease such as rheumatoid arthritis (RA) or systemic lupus erythematosus (SLE). The secondary form of SS is the focus of this chapter. The current nomenclature struggles to classify patients with mixed features of SS and another autoimmune condition. The term "Sjögren's overlap" has been proposed to describe such patients.

In patients with RA who develop sicca symptoms, the term "secondary" Sjögren's syndrome (sSS) is an accurate description. The sicca symptoms in such patients typically occur years after the onset of the RA and are generally milder than those of primary SS (pSS). Furthermore, there a number of clinical, pathological, serological, and genetic differences between pSS and RA with secondary SS (RA-SS). These are explored in detail below (see also Table 32.1). However, these observations do not hold true for other autoimmune diseases such as SLE and systemic sclerosis. SS in these diseases is much more similar to pSS, and the term 'associated SS' may be preferable to 'secondary'. The importance of the distinction is that grouping together discrete clinical entities as 'secondary SS' may hamper research into pathogenesis and new therapies. Patients with clearly defined pSS may later develop another autoimmune disease. Using the current classification criteria, these patients are often then considered to have 'secondary' SS, although the 'primary' autoimmune disease developed after the SS [1].

The physician is wise to recall the mantra 'autoimmune diseases hunt in packs'. The frequency of both organ-specific and systemic autoimmune diseases is significantly higher in pSS than in the general population, reflecting some common etiological factor. A retrospective study of 114 patients with pSS found that 38 patients had another autoimmune disorder, and 9 had two or more [2]. The additional autoimmune disorder was equally likely to have been diagnosed after the pSS as before it, although it is worth noting that patients with pSS are typically symptomatic for years before diagnosis. However, some autoimmune diseases described in that study such as renal tubular acidosis or interstitial lung disease are not perhaps truly independent diseases but were rather extra-glandular manifestations of pSS.

Studies in this area require cautious interpretation. The several classification systems for SS have led to heterogeneity between study groups and probably account for some of the variation in outcome. There may be genetic differences between the various populations studied. Many studies have been small and retrospective. Some studies may contain selection bias, with overrepresentations of patients with more severe disease under the care of specialist units.

32.2   SS Associated with Systemic Lupus Erythematosus (SLE)

The relationship between SLE and SS was first described 50 years ago [3]. In that original description, SS was felt to be a mild form of SLE. Only later were pSS and SS secondary to SLE recognized as distinct entities. Estimates of the prevalence of

Table 32.1 Comparison of SS accompanying other autoimmune diseases with pSS

	Frequency of SS (%)	Sicca symptoms compared to pSS	Presence of antibodies to Ro and La compared to pSS	Extra-glandular features	Genetic associations	References
SLE	2–30	Similar	Similar	Generally similar-more CNS involvement	Similar to pSS HLA DRB1*0301	[4, 11, 12, 14]
RA	5–31	Less	Fewer	Fewer	HLA-DR4 HLA-DRB*15	[19, 23, 32]
SSc	17–29	Similar Xerostomia> xerophthalmia	Ro similar La fewer RF fewer	Arthritis and peripheral neuropathy more common		[46, 47]
MCTD	41.8–56	Similar	Fewer	Raynaud's, lung fibrosis, myositis, arthritis more common		[54, 55]
Autoimmune thyroiditis	2–20	Similar	Fewer		HLA-DR3 (similar to pSS)	[65, 66, 69]
Primary biliary cirrhosis	3–25	Milder than pSS Xerostomia predominant	Fewer		Similar to RA-SS	[78, 79]

SLE: systemic lupus erythematosus; RA: rheumatoid arthritis; SSc: systemic sclerosis; MCTD: mixed connective tissue disease; pSS: primary Sjögren syndrome; CNS: central nervous system; RF: rheumatoid factor.

secondary SS in SLE (SLE-SS) vary between 8% and 30% [4]. This variation probably reflects the differing classification criteria used for SS and differences in the populations studied. In one study, 15% of 1,138 SLE patients were suspected of having sSS. However, this study relied heavily on self-reporting, and not all of the patients identified necessarily met the American European Consensus Group (AECG) criteria [5]. A study of 542 consecutive Chinese SLE patients reported that 6.5% had SLE-SS [6].

Moutsopoulos et al. evaluated 24 patients with SLE [7]. Twenty-one percent of these patients had subjective complaints of dry eyes, but only one patient spontaneously volunteered that symptom. Twenty-one percent also had abnormal Schirmer's tests, but none had an abnormal slit lamp examination. Thirty percent had symptoms of dry mouth, but 58% had abnormal parotid scintigraphy. Half of patients had lymphocytic infiltration on salivary gland biopsy, of whom 42% had Tarpley's scores of 2+ and the remainder had a score of 1+ (usually considered non-specific). Among the patients with positive lip biopsies, 58% had antibodies to Ro. No patient with a normal lip biopsy had anti-Ro antibodies. Anti-La antibodies were present in one patient with a positive biopsy, and absent in patients with a negative biopsy.

Eleven of 66 patients (16%) with SLE had a lymphocytic sialadenitis with a Chisholm and Mason score of ≥3 [8] (see Chap. 25). Among those 11 patients, dry eyes, decreased parotid flow, parotid swelling, lymphadenopathy, RF, and antibodies to La were more common than in patients with a negative biopsy. Five of these 11 patients had keratoconjunctivitis sicca on Rose Bengal staining. Thus, the prevalence of SS in this group of SLE patients was approximately 8%. There were no other significant differences in SLE features between those with and without sSS.

In a Swedish prospective population-based study of 133 patients with probable or definite SLE (86 with definite SLE), 79 (60%) reported sicca symptoms and 12 (9%) had sSS (defined as subjective dry eyes and/or mouth, plus either a positive Rose Bengal stain, or a positive lip biopsy) [9]. This figure may be more accurate than estimates based on selected patient populations, but may not apply to countries where a greater proportion of the population is non-Caucasian. Patients with sicca symptoms were older than those without, but otherwise there were no clinical differences. The study found an association between SLE-SS and antibodies to Ro and La, but there were no other immunological differences between patients with and without sSS. In particular, the frequency of dsDNA antibodies was the same.

A prospective study by Nossent et al. followed 138 patients who fulfilled the 1982 American College of Rheumatology revised criteria for SLE and evaluated them for the presence of sSS (by the 1993 European Study Group criteria) [10]. After a mean follow-up period of 90.5 months, sSS had been diagnosed in 20% of the patients. There was a gradual increase in prevalence of sSS over time after SLE onset. Patients with sSS were older and had less renal disease than those without, a finding reproduced in a large Chinese study [6]. Nossent et al. reported more thrombocytopenia but lower overall mortality in SLE-SS compared to SLE alone. The patients with and without sSS had similar serological profiles. In particular, there was no association between sSS and anti-Ro or anti-La antibodies, in contrast to other studies [7–9, 11].

Although traditionally thought to be most common in rheumatoid arthritis, Gilboe et al. found that sSS is in fact more common in SLE than RA, with frequencies of 11% and 4% respectively [4]. However, 60% of SLE patients had sicca symptoms. Fatigue, the subjective sensation of dry eyes, and objective measurements of reduced tear production were more marked in SLE-SS than RA-SS, but prevalence of dry mouth symptoms was the same. Antibodies to Ro and La were more common in patients with SLE-SS, compared to SLE alone. There was no renal disease in patients with SLE-SS, versus 14% in SLE alone. There was no statistically significant difference in the number of patients with antibodies to dsDNA and hypocomplementemia between the two groups. Thus, SLE-SS is evidently more similar to pSS than to RA-SS. Manthorpe et al. found that anti-La antibodies are more common in SLE-SS than SLE alone or RA-SS, supporting this hypothesis [12]. In another study of SLE, 72 consecutive patients underwent labial salivary gland biopsy, regardless of whether or not sicca symptoms were present [13]. Fifty-one percent of these patients had a normal biopsy (group A); 24% had mild lymphocytic infiltration (15–20 lymphocytes per focus) (group B); and 25% had heavy lymphocytic infiltration (>50 lymphocytes per focus) (group C). Objective keratoconjunctivitis sicca occurred in 41% and 44% of group B and C respectively, but in no patients with a normal biopsy. In group B, the infiltrate was perivascular, principally in vessels adjacent to ducts. In group C, the infiltrate was located in the center of the gland close to the interlobular septae, with additional perivascular peripheral lobule involvement in 5 of the 18 patients. Salivary duct dilatation and acinar tissue destruction, which often occur in pSS, were not present. Patients with perivascular infiltrates did not exhibit more frequent vasculitis in other organs. Patients with heavy lymphocytic infiltration had less renal involvement, but more frequent lymphadenopathy, rheumatoid factors, anti-Ro/La antibodies, and cryoglobulinemia, than those with mild or no lymphocytic sialadenitis. There was no correlation between biopsy findings and the frequencies of antibodies to dsDNA or RNP, or with serum complement levels. This study suggests that the characteristic histological lesion of SLE-SS is perivascular lymphocytic infiltration. In contrast, in pSS the infiltrate is in the acinar proper (see Fig. 32.1). Manoussakis et al. found similar differences in salivary gland histopathology between SLE-SS and pSS [11] (see below).

A Hungarian study compared 56 patients with SLE-SS to 50 patients with SLE alone, and 50 with pSS [14]. Patients with SLE-SS were significantly older than patients with SLE alone, but younger than patients with pSS. Central nervous system, renal and pulmonary involvement, and anti-dsDNA and antiphospholipid antibodies were more common in SLE-SS than pSS. Anti-Ro and anti-La antibodies were more common in SLE-SS than in pSS or SLE alone. There was no difference in salivary gland histopathology or major histocompatibility complex alleles between SLE-SS and pSS. Interestingly, autoimmune thyroiditis occurred more commonly in SLE-SS than in either pSS or SLE alone. Another group has reproduced this finding, with autoimmune thyroiditis occurring in 27% of SLE-SS patients versus 12% of patients with SLE alone [5].

Of 283 Greek SLE patients, 18% had subjective sicca symptoms, 12.4% had objective signs of ocular or oral dryness, and 9.2% fulfilled the AECG criteria for

Fig. 32.1 Minor labial salivary gland biopsies (stain H + E) taken from: (**a**) a patient with primary Sjögren's syndrome, infiltrates are located around ducts (*arrowhead*); (**b**) a patient with systemic lupus erythematosus and Sjögren's syndrome, infiltrates surrounds vessels (*arrow*). Original magnification: ×200 (Kindly supplied by and used with permission from Prof. H. M. Moutsopoulos, School of Medicine, University of Athens)

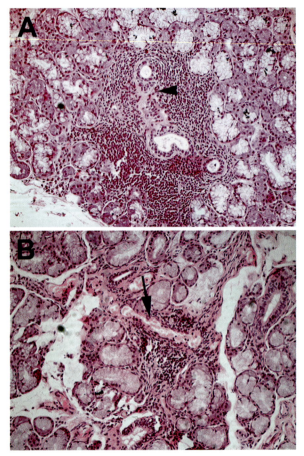

SLE-SS [11]. Sicca symptoms preceded the diagnosis of lupus in 70% of those with SLE-SS, whereas sSS in RA typically develops in patients with long-standing disease. Comparison of SLE-SS with SLE alone and with pSS revealed broadly similar findings to Szanto et al. Mean age in SLE-SS was greater than in SLE alone but less than in pSS. Objective keratoconjunctivitis sicca was more common in pSS than in SLE-SS, and vice versa for dyspareunia. Otherwise the clinical expression of sicca symptoms was similar between pSS and SLE-SS, including the presence of salivary gland enlargement (which in contrast is infrequent in RA-SS). In the majority of both pSS and SLE-SS patients, salivary gland biopsy revealed periductal lymphocytic infiltrates. However, a predominantly perivascular location of the infiltrate was much more common in SLE-SS (in 39%, versus 2% of pSS patients). Patients with perivascular infiltrates had a longer duration of both SLE and sicca symptoms. This may indicate a time-dependent effect, but a longitudinal study would be required to determine this. Perivascular infiltrates were strongly associated with the presence of anticardiolipin antibodies. The SLE-SS group had more arthritis, serositis, Raynaud's phenomenon and CNS involvement, but less lymphadenopathy, than the pSS group. SLE-SS patients were less likely to have thrombocytopenia, lymphadenopathy, and renal involvement, but more likely to have Raynaud's phenomenon than were those with SLE alone. CNS involvement was equally common in SLE-SS as SLE alone. Rheumatoid factors and anti-Ro and -La antibodies were more prevalent in SLE-SS patients than in those with SLE alone. There was no difference in the prevalence of these antibodies between SLE-SS and pSS, in contrast to Szanto's findings. Antibodies to dsDNA, nRNP, and anticardiolipin were less common in pSS. SLE-SS and pSS patients both had a high frequency of the DRB1*0301 allele, whereas the SLE alone group had an increased frequency of DRB1*1501 and DQB1*0602 alleles.

Two smaller studies have produced conflicting results on serological differences between SLE-SS and pSS. Moutsopoulos et al. found that La antibodies were rarer, but Ro antibodies equally common, in SLE-SS compared to pSS [7]. Turkcapar et al. found La antibodies were equally common in these disorders, but Ro antibodies were more common in SLE-SS [15].

In summary, these findings suggest that patients with SLE-SS represent an older subset of lupus patients who have milder disease, less renal involvement, and a predominance of the Sjögren-type features. The presence of the sicca syndrome prior to the development of lupus features in the majority of these patients suggests that 'secondary SS' is not an appropriate label. 'SLE-SS overlap syndrome' or 'SLE with accompanying SS' is a more accurate description. Most studies suggest that anti-Ro and anti-La antibodies occur more frequently in SLE-SS than SLE alone. The clinical expression and genetic associations are similar in patients with SLE-SS compared to patients with pSS. The shared immunogenetic background of pSS and SLE-SS differs from that of SLE without SS. Perivascular infiltrates on minor salivary gland biopsy are distinct to SLE-SS, and differ from the classic periductal acinar infiltrates in pSS. The prevalence of anti-Ro and anti-La antibodies is similar in pSS and SLE-SS. There is no difference in the nature of the Ro and La antibodies in the two diseases [16], suggesting that these antibodies reflect common immunopathogenic mechanisms. Thus, differentiation between pSS and SLE-SS can be difficult. Central nervous system and renal involvement, or the presence of dsDNA, Sm or anticardiolipin autoantibodies favor the latter diagnosis. Patients with well-defined pSS but with positive anti-dsDNA antibodies have been described, but they tend to fulfill SLE criteria over time [16].

32.3   SS Associated with Rheumatoid Arthritis (RA)

Bloch et al. reported secondary SS in 50% of patients with RA [17]. Coll et al. identified SS in 62% of RA patients [18]. Objective keratoconjunctivitis sicca occurred in 24%, and objective xerostomia in 52%. However, a large, population-based study found that the percentage of RA patients who fit the diagnostic criteria for SS was only 7%, despite the fact that up to 50% had sicca symptoms. In RA, sicca symptoms have only weak correlations with objective measurements of tear and saliva production [19].

A series of 143 consecutive patients with RA were prospectively evaluated for SS; 111 underwent salivary gland biopsy [20]. A diagnosis of SS was made when a patient had a positive lip biopsy ($\geq$2+ on Tarpley's classification [see Chap. 25]) plus at least of one of the following: (a) a positive Rose Bengal test; (b) the combination of subjective dry eyes and an abnormal Schirmer's test; or (c) subjective xerostomia and decreased parotid flow rate. Forty percent of patients who underwent biopsy had salivary gland histopathology with a Tarpley's score $\geq$2+, 25% had a score of 1+, and 35% had a negative biopsy. Thirty-four patients fit the authors' criteria for sSS, suggesting a prevalence in RA of 20%. Parotid enlargement was unusual, in contrast to pSS, as were other extra-glandular features with the exception of interstitial lung disease. Twenty-four percent of patients had antibodies to Ro, the presence of which was associated with a positive lip biopsy.

The prevalence of sicca symptoms in RA increases with disease duration. In a Spanish multicentre study of 788 randomly selected RA patients, the cumulative prevalence of sSS was 17% at 10 years' disease duration and 25% after 30 years [21]. sSS in RA is thought to result from the accumulation of chronically activated lymphocytes in exocrine tissues leading to glandular destruction [7]. Although the prevalence of sicca symptoms also increases with disease duration in SLE, sSS tends to occur after relatively fewer years of disease than in RA. Nossent et al. found the mean duration of SLE prior to development of sSS was 39 months (range 1–130) [10].

32.3.1   Clinical and Serological Differences Between pSS and RA-SS

Patients presenting with polyarthritis, sicca symptoms, and positive RF present a classification challenge. Should they be considered to have RA with sSS, or pSS with articular involvement? Gottenberg et al. found that 10% of pSS patients also fulfilled the diagnostic criteria for RA, although only 40% of them had an erosive arthritis [22]. Anti-CCP antibodies or rheumatoid nodules in such patients favor a diagnosis of RA with secondary SS. Mild, non-erosive disease and marked polyclonal hypergammaglobulinemia favors pSS.

Moutsopoulos et al. first described the distinct clinical differences between pSS and RA-SS in a retrospective study of 22 pSS patients and 21 RA-SS patients [23]. Parotiditis, lymphadenopathy, purpura, Raynaud's phenomenon, renal involvement and myositis occurred more frequently in pSS. There were no differences in the salivary gland histopathology, the frequency of rheumatoid factors, or levels of serum immunoglobulins or C3. The mean age of diagnosis of sicca symptoms was the same in both groups. In contrast, a Japanese study found that the average age for development of pSS was 12 years less than that in RA [24]. This study confirmed more frequent parotiditis, lymphadenopathy and purpura in pSS than in RA-SS.

Table 32.2 Alpha-fodrin antibody determination in patients with systemic autoimmune diseases (Turkcapar et al, 15).

	pSS (n = 20)	RA-SS (n = 10)	SLE-SS (n = 10)	RA alone (n = 10)	SLE alone (n = 10)	Healthy controls (n = 20)
α fodrin IgA abs (%)	20	10	20	0	0	0
α fodrin IgG abs (%)	10	0	10	0	0	0

Table 32.3 Alpha-fodrin antibody determination in patients with systemic autoimmune diseases (Witte et al, 27).

	pSS (n = 85)	RA-SS (n = 7)	SLE-SS (n = 15)	RA alone (n = 12)	SLE alone (n = 50)	Healthy controls (n = 160)
α fodrin IgA abs (%)	64	86	47	17	2	<1
α fodrin IgG abs (%)	55	43	40	40	2	2

Table 32.4 Alpha-fodrin antibody determination in patients with systemic autoimmune diseases (Ruiz-Tiscar et al, 29).

	pSS[a] (n = 216)	RA-SS[a] (n = 198)	SLE-SS[a] (n = 41)	Controls (n = 100)
α fodrin IgG abs (%)	1.4	1	2.4	0

Ruiz-Tiscar et al. [29]

[a]SS defined by European Community Study Group criteria

Anti-nuclear antibodies were more common in pSS. Nearly half the patients with pSS had arthritis, but none developed erosive changes, a finding confirmed by other investigators [25]. Both patients with RA alone, and RA-SS develop erosive changes, but these are more severe in the patients with RA alone [25].

Despite the presence of sSS in 20% of RA patients in Andonopoulos et al.'s series, no patient volunteered sicca symptoms until directly questioned suggesting that these symptoms are less severe in RA-SS than in pSS [20]. A small study found more pronounced salivary gland inflammation and reduced salivary flow in pSS than in RA-SS [26]. The CD4/CD8 ratios in both peripheral blood and salivary gland lesions were significantly lower in the former.

Most studies have found that antibodies to Ro and La occur less commonly in RA-SS than pSS [12, 20, 23]. Turkcapar et al. did not find a difference, but the study was small [15].

α-fodrin antibodies have been described in pSS. Data presented in the Tables 32.2–32.4 show that these antibodies also occur in secondary SS in both RA and SLE. Turkcapar et al. did not find these antibodies in any patients with RA or SLE alone [15], although Witte et al. did [27]. The numbers in the studies were too small to reliably establish a difference in antibody profiles between the various forms of SS. In a more recent paper the prevalence of anti-α-fodrin IgA and IgG antibodies in pSS was 35% and 31% respectively, compared to 29% and 21% in sSS, although this paper grouped sSS due to different autoimmune diseases as one entity [28]. A large study found a low prevalence of anti-α-fodrin IgG antibodies in

SS, with no difference in frequency between pSS, SS-RA, and SS-SLE [29]. It has been suggested that antibodies to the N-terminal of alpha fodrin (α-N46PA) [30] and antibodies to NA14 (nuclear autoantigen of 14 kDa) [31] may occur more commonly in pSS than sSS, but further studies are required before these reports can be confirmed.

32.3.2 Genetic Differences Between pSS and RA-SS

Several studies (described in detail in Chap. 2) have shown an association between genes of the HLA region and pSS. They include HLA-B8, HLA-Dw3 and HLA-DR3 [32]. The HLA associations vary according to ethnic group, with an increased frequency of HLA-DR5 in Greeks and Israelis, HLA-DRw53 in Japanese, and DQA1*0501 and DQB1*201 in US populations.

The primary and secondary forms of SS are associated with different HLA genes. Moutsopoulos et al. showed that HLADR3 is associated with pSS (subsequently confirmed by others including Vitali et al. [33]), whereas HLADR4 is associated with RA-SS [34]. However, the same author did not find either of these associations when a Greek population was examined, suggesting there is ethnic variation in susceptibility genes for both primary and secondary SS [35]. This study found an association between HLA-DR5 and pSS. Wilson et al. also confirmed the association between pSS and HLA-DR3, but found no association between this gene and sSS in RA, SLE or mixed connective tissue disease [36]. There was an association between HLA-DR3 and DR2 and the presence of antibodies to Ro. Antibodies to La were correlated only with DR3. The HLA-DS MT2 specificity was more common in both primary and secondary SS than in either controls or patients with rheumatic disease without sSS. A Danish study showed a significantly increased frequency of HLA-Dw2 in pSS compared to controls, whilst this was non-significantly decreased in RA-SS [37]. There was an association between HLA-Dw4 and RA-SS, but not pSS. Warlow et al. found associations between RA-SS and HLA-Bw62, DR4, C4B2.9, and C4A8 [38].

Most studies have not determined whether the HLA associations in sSS syndrome simply reflect the association of the HLA type with the underlying autoimmune disease; for example, the association between RA and HLA-DR4 is well-described. Mattey et al. were able to dissect out the nature of the association between HLA genes and sSS in RA. They evaluated 179 Spanish RA patients, of whom 12.3% had sSS [32]. The frequency of DRB1*15*16 was significantly increased in patients with sSS compared to those with RA alone, and that of DRB1*04 was reduced in patients with sSS. To test whether the association of HLA DRB*15 was purely related to the secondary SS, or whether there was an association between RA and DRB*15 independent of sSS, all RA patients were compared to a control group. Overall there was no association between DRB*15 and RA, but subgroup analysis showed that in RA patients who lack the RA 'shared epitope' there was an association independent of sSS.

32.4   SS Associated with Systemic Sclerosis (SS-SSc)

Up to 70% of patients of patients with systemic sclerosis (SSc) have sicca symptoms, but this is due mainly to salivary gland fibrosis resulting from the primary disease process. The prevalence of true sSS with lymphocytic sialadenitis is lower, between 14% and 29% [18, 39–41]. These estimates are controversial because they come principally from small studies performed without consensus on the definition of sSS. These studies are presented below.

Six of 35 (17%) prospectively evaluated SSc patients had sSS [39]. Of 58 SSc patients, 38% and 34% had subjective dry eyes and dry mouth respectively, 34% had an abnormal Schirmer's test, and 4% parotid enlargement [40]. Twenty-nine percent had lymphocytic infiltration characteristic of SS on biopsy, 33% had fibrosis without inflammation, and 38% no abnormality. Patients with a purely fibrotic biopsy had more severe SSc. The presence of Ro-antibodies is associated with sSS in SSc. Anti-Ro or La antibodies occurred in half of patients with lymphocytic infiltration on biopsy, versus in only 1 of 22 patients with normal biopsy, and in no patients with a purely fibrotic biopsy.

Ten of 44 (23%) prospectively evaluated SSc patients had a salivary gland biopsy with Tarpley's score of 2+ [41]. Thirty-nine percent had pure fibrosis without lymphocytic infiltration. Parotid enlargement occurred in 44% of patients with SS-SSc, but was very rare in patients with fibrotic or normal biopsies. Anti-Ro antibodies were found in a third of patients with SS-SSc and in 11% of those with a fibrotic biopsy.

Twenty-five consecutive patients with SSc were evaluated clinically, and with Schirmer's test, Rose-Bengal staining, parotid sialography, [99-m]Tc-scintigraphy, and salivary gland biopsy [42]. Seventy-two percent had subjective dry eyes, 40% an abnormal Schirmer's test, and 44% abnormal Rose-Bengal staining. Eighty-four percent had xerostomia. Sixty-five percent of salivary gland biopsies showed lymphocytic infiltration (35% showed a lymphocytic score of ≥2+), and 80% showed fibrosis.

Sixty-nine percent of 16 patients with SSc had SS [18]. Nineteen percent had objective keratoconjunctivitis sicca and 69% of patients had objective xerostomia with lymphocytic sialadenitis on salivary gland biopsy. Sixty percent of 23 patients with the CREST variant (calcinosis, Raynaud's, esophageal dysmotility, sclerodactyly, telangiectasia) of SSc had SS [43]. There were no other differences between patients with and without associated SS. Anti-Ro antibodies were rare in CREST patients. Parotid enlargement was more common in patients with pSS than in the CREST patients. Six out of seven patients with CREST accompanied by vasculitis also had SS [44].

Andonopoulos et al. prospectively evaluated 111 RA patients and 44 SSc patients [45]. Forty percent of RA patients and 23% of SSc patients had a positive lip biopsy. Thirty-one percent of RA patients and 21% of SSc patients met the criteria for sSS (defined as a lip biopsy with focal lymphocytic infiltration of ≥2+ on Tarpley's scale, plus keratoconjunctivitis sicca and/or xerostomia). In contrast, a higher proportion of patients with SSc than RA spontaneously volunteered sicca symptoms

(11% dry eyes and 22% dry mouth in SSc compared to 6% dry eyes in RA). On direct questioning dry eyes and dry mouth occurred in 38% and 6% of RA patients respectively, compared to 56% and 67% in SSc. Parotid gland enlargement occurred more frequently in SSc (44%) than in RA (21%). Anti-Ro antibodies occurred in 24% of RA and 33% of SSc patients. Extra-glandular features were uncommon in both groups. This study suggests that SS in RA tends to be less symptomatic, whilst the SS that occurs in SSc has more in common with pSS. The authors argue that the term 'secondary SS' for the syndrome accompanying SSc, as it has been applied to that accompanying RA, is not an accurate description.

Since the introduction of the AECG criteria in 2002, the definition of secondary SS has been clarified. Only two studies have looked at the prevalence of sSS in SSc using these criteria [46, 47]. Avouac et al. examined 133 consecutive SSc patients, of whom 81 had limited cutaneous SSc [46]. Ninety-one patients (68%) had sicca symptoms. Salivary gland biopsy revealed fibrosis in 50 out of 91 patients, and lymphocytic infiltration in 19. The prevalence of true sSS in this cohort was 14%. Three patients had anti-Ro antibodies and another had both anti-Ro and anti-La antibodies; all of these patients had a lymphocytic biopsy. SS was strongly associated with the limited form of the disease. Ninety-five percent of the patients with sSS had limited cutaneous SSc and anti-centromere antibodies, whereas limited cutaneous SSc occurred in only 12% of patients without sicca symptoms, and in 26% of those with sicca symptoms without lymphocytic sialadenitis.

A retrospective multicentre study compared 27 patients with SS-SSc, 202 patients with pSS (fulfilling AECG criteria), and 94 patients with SSc alone [47]. There was no difference in subjective xerostomia or xerophthalmia, or in tear production measured by Schirmer's test, between SS-SSc and pSS. Objective xerostomia (assessed by unstimulated salivary flow, parotid sialography or salivary gland $^{99\text{-m}}$Tc scintigraphy) was more common is SS-SSc than pSS. There was no significant difference in salivary gland histopathology or in the prevalence of anti-Ro/anti-La or RF antibodies between pSS and SS-SSc, although the study may have been underpowered to detect a difference. Overall, there was no statistically significant difference in the proportion of pSS and SS-SSc patients with extra-glandular features, although there was a trend to a higher percentage in the SS-SSc group. Arthritis and peripheral neuropathy occurred more frequently in SS-SSc. 18.5% out of SS-SSc patients had an additional autoimmune disease, compared to only 3.9% of pSS patients, consistent with the idea that sSS accompanying another autoimmune rheumatic disease represents the 'spreading of autoimmunity'. The prevalence of other antibodies (other than Ro, La, centromere and anti-Scl70 antibodies) was higher in the SS-SSc. Cryoglobulinemia was more frequent in SS-SSc (in 20%, versus 1.5% in pSS). However, this was not associated with an increased frequency of lymphoma; lymphoma occurred in 10 of the 202 pSS patients and in no patient with SS-SSc. There was no difference in the frequency of monoclonal gammopathy, decreased C4 complement level, or parotid enlargement, or in mean ESR, CRP, serum gammaglobulins or α-2 microglobulin levels between the two groups. SS-SSc was less severe than SSc alone, with less renal crises, lung fibrosis, cardiac involvement and pulmonary artery hypertension in the former. The comparison group of patients with SSc alone was selected so it contained the same proportion of patients with limited and diffuse SSc in order to prevent the type of SSc skewing the results.

A criticism of most case series is that they consist of selected patients in specialist centers, and may over-represent patients with more severe disease. An Australian group used a regional scleroderma register to perform a population-based study [48]. Questionnaires were sent all 240 patients on the register, of whom 80% responded. Overall sicca symptoms were present in 52%. They were most frequent in patients with limited SSc, occurring in 59%, whilst they occurred in 49%, 40%, and 29% of patients with diffuse SSc, overlap SSc and unspecified SSc respectively. The results of ENA testing were available for 147 patients. Eight patients were Ro positive; sicca symptoms were independent of Ro antibody status. Biopsy data was not available, consequently this study could not differentiate sicca symptoms due to fibrosis from true sSS.

A Thai study examined RA, SLE and SSc patients along with age-matched controls [49]. They found ocular sicca symptoms occurred in 38% of RA patients, 36% of SLE patients and 54% of SSc patients, all of which were significantly higher than controls. However, only patients with RA had a significantly higher proportion of patients with abnormal Schirmer's test compared to controls. Oral sicca symptoms were more frequent in patients with SLE (22%) and SSc (16%) than controls. There was no correlation between sicca symptoms and other clinical or laboratory data, including Ro or La autoantibodies.

0.9% of a British cohort of pSS patients had scleroderma at the time of diagnosis, and 3.5% subsequently developed it [2]. In primary SS, anticentromere antibodies have been reported in 14% [50]. Patients with these antibodies often have Raynaud's phenomenon and may develop coexistent limited cutaneous SSc [51, 52].

In summary, sicca symptoms are common in SSc, but are often due to salivary gland fibrosis rather than true SS with lymphocytic sialadenitis. SS in SSc (SS-SScSS-SSc) has more in common with pSS than RA-SS, and the terms 'associated' or 'accompanying' better describe it than 'secondary'. Sicca symptoms are more severe and parotid swelling more common in SS-SScSS-SSc than in RA-SS. Sicca symptoms in SS-SScSS-SSc are generally similar to those in pSS, but xerostomia may be more marked in SS-SSc. Salivary gland histopathology is similar in the two diseases. SS-SSc is associated with the limited form of SSc and anticentromere antibodies. Most studies suggest an association with anti-Ro antibodies. Patients with SS-SSc have less severe systemic disease than those with SSc alone. The overall frequency of extra-glandular features is similar in SS-SSc and pSS, but arthritis and peripheral neuropathy occur more frequently in the former. Other autoimmune diseases and autoantibodies are more common in SS-SSc than pSS. This is consistent with the concept that the presence of SS in SSc represents the 'spreading of autoimmunity' or an overlap syndrome.

32.5   SS Associated with Other Systemic Autoimmune Diseases

32.5.1   Mixed Connective Tissue Disease

Mixed connective tissue disease (MCTD) is a controversial entity [53]. The original description was of a relatively mild disorder with overlapping features of SLE, polymyositis and SSc in association with antibodies to nRNP. However, it has become clear that antibodies to nRNP are relatively common in SLE, and many patients presenting with the above features tend to differentiate over time into a phenotype where the features of one of the three diseases predominates over the other two. Therefore, the evaluation of any association with SS is difficult, particularly as clinical features such as Raynaud's and non-erosive arthritis are common to both conditions.

Ohtsuka et al. reported that 'secondary SS' and sialectasia are more common in MCTD than in any other autoimmune disease [54]. Raynaud's phenomenon, arthritis, myositis, sclerodactyly, fever, cutaneous erythema, and lymphadenopathy occurred more frequently in MCTD than in pSS. The frequency of these manifestations was no different in MCTD with sSS than in MCTD alone. The ESR and CRP level were higher in MCTD than pSS. Antinuclear antibodies, anti-dsDNA antibodies and anti-RNP antibodies were more prevalent in the former. However, there were no differences in inflammatory markers or autoantibody profile between MCTD without and without sSS. There was a strict dissociation between the presence of anti-RNP antibodies and anti-La antibodies in both MCTD and pSS patients.

A longitudinal study of 55 patients with MCTD, all of whom had antibodies to RNP, found that sicca symptoms (defined as daily oral dryness, frequent use of liquid because of oral dryness, or daily ocular dryness) occurred in 41.8% of patients [55]. The length of the follow period ranged from 3 to 30 years (mean 9 years). Common clinical characteristics of the patients included Raynaud's phenomenon, swollen hands, gastro-esophageal reflux, arthralgia, myalgia, serositis, lymphopenia and reduced gas transfer on pulmonary function testing. Patients were not assessed with more quantitative methods such as Schirmer's test, salivary gland biopsy, unstimulated salivary flow or sialography, so how many met the AECG criteria for sSS is unknown. 32.7% of patients had antibodies to Ro, but only 2 patients (3.6%) had antibodies to La. Anti-Ro antibodies were strongly associated with malar rash and photosensitivity, in keeping with previous observations. There was no association between sicca symptoms and anti-Ro antibodies.

The authors stated, rather surprisingly, that no patients evolved into a diagnosis of SLE or SSc over the follow-up period. However, many of the clinical features of the patients described occur in both SLE and primary SS. Given that the patients were not fully assessed for SS, one can speculate that at least some of their patients would fit the criteria for pSS. Furthermore, MCTD is an overlap syndrome; it is therefore debatable whether patients with MCTD and features of the SS should be considered to have sSS. Rather, the presence of sicca symptoms could be considered a manifestation of the overlap syndrome, and not the development of a second autoimmune disease.

32.5.2 Systemic Vasculitis

Vasculitis occurring in pSS is typically considered as a manifestation of the primary disease and is strongly associated with cryoglobulinemia. This is detailed in Chap. 12. True co-existence of a well-defined primary systemic vasculitis with pSS is very rare, and limited to a handful of cases [56, 57]. Positive ANCA immunofluorescence tests are often found in pSS [16], but do not by themselves indicate the presence of an ANCA-associated vasculitis.

32.5.3 Antiphospholipid Syndrome (APS)

Antiphospholipid antibodies are detectable in 13% of pSS patients, but only 1% have the antiphospholipid syndrome itself [51]. A small number of pSS patients with antiphospholipid antibodies not meeting the criteria for APS nevertheless have certain APS-like features including thrombocytopenia, livedo reticularis and hemolytic anemia.

32.5.4 Sarcoidosis

Sarcoidosis is a systemic autoimmune process characterized pathologically by the presence of non-caseating granulomata. It can present with parotid swelling and sicca symptoms, making it difficult to distinguish from pSS clinically. A firm diagnosis depends on demonstrating the characteristic histological findings on biopsy, and may be difficult to achieve. Drosos et al. reported five cases of sarcoidosis presenting with sicca symptoms [58]. All five patients had abnormal Rose-Bengal staining, four had an abnormal Schirmer's test, and three had reduced parotid flow rate. Minor salivary gland biopsy revealed scattered lymphoplasmacytic infiltrates in all patients, with concurrent non-caseating granulomata in three. In the remaining two patients, the diagnosis of sarcoidosis was made by demonstrating non-caseating granulomata on transbronchial lung biopsy.

The currently accepted AECG criteria for pSS has sarcoidosis as an exclusion criterion. Therefore, by this definition, the two disorders cannot co-exist. However, Ramos-Casals and colleagues [59] have reported five cases of sarcoidosis with coexistent pSS (as defined by the previously used and less restrictive European Consensus Criteria). All five patients had the typical focal lymphocytic sialadenitis of pSS and biopsy–proven sarcoidosis. None of the five patients had antibodies to Ro and La, which is rather surprising if they had true pSS. Perhaps rather than there being two coexistent autoimmune diseases, the sialadenitis in these patients was a manifestation of the sarcoidosis. Certainly, early pulmonary sarcoidosis can present histopathologically as alveolitis with lymphocytic foci prior to the development of granulomata. It is not unreasonable to assume that an analogous sequence of events could occur in the salivary glands. A further 28 cases from the literature have been identified in which the histology suggested co-existence of pSS and sarcoidosis [59]. The patients said to have both pSS and sarcoidosis had more frequent articular symptoms, uveitis, and positive RF, ANA and anti-Ro antibodies, than patients with a single diagnosis of sarcoidosis mimicking pSS.

Drosos' case series detailed above demonstrated that lymphoplasmacytic salivary gland infiltrates do occur in sarcoidosis. However, the same group have shown that, at least when interpreted by expert histopathologists, salivary gland biopsy is a reliable discriminator between pSS and sarcoidosis [60]. Sixty labial minor salivary gland biopsies (from 32 patients with definite sarcoidosis and 28 with pSS) were retrospectively reviewed by a histopathologist unaware of the diagnosis or clinical details. Non-caseating granulomata were identified on six biopsies, all of which were from sarcoidosis patients. Twelve biopsies, again all from sarcoidosis patients, showed scattered lymphocytic infiltrates with a Tarpley's score of ≤1+. The remainder of the sarcoidosis patients had normal biopsies. All 28 pSS patients had a Tarpley's score of ≥2+. Thus, although lip biopsy has a low sensitivity for diagnosing sarcoidosis, it can reliably distinguish it from pSS.

32.6   SS Associated with Organ-Specific Autoimmune Diseases

32.6.1   SS Associated with Autoimmune Thyroiditis

The literature in this area is confused. There is debate as to whether the development of SS symptoms in patients with autoimmune thyroiditis is a form of secondary SS, an overlap syndrome, or the co-existence of two separate autoimmune diseases. When autoimmune thyroiditis develops in a patient with pSS there is again dispute as to whether this represents two separate diagnoses, or a manifestation of the primary SS.

There is a strong association between pSS and thyroid disease, particularly autoimmune hypothyroidism [61]. Subclinical hypothyroidism is the most common endocrine abnormality. A study of 33 pSS patients found autoimmune thyroiditis in 24% and autoimmune hyperthyroidism in 6% [62]. Autoantibodies against thyroid peroxidase and thyroglobulin were detected in 45% and 15% respectively. A British prospective longitudinal study of 100 pSS patients found that 14% also had thyroid disease [63]. Another UK study involving a retrospective case review of 114 patients with pSS found that hypothyroidism occurred in a similar proportion [2]. In the latter study, hypothyroidism was diagnosed prior to the pSS in 12 cases, concurrently in 1 case, and a year or more after the time of pSS diagnosis in 3 patients. Only 2 patients (1.8%) had Grave's disease. A French study prospectively followed 137 patients with pSS, all female, for a mean duration of 6 years [64]. They found 22% of cases had thyroid dysfunction at diagnosis, compared to only 6% in a control group. The commonest thyroid disease was Hashimoto's thyroiditis. The presence of rheumatoid factor and anti-Ro antibodies were associated with increased risk of thyroid disease. Of the pSS patients with normal thyroid function at initial diagnosis, 12 developed thyroid disease during the follow up period; most frequently Hashimoto's thyroiditis. Most of these patients had antibodies to thyroid peroxidase and/or thyroglobulin at initial evaluation. Ramos-Casels et al. found that 20% of pSS had autoimmune thyroid disease, but this was no higher than in their controls [65]. They confirmed the association between thyroid disease and antibodies to thyroid peroxidase and thyroglobulin, as well as anti-parietal cell antibodies.

Eighteen percent of 28 pSS patients had autoimmune thyroiditis, and 35% had thyroglobulin and/or antimicrosomal autoantibodies [66]. Ten percent of 400 Hungarian pSS patients had autoimmune thyroid disease: 7% Hashimoto's thyroiditis and 3% Graves' disease [67]. In contrast, a study of 53 Turkish patients did not find an association between pSS and autoimmune thyroid disease or thyroid autoantibodies [68].

The converse relationship between the two diseases also holds true, with pSS occurring ten times more frequently in patients with autoimmune thyroid disease than in the general population. Of 63 prospectively evaluated patients with autoimmune thyroiditis, 4 had autoimmune sialadenitis and 6 had objective keratoconjunctivitis sicca and xerostomia [66]. Only one patient had anti-Ro antibodies and none had anti-La antibodies. This association may reflect common pathogenic mechanisms. There are shared immunogenetic influences in autoimmune hypothyroidism and pSS, with both diseases associated with HLA-DR3 [69], and similarities between the target organ antigens. Anti-α-fodrin antibodies occur in Hashimoto's thyroiditis. A study of 61 patients with pSS, 27 with Hashimoto's thyroiditis alone, and 31 patients with SS associated with thyroiditis found no difference in the prevalence of these antibodies between the groups [70].

Thus, thyroid autoantibodies should be checked at the time the diagnosis of pSS is made and regular measurement of thyroid function at follow-up clinic visits is advised. Conversely, patients with autoimmune hypothyroidism should be evaluated for clinical and immunological evidence of SS.

32.6.2   SS Associated with Autoimmune Liver Disease

The association between liver disease and SS was first identified in 1954 [71], and is discussed in detail in Chap. 17. Debate exists as to whether SS occurring in the context of autoimmune liver disease (particularly primary biliary cirrhosis) is 'secondary' in the way that sSS occurs in RA, or whether it reflects co-existence of two autoimmune conditions (pSS and autoimmune liver disease).

32.6.3   Association of SS with Coeliac Disease

Several studies have found an increased incidence of coeliac disease in pSS. Fifteen percent of 34 pSS patients investigated prospectively had coeliac disease [72]. 4.5% of 111 Hungarian patients with pSS had coeliac disease, compared to 0.5% in the general population [73]. A UK cohort had a lower prevalence of coeliac disease at 0.9% [2]. Three of 141 pSS patients had coeliac disease in a Mexican study [74]. Luft et al. found that 6 of 50 (12%) patients with pSS had antibodies to tissue trans-glutaminase (TTG), with 5 of the 6 having histological evidence of coeliac disease [74]. This contrasts with a study by Roth et al. who found that only 2 of 77 patients with pSS had IgA antibodies to transglutaminase, and none had IgG antibodies [75]. A study of 334 patients with coeliac disease found that 3.3% of patients had SS, compared to 0.3% of controls [76].

32.7   Conclusions

The key messages to emerge from this chapter include:
1. Although SS is principally a disease of the exocrine glands, it may can a variety of tissues beyond the exocrine glands and lead to significant cumulative co-morbidity. A wide range of clinical features have been linked to SS, and other autoimmune diseases frequently co-exist with this condition. Autoimmune hypothyroidism is the organ-specific autoimmune disease that is most commonly associated with SS, followed by autoimmune liver disease. Thus, making a diagnosis of SS is not the 'end of the story'. Life-long follow-up is required, with vigilance for the development of extra-glandular manifestations, other autoimmune diseases, and lymphoma. In particular, anti-thyroid antibodies should be checked at diagnosis, and thyroid function measured regularly thereafter.
2. The terminology of 'secondary', 'associated' and 'overlap' SS needs clarification.
3. SS secondary to RA is milder than the primary form of the disease, with different genetic associations. SS accompanying SLE (SLE-SS) and primary SS are clini-cally, serologically, and genetically similar. Patients with SLE-SS tend to be older and have milder lupus than patients with SLE alone. Sicca symptoms are frequent in SSc, but are often due to pure glandular fibrosis. SS accompanying SLE and SSc may be better described as 'associated' than 'secondary'. By contrast, in RA 'secondary SS' is an accurate description.

References

1. Theander E, Jacobsson LTH. Relationship of Sjögren's syndrome to other connective tissue and autoimmune disorders. Rheum Dis Clin North Am. 2008;34:935–47.
2. Lazarus MN, Isenberg DA. Development of additional autoimmune diseases in a population of patients with primary Sjögren's syndrome. Ann Rheum Dis. 2005;64:1062–4.
3. Heaton J. Sjögren's syndrome and systemic lupus erythematosus. BMJ. 1959;1:466–9.

4. Gilboe I, Kvien T, Uhlig T, et al. Sicca symptoms and secondary Sjögren's syndrome in systemic lupus erythematosus: comparison with rheumatoid arthritis and correlation with disease variables. Ann Rheum Dis. 2001;60:1103–9.
5. Scofield RH, Bruner GR, Harley JB, et al. Autoimmune thyroid disease is associated with a diagnosis of secondary Sjögren's syndrome in familial systemic lupus. Ann Rheum Dis. 2007;66:410–3.
6. Pan HF, Ye DQ, Wang Q, et al. Clinical and laboratory profiles of systemic lupus erythematosus associated with Sjögren syndrome in China: a study of 542 patients. Clin Rheumatol. 2008;27:339–43.
7. Moutsopoulos HM, Klippel JH, Pavlides N, et al. Correlative histopathologic and serologic findings of sicca syndrome in patients with systemic lupus erythematosus. Arthritis Rheum. 1980;23:36–40.
8. Andonopoulos AP, Skopuli FN, Dimou GS, et al. Sjögren's syndrome in patients with systemic lupus erythematosus. J Rheumatol. 1990;17:201–4.
9. Jonsson H, Nived O, Sturfeld G. Outcome in systemic lupus erythematosus: a prospective study in patients from a defined population. Medicine (Baltimore). 1989;68:141–50.
10. Nossent JC, Swaak A. Systemic lupus erythematosus VII: impact and frequency of secondary Sjögren's syndrome. Lupus. 1998;7:231–4.
11. Manoussakis MN, Georgopoulou C, Zintzaras E, et al. Sjögren's syndrome associated with systemic lupus erythematosus: clinical and laboratory profiles and comparison with primary Sjögren's syndrome. Arthritis Rheum. 2004;50:882–91.
12. Manthorpe R, Teppo AM, Bendixen G, et al. Antibodies to SS-B in chronic inflammatory connective tissue diseases. Relationship with HLA-Dw2 and HLA-Dw3 antigens in primary Sjögren's syndrome. Arthritis Rheum. 1982;25:662–7.
13. Skopuli FN, Siouna-Fatourou H, Dimou GS, et al. Histologic lesion in labial salivary glands of patients with systemic lupus erythematosus. Oral Surg Oral Med Oral Pathol. 1991;72: 208–12.
14. Szanto A, Szodoray P, Kiss E, et al. Clinical, serological, and genetic profiles of patients with associated Sjögren's syndrome and systemic lupus erythematosus. Hum Immunol. 2006;67: 924–30.
15. Turkcapar N, Olmez U, Tutkak H, et al. The importance of alpha-fodrin antibodies in the diagnosis of Sjögren's syndrome. Rheumatol Int. 2006;26:354–9.
16. Ramos-Casals M, Brito-Zerón P, Font J. The overlap of Sjögren's syndrome with other systemic autoimmune diseases. Semin Arthritis Rheum. 2007;36:246–55.
17. Bloch KJ, Buchanan WW, Wohl MJ, et al. Sjögren's syndrome. A clinical, pathological and serological study of sixty-two cases. Medicine (Baltimore). 1965;44:187–228.
18. Coll J, Rives A, Grino MC, et al. Prevalence of Sjögren's syndrome in autoimmune diseases. Ann Rheum Dis. 1987;46:286–9.
19. Uhlig T, Kvien TK, Jensen JL, et al. Sicca symptoms, saliva and tear production, and disease variables in 636 patients with rheumatoid arthritis. Ann Rheum Dis. 1999;58:415–22.
20. Andonopoulos AP, Drosos AA, Skopuli FN, et al. Secondary Sjögren's syndrome in rheumatoid arthritis. J Rheumatol. 1987;14:1098–103.
21. Carmona L, Gonzalez-Alvaro I, Balsa A, et al. Rheumatoid arthritis in Spain: occurrence of extra-articular manifestations and estimates of disease severity. Ann Rheum Dis. 2003;62: 897–900.
22. Gottenberg J, Mignot S, Nicaise-Rolland P, et al. Prevalence of anti-cyclic citrullinated peptide and anti-keratin antibodies in patients with primary Sjögren's syndrome. Ann Rheum Dis. 2005;64:114–7.
23. Moutsopoulos HM, Webber BL, Vlagopoulos TP, et al. Differences in the clinical manifestations of sicca syndrome in the presence of absence of rheumatoid arthritis. Am J Med. 1979;66:733–6.
24. Kawashima K, Yoshino S. Differences in the clinical features of Sjögren syndrome in the presence and absence of rheumatoid arthritis. Nippon Ika Daigaku Zasshi – J Nippon Med Sch. 1989;56:31–8.

25. Tsampoulas CG, Skopouli FN, Sartoris DJ, et al. Hand radiographic changes in patients with primary and secondary Sjögren's syndrome. Scand J Rheumatol. 1986;15:333–9.
26. Kroneld U, Halse AK, Jonsson R, et al. Differential immunological aberrations in patients with primary and secondary Sjögren's syndrome. Scand J Immunol. 1997;45:698–705.
27. Witte T, Matthias T, Arnett FC, et al. IgA and IgG autoantibodies against alpha-fodrin as markers for Sjögren's syndrome. Systemic lupus erythematosus. J Rheumatol. 2000;27:2617–20.
28. Willeke P, Gaubitz M, Schotte H, et al. Clinical and immunological characteristics of patients with Sjögren's syndrome in relation to alpha-fodrin antibodies. Rheumatology. 2007;46: 479–83.
29. Ruiz-Tiscar JL, Lopez-Longo FJ, Sanchez-Ramon S, et al. Prevalence of IgG anti-alpha-fodrin antibodies in Sjögren's syndrome. Ann N Y Acad Sci. 2005;1050:210–6.
30. Chen Q, Li X, Zhang H, et al. The epitope study of alpha-fodrin autoantibody in primary Sjögren's syndrome. Clin Exp Immunol. 2007;149:497–503.
31. Nozawa K, Ikeda K, Satoh M, et al. Autoantibody to NA14 is an independent marker primarily for Sjögren's syndrome. Front Biosci. 2009;14:3733–9.
32. Mattey DL, Gonzalez-Gay MA, Hajeer AH, et al. Association between HLA-DRB1*15 and secondary Sjögren's syndrome in patients with rheumatoid arthritis. J Rheumatol. 2000;27:2611–6.
33. Vitali C, Tavoni A, Rizzo G, et al. HLA antigens in Italian patients with primary Sjögren's syndrome. Ann Rheum Dis. 1986;45:412–6.
34. Moutsopoulos HM, Mann DL, Johnson AH, et al. Genetic differences between primary and secondary sicca syndrome. N Engl J Med. 1979;301:761–3.
35. Papasteriades CA, Skopouli FN, Drosos AA, et al. HLA-alloantigen associations in Greek patients with Sjögren's syndrome. J Autoimmun. 1988;1:85–90.
36. Wilson RW, Provost TT, Bias WB, et al. Sjögren's syndrome: influence of multiple HLA-D region allogens on clinical and serological expression. Arthritis Rheum. 1984;27:1245–53.
37. Manthorpe R, Morling N, Platz P, et al. HLA-D antigen frequencies in Sjögren's syndrome. Differences between the primary and secondary form. Scand J Rheumatol. 1981;10:124–8.
38. Warlow RS, Kay PH, McCluskey J, et al. Secondary Sjögren's syndrome and chromosome six markers. Tissue Antigens. 1985;25:247–54.
39. Cipoletti JF, Buckingham RB, Barnes EL, et al. Sjögren's syndrome in progressive systemic sclerosis. Ann Intern Med. 1977;87:535–41.
40. Osial Jr TA, Whiteside TL, Buckingham RB, et al. Clinical and serological study of Sjögren's syndrome in patients with progressive systemic sclerosis. Arthritis Rheum. 1983;26:500–8.
41. Drosos AA, Andonopoulos AP, Costopoulos JS, et al. Sjögren's syndrome in progressive systemic sclerosis. J Rheumatol. 1988;15:965–8.
42. Alarcon-Segovia D, Ibañez G, Hernandez-Ortiz J, et al. Sjögren's syndrome in progressive systemic sclerosis. Am J Med. 1974;57:78–85.
43. Drosos AA, Pennec YL, Elisaf M, et al. Sjögren's syndrome in patients with the CREST variant of progressive systemic scleroderma. J Rheumatol. 1991;18:1685–8.
44. Oddis CV, Eisenbeis Jr CH, Reidbord HE, et al. Vasculitis in systemic sclerosis: association with Sjögren's syndrome and the CREST syndrome variant. J Rheumatol. 1987;14:942–8.
45. Andonopoulos AP, Drosos AA, Skopuli FN, et al. Sjögren's syndrome in rheumatoid arthritis and progressive systemic sclerosis: a comparative study. Clin Exp Rheumatol. 1989;7:203–5.
46. Avouac J, Sordet C, Depinay C, et al. Systemic sclerosis-associated Sjögren's syndrome and relationship to the limited cutaneous subtype: results of a prospective study of sicca syndrome in 133 consecutive patients. Arthritis Rheum. 2006;54:2243–9.
47. Salliot C, Mouthon L, Ardizzone M, Sibilia J, et al. Sjögren's syndrome is associated with and not secondary to systemic sclerosis. Rheumatology. 2007;46:321–6.
48. Swaminathan S, Goldblatt F, Dugar M, et al. Prevalence of sicca symptoms in a South Australian cohort with systemic sclerosis. Intern Med J. 2008;38:897–903.
49. Wangkaew S, Kasitanon N, Sivasomboon C, et al. Sicca symptoms in Thai patients with rheumatoid arthritis, systemic lupus erythematosus and scleroderma: a comparison with age-matched controls and correlation with disease variables. Asian Pac J Allergy Immunol. 2006;24:213–21.

50. Hida A, Kawabe Y, Kawakami A, et al. HTLV-I associated Sjögren's syndrome is aetiologically distinct from anti-centromere antibodies positive Sjögren's syndrome. Ann Rheum Dis. 1999;58:320–2.

51. Ramos-Casals M, Nardi N, Brito-Zeron P, et al. Atypical autoantibodies in patients with primary Sjögren syndrome: clinical characteristics and follow-up of 82 cases. Semin Arthritis Rheum. 2006;35:312–21.

52. Salliot C, Gottenberg JE, Bengoufa D, et al. Anticentromere antibodies identify patients with Sjögren's syndrome and autoimmune overlap syndrome. J Rheumatol. 2007;34:2253–8.

53. Black C, Isenberg DA. Mixed connective tissue disease – goodbye to all that. Rheumatology. 1992;31:695–700.

54. Ohtsuka E, Nonaka S, Shingu M, et al. Sjögren's syndrome and mixed connective tissue disease. Clin Exp Rheumatol. 1992;10:339–44.

55. Setty YN, Pittman CB, Mahale AS, et al. Sicca symptoms and anti-SSA/Ro antibodies are common in mixed connective tissue disease. J Rheumatol. 2002;29:487–9.

56. Young C, Hunt S, Watkinson A, et al. Sjögren's syndrome, cavitating lung disease and high sustained levels of antibodies to serine proteinase 3. Scand J Rheumatol. 2000;29:267–9.

57. Radaelli F, Meucci G, Spinzi G, et al. Acute self-limiting jejunitis as the first manifestation of microscopic polyangiitis associated with Sjögren's disease: report of one case and review of the literature. Eur J Gastroenterol Hepatol. 1999;11:931–4.

58. Drosos AA, Constantopoulos SH, Psychos D, et al. The forgotten cause of sicca complex; sarcoidosis. J Rheumatol. 1989;16:1548–51.

59. Ramos-Casals M, Brito-Zeron P, Garcia-Carrasco M, et al. Sarcoidosis or Sjögren syndrome? Clues to defining mimicry or coexistence in 59 cases. Medicine (Baltimore). 2004;83: 85–95.

60. Giotaki H, Constantopoulos SH, Papadimitriou CS, et al. Labial minor salivary gland biopsy: a highly discriminatory diagnostic method between sarcoidosis and Sjögren's syndrome. Respiration. 1986;50:102–7.

61. Jara L, Navarro C, Brito-Zerón P, et al. Thyroid disease in Sjögren's syndrome. Clin Rheumatol. 2007;26:1601–6. Epub 2007 Jun 9.

62. Pérez EB, Kraus A, López G, et al. Autoimmune thyroid disease in primary Sjögren's syndrome. Am J Med. 1995;99:480–4.

63. Kelly C, Foster H, Pal B, et al. Primary Sjögren's syndrome in north east England – a longitudinal study. Br J Rheumatol. 1991;30:437–42.

64. D'Arbonneau F, Ansart S, Le Berre R, et al. Thyroid dysfunction in primary Sjögren's syndrome: a long-term follow-up study. Arthritis Rheum. 2003;49:804–9.

65. Ramos-Casals M, Garcia-Carasco M, Cervera R, et al. Thyroid disease in primary Sjögren syndrome. Study in a series of 160 patients. Medicine (Baltimore). 2000;79:103–8.

66. Hansen BU, Ericsson UB, Henricsson V, et al. Autoimmune thyroiditis and primary Sjögren's syndrome: clinical and laboratory evidence of the coexistence of the two diseases. Clin Exp Rheumatol. 1991;9:137–41.

67. Biro E, Szekanecz Z, Czirjak L, et al. Association of systemic and thyroid autoimmune diseases. Clin Rheumatol. 2006;25:240–5.

68. Tunc R, Gonen MS, Acbay O, et al. Autoimmune thyroiditis and anti-thyroid antibodies in primary Sjögren's syndrome: a case-control study. Ann Rheum Dis. 2004;63:575–7.

69. Tandon N, Zhang L, Weetman AP. HLA associations with Hashimoto's thyroiditis. Clin Endocrinol. 1991;34:383–6.

70. Szanto A, Csipo I, Horvath I, et al. Autoantibodies to alpha-fodrin in patients with Hashimoto thyroiditis and Sjögren's syndrome: possible markers for a common secretory disorder. Rheumatol Int. 2008;28:1169–72.

71. Cristiansson J. Corneal changes in a case of hepatitis. Acta Ophthalmol. 1954;32:161.

72. Iltanen S, Collin P, Korpela M, et al. Celiac disease and markers of celiac disease latency in patients with primary Sjögren's syndrome. Am J Gastroenterol. 1999;94:1042–6.

73. Szodoray P, Barta Z, Lakos G, et al. Coeliac disease in Sjögren's syndrome – a study of 111 Hungarian patients. Rheumatol Int. 2004;24:278–82.

74. Luft LM, Barr SG, Martin LO, et al. Autoantibodies to tissue transglutaminase in Sjögren's syndrome and related rheumatic diseases. J Rheumatol. 2003;30:2613–9.
75. Roth E, Theander E, Londos E, et al. Pathogenesis of autoimmune diseases: antibodies against transglutaminase, peptidylarginine deiminase and protein-bound citrulline in primary Sjögren's syndrome, multiple sclerosis and Alzheimer's disease. Scand J Immunol. 2008;67:626–31.
76. Collin P, Reunala T, Pukkala E, et al. Coeliac disease–associated disorders and survival. Gut. 1994;35:1215–8.

Chapter 33
Cancer

Elke Theander and Eva Baecklund

Contents

E. Theander (✉)
Department of Rheumatology, Skåne University Hospital,
Malmö, Sweden

E. Baecklund
Rheumatology Unit, Department of Medical Sciences, Uppsala University,
Uppsala, Sweden

M. Ramos-Casals et al. (eds.), *Sjögren's Syndrome*,
DOI 10.1007/978-0-85729-947-5_33, © Springer-Verlag London Limited 2012

33.1 Introduction

Sjögren's syndrome (SS) is a chronic, systemic, inflammatory rheumatic disease that demonstrates features of organ-specific and non-organ-specific autoimmunity [1]. SS can occur in a primary form (pSS) or in secondary form (sSS) in association with various other rheumatic diseases, primarily rheumatoid arthritis (RA) and systemic lupus erythematosus (SLE) [2]. In SLE, the term "associated disorder" or overlap syndrome may be more appropriate than "secondary" SS because of the similarities of pathogenic processes and clinical manifestations in the two diseases and the difficulties in differentiating reliably between them in a considerable number of patients [2].

This chapter outlines what is known about SS and cancer. We will summarize present knowledge on incidence and prevalence of cancer in SS, clinical risk factors and predictors, types and subtypes of malignancies, and prognosis. The focus will be on hematological malignancies, because lymphoma development is the major threat for patients with SS and one of the few factors that contribute to premature mortality in this disease [3]. Therapy of these cancers is dealt with in another chapter of this book (Chap. 37). With the exception of the most important classic papers, we focus this review on studies that have applied the American European Consensus Criteria (AECC) [4] for case definitions of pSS and sSS.

The association between autoimmune disease and malignancy risk, especially hematological malignancy, is not restricted to SS [5]. Heightened risks of cancer accompany states of chronic inflammation associated with autoimmunity in general and may be further increased by certain treatments [6]. Thus, we also review the results of recent important studies in SLE and RA in order to understand the risk of malignancy in SS in a fuller context. Patients with autoimmune disease constitute only a small part of patients with lymphoma.

33.2 Methodological Considerations

Malignancy is a common phenomenon in human life. However, some types of malignancy (and in particular those that pertain to autoimmune diseases, e.g., hematological malignancies) are quite rare. Estimates of the prevalence of pSS have ranged widely, from as high as 0.3% [7] to as low as 0.05% [8]. Prevalence estimates for sSS and associated disorders are difficult to obtain because this condition has seldom been studied systematically. Thus, evaluations of the association between special types of malignancies and SS require studies within large, representative unselected patient cohorts with reliable case definition. Further, such studies require many years of follow-up time on individual patients, preferably decades, as well as registry data available for the relevant malignancies within the cohort and background population. Case reports and case series may give hints for additional rare associations. However, there is a strong risk of selection bias in such reports towards

Table 33.1 Selection of studies of lymphoma incidence in patients with Sjögren's syndrome

Author	Year	Country	SIR (95% CI)	No. of pSS patients	No. of lymphomas
Kassan et al. [12]	1978	United States	44.4 (16.7–118.4)	142	7
Kauppi et al. [48]	1997	Finland	8.7 (4.3–15.5)	676	11
Pertovaara et al. [31]	2001	Finland	13 (2.7–38.0)	110	3
Zintzaras et al.[16]	2005	Meta-analysis 5 studies	18.8 (9.5–37.3)	1,323	30
Lazarus et al. [50]	2006	United Kingdom	37.5 (20.7–67.6)	112	11
Theander et al. [10]	2006	Sweden	15.6 (7.8–27.9)	507	11
Zhang et al.[17]	2010	China	48.1 (20.7–94.8)	1,320	8

SIR Standardized incidence ratio

more severe cases. This chapter therefore confines its conclusions to studies that have employed with case verification procedures based upon the AECC 2002 [4].

Another methodological concern is the possibility of reverse causality; that is, the chance that cancer or lymphoma might induce autoimmune phenomena and mimic the rheumatic disease in question. However, in the case of SS, disease onset is difficult to define and median delays of 8 years between first symptoms and diagnosis have been registered (personal communications and own unpublished experience). Short observation times may lead to underestimation of the risk of malignancy because in pSS, lymphoma frequently appears late instead of early [9, 10].

Lymphomas, the main type of malignancy associated with SS, have been classified according to various systems. Major advances in understanding of the biology of these diseases have led to the now universally accepted World Health Organization (WHO) classification [11]. The WHO classification separates the lymphomas into either B-cell or T/NK-cell neoplasms (previously "non-Hodgkin lymphoma" (NHL)) or Hodgkin lymphoma (HL), and each of these entities is then divided into a number of specific subtypes.

33.3   Primary Sjögren's Syndrome and Lymphoma

33.3.1   Risk Levels

An increased risk for malignant lymphoma in patients with pSS has been observed in a number of studies (Table 33.1). Kassan et al. reported in their classic 1978 paper that 15 patients within their National Institute of Health (NIH) cohort of 142 patients with sicca syndrome had developed malignancies other than skin cancer, among whom seven patients had 7 NHL [12]. Although the incidence of the eight other types of cancer reported were within the expected range for the comparison population, the incidence of lymphomas was not. The Standardized Incidence Ratio (SIR) for NHL in the patients with pSS was calculated to be 44.4, and for those with SS secondary to RA 42.9. The risk for patients with parotid enlargement was considerably higher (relative risk 66.7) than for those without (relative risk 12.5), and parotid radiation enhanced the risk (relative risk 300). This important first observation, though probably influenced by selection of patients with severe disease manifestations into the NIH cohort, stimulated research on SS and lymphoma.

More than 20 years after this study, registry-linkage studies gave more reliable estimations of the risk of malignancy in the pSS population [10, 13–15]. The magnitude of the association between lymphoma and SS shows wide variation among studies. Zintzaras et al. reported in a meta-analysis that the SIRs for NHL in SS cohorts varied between 8.7 and 44.4. The pooled analysis resulted in an SIR of 18.8 (95% CI 9.5–37.3) [16]. The results of our own cohort study, in which an SIR for NHL of 15.6 (95% CI 7.8–27.9) [10] was reported, were concordant with this meta-analysis.

A study by Zhang et al. that involved 1,320 Chinese pSS patients found an SIR for NHL of 48.1 (95% CI: 20.7–94.8) [17]. The mean age of these patients was only 39 years – very young for a pSS cohort. The high SIR in this study may pertain both to the lower mean age of the patients and also to selection bias of a patient cohort with more severe disease [17, 18]. The other investigations have revealed more modest risk increases. A recent study by Andersson et al. compared 44,350 patients with lymphoproliferative malignancies with 120,531 individuals without malignancies. All subjects in the study were older than 67 years. One hundred and forty-two patients in the malignancy group had SS, versus 255 subjects in the comparison group, for an odds ratio (OR) for having SS of 1.9 (95% CI: 1.5–2.3) [15].

The cumulative incidence of lymphoma in pSS was reported to be 18% after 20 years of observation in one study [19]. Most studies report a lifetime risk of lymphoma in pSS of approximately 5–10% [9].

33.3.2   Lymphoma Subtypes

Various subtypes of lymphoma have been described in pSS. Extranodal marginal zone lymphoma of mucosa-associated lymphoid tissue (i.e., MALT lymphomas) were once considered to be the only lymphoma subtype associated with pSS. However, in recent years, appreciation has grown for the development of other subtypes, particularly diffuse large B-cell lymphomas (DLBCL) (Fig. 33.1). Smedby et al. presented risk ratios for the different subtypes and noted a 28-fold increased risk for marginal zone B-cell lymphoma (MZBCL) (including MALT lymphoma) and an 11-fold increase of DLBCL [13].

Taking into account that DLBCL is the most frequent lymphoma in the general population, the DLBCL is numerically more important in pSS than the MALT lymphoma [20]. Anderson et al. found in their nested case control study that patients with DLBCL had a twofold increase of SS compared to patients without

Fig. 33.1 Diffuse large B-cell lymphoma in a salivary gland. Hematoxylin and eosin staining

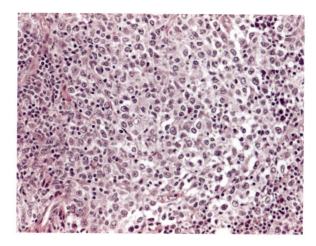

DLBCL (95% CI: 1.5–2.8) and patients with MZBCL had an odds ratio (OR) of 6.6 (95% CI: 4.6–9.5) for SS. Patients with other types of lymphomas, including Hodgkin lymphoma, did not have increased risks of SS [15]. However, in patients with salivary gland lymphomas and salivary gland MALT lymphomas, the ORs for SS were 22 (95% CI: 14–36) and OR 71 (95% CI: 40–120), respectively [15]. Among 40 pSS patients with lymphoma, Baimpa found 52.5% MALT lymphomas, 12.5% nodal MZBCLs, 17.5% DLBCLs, and 17.5% lymphomas of other subtypes (lymphoplasmocytic, follicular, polymorphic B cell, peripheral B cell, and Hodgkin disease) [21].

The features of MALT lymphomas in pSS are reviewed in detail recently [22]. MALT lymphomas may appear in salivary glands as the predominant site, but also in the stomach, nasopharynx, skin, kidney, and lungs. MALT lymphomas present at more than one extranodal site in 20% of patients, emphasizing the need for complete staging at diagnosis [22]. Bone marrow infiltration is rare (10%).

MALT lymphomas may transform into DLBCL in the course of the disease, but precisely what percentage of DLBCL arise from pre-existing MALT or follicular lymphomas is not known [22]. However, the histological transformation into a DLBCL is a poor prognostic sign, as survival in de novo or secondary DLBCL is poor [9, 10]. With the possible exception of vasculitis, lymphoma is the only cause of death conferring premature mortality to pSS patients, adding an excess death rate of 9.4 cases per 1,000 patient years at risk [3]. The median survival time for low-grade lymphomas was 76 months, in contrast to that of only 31 months for high-grade lymphomas [10]. However, most of these cases were treated before rituximab was widely used in the treatment of lymphomas. In 2006, Friedman et al. proposed T-cell (CD3+) large granular lymphocyte (LGL) leukemia as an under-recognized association with pSS. Twelve of 48 patients with T-cell (CD3+) LGL leukemia met criteria for SS [23].

33.4 Prediction of Lymphoma

33.4.1 Can We Tell Who Will Develop Lymphoma and When This May Occur?

Primary SS is a bothersome but often benign disorder. In contrast, the development of lymphoma has a considerable impact on survival [3]. Still, the threat of NHL applies to only 10–20% of SS patients depending on selection criteria and observation time. In order to deliver optimal care and follow-up, it is of utmost importance to be able to differentiate between patients at risk for NHL development and those without. Patients at high risk could be assigned to screening programmes for early detection and possibly preventive therapy.

Proposals of dividing SS into type I (high risk for lymphoma) and type II (low risk) have been made from Greece [14]. Patients with low complement factor 4 (C4), parotid gland enlargement, or palpable purpura at presentation constitute type I pSS. These factors are easily assessed during the primary diagnostic process. However, these three factors alone are insufficient to predict subsequent progression to malignant lymphoma reliably [21].

When does the lymphoma arise? Very early research proposed that a decrease in the level of serum immunoglobulins and disappearance of RF from the serum heralded progression to lymphoma [24, 25]. In fact, these findings are probably indicators of early lymphoma rather than predictors of imminent transformation from a benign to a malignant B-cell disorder. Longitudinal studies of BAFF levels or cytokine patterns in relationship to lymphoma development might reveal useful information about the time course of lymphoma formation. Barone et al. demonstrated differential chemokine expression in salivary glands depending on the presence of benign or malignant lymphoepithelial proliferation [26]. Repeated biopsies for analyses of the local cytokine milieu are difficult to perform, but correlations between saliva concentrations and tissue sampling are potential surrogates that might have therpeutic implications in the future.

33.4.2 Established Risk Factors

A number of predictors of lymphoma have been confirmed repeatedly. Those reported most commonly are recurrently or persistently swollen salivary glands [9, 10, 12, 14, 17, 19] (Fig. 33.2), lymphadenopathy [9, 10, 17, 19, 21], cryoglobulinemia [14, 21, 27, 28], splenomegaly [21], low serum C4 concentrations [10, 14, 21, 27, 29], low serum C3 concentrations [10, 29], lymphopenia [9], cutaneous vasculitis [9, 10, 14, 27], monoclonal bands within the serum or urine [9, 30], peripheral neuropathy [9], and high serum beta2-microglobulin levels [25, 31]. Two recent studies demonstrated a "dose effect", with greater numbers of risk factors associated with an increased risk of lymphoma development [17, 21]. In one study, 12% of patients with only one risk factor developed NHL [21]. In contrast, in patients with four known study risk factors,

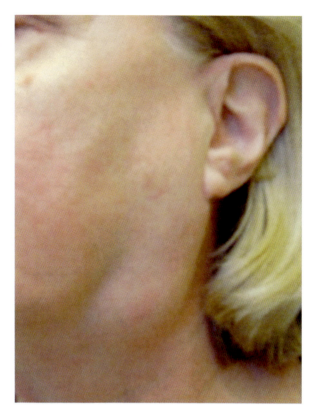

Fig. 33.2 Patient with primary Sjögren's syndrome and persistent severe parotid gland enlargement, histologically with germinal center-like formation but without lymphoma (Published with patient's permission)

the likelihood of lymphoma development was 100%. In another Chinese study, patients with three or more risk factors had a risk of malignancy that was increased approximately 30-fold compared to those without risk factors [17].

33.4.3 Recently Proposed Newer Risk Factors

Having observed a number of pSS patients presenting with CD4+ T-lymphocytopenia [32], mainly in association with autoantibodies to SSA [33], we documented that CD4+ T-lymphocytopenia is a strong predictor of lymphoma development [10]. The classic cause of CD4+ T-lymphocytopenia, HIV infection, is well-known to be associated with a 20-fold increased risk of NHL. Furthermore, there are case reports of lymphoma development in association with idiopathic CD4+ T-lymphocytopenia [34–36]. The association between CD4+ T-lymphocytopenia in pSS with lymphoma development has, however, not yet been confirmed by others.

The occurrence of forkhead/winged-helix transcription factor 3 positive (Foxp3+) (CD4+ 25^{high}) T-cells in the salivary glands showed a bimodal distribution [37]. The number of Foxp3+ regulatory T cells increased with the intensity of the inflammatory infiltrate but decreased in the most severe lesions and correlated with markers of lymphoma development such as low complement levels. No lymphoma patients

Fig. 33.3 Germinal
center-like structures in lower
lip salivary gland biopsy

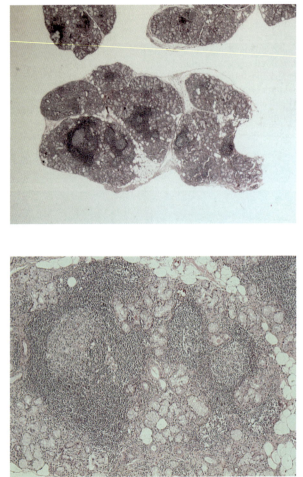

Fig. 33.4 Germinal
center-like structures in lower
lip salivary gland biopsy,
detail

were included in the study, but these findings might indicate an inability by regulatory T cells to exert sufficient control of local immune responses.

Another new marker of lymphoma in pSS is the presence of germinal center-like structures in the salivary gland biopsy [38]. Although T-cell subsets are seldom included in routine diagnostic evaluations, the lower lip salivary gland biopsy is part of the AECC classification criteria set [4] and easily performed in all patients if suitable for risk stratification. Germinal centers have been detected in lip biopsies from 20% to 30% of patients with pSS [39] (Figs. 33.3 and 33.4). Germinal centers are proposed as important sites of intensive cellular, molecular, and genetic activity leading to extensive clonal expansion of B cells, somatic hypermutation, and class-switch recombination of immunoglobulin genes [40]. Germinal center reactions have been linked to the occurrence or initiation of malignant B-cell transformation [41] (Fig. 33.5) and termed the condition "sine qua non" for lymphoma

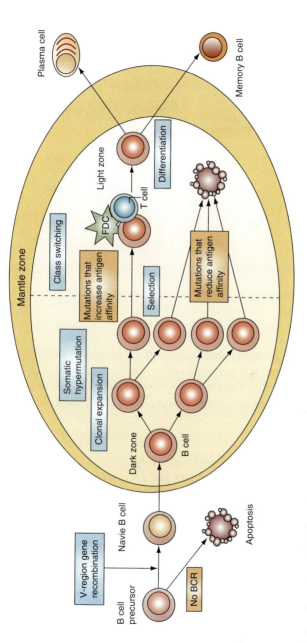

Fig. 33.5 Transformation of B cells and possible lymphoma development in germinal centers (Reproduced from [40] with author's permission, permission from journal pending)

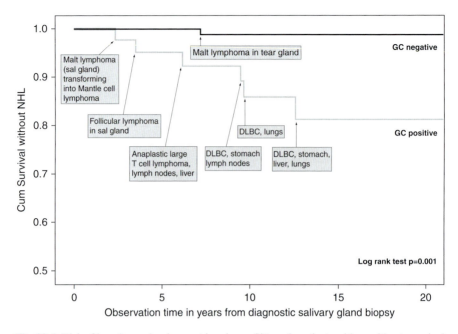

Fig. 33.6 Risk of lymphoma development in primary Sjögren's patients with or without germinal center-like structures. Kaplan–Meier curve [38]

development. We observed that six out of seven pSS patients who eventually developed lymphoma had germinal center-like structures in their salivary gland biopsies [38] (Fig. 33.6). The predictive power of the presence of germinal centers for lymphoma development needs to be explored in further clinical and epidemiologic studies.

33.4.4   Are There Risk Factors for Distinct Subtypes of SS-Associated Lymphomas?

Treatment approaches and outcome are different between the low-grade MALT lymphomas and high-grade DLBCL. Consequently, early detection of DLBCL or transformation of MALT into DLBCL is important because these clinical developments require aggressive intervention. In one study, the age of patients with DLBCL was higher than that of patients with marginal zone B cell lymphomas (MZBCL). In addition, the time between diagnosis of SS and lymphoma was longer for DLBCL – a median of 7 versus 1.5 years. However, the range of the time before lymphoma development overlapped considerably, being up to 15 years for DLBCL and up to 26 years for MZBCL [21]. The same study identified cryoglobulinemia, neutropenia, low C4 levels, lymphadenopathy, and splenomegaly as independent risk factors for

MZBCL, while only lymphocytopenia was retained as a risk factor for non-MZBCL [21]. Between various studies there are inconsistencies regarding the frequency of the different subtypes of lymphomas. Baimpa et al. proposed a diversity of triggering stimuli of lymphomagenesis in different geographic areas as one reason [21]. Another might be that low-grade MALT lymphomas can be difficult to detect in some patients without active searches and may come to medical attention only at the time they transform into DLBCL [42].

33.5 Pathogenetic Mechanisms

The underlying mechanisms for the inter-relationship of autoimmune disease and lymphoproliferative neoplasias are still insufficiently understood. Both situations occur in hosts with altered immune responses and surveillance mechanisms. The interplay of genetic, environmental, and infectious agents may be regarded as critical to the development of both autoimmunity and malignancy.

Certain risk factors for malignancy in pSS (e.g., hypergammaglobulinemia, chronic lymphocytic infiltration into salivary glands, germinal centre formation) are consistent with the hypothesis of chronic antigenic stimulation of B-cell subsets within the salivary glands. Other risk factors, e.g., lymphopenia and neutopenia, suggest the importance of decreased immune surveillance. Still others (monoclonal immunoglobulin) imply the survival of B cells with potential for malignancy supported by factors such as BAFF or APRIL. BAFF levels have not yet been directly associated with lymphoma development in pSS, but are known to play a role in the evolution of idiopathic NHLs and in hepatitis C-associated NHLs [43, 44]. Among the autoimmune diseases, BAFF levels are highest in pSS, both in the systemic circulation and in salivary glands; higher even than in SLE and RA. Increased B cell survival is favored further by upregulation of the anti-apoptotic mediator Bcl-2.

Although such predictors of lymphoma are present at the time of SS diagnosis and thus often many years before the clinical appearance of the lymphoma, additional triggers – possibly local aberrant genetic events within the GCs – must be necessary to induce the final multistep transition resulting in lymphomagenesis [41, 45]. Understanding these additional triggers might permit more accurate predictions of the time when lymphoma will appear. The availability of therapeutic B-cell depletion makes precise prediction of when and in whom a lymphoma will develop particularly important.

In RA, disease activity and chronic inflammation have been identified as the major risk factors for lymphoma development. In pSS, measurement instruments for disease activity have been lacking until very recently, but are now available as the EULAR Sjögren's Syndrome Disease Activity Index (ESSDAI) instrument [46]. We have observed an association between higher ESSDAI scores in SS and germinal center-like structures in pSS lower lip salivary gland biopsies [38]. This may indicate that higher disease activity burden is also accompanied by increased lymphoma risk in pSS.

33.6   Medication and Risk of Lymphoma in SS

The question of medication-induced lymphoma has been addressed in a number of publications in other rheumatic diseases, especially RA and SLE. Similar considerations are of interest in sSS associated with RA or SLE, but data on such questions are lacking. Immunosuppression is generally considered unnecessary or ineffective in pSS, at least with regard to traditional Disease Modifying Anti-Rheumatic Drugs (DMARDs) and TNF-alpha blocking agents, and is therefore avoided. A question important for pSS, however, is the potential efficacy of newer therapies directed against B cells and whether or not such interventions reduce the risk of lymphomagenesis. The short-term effects of B cell depletion in pSS, such as the reduction of the number of extraglandular manifestations [47] or the reduction in the number of germinal centers in the parotid gland [48], support such a strategy, but further studies are required. Long follow-up periods and use of surrogate biomarkers for lymphoma risk profile changes will be necessary before this question can be answered definitively.

33.7   Associated Sjögren's Syndrome and Lymphoma

Very little is known about the risk of lymphoproliferative disease in sSS or to what extent sSS enhances the risks of lymphoma known to exist for RA and SLE. A study by Kauppi et al. from Finland demonstrated a twofold increased risk of lymphoma for RA patients with sSS compared to RA alone [49]. The large InterLymph Consortium Study observed higher lymphoma risks for sSS than for pSS, with odds ratios of 9.57 and 4.75, respectively [20]. Löfström et al. documented that sicca symptoms constitute a risk factor for lymphoma development in SLE [50].

33.8   Other Cancers in SS

Information about risk of other malignancies than lymphoproliferative disorders in pSS is scarce. In a Swedish cohort study including 286 pSS patients who fulfilled the AECC criteria, we found 33 malignancies compared to the expected number of 23, resulting in a SIR for all malignancies of 1.42 (95% CI 0.98–2.00). However, instead of the expected 0.71 cases of NHL, we detected 11. Thus, ten excess malignancies were attributable to an increased risk of NHL in pSS [10].

Lazarus confirmed in a British SS cohort a lack of increased cancer risk for other malignancies than hematological ones: SIR 1.5 (95% CI 0.9–2.6) [51]. In contrast, the recently published cohort study investigating cancer risk in young Chinese SS patients revealed a SIR for all tumors of 3.25 (95% CI 2.12–4.52), and for non-hematological tumors the SIR was 2.12 (95% CI 1.27–3.31) [17]. There is not much information about risk factors or predictors for development of other cancers than lymphoma in pSS. In the Swedish cohort described above [10], a trend towards lower percentage of CD4+ T cells, but no other marker of lymphoma development seemed to predict other malignancy as well. Anticipating similarities between SLE and SS one might speculate that hormonal and reproductive factors would influence the risk of breast, cervix, uterus and ovarian cancer in a similar way as in the general population, as does smoking with regard to lung cancer [52]. Do several cancers appear in the same patient, or do other cancers increase the risk of lymphoma development? In the British cohort nine patients had two or more cancers [51], and in the Swedish cohort there seemed to be an increased risk of lymphoproliferative diseases in patients with concomitant skin cancer [10], in concordance with general findings of increased risks for other cancers in patients with skin cancers [53–55].

33.9 Conclusion

Patients with pSS who have persistent salivary gland swelling, hypocomplementemia, cytopenia or germinal center-like structures within their salivary glands should be followed more closely than others. Recent research supports the opinion that increasing number or risk factors increase the lymphoma risk, but the ability to predict lymphomagenesis from these identified risk factors remains imperfect. The increased risk in patients with other cancers, especially skin cancers, and concomitant lymphoma associated autoimmune diseases, requires further prospective studies. Regular follow-up of high-risk groups with longitudinal assessments of all known risk factors, including increased disease activity as assessed by the ESSDAI instrument, will facilitate understanding of these questions. Research must now be directed towards understanding the mechanism of lymphomagenesis in SS and in designing intervention strategies to prevent such events.

Acknowledgments The authors are grateful to Prof. Otto Ljungberg and Dr. Malin V. Jonsson for providing photographs of B cell lymphomas and germinal center-like structures in the salivary glands and Prof. Küppers for allowing the reproduction of the cartoon on B cell development within the Germinal Centers.

References

1. Jonsson R, Bolstad AI, Brokstad KA, Brun JG. Sjogren's syndrome – a plethora of clinical and immunological phenotypes with a complex genetic background. Ann N Y Acad Sci. 2007;1108: 433–47.
2. Theander E, Jacobsson LT. Relationship of Sjogren's syndrome to other connective tissue and autoimmune disorders. Rheum Dis Clin North Am. 2008;34:935–47.
3. Theander E, Manthorpe R, Jacobsson LTH. Mortality and causes of death in primary Sjögren's syndrome. Arthritis Rheum. 2004;50:1262–9.
4. Vitali C, Bombardieri S, Jonsson R, et al. Classification criteria for Sjögren's syndrome: a revised version of the European criteria proposed by the American-European Consensus Group. Ann Rheum Dis. 2002;61:554–8.

5. Smedby KE, Baecklund E, Askling J. Malignant lymphomas in autoimmunity and inflammation: a review of risks, risk factors, and lymphoma characteristics. Cancer Epidemiol Biomarkers Prev. 2006;15:2069–77.

6. Baecklund E, Iliadou A, Askling J, et al. Association of chronic inflammation, not its treatment, with increased lymphoma risk in rheumatoid arthritis. Arthritis Rheum. 2006;54: 692–701.

7. Bowman SJ, Ibrahim GH, Holmes G, Hamburger J, Ainsworth JR. Estimating the prevalence among Caucasian women of primary Sjögren's syndrome in two general practices in Birmingham, UK. Scand J Rheumatol. 2004;33:39–43.

8. Goransson LG, Haldorsen K, Brun JG, et al. The point prevalence of clinically relevant primary Sjogren's syndrome in two Norwegian counties. Scand J Rheumatol 2011;40: 221–4.

9. Voulgarelis M, Dafni UG, Isenberg DA, Moutsopoulos HM. Malignant lymphoma in primary Sjogren's syndrome: a multicenter, retrospective, clinical study by the European Concerted Action on Sjogren's Syndrome. Arthritis Rheum. 1999;42:1765–72.

10. Theander E, Henriksson G, Ljungberg O, Mandl T, Manthorpe R, Jacobsson LT. Lymphoma and other malignancies in primary Sjögren's syndrome: a cohort study on cancer incidence and lymphoma predictors. Ann Rheum Dis. 2006;65:796–803.

11. Swerdlow SH, Campo E, Harris NL, et al., editors. Pathology and genetics: tumours of the haematopoietic and lymphoid tissue. Lyon: IARC Press; 2008.

12. Kassan SS, Thomas TL, Moutsopoulos HM, et al. Increased risk of lymphoma in sicca syndrome. Ann Intern Med. 1978;89:888–92.

13. Smedby KE, Hjalgrim H, Askling J, et al. Autoimmune and chronic inflammatory disorders and risk of non-Hodgkin lymphoma by subtype. J Natl Cancer Inst. 2006;98:51–60.

14. Ioannidis JP, Vassiliou VA, Moutsopoulos HM. Long-term risk of mortality and lymphoproliferative disease and predictive classification of primary Sjögren's syndrome. Arthritis Rheum. 2002;46:741–7.

15. Anderson LA, Gadalla S, Morton LM, et al. Population-based study of autoimmune conditions and the risk of specific lymphoid malignancies. Int J Cancer. 2009;125:398–405.

16. Zintzaras E, Voulgarelis M, Moutsopoulos HM. The risk of lymphoma development in autoimmune diseases: a meta-analysis. Arch Intern Med. 2005;165:2337–44.

17. Zhang W, Feng S, Yan S, et al. Incidence of malignancy in primary Sjogren's syndrome in a Chinese cohort. Rheumatology (Oxford). 2010;49:571–7.

18. Ramos-Casals M, Cervera R, Font J, et al. Young onset of primary Sjogren's syndrome: clinical and immunological characteristics. Lupus. 1998;7:202–6.

19. Sutcliffe N, Inanc M, Speight P, Isenberg D. Predictors of lymphoma development in primary Sjögren's syndrome. Semin Arthritis Rheum. 1998;28:80–7.

20. Ekstrom Smedby K, Vajdic CM, Falster M, et al. Autoimmune disorders and risk of non-Hodgkin lymphoma subtypes: a pooled analysis within the InterLymph Consortium. Blood. 2008;111:4029–38.

21. Baimpa E, Dahabreh IJ, Voulgarelis M, Moutsopoulos HM. Hematologic manifestations and predictors of lymphoma development in primary Sjogren syndrome: clinical and pathophysiologic aspects. Medicine (Baltimore). 2009;88:284–93.

22. Voulgarelis M, Moutsopoulos HM. Mucosa-associated lymphoid tissue lymphoma in Sjögren's syndrome: risks, management, and prognosis. Rheum Dis Clin North Am. 2008;34: 921–33.

23. Friedman J, Schattner A, Shvidel L, Berrebi A. Characterization of T-cell large granular lymphocyte leukemia associated with Sjogren's syndrome-an important but under-recognized association. Semin Arthritis Rheum. 2006;35:306–11.

24. Anderson LG, Talal N. The spectrum of benign to malignant lymphoproliferation in Sjögren's syndrome. Clin Exp Immunol. 1972;10:199–221.

25. Anaya JM, McGuff S, Banks PM, Talal N. Clinicopathological factors relating malignant lymphoma with Sjögren's syndrome. Semin Arthritis Rheum. 1996;25:337–46.

26. Barone F, Bombardieri M, Rosado MM, et al. CXCL13, CCL21, and CXCL12 expression in salivary glands of patients with Sjogren's syndrome and MALT lymphoma: association with reactive and malignant areas of lymphoid organization. J Immunol. 2008;180:5130–40.

27. Skopouli FN, Dafni U, Ioannidis JPA, Moutsopoulos HM. Clinical evolution, and morbidity and mortality of primary Sjögren's syndrome. Semin Arthritis Rheum. 2000;29:296–304.

28. Tzioufas AG, Boumba DS, Skopouli FN, Moutsopoulos HM. Mixed monoclonal cryoglobulinemia and monoclonal rheumatoid factor cross-reactive idiotypes as predictive factors for the development of lymphoma in primary Sjögren's syndrome. Arthritis Rheum. 1996;39:767–72.

29. Ramos-Casals M, Brito-Zeron P, Yague J, et al. Hypocomplementaemia as an immunological marker of morbidity and mortality in patients with primary Sjögren's syndrome. Rheumatology (Oxford). 2005;44:89–94.

30. Walters MT, Stevenson FK, Herbert A, Cawley MI, Smith JL. Urinary monoclonal free light chains in primary Sjogren's syndrome: an aid to the diagnosis of malignant lymphoma. Ann Rheum Dis. 1986;45:210–9.

31. Pertovaara M, Pukkala E, Laippala P, Miettinen A, Pasternack A. A longitudinal cohort study of Finnish patients with primary Sjögren's syndrome: clinical, immunological, and epidemiological aspects. Ann Rheum Dis. 2001;60:467–72.

32. Kirtava Z, Blomberg J, Bredberg A, Henriksson G, Jacobsson L, Manthorpe R. CD4+ T-lymphocytopenia without HIV infection: increased prevalence among patients with primary Sjögren's syndrome. Clin Exp Rheumatol. 1995;13:609–16.

33. Mandl T, Bredberg A, Jacobsson LT, Manthorpe R, Henriksson G. CD4+ T-lymphocytopenia – a frequent finding in anti-SSA antibody seropositive patients with primary Sjogren's syndrome. J Rheumatol. 2004;31:726–8.

34. Hanamura I, Wakita A, Harada S, et al. Idiopathic CD4+ T-lymphocytopenia in a non-Hodgkin's lymphoma patient. Intern Med. 1997;36:643–6.

35. Cook M, Bareford D, Kumararatne D. Non-Hodgkin's lymphoma: an unusual complication of idiopathic CD4+-lymphocytopenia. Hosp Med. 1998;59:582.

36. Guilloton L, Drouet A, Bernard P, Berbineau A, Berger F, Kopp N. Cerebral intravascular lymphoma during T-CD4+ idiopathic lymphopenia syndrome. Presse Med. 1999;28:1513–5.

37. Christodoulou MI, Kapsogeorgou EK, Moutsopoulos NM, Moutsopoulos HM. Foxp3+ T-regulatory cells in Sjogren's syndrome: correlation with the grade of the autoimmune lesion and certain adverse prognostic factors. Am J Pathol. 2008;173:1389–96.

38. Theander E, Vasaitis L, Baecklund E, et al. Lymphoid organisation in labial salivary gland biopsies is a possible predictor for the development of malignant lymphoma in primary Sjogren's syndrome. Ann Rheum Dis 2011;70:1363–68.

39. Jonsson MV, Skarstein K, Jonsson R, Brun JG. Serological implications of germinal center-like structures in primary Sjögren's syndrome. J Rheumatol. 2007;34:2044–9.

40. Küppers R, Klein U, Hansmann M-L, Rajewsky K. Cellular origin of human B-cell lymphomas. N Engl J Med. 1999;341:1520–9.

41. Hansen A, Lipsky PE, Dorner T. B-cell lymphoproliferation in chronic inflammatory rheumatic diseases. Nat Clin Pract Rheumatol. 2007;3:561–9.

42. Ghesquieres H, Berger F, Felman P, et al. Clinicopathologic characteristics and outcome of diffuse large B-cell lymphomas presenting with an associated low-grade component at diagnosis. J Clin Oncol. 2006;24:5234–41.

43. Novak AJ, Grote DM, Stenson M, et al. Expression of BLyS and its receptors in B-cell non-Hodgkin lymphoma: correlation with disease activity and patient outcome. Blood. 2004;104:2247–53.

44. De Vita S, Quartuccio L, Fabris M. Hepatitis C virus infection, mixed cryoglobulinemia and BLyS upregulation: targeting the infectious trigger, the autoimmune response, or both? Autoimmun Rev. 2008;8:95–9.

45. Mariette X. Lymphomas complicating Sjögren's syndrome and hepatitis C virus infection may share a common pathogenesis: chronic stimulation of rheumatoid factor B cells. Ann Rheum Dis. 2001;60:1007–10.

46. Seror R, Ravaud P, Bowman S, et al. EULAR Sjogren's syndrome disease activity index (ESSDAI): development of a consensus systemic disease activity index in primary Sjogren's syndrome. Ann Rheum Dis. 2010;69:1103–9.
47. Meijer J, Meiners P, Vissink A, et al. Effective rituximab treatment in primary Sjogren's syndrome: a randomised, double-blind, placebo-controlled trial. Arthritis Rheum. 2010;62: 960–8.
48. Pijpe J, Meijer JM, Bootsma H, et al. Clinical and histologic evidence of salivary gland restoration supports the efficacy of rituximab treatment in Sjogren's syndrome. Arthritis Rheum. 2009;60:3251–6.
49. Kauppi M, Pukkala E, Isomäki H. Elevated incidence of hematologic malignancies in patients with Sjögren's syndrome compared with patients with rheumatoid arthritis (Finland). Cancer Causes Control. 1997;8:201–4.
50. Löfström B, Backlin C, Sundstrom C, Ekbom A, Lundberg I. A closer look at non-Hodgkin's lymphoma cases in a national Swedish systemic lupus erythematosus cohort: a nested case-control study. Ann Rheum Dis. 2007;66:1627–32.
51. Lazarus MN, Robinson D, Mak V, Moller H, Isenberg DA. Incidence of cancer in a cohort of patients with primary Sjogren's syndrome. Rheumatology (Oxford). 2006;45:1012–5.
52. Bernatsky S, Boivin JF, Joseph L, et al. Prevalence of factors influencing cancer risk in women with lupus: social habits, reproductive issues, and obesity. J Rheumatol. 2002;29:2551–4.
53. Frisch M, Melbye M. New primary cancers after squamous cell skin cancer. Am J Epidemiol. 1995;141:916–22.
54. Frisch M, Hjalgrim H, Olsen JH, Melbye M. Risk for subsequent cancer after diagnosis of basal-cell carcinoma. A population-based, epidemiologic study. Ann Intern Med. 1996;125: 815–21.
55. Wassberg C, Thorn M, Yuen J, Ringborg U, Hakulinen T. Second primary cancers in patients with squamous cell carcinoma of the skin: a population-based study in Sweden. Int J Cancer. 1999;80:511–5.

Chapter 34
Prognostic Factors and Survival

Andreas V. Goules and Fotini N. Skopouli

Contents

34.1 Introduction

The histological hallmark of primary Sjögren's syndrome (pSS) is the focal lymphocytic infiltrates that slowly and steadily replace the epithelium of salivary and lacrimal glands and produce exocrine gland dysfunction, manifested mainly by xerostomia and xerophthalmia [1]. These two clinical manifestations are determinants for the term "exocrinopathy" in SS. Studies in the last 20 years have delineated the type and spectrum of other organ involvement in SS. Lungs, liver and the kidneys are usually affected in pSS. The histology and the evolution of the lesion in the above parenchymal tissues do not differ from that observed in salivary and lacrimal glands. These extragrandular manifestations are mild in severity in most cases, evolve slowly, and do not appear to respond to glucocorticoids or other immunosuppressive agents. The central role of the epithelial cell as the main target of the immune injury in the exocrine glands as well as in the lungs, the liver and the kidneys has led to the introduction of the term "autoimmune epithelitis" [1].

A.V. Goules
Department of Pathophysiology, School of Medicine, University of Athens, Athens, Greece

F.N. Skopouli (✉)
Department of Dietetics and Nutritional Science, Harokopio University of Athens,
Athens, Greece

M. Ramos-Casals et al. (eds.), *Sjögren's Syndrome*,
DOI 10.1007/978-0-85729-947-5_34, © Springer-Verlag London Limited 2012

A subset of patients, in addition to epithelitis develop extraepithelial manifestations such as palpable purpura, glomerulonephritis, and peripheral neuropathy. These findings are attributed to an immune complex-mediated process [2–4]. This group of pSS patients constitutes a specific subcategory: the vasculitic form of the disease. Patients with the vasculitic form of pSS are characterized by higher morbidity and mortality rates and an increased risk of lymphoproliferative malignancies [2, 3, 5].

The impact of treatment on morbidity and mortality in pSS patients is minimal. Most pSS patients are not treated with glucocorticoids because of their substantial side effect profile as well as their lack of efficacy in most settings. The same is true for conventional immunomodulating agents. In contrast, the introduction of anti-CD20 interventions to the treatment of pSS-associated lymphoma has improved patients' survival [6–8]. Finally, an issue that remains poorly addressed to date is the impact of patients' psychological distress on morbidity and mortality.

34.2 Mortality and Causes of Death in pSS

The association between pSS and lymphoma and the impact of lymphoproliferative malignancies on patients' survival are important issues. In the early 1950s, Rothman et al. first described a patient with rheumatoid arthritis and SS who died of malignant lymphoma [9]. Talal et al. reported four cases of pSS who developed lymphoproliferative disorders and, based on the sequence of clinical and pathological events, supported the notion that lymphomas could be late sequelae of SS [10]. In a systematic study of 142 patients conducted at the National Institutes of Health [11], the relative risk of lymphoma was estimated to be 44-fold higher than that of the general population. Since then, several studies have confirmed this association. In a recent meta-analysis, the estimated standardized incidence ratio (SIR) of lymphoma in pSS was found to be 18.9 (95% CI 9.4–37.9) [12]. The lifetime risk of developing lymphoma for a patient with pSS is approximately 5–10% [4, 5, 13, 14] (Table 34.1).

Extranodal marginal zone B-cell lymphomas of mucosa associated lymphoid tissue (MALT), known as MALT lymphomas, comprise the most common histologic type of malignancy in pSS. Other lymphoma subtypes have been also described, however, including lymphoplasmacytoid, follicular, and diffuse large B cell lymphomas (DLBC) [4, 11, 15–18]. MALT lymphomas are usually low grade, indolent, and carry a favorable outcome [4, 19]. In contrast, DLBC lymphomas have a poorer prognosis [20]. Lymphomas are often the cause of death among SS patients and have been the leading cause of death in some large series [9, 10, 21, 22]. In a study of 261 pSS patients followed for a mean of 3.6 years the standardized mortality ratio (SMR) was 2.07 (95% CI 1.03–3.71) [2]. The increased mortality rate among pSS patients was attributed to lymphoma.

In a longitudinal cohort study of 110 Finnish pSS patients with a median follow-up of 9 years, 17 deaths occurred, for an SMR of 1.2 compared to the general Finnish population [23]. Two of the 17 deaths in this series were

Table 34.1 Causes and number of reported deaths in pSS

	Reported number of deaths in each study							
	Kruize [21]	Martens [22]	Skopouli [2]	Pertovaara [23]	Ioannidis [5]	Theader [24]	Alamanos [25]	Brito-Zeron [26]
Total number of deaths	8	11	11	17	39	34	47	25
Malignancies	3	2	4	4	17	6	NR	5
Lymphoma	3	–	3	2	7	6	3	2
Vascular causes	–	5	4	9	12	11	NR	9
Infection	1	–	–	3	3	–	NR	8
Pulmonary	–	3	2	–	2	–	–	–
Drug toxicity	–	–	–	–1	–	–	–	–
Other	4	1	1	–	5	17	–	–

attributable to lymphoma. Although the number of lymphoma cases in this series was small, the SIR for non-Hodgkin's lymphoma (NHL) was 13 (95% CI, 2.07–38).

Ioannidis et al. analyzed the records of 723 consecutive Geek patients with pSS who were followed for a mean of 6.1 years (4.4 patient-years) [5]. The SMR was 1.15 (95% CI 0.86–1.73) and 39 deaths were observed, of which 7 were attributable to lymphoma. Although the 10-year risk of developing lymphoma was only 4%, the slight increase of mortality compared to the general population was attributed to lymphoproliferative disease. Other mortality studies have confirmed this finding [5, 24]. Theader et al. found that the specific SMR for lymphoproliferative disorders was 7.89 (95% CI 2.89–17.18) [24]. Nevertheless in more recent studies, the risk of death from lymphoma among pSS patients was not found increased [25, 26].

Besides lymphomas, other causes of death related to the syndrome have been also reported in patients with pSS. Progressive renal involvement occurs in less than 5% of pSS patients and may cause significant renal impairment. In some cases, glomerulonephritis due to cryoglobulinemia may lead to end-stage renal failure that requires hemodialysis [27]. On the other hand, patients with interstitial nephritis and renal tubular acidosis usually present with alkaline urinary pH, a low urine specific gravity, and perhaps slight renal impairment that remains stable for long periods of time. In rare cases, renal tubular dysfunction presents with severe hypokalemia, a potentially lethal electrolyte disorder [28–30].

Vascular involvement in the form of small vessel vasculitis, due to cryoglobulinemia, is usually treatable. However, vasculitis affecting organs such as the peritoneum or the gallbladder is difficult to diagnose and sometimes leads to death [31]. Interstitial lung disease, a rare complication of pSS, occasionally leads to respiratory failure and death [2, 5, 23].

Secondary causes of death in pSS patients can pertain to immunosuppressive treatment. Cyclophosphamide and glucocorticoids are reserved for the minority of pSS patients who develop systemic vasculitis, glomerulonephritis, or interstitial lung disease. Predisposition to infections is the greatest concern with these patients [5, 23]. Death as the result of direct drug toxicity is much less common [23].

Cardiovascular disease is not a common cause of death among patients with pSS. In contrast to other systemic autoimmune diseases such as rheumatoid arthritis and systemic lupus erythematosus, pSS does not seem to induce a chronic inflammatory or hypercoagulable state and is not associated with an increased cardiovascular risk from atherosclerosis or thrombosis.

34.3   Clinical and Immunological Prognostic Factors: Classification of SS (Types I and II)

Lymphoma development and the systemic form of the disease are observed in less than 10% of pSS patients. However, pSS patients whose clinical courses evolve in this manner have increased morbidity, greater numbers of hospital admissions, and premature mortality. Do these patients express any clinical or serological characteristic that may predict this evolution?

In 1971, Anderson et al. showed that the decline of serum immunoglobulin levels and the disappearance of rheumatoid factors (RF) coincided with the time of any progression lymphoma [32]. In 1978, Kassan et al. demonstrated that patients with lymphadenopathy, splenomegaly, parotid gland enlargement and history of low-dose irradiation or chemotherapy had an increased risk of lymphoma development [11]. In addition, it was demonstrated that the expression of a monoclonal B-cell population in salivary glands and the presence of serum monoclonal immunoglobulins appeared before lymphoma became clinically apparent [11].

In 1986, Tzioufas et al. demonstrated that in patients with pSS, serum monoclonality was expressed by cryoprecipitable IgM-kappa RF [33]. Ten years later, the same investigators showed that patients with pSS and mixed monoclonal cryoglobulinemia were at increased risk for non-Hodgkin's lymphoma development compared to pSS patients without cryoglobulins [3]. In addition, some of these patients had evidence of immune complex-mediated disease such as purpura, glomerulonephritis, and low C4 complement levels. Recurrent parotid gland enlargement was also a consistent finding. In these patients, cryoglobulinemia heralded the onset of lymphoma by 1–16 months [3].

Lymphoma development was linked in our study to the presence of palpable purpura, low C4 levels, and mixed monoclonal cryoglobulinemia (MMC) [2]. In that investigation, low levels of C4 at diagnosis were the strongest predictor of mortality after adjustments for age (relative risk, 6.5; $P = .0041$) [2]. Unpublished data from the same study demonstrated that serological evidence of monoclonality

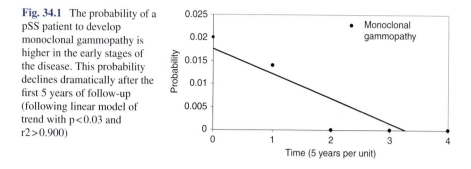

Fig. 34.1 The probability of a pSS patient to develop monoclonal gammopathy is higher in the early stages of the disease. This probability declines dramatically after the first 5 years of follow-up (following linear model of trend with $p < 0.03$ and $r2 > 0.900$)

can be present in the early stages of SS despite the fact that lymphoproliferative disorders have a late clinical expression (Fig. 34.1).

Because monoclonality in pSS is expressed mainly by circulating cryoglobulins, the evaluation for cryoglobulinemia at the first patient visit and periodically during follow-up is a valuable tool in determining disease prognosis. The evaluation of cryoglobulins and their analysis are neither difficult nor expensive to be performed. The blood should be immediately allowed to clot and subsequently centrifuged at 37°C. This is the most critical step of the procedure and unfortunately it is not done properly, even in the best clinical units. The serum obtained after centrifugation of the blood should be placed in a refrigerator at 4°C for 1–7 days. The cryoprecipitated proteins, if present, should be analyzed with high-resolution electrophoresis and immunofixation. The presence of cryoglobulins tends to correlate with a depression in serum C4 levels (out of proportion to depression in C3 levels). Thus, evaluations of complement components are also important in gauging the prognosis of patients with SS. Hypocomplementemia is often identified as the strongest predictor of mortality.

Ioannidis et al. confirmed that parotid gland enlargement, the presence of purpura, and low serum C4 complement levels at the first patient visit were independent risk factors for lymphoma development. Patients without any of these factors are at negligible risk for lymphoma. Mortality was strongly associated with low C4 complement levels [5]. Subsequent studies confirmed the prognostic value of hypocomplementemia in lymphoma development and death [18, 24, 26, 34]. Based on the above findings, a predictive classification of pSS was proposed: patients with parotid gland enlargement or palpable purpura and/or cryoglobulinemia or hypocomplementinemia are classified to be at high risk (type I autoimmune epithelitis with increased risk of lymphoma and early mortality), while those without such manifestations are classified as low-risk patients (type II autoimmune epithelitis with no risk of lymphoma development and early mortality). Only 20% of all pSS patients are classified as type I. Hence, early detection of these poor prognostic factors should lead the physicians to follow these patients carefully, with an eye toward early therapeutic intervention in the event of disease complications. Anecdotal data from our department suggest that administration of anti-CD 20 monoclonal antibodies in patients with high-risk markers can alter the clinical and serological negative prognostic factors. However, large prospective studies are needed to determine whether anti-CD20 treatment in the poor prognosis group of patients has a preventive effect for lymphoma development.

34.4   Conclusions

Careful clinical evaluation (parotid gland enlargement, palpable purpura) and routine blood testing (hypocomplementemia, cryoglobulinemia) at the first patient evaluation can identify a subgroup of patients at risk for higher morbidity and lymphoma development. Overall mortality of pSS patients do not differ significantly from age- and sex- matched unaffected individuals. However, pSS patients with lymphoma have higher morbidity and mortality.

References

1. Moutsopoulos HM. Sjogren's syndrome: autoimmune epithelitis. Clin Immunol Immunopathol. 1994;72:162–5.
2. Skopouli FN, Dafni U, Ioannidis JP, Moutsopoulos HM. Clinical evolution, and morbidity and mortality of primary Sjogren's syndrome. Semin Arthritis Rheum. 2000;29:296–304.
3. Tzioufas AG, Boumba DS, Skopouli FN, Moutsopoulos HM. Mixed monoclonal cryoglobulinemia and monoclonal rheumatoid factor cross-reactive idiotypes as predictive factors for the development of lymphoma in primary Sjogren's syndrome. Arthritis Rheum. 1996;39:767–72.
4. Voulgarelis M, Dafni UG, Isenberg DA, Moutsopoulos HM. Malignant lymphoma in primary Sjogren's syndrome: a multicenter, retrospective, clinical study by the European Concerted Action on Sjogren's syndrome. Arthritis Rheum. 1999;42:1765–72.
5. Ioannidis JP, Vassiliou VA, Moutsopoulos HM. Long-term risk of mortality and lymphoproliferative disease and predictive classification of primary Sjogren's syndrome. Arthritis Rheum. 2002;46:741–7.
6. Voulgarelis M, Giannouli S, Anagnostou D, Tzioufas AG. Combined therapy with rituximab plus cyclophosphamide/doxorubicin/vincristine/prednisone (CHOP) for Sjogren's syndrome-associated B-cell aggressive non-Hodgkin's lymphomas. Rheumatology (Oxford). 2004;43:1050–3.
7. Voulgarelis M, Giannouli S, Tzioufas AG, Moutsopoulos HM. Long term remission of Sjogren's syndrome associated aggressive B cell non-Hodgkin's lymphomas following combined B cell depletion therapy and CHOP (cyclophosphamide, doxorubicin, vincristine, prednisone). Ann Rheum Dis. 2006;65:1033–7.
8. Voulgarelis M, Moutsopoulos HM. Mucosa-associated lymphoid tissue lymphoma in Sjögren's syndrome: risks, management, and prognosis. Rheum Dis Clin North Am. 2008;34:921–33, viii.
9. Rothman S, Block M, Hauser FV. Sjogren's syndrome associated with lymphoblastoma and hypersplenism. AMA Arch Derm Syphilol. 1951;63:642–3.
10. Talal N, Bunim JJ. The development of malignant lymphoma in the course of Sjogren's syndrome. Am J Med. 1964;36:529–40.
11. Kassan SS, Thomas TL, Moutsopoulos HM, Hoover R, Kimberly RP, Budman DR, et al. Increased risk of lymphoma in sicca syndrome. Ann Intern Med. 1978;89:888–92.
12. Zintzaras E, Voulgarelis M, Moutsopoulos HM. The risk of lymphoma development in autoimmune diseases: a meta-analysis. Arch Intern Med. 2005;165:2337–44.
13. Kauppi M, Pukkala E, Isomaki H. Elevated incidence of hematologic malignancies in patients with Sjogren's syndrome compared with patients with rheumatoid arthritis (Finland). Cancer Causes Control. 1997;8:201–4.

14. Pariente D, Anaya JM, Combe B, Jorgensen C, Emberger JM, Rossi JF, et al. Non-Hodgkin's lymphoma associated with primary Sjogren's syndrome. Eur J Med. 1992;1:337–42.
15. Baimpa E, Dahabreh IJ, Voulgarelis M, Moutsopoulos HM. Hematologic manifestations and predictors of lymphoma development in primary Sjogren syndrome: clinical and pathophysiologic aspects. Medicine (Baltimore). 2009;88:284–93.
16. Mariette X. Lymphomas in patients with Sjogren's syndrome: review of the literature and physiopathologic hypothesis. Leuk Lymphoma. 1999;33:93–9.
17. Royer B, Cazals-Hatem D, Sibilia J, Agbalika F, Cayuela JM, Soussi T, et al. Lymphomas in patients with Sjogren's syndrome are marginal zone B-cell neoplasms, arise in diverse extranodal and nodal sites, and are not associated with viruses. Blood. 1997;90:766–75.
18. Theander E, Henriksson G, Ljungberg O, Mandl T, Manthorpe R, Jacobsson LT. Lymphoma and other malignancies in primary Sjogren's syndrome: a cohort study on cancer incidence and lymphoma predictors. Ann Rheum Dis. 2006;65:796–803.
19. Ambrosetti A, Zanotti R, Pattaro C, Lenzi L, Chilosi M, Caramaschi P, et al. Most cases of primary salivary mucosa-associated lymphoid tissue lymphoma are associated either with Sjogren syndrome or hepatitis C virus infection. Br J Haematol. 2004;126:43–9.
20. Coiffier B, Lepage E, Briere J, Herbrecht R, Tilly H, et al. CHOP chemotherapy plus rituximab compared with CHOP alone in elderly patients with diffuse large-B-cell lymphoma. N Engl J Med 2002;346:235–42.
21. Kruize AA, Hene RJ, van der Heide A, Bodeutsch C, de Wilde PC, van Bijsterveld OP, et al. Long-term followup of patients with Sjogren's syndrome. Arthritis Rheum. 1996;39:297–303.
22. Martens PB, Pillemer SR, Jacobsson LT, O'Fallon WM, Matteson EL. Survivorship in a population based cohort of patients with Sjogren's syndrome, 1976-1992. J Rheumatol. 1999;26:1296–300.
23. Pertovaara M, Pukkala E, Laippala P, Miettinen A, Pasternack A. A longitudinal cohort study of Finnish patients with primary Sjogren's syndrome: clinical, immunological, and epidemiological aspects. Ann Rheum Dis. 2001;60:467–72.
24. Theander E, Manthorpe R, Jacobsson LT. Mortality and causes of death in primary Sjogren's syndrome: a prospective cohort study. Arthritis Rheum. 2004;50:1262–9.
25. Alamanos Y, Tsifetaki N, Voulgari PV, Venetsanopoulou AI, Siozos C, Drosos AA. Epidemiology of primary Sjogren's syndrome in north-west Greece, 1982-2003. Rheumatology (Oxford). 2006;45:187–91.
26. Brito-Zeron P, Ramos-Casals M, Bove A, Sentis J, Font J. Predicting adverse outcomes in primary Sjogren's syndrome: identification of prognostic factors. Rheumatology (Oxford). 2007;46:1359–62.
27. Goules A, Masouridi S, Tzioufas AG, Ioannidis JP, Skopouli FN, Moutsopoulos HM. Clinically significant and biopsy-documented renal involvement in primary Sjogren syndrome. Medicine (Baltimore). 2000;79:241–9.
28. Aygen B, Dursun FE, Dogukan A, Ozercan IH, Celiker H. Hypokalemic quadriparesis associated with renal tubular acidosis in a patient with Sjogren's syndrome. Clin Nephrol. 2008;69:306–9.
29. Dowd JE, Lipsky PE. Sjogren's syndrome presenting as hypokalemic periodic paralysis. Arthritis Rheum. 1993;36:1735–8.
30. Zimhony O, Sthoeger Z, Ben David D, Bar Khayim Y, Geltner D. Sjogren's syndrome presenting as hypokalemic paralysis due to distal renal tubular acidosis. J Rheumatol. 1995;22: 2366–8.
31. Tsokos M, Lazarou SA, Moutsopoulos HM. Vasculitis in primary Sjogren's syndrome. Histologic classification and clinical presentation. Am J Clin Pathol. 1987;88:26–31.
32. Anderson LG, Talal N. The spectrum of benign to malignant lymphoproliferation in Sjogren's syndrome. Clin Exp Immunol. 1972;10:199–221.
33. Tzioufas AG, Costello R, Manoussakis MN, Papadopoulos NM, Moutsopoulos HM. Cryoglobulinemia in primary Sjogren's syndrome: a monoclonal process. Scand J Rheumatol Suppl. 1986;61:111–3.
34. Ramos-Casals M, Brito-Zeron P, Yague J, Akasbi M, Bautista R, Ruano M, et al. Hypocomplementaemia as an immunological marker of morbidity and mortality in patients with primary Sjogren's syndrome. Rheumatology (Oxford). 2005;44:89–94.

Chapter 35
Primary Sjögren Syndrome in Primary Health Care

Antoni Sisó-Almirall, Jaume Benavent, Xavier Bosch,
Albert Bové, and Manuel Ramos-Casals

Contents

A.S. Almirall (✉) • J. Benavent
Research Group on Primary Care, Institut d'Investigacions Biomèdiques August Pi i Sunyer
(IDIBAPS), CAP Les Corts, GesClínic, University of Barcelona, Barcelona, Spain

X. Bosch
Department of Internal Medicine, ICMiD, Hospital Clínic, Barcelona, Spain

A. Bové • M. Ramos-Casals
Sjögren Syndrome Research Group (AGAUR), Laboratory of Autoimmune Diseases Josep Font,
Institut d'Investigacions Biomèdiques August Pi i Sunyer (IDIBAPS), Department of
Autoimmune Diseases, Hospital Clínic, Barcelona, Spain

M. Ramos-Casals et al. (eds.), *Sjögren's Syndrome*,
DOI 10.1007/978-0-85729-947-5_35, © Springer-Verlag London Limited 2012

35.1 Introduction

Sjogren's syndrome (SjS) is a slowly progressive autoimmune disease that predominantly affects middle-aged women, with a female to male ratio on the order of 9:1. SS is characterized by lymphocytic infiltration of the exocrine glands, mainly the lacrimal and salivary glands, resulting in reduced secretory function and oral and ocular dryness. The syndrome can present alone as primary SjS (pSjS) or in the context of underlying connective tissue disease as secondary SjS (sSjS). Although the pathogenesis of the disease remains elusive, environmental, genetic and hormonal factors all appear to contribute [1]. The clinical manifestations of pSjS patients are mainly those of an autoimmune exocrinopathy, but almost half of patients develop extraglandular disease, which may be manifested by liver, lung, kidney, skin, or nervous system problems. In addition, the disease spectrum of SjS can also be complicated by the development of lymphoma. Patients with pSjS present a broad spectrum of laboratory (cytopenias, hypergammaglobulinemia, elevated erythrocyte sedimentation rate) and serological features, of which antinuclear antibodies (ANA) are the most frequently detected. Anti-Ro/SS-A antibodies are the most specific autoantibody. Cryoglobulins and hypocomplementemia are the main prognostic markers [2].

35.2 General Considerations

Primary care is the first level of access to the health care system for patients and the main entry point for public health services. Primary care, underpinned by the attributes espoused by Alma-Ata (accessibility, continuity, longitudinality, quality and efficiency), includes preventive and curative care, health promotion, and health education [3]. Problems such as oral or ocular dryness present to community-based primary care practitioners very differently than they do to specialists. The prevalence and incidence of illnesses are different from those that occur in hospital settings and serious disease presents less often in general practice because there is no prior selection. Choices about test ordering require a probability-based decision-making process that is informed by a knowledge of patients and the community [4]. The positive and negative predictive values of oral or ocular dryness and of immunological tests carry different weights in primary care as opposed to the hospital or specialist settings. Primary care practitioners often must reassure individuals with anxieties about illness after determining that the likelihood of illness is low [5].

The diagnosis of SjS is difficult at early stages of the disease, when patients present with nonspecific complaints and findings such as ocular or oral dryness, conjunctivitis, corneal damage, dental disease, oral ulcerations, angular cheilitis, fatigue or other general symptoms [6]. Thus, important decisions must be undertaken on the basis of limited information in a setting in which the predictive values of clinical examination

Table 35.1 Non-sicca manifestations suggestive of Sjögren syndrome

(a) *Clinical features*
Chronic fatigue
Fever of unknown origin
Leukocytoclastic vasculitis
Parotid or submandibular gland swelling
Raynaud phenomenon
Peripheral neuropathy
Pulmonary fibrosis
Mother of a baby born with congenital cardiac block

(b) *Analytical features*
Elevated erythrocyte sedimentation rate
Hypergammaglobulinemia
Leukopenia, thrombocytopenia
Serum and/or urine monoclonal band
Positive antinuclear antibodies or rheumatoid factor in an
   asymptomatic patient

findings, ocular or oral test results, and immunological assays are frequently unclear. Risk management under these circumstances is a key feature of primary care. Having excluded an immediately serious outcome, the appropriate decision may be to review at a later time and await further developments (if any) [7].

35.3 Symptoms That Aid Early Identification

A variety of clinical and laboratory features may indicate undiagnosed SjS (Table 35.1). Many SjS patients present with sicca symptoms, but the variability in SjS presentations partially explains the fact that delays in diagnosis of many years after the onset of symptoms are common in this condition [8]. The disease may occur at all ages but typically has its onset in the fourth to sixth decades of life. When sicca symptoms appear in a previously healthy person, the syndrome is classified as primary SjS. When sicca features are found in association with another systemic autoimmune disease, most commonly rheumatoid arthritis (RA), systemic sclerosis (SjSc) or systemic lupus erythematosus (SLE), it is classified as associated SjS.

35.3.1 *Keratoconjunctivitis Sicca*

Dry eyes are the most prominent ocular manifestation of SjS, has a long differential diagnosis (Table 35.2). Symptoms of dry eye, which include sensations of pruritus, grittiness, or soreness, may occur when the appearance of the eyes is normal. Other

Table 35.2 Causes of dry eyes

- Allergic conjunctivitis: burning eyes, mucoid secretion, and conjunctival erythema
- Blepharitis: eyelid margins are erythematous and thickened with crusts and debris within the lashes; usually worse in the morning and improves as the day goes on; does not respond to lubricant drops
- Blepharospasm: uncontrolled blinking due to an increased local neural reflex circuit
- Iritis/uveitis: in most cases associated with pronounced photosensitivity
- Herpetic keratitis: generally with ophthalmic distribution of shingles
- Environment: dryness caused by prolonged exposure to low humidity, dust, or sun
- Lifestyle: dryness caused by diminished blinking during long periods of reading, driving, or computer use
- Medications: diuretics and anticholinergic medications, including treatments for Parkinson disease, Alzheimer disease, multiple sclerosis, depression, allergic rhinitis, and incontinence
- Rosacea: ocular symptoms (e.g., itchy, burning, dry eyes with eyelid swelling and erythema) occur in 50% of patients with rosacea

Table 35.3 Causes of dry mouth

- Diabetes: dryness worsens with poor glycemic control
- Periodontal gingivitis
- Head and neck radiation: external beam radiation damages salivary glands
- Hepatitis C: sialadenitis results in dry mouth in 15% of persons with hepatitis C
- HIV infection: Oral candidosis, and HIV-related salivary gland disease exhibits clinical manifestations similar to Sjögren syndrome
- Medications: the same that cause dry eyes
- Obstructed nasal passages: dryness caused by mouth breathing
- Sarcoidosis: decreased salivary flow results from non-caseating granulomas in salivary glands

ocular complaints include photosensitivity, erythema, eye fatigue or decreased visual acuity, and the sensation of a film across the visual field [9]. Environmental irritants such as smoke, wind, air conditioning, and low humidity can exacerbate ocular symptoms. Diminished tear secretion may lead to chronic irritation and destruction of the corneal and bulbar conjunctival epithelium (keratoconjunctivitis sicca). In addition, because tears possess an inherent antimicrobial activity, SjS patients are more susceptible to ocular infections such as blepharitis, bacterial keratitis, and conjunctivitis. Severe ocular complications of SjS include ulceration, vascularization, and opacification of the cornea [10].

35.3.2 Xerostomia

Xerostomia, a key feature in the diagnosis of primary SjS, occurs in more than 95% of patients [11, 12]. However, a broad differential diagnosis must be considered in the evaluation of dry mouth symptoms (Table 35.3). Dry mouth lasting longer than 3 months is one of the sicca symptoms reported most often. In the early stages of SjS, the mouth may appear moist. As the disease progresses, the usual pooling of saliva in the floor of the mouth becomes absent and lines of contact between frothy saliva and the oral soft tissue are seen. The surface of the tongue becomes red and lobulated, with partial or complete depapillation. Early restoration of salivary function can relieve dry mouth symptoms and prevent or slow the progression of oral complications, including dental caries, oral candidiasis, and periodontal disease. Reduced salivary volume interferes with basic functions such as speaking or eating, and the lack of saliva components (lysozyme, lactoferrin or lactoperoxidase) that inhibit bacteria and fungi may accelerate infections by *Streptococcus mutans* and *Candida albicans*. Dental care utilization is significantly greater among patients with pSjS compared with control subjects [13].

35.3.3 Systemic Dryness

Reduction or absence of respiratory tract glandular secretions can lead to dryness of the nose, throat, and trachea, resulting in persistent hoarseness and chronic, nonproductive cough. Involvement of the exocrine glands of the skin also leads to cutaneous dryness. In female patients with SjS, dryness of the vagina and vulva may result in dyspareunia and pruritus [14].

35.3.4 Extraglandular Manifestations

Patients with primary SjS often present with general symptomatology that includes fever, generalized pain, fatigue, weakness, sleep disturbances, and anxiety and depression, which may have a much greater impact on the quality of life of patients than do sicca features. Fatigue occurs in 50% of patients with pSjS, and fibromyalgia has been reported in 22% [15]. Joint disease in pSjS is typically an intermittent, polyarticular problem that affects small joints in an asymmetric manner. Arthralgias exist in 48% of patients and arthritis in 15% [2]. Dry skin, another exocrine manifestation of SjS, affects 55% of patients.

Two major forms of vascular disease occur in SjS: Raynaud phenomenon, which affects 20–30% of patients; and vasculitis of small- or medium-sized vessels, which affects 10%. Up to 30% of patients with SjS have subclinical pulmonary disease. Cough, the main manifestation of respiratory tract disease, is usually a symptom of xerotrachea. Other systemic involvement includes esophageal dysmotility, tubulointerstitial nephritis, and a peripheral neuropathy with principally sensory features.

Table 35.4 Classification criteria of Sjögren syndrome

I. Ocular symptoms: a positive response to at least one of the following questions:
  (a) Have you had daily, persistent, troublesome dry eyes for more than 3 months?
  (b) Do you have a recurrent sensation of sand or gravel in the eyes?
  (c) Do you use tear substitutes more than 3 times a day?

II. Oral symptoms: a positive response to at least one of the following questions:
  (a) Have you had a daily feeling of dry mouth for more than 3 months?
  (b) Have you had recurrently or persistently swollen salivary glands as an adult?
  (c) Do you frequently drink liquids to aid in swallowing dry food?

III. Ocular signs, that is, objective evidence of ocular involvement defined as a positive result for at least one of the following two tests:
  (a) Schirmer's I test, performed without anesthesia (5 mm in 5 min)
  (b) Rose Bengal score or other ocular dye score (4 according to van Bijsterveld's scoring system)

IV. Histopathology: In minor salivary glands (obtained through normal-appearing mucosa) focal lymphocytic sialoadenitis, evaluated by an expert histopathologist, with a focus score 1, defined as a number of lymphocytic foci (which are adjacent to normal-appearing mucous acini and contain more than 50 lymphocytes) per 4 mm^2 of glandular tissue

V. Salivary gland involvement: objective evidence of salivary gland involvement defined by a positive result for at least one of the following diagnostic tests:
  (a) Unstimulated whole salivary flow (1.5 mL in 15 min)
  (b) Parotid sialography showing the presence of diffuse sialectasias (punctate, cavitary or destructive pattern), without evidence of obstruction in the major ducts
  (c) Salivary scintigraphy showing delayed uptake, reduced concentration and/or delayed excretion of tracer

VI. Autoantibodies: presence in the serum of the following autoantibodies:
  (a) Antinuclear antibodies
  (b) Rheumatoid factor
  (c) Antibodies to Ro/SjS-A or La/SjS-B antigens, or both

Patients are classified as having primary SjS when they fulfill four or more of the six classification criteria (1993 European Classification Criteria)
According to the recently proposed 2002 American-European Classification Criteria, either criteria IV (salivary gland biopsy) or criteria VIc (anti-Ro/La antibodies) are mandatory

35.4 Diagnosis

35.4.1 Classification Criteria

The diagnosis of SjS is based on the fulfillment of a specific set of classification criteria, with the 1993 European criteria being the most frequently used and the American-European criteria the most recently proposed (Table 35.4). The 1993 European criteria [16] permit the inclusion of patients with a sicca syndrome with negative salivary gland biopsy and no demonstrable autoantibodies. In contrast, the 2002 criteria [17] are more restrictive (positive salivary gland biopsy or positive anti-Ro/SSA or anti-La/SSB antibodies are obligatory criteria). As a result, subsets of patients unlikely to have these autoantibodies (e.g., males, the elderly, and patients with a sicca-limited disease) are not classifiable as primary SjS using these criteria.

Patients who fulfill the 2002 criteria who have either a specific histological diagnosis (lymphocytic infiltration) or possess highly specific autoantibodies within their sera might be regarded as having Sjögren's "disease." It is possible that etiopathogenic mechanisms other than lymphocytic-mediated epithelial damage are involved in patients with negative minor salivary gland biopsies and negative autoantibody assays. For those patients, the term Sjögren's "syndrome" seems more appropriate [18]. The heterogeneity in the clinical presentation of primary SjS observed in the largest series of patients [11, 12] shows that our understanding of how to diagnose this systemic autoimmune disease is still evolving.

35.4.2 Diagnostic Methods

35.4.2.1 Keratoconjunctivitis Sicca

The main ocular tests are Schirmer test and rose Bengal staining. The Schirmer test for the eye quantitatively measures tear formation via placement of filter paper in the lower conjunctival sac. The test result is positive when less than 5 mm of paper is wetted after 5 min. This test is simple to perform in primary care. Rose bengal scoring involves the placement of 25 mL of rose Bengal solution in the inferior fornix of each eye and having the patient blink twice. Rose bengal staining of the ocular surface is an important observation in the detection of SjS and important in differentiating the keratoconjunctivitis sicca of primary SjS from other causes of dry eye [10]. A staining score of 4 or more on the van Bijsterveld scoring system is considered to be significant [16]. Because of the irritative nature of Rose Bengal staining, lissamine green is now often used in its place.

35.4.2.2 Xerostomia

Several methods to assess oral involvement have been proposed [6, 8], such as measurement of the salivary flow rate, sialochemistry, sialography or scintigraphy. Measurement of the salivary flow, with or without stimulation, is the simplest method in evaluating xerostomia. The procedure is acceptable to patients and requires no special equipment [19]. Normal unstimulated salivary flow should be greater than 1.5 mL in 15 min. Salivary gland scintigraphy using intravenous injection of 5 mCi of sodium pertechnetate (^{99m}Tc) is a functional test performed primarily in specialty centers and tertiary care hospitals.

35.4.2.3 Salivary Gland Biopsy

Minor salivary gland biopsy remains a highly specific test for the diagnosis of SjS. However, it is an invasive technique that can lead to local side effects if not performed correctly. Thus, the procedure should be performed only by an individual experienced in this technique.

35.4.2.4 Immunological Tests

The main immunological markers found in primary SjS are ANA, anti-Ro/SS-A or anti-La/SS-B autoantibodies, rheumatoid factor, hypocomplementemia, and cryoglobulins. ANA are detected in more than 80% of cases of primary SjS. Titers ≥1/80 play a central role in differentiating SjS from non-autoimmune causes of sicca syndrome. Anti-Ro/SS-A and La/SS-B antibodies, detected in 40–60% of patients, are closely associated with most extraglandular features [2]. In nearly 50% of cases, patients with primary SjS also present with positive assays for rheumatoid factor [4]. Hypocomplementemia and cryoglobulinemia are two closely related immunological markers that have been linked with more severe SjS. Low complement levels are associated with chronic HCV infection, lymphoma development, and mortality [20–22].

35.4.2.5 Other Laboratory Findings

The most frequent routine laboratory features are asymptomatic cytopenias (33%), an elevated erythrocyte sedimentation rate >50 mm/h (22%), and hypergammaglobulinemia (22%) [23]. The most frequent cytopenias detected are normocytic anemia (20%), leukopenia (16%), and thrombocytopenia (13%). The erythrocyte sedimentation rate correlates closely with the percentage of circulating gammaglobulins (hypergammaglobulinemia). Serum C-reactive protein concentrations are usually normal even in the setting of substantial erythrocyte sedimentation rate elevations. Circulating monoclonal immunoglobulins are detected in nearly 20% of patients with primary SjS. Monoclonal IgG is detected most often [24].

35.5 Comorbidities and Occupational Disability

The adverse effects on general health, functional status, and quality of life of comorbidity in chronic illness have been amply demonstrated in SjS. Although multiple extraglandular conditions have been recognized in SjS, many of these diseases have been reported only sporadically. Patients with pSjS experience a high prevalence of fatigue, pain, and depression, which could be associated with coexisting comorbidities. Those with primary SjS have a twofold higher risk of diabetes mellitus and a 1.5-fold higher prevalence of hypertriglyceridemia compared with primary care patients [25]. Patients with pSjS are also more likely to have hyperlipidemia (odds ratio [OR] 1.42), cardiac arrhythmias (OR 1.32), headaches (OR 1.47), migraine headaches (OR 1.86), fibromyalgia (OR 1.71), asthma (OR 1.54), pulmonary circulation disorders (OR 1.42), hypothyroidism (OR 2.37), liver disease (OR 1.89), peptic ulcers (OR 1.88), depression (OR 2.57), and psychoses (OR 2.15) [26]. Thus, the impact of SjS on health-related quality of life is substantial.

Primary SjS patients are more likely than the non-SjS adults to not be working due to disability [27]. Furthermore, the prevalence of pain, fatigue, depressed mood, and cognitive symptoms are significantly higher in SjS patients compared to controls, and both depression and fatigue predict negative impacts on emotional well-being and general health. Health care utilization among pSjS patients is high and significantly more likely than general population to have been hospitalized in the last 5 years. They experience more frequent infections, including urinary tract, pneumonia, and vaginal infections and are more likely to use multiple medications and spending for dental care [26–28].

35.6 Treatment

The therapeutic approach in primary care is based on symptomatic replacement for patients with mild or moderate symptoms and is intended to limit the damage resulting from chronic involvement. The use of anticholinergic medications, alcohol, and smoking should be curtailed whenever possible.

35.6.1 Keratoconjunctivitis Sicca

Six studies (five randomized, controlled trials and one prospective study) have analyzed the use of topical eye drops [29–34]. Five of these studies have investigated sodium hyaluronate as the active principle, and one studied hydroxyl-propyl-methylcellulose [29–34]. A total of 221 patients were included. Three studies [29–31] also included non-SjS patients with keratoconjunctivitis sicca. All studies found significant improvements with respect to baseline subjective and objective measures. Topical ocular non-steroidal anti-inflammatory drugs (NSAIDs) or topical ocular glucocorticoids should be avoided.

35.6.2 Xerostomia

For patients with SjS who have residual salivary gland function, stimulation of saliva flow with a secretagogue is the treatment of choice. Two muscarinic agonists, pilocarpine and cevimeline, have been approved for the treatment of sicca symptoms in SjS. These agents stimulate the M1 and M3 receptors present on salivary glands, leading to increased secretory function. Pilocarpine, administered at a doses of 5 and 7.5 every 6 h while awake, improves dry mouth and dry eye symptoms; nasal, vaginal, and skin dryness; and salivary flow rates [35–37]. However, pilocarpine is associated with a significantly higher frequency of adverse events in comparison with placebo, including sweating, increased urinary frequency, flushing, increased salivation, and chills. Cevilimine achieves the best results with a dose of 30 mg/8 h, including significant improvements in visual analogue scale measurements of dry mouth

Table 35.5 Key recommendations for practice in primary care

Clinical recommendations

Sjogren's syndrome (SjS) is a chronic autoimmune disorder affecting middle aged women characterized by dry eyes and dry mouth

Major clinical manifestations of Sjögren's syndrome may be detected in primary health care

Extraglandular disease can affects lung, liver, kidney (interstitial nephritis), skin vasculitis, peripheral neuropathy, glomerulonephritis, and low C4 levels (immune complex disease)

Complete blood cell count, erythrocyte sedimentation rate, liver function tests, proteinogram, electrolytes and urinalysis, ANA and rheumatoid factor may be the first step for the immunological evaluation in primary health care

The presence of purpura, peripheral neuropathy, low complement levels, neutropenia and lymphopenia define a high-risk group for lymphoma development

Treatment recommendations

The muscarinic agonists pilocarpine and cevimeline can be used to relieve the symptoms of dry eyes and keratoconjunctivitis sicca

Muscarinic agonists improve subjective and objective signs and symptoms of xerostomia

Management of extraglandular manifestations is mainly empirical: steroids and immunosuppressive agents are of some benefit; anti-B-cell therapy shows promising results

and dry eyes, salivary flow rates, and ocular tests [38–41]. Cevilimine also significantly reduces candidiasis, dental plaque, and gingival bleeding. In randomized, controlled trials, however, this medication is associated with sweating and nausea, rigors, and diarrhea in significant subsets of patients [38, 40, 41].

35.6.3 *Management of Extraglandular Features*

Hydroxychloroquine may be used in patients with fatigue, arthralgias, and myalgias. NSAIDs can relieve the minor musculoskeletal symptoms of SjS as well as the painful parotid swelling that occurs in some patients. Glucocorticoids, immunosuppresive drugs, and biological agents are limited to patients with severe extraglandular manifestations.

35.7 When to Refer to a Specialist

The goal of the evaluation for SjS in primary care is to know key recommendations (Table 35.5). This workup involves the coordination of various specialists in order to assess the different mucosal surfaces and internal organs involved. Primary SjS is a benign disease in the majority of cases but the prognosis depends on associated diseases and three potential complications of alarm for the family doctor:

(a) Eye pain due to corneal ulcer.
(b) Vasculitis.
(c) A change in lymphocyte proliferation the potential for the development of non-Hodgkin's lymphoma. Patients with SjS have a relative risk of lymphoma

Table 35.6 Information from your family doctor

Information is available from the AAFP online at http://familydoctor.org. and http://www.aafp.
  org/afp/2009/0315/p472.html

What is Sjögren syndrome?

Sjögren syndrome is a disease that causes a dry mouth and dry eyes. It is an autoimmune
  disease, which happens when your body's immune system attacks your own cells. Most
  people with Sjögren syndrome have very mild symptoms, but it may affect other organs,
  such as the bowel, joints, kidneys, lungs, nervous system, and skin

Who gets it and why?

Sjögren syndrome is one of the most common autoimmune diseases. It usually affects women
  in their late 40s and early 50s. People with Sjögren syndrome may have other autoimmune
  diseases, such as rheumatoid arthritis or lupus. Doctors do not know what causes Sjögren
  syndrome

How do I know if I have Sjögren syndrome?

Most people with Sjögren syndrome have dry eyes and a dry mouth for months. Your eyes may
  feel gritty or itchy. Your mouth will be dry, and you may have trouble swallowing, eating
  dry foods, or even speaking. You should see your doctor if you think you might have
  Sjögren syndrome

How is it treated?

There are several artificial tear and saliva substitutes that may help your symptoms. Your doctor
  can prescribe other medicines that will help your body make more tears and saliva.
  Depending on your symptoms, you might also need medicines for your immune system

Is there a cure?

No, Sjögren syndrome is a lifelong disease

Where can I get more information?

Your doctor

The Sjögren's Syndrome Foundation

Web site: http://www.sjogrens.org/

elevated substantially over that of the general population, and clinically identifiable lymphomas occur in approximately 5% of patients. The predictors of lymphoma development in SjS are persistent enlargement of parotid glands, splenomegaly, lymphadenopathy, palpable purpura, leg ulcers, low levels of C4, mixed monoclonal cryoglobulinemia, and cross-reactive idiotypes of monoclonal rheumatoid factors [42]. When a lymphoproliferative process is suspected, the patient should be referred to a hematologist in order to confirm the diagnosis.

Three specialists, the ophthalmologist, gynecologist, and odontologist, should be routinely involved in the follow-up of the corresponding dryness (ocular, vaginal, and oral) and be available to consult on local complications. The main extraglandular involvements require cooperation with the corresponding specialist (nephrologist, neurologist, and hepatologist) [6].

Due to the heterogeneity and often non-specific nature of its clinical manifestations, SjS is probably the autoimmune disease most frequently undiagnosed. Primary care practitioners play an important role in identifying patients with possible SjS, by ordering specific tests to confirm the diagnosis, by making appropriate referrals, and by working with specialists to explain the disease and direct the patient to accurate information (Table 35.6) [43].

References

1. Mavragani CP, Moutsopoulos HM. The geoepidemiology of Sjögren's syndrome. Autoimmunity Reviews 2010;9:A305–A310.
2. Ramos-Casals M, Solans R, Rosas J, et al. Primary Sjögren syndrome in Spain. Clinical and immunologic expression in 1010 patients. Medicine. 2008;87:210–9.
3. Lawn JE, Rohde J, Rifkin S, et al. Alma-Ata 30 years on: revolutionary, relevant, and time to revitalise. Lancet. 2008;372(9642):917–27.
4. Sisó A, Aymamí A, Campoy A, et al. Síndrome de Sjögren primario: ?Una entidad infradiagnosticada por el Médico de Familia? 18° Congreso Nacional de la Sociedad Española de Medicina Familiar y Comunitaria. Zaragoza 1998. Aten Primaria. 1998;22 Suppl 1:390.
5. Allen J, Gay B, Crebolder H et al. The European definitions of general practice/family medicine. The key features of the discipline of general practice. EURACT 2005 (2005). Available in http://www.euract.org/index.php?folder_id=25 Accessed Date: [11-October-2010].
6. Kassan SjS, Moutsopoulos HM. Clinical manifestations and early diagnosis of Sjögren syndrome. Arch Intern Med. 2004;164:1275–84.
7. Sorlí JV, Doménech IE, Zurián FJ, et al. Sjögren syndrome. Aten Primaria. 2009;41(7): 417–9.
8. Fox RI. Sjogren's syndrome. Lancet. 2005;366:321–31.
9. Al-Hashimi I. The management of Sjogren's syndrome in dental practice. J Am Dent Assoc. 2001;132:1409–14.
10. Caffery B, Simpson TL, Wang S, et al. Rose bengal staining of the temporal conjunctiva differentiates Sjögren's syndrome from keratoconjunctivitis sicca. Invest Ophthalmol Vis Sci. 2010;51(5):2381–7.
11. García-Carrasco M, Ramos-Casals M, Rosas J, et al. Primary Sjögren syndrome: clinical and immunologic disease patterns in a cohort of 400 patients. Medicine. 2002;81:270–80.
12. Skopouli FN, Dafni U, Ioannidis JP, Moutsopoulos HM. Clinical evolution, and morbidity and mortality of primary Sjogren's syndrome. Semin Arthritis Rheum. 2000;29:296–304.
13. Fox PC, Bowman SJ, Segal B, et al. Oral involvement in primary Sjögren syndrome. J Am Dent Assoc. 2008;139:1592–601.
14. Belenguer R, Ramos-Casals M, Brito-Zeron P, et al. Influence of clinical and immunological parameters on the health-related quality of life of patients with primary Sjögren's syndrome. Clin Exp Rheumatol. 2005;23:351–6.
15. Ostuni P, Botsios C, Sfriso P, et al. Prevalence and clinical features of fibromyalgia in systemic lupus erythematosus, systemic sclerosis, and Sjögren's syndrome. Minerva Med. 2002;93:203–9.
16. Vitali C, Bombardieri S, Moutsopoulos HM, et al. Preliminary criteria for the classification of Sjogren's syndrome. Results of a prospective concerted action supported by the European community. Arthritis Rheum. 1993;36:340–7.
17. Vitali C, Bombardieri S, Jonsson R, et al. Classification criteria for Sjögren's syndrome: a revised version of the European criteria proposed by the American-European Consensus Group. Ann Rheum Dis. 2002;61:554–8.
18. Ramos-Casals M, Brito-Zerón P, Pérez-de-Lis M, et al. Sjögren syndrome or Sjögren disease? the histological and immunological bias caused by the 2002 criteria. Clin Rev Allergy Immunol. 2010;38(2–3):178–85.
19. Rosas J, Ramos-Casals M, Ena J, et al. Usefulness of basal and pilocarpine-stimulated salivary flow in primary Sjögren's syndrome. Correlation with clinical, immunological and histological features. Rheumatology. 2002;41:670–5.
20. Theander E, Manthorpe R, Jacobsson LT. Mortality and causes of death in primary Sjögren's syndrome: a prospective cohort study. Arthritis Rheum. 2004;50:1262–9.
21. Ioannidis JP, Vassiliou VA, Moutsopoulos HM. Long-term risk of mortality and lymphoproliferative disease and predictive classification of primary Sjogren's syndrome. Arthritis Rheum. 2002;46:741–7.

22. Ramos-Casals M, Brito-Zeron P, Yague J, Akasbi M, Bautista R, Ruano M, et al. Hypocomplementaemia as an immunological marker of morbidity and mortality in patients with primary Sjogren's syndrome. Rheumatology (Oxford). 2005;44:89–94.
23. Ramos-Casals M, Font J, Garcia-Carrasco M, et al. Primary Sjogren syndrome: hematologic patterns of disease expression. Medicine. 2002;81:281–92.
24. Brito-Zeron P, Ramos-Casals M, Nardi N, et al. Circulating monoclonal immunoglobulins in Sjogren syndrome: prevalence and clinical significance in 237 patients. Medicine. 2005;84: 90–7.
25. Pérez-de-Lis M, Akasbi M, Sisó A, et al. Cardiovascular risk factors in primary Sjögren's syndrome: a case-control study in 624 patients. Lupus. 2010;19(8):941–8.
26. Kang JH, Lin HC. Comorbidities in patients with primary Sjögren's Syndrome: a registry-based case-control study. J Rheumatol. 2010;37:1188–94.
27. Segal B, Bowman SJ, Fox PC, et al. Primary Sjögren's Syndrome: health experiences and predictors of health quality among patients in the United States. Health Qual Life Outcomes. 2009;7:46.
28. Meijer JM, Meiners PM, Huddleston Slater JJ, et al. Health-related quality of life, employment and disability in patients with Sjogren's syndrome. Rheumatology. 2009;48(9): 1077–82.
29. Aragona P, Di Stefano G, Ferreri F, Spinella R, Stilo A. Sodium hyaluronate eye drops of different osmolarity for the treatment of dry eye in Sjögren's syndrome patients. Br J Ophthalmol. 2002;86(8):879–84.
30. Aragona P, Papa V, Micali A, Santocono M, Milazzo G. Long term treatment with sodium hyaluronate-containing artificial tears reduces ocular surface damage in patients with dry eye. Br J Ophthalmol. 2002;86(2):181–4.
31. Brignole F, Pisella PJ, Dupas B, Baeyens V, Baudouin C. Efficacy and safety of 0.18% sodium hyaluronate in patients with moderate dry eye syndrome and superficial keratitis. Graefes Arch Clin Exp Ophthalmol. 2005;243(6):531–8.
32. Condon PI, McEwen CG, Wright M, Mackintosh G, Prescott RJ, McDonald C. Double blind, randomised, placebo controlled, crossover, multicentre study to determine the efficacy of a 0.1% (w/v) sodium hyaluronate solution (Fermavisc) in the treatment of dry eye syndrome. Br J Ophthalmol. 1999;83(10):1121–4.
33. McDonald CC, Kaye SB, Figueiredo FC, Macintosh G, Lockett C. A randomised, crossover, multicentre study to compare the performance of 0.1% (w/v) sodium hyaluronate with 1.4% (w/v) polyvinyl alcohol in the alleviation of symptoms associated with dry eye syndrome. Eye (Lond). 2002;16(5):601–7.
34. Toda I, Shinozaki N, Tsubota K. Hydroxypropyl methylcellulose for the treatment of severe dry eye associated with Sjögren's syndrome. Cornea. 1996;15(2):120–8.
35. Papas AS, Sherrer YS, Charney M, et al. Successful treatment of dry mouth and dry eye symptoms in Sjögren's syndrome patients with oral pilocarpine: a randomized, placebo-controlled, dose-adjustment study. J Clin Rheumatol. 2004;10(4):169–77.
36. Vivino FB, Al-Hashimi I, Khan Z, et al. Pilocarpine tablets for the treatment of dry mouth and dry eye symptoms in patients with Sjögren syndrome: a randomized, placebo-controlled, fixed-dose, multicenter trial. P92-01 Study Group. Arch Intern Med. 1999;159(2): 174–81.
37. Wu CH, Hsieh SC, Lee KL, Li KJ, Lu MC, Yu CL. Pilocarpine hydrochloride for the treatment of xerostomia in patients with Sjögren's syndrome in Taiwan – a double-blind, placebo-controlled trial. J Formos Med Assoc. 2006;105(10):796–803.
38. Fife RS, Chase WF, Dore RK, et al. Cevimeline for the treatment of xerostomia in patients with Sjögren syndrome: a randomized trial. Arch Intern Med. 2002;162(11):1293–300.
39. Leung KC, McMillan AS, Wong MC, Leung WK, Mok MY, Lau CS. The efficacy of cevimeline hydrochloride in the treatment of xerostomia in Sjögren's syndrome in southern Chinese patients: a randomised double-blind, placebo-controlled crossover study. Clin Rheumatol. 2008;27(4):429–36.

40. Ono M, Takamura E, Shinozaki K, et al. Therapeutic effect of cevimeline on dry eye in patients with Sjögren's syndrome: a randomized, double-blind clinical study. Am J Ophthalmol. 2004;138(1):6–17.
41. Petrone D, Condemi JJ, Fife R, Gluck O, Cohen S, Dalgin P. A double-blind, randomized, placebo-controlled study of cevimeline in Sjögren's syndrome patients with xerostomia and keratoconjunctivitis sicca. Arthritis Rheum. 2002;46(3):748–54.
42. Voulgarelis M, Moutsopoulos HM. Malignant lymphoma in primary Sjögren's syndrome. Isr Med Assoc J. 2001;3:761–6.
43. Kruszka P, O'Brian RJ. Diagnosis and management of Sjögren syndrome. Am Fam Physician. 2009;79(6):465–70.

Part IV
Therapeutic Aspects

Chapter 36
Therapy of Oral and Cutaneous Dryness Manifestations in Sjögren's Syndrome

Robert I. Fox and Carla M. Fox

Contents

36.1 Background

Sjögren's syndrome (SjS) is characterized by dry eyes and dry mouth. This chapter will concentrate on the treatment of dry mouth and other mucosal surfaces, particularly skin and vaginal tissues.

R.I. Fox (✉) • C.M. Fox
Chief, Rheumatology Clinic, Scripps Memorial Hospital and Research Foundation,
9850 Genesee Ave, La Jolla, CA 92037, USA
email: robertfoxmd@mac.com

M. Ramos-Casals et al. (eds.), *Sjögren's Syndrome*,
DOI 10.1007/978-0-85729-947-5_36, © Springer-Verlag London Limited 2012

The importance of oral dryness extends far beyond simple difficulty in eating certain foods or increased frequency/expense of dental problems. Women, who are disproportionately affected by this disorder compared with men, socialize around eating. The inability to eat the same foods with family and friends impact on their overall quality of life, as measured by the "Oral Health Quality/Assessment Scales" [1, 2].

Women increasingly engage in "working" breakfast, lunch, and dinner meetings, as well as the need to give oral presentations. All of these activities are profoundly impacted by dry mouth and difficulty with talking due to oral dryness. For example, it may be necessary to pause for a sip of water every few sentences in order to be able to spend hours on the phone or give public presentations. Tooth loss leads to expensive and often painful dental restorations, but also may alter the nutritional intake, as the patient is unable to chew or swallow particular foods.

A first step in the effective management of SjS is the recognition of medications with drying anticholinergic side effects. These include blood pressure medications, sleeping aids, anti-convulsant medications, and drugs designed to treat symptoms of neuropathy. Indeed, more than 40% of prescription medications are listed to have anticholinergic side effects [3].

The use of anticholinergic medications at bedtime may play a large role in sleep disturbances and the accompanying symptoms of fatigue often associated with SjS. The interruption of sleep due to dryness may result from a vicious cycle of drinking more water and resulting polyuria that leads to morning fatigue. Thus, patients might be encouraged to drink less water after dinner and use oral lubricants and lip balm to soothe dry lips, in order to avoid sleep disruption due to need for urination.

The treatment of dryness symptoms remains unsatisfactory, due in part to the poor correlation of patient symptoms of oral discomfort with objective measurement of salivary flow rates [4]. There is a general misconception that dryness results from the destruction of the salivary glands, when only about 50% of the acini/ductal cells are destroyed in patients with severe dryness. This points out the importance of the inflammatory process on the neural innervation and post-neural salivary gland function induced by local production of cytokines and metalloproteinases. Further, there are changes in the qualitative and quantitative content of salivary proteins and mucins which influence the "viscosity" of membranes and the mucosal integrity of the mouth [5].

In addition, symptoms of dry mouth (like dry eyes) are highly dependent on a "functional circuit" in which afferent nerves from the mucosal surface travel to the midbrain (salivatory nucleus) [6]. The midbrain also receives input from higher cortical regions [7] that mediate including taste, smell, hearing, and anxiety. Careful studies of the fifth cranial nerve's sensory afferents localize the problem to the level of the gasserian ganglia rather than the trigeminal ganglia [8].

The discrepancy between signs and symptoms of dry mouth is extremely important clinically. It is most apparent in those patients with "burning mouth" syndrome, where severe symptoms are not accompanied by objective evidence of oral dryness on exam or a dramatic decrease in the flow salivary flow rate by scanning technique [9–13]. This emphasizes the role of the central nervous system (central sensitization) or localized neuropathy in the generation of symptoms and how the patient perceives the severity of "dryness."

Patients with clinical depression, anxiety, neuropathy, Alzheimer's disease (even in the presence of drooling), and multiple sclerosis frequently have complaints of dryness [14, 15]. This indicates the importance of cortical influence and cholinergic white matter (cholinergic) outflow tracts.

The first line of treatment for dry mouth includes topical agents to lubricate and facilitate swallowing and talking, as well as lip balms to moisturize and soothe the lips. In addition, over the past 20 years, a variety of mechanical and electrical devices placed in the mouth have been shown to stimulate basal saliva flow [16, 17]. For the past 20 years, a variety of electrical devices (such as the Salitron) have been approved by FDA but have not proven cost-effective [18]. However, these devices do establish the role of mechanical stimulation in stimulation of saliva. As such, patients need to recognize the importance of mechanical stimulation in saliva stimulation and the importance of brushing their tongue and buccal mucosa when brushing their teeth, as well as frequent use of sugar-free lozenges.

In addition, other sicca symptoms include dryness of the skin (xerosis), nasal dryness, and vaginal dryness [19]. The need to keep the nasal passages clear and moist will prevent mouth breathing, particularly at night, when the basal secretory rate is diminished. The role of smell is closely linked to gustatory stimulation [20].

36.2   General Approach to Dry Mouth

36.2.1   Oral Hygiene and Self-Care by the Patient

Approaches to clinical management of oral sicca symptoms are generally the same for primary or secondary SjS. The quality of information available from resources on the Internet or from patient support groups varies widely.

Current recommendations by the American Dental Association [21–23] include:

- Use of dental floss after EACH meal, AND fluoride – either as toothpaste or a mouth rinse daily.

  - Carrying portable toothbrush and fluoride toothpaste is a very worthwhile practice for patients with SjS.

- Avoidance of sucrose, carbonated beverages, juices, and water with "sweetener" additives.
- Avoidance of oral irritants (e.g., coffee, alcohol, and nicotine).
- Maintenance of good hydration by taking regular sips of water and drinking sugar-free liquids (see "Fluids" below).
- Use of toothpastes specifically designed for dry mouth, which lack detergents (such as sodium laurel sulfate, which is the foaming agent in most toothpastes). These substances, present in many types of toothpaste, can irritate dry mouths.

Some fluoride-containing toothpastes may lead to brown discoloration of the teeth. Many of these "dry mouth" toothpastes are widely advertised, but have not been carefully studied in terms of their outcome for dental caries or tooth loss.

- One commercially available toothpaste (Biotene®) was found to give improved symptomatic relief in SjS patients, although no change in the microbacterial composition of the biofilm was noted [24, 25].

We strongly encourage our patients to use toothbrushes with features that improve effectiveness, such as interdental brushes (for cleaning between teeth) and electric toothbrushes. Table 3 includes suggestions for dental hygiene and suggestions that are helpful to patients with SjS.

A number of basic measures are used to prevent as well as treat dry mouth in those with SjS. The published evidence supporting these measures consists largely of clinical experience and small case series [25]. Several older double-blind studies in SjS patients demonstrated that the addition of mucins or lactoperoxidase to carboxymethylcellulose (CMC) was superior to CMC alone [24, 26]. A small single-blinded study using a commercially available product (Oral Balance®) also showed symptomatic benefit [24].

The following measures for prevention of dryness, stimulation of secretions, dental prophylaxis, and attention to complications should be used in all patients with dry mouth due to SjS, regardless of symptom severity:

1. Avoidance of drying medications that may worsen oral dryness, especially those with anticholinergic side effects. These include over-the-counter antihistamines, cold and sleep remedies.
2. Avoidance of smoking and alcohol.
3. Maintenance of open nasal passages to avoid mouth breathing (see 'Nasal Dryness' below).
4. Use of room cold humidifiers, particularly at night, in areas that are dry or windy.
5. Stimulation of salivary secretions, using sugar-free salivary stimulants (e.g., chewing gums and lozenges).
6. Careful chewing of food before swallowing (see 'Topical Stimulation of Salivary Flow' below).
7. Meticulous oral hygiene and regular dental care, and avoidance of pre-processed "soft" foods that may be high in sugar content (see 'Basic Dental Care' below and 'Prevention of Dental Caries' below).
8. Recognition of oral candidiasis that may mimic or exacerbate dry mouth symptoms (see 'Oral Candidiasis' below).

Various solutions – ranging from water to forms of artificial saliva – can be used to replace oral secretions. We suggest frequent sips of water, because of convenience, low cost, and efficacy. The water does not have to be swallowed, but can be rinsed around the mouth and expectorated. Although water provides temporary moisture, it does not provide the lubricating properties that are characteristic of the mucin/water mixtures that constitute normal saliva.

Patients should be aware that excessive water sipping might actually reduce the mucus film in the mouth and increase symptoms. If water consumption is excessive, especially in the evening, nocturia can occur, resulting in sleep disturbance that may worsen fatigue, cognitive difficulties, and pain that some patients experience.

We advise patients to avoid acidic beverages, which may adversely affect dental enamel. Examples of common beverages and their relative acidity include:

- Carbonated waters have high acidity
- "Energy drinks" are usually acidic
- Flavored waters are often acidic
- Cola drinks pH 2.6 (Black Cherry soda: highest acidity and sugar)
- Tea, herbal pH 3.2
- Coffee pH 5.0
- Tea, black pH 5.7–7.0
- Water from tap pH 7.0 (neutral)

The maintenance of pH in the oral cavity is highly important [27]. When the pH in the oral cavity is stable, there is a decrease in the amount of demineralization that takes place. Further, the pH of the oral cavity affects the microflora [28], the biofilm, and the ability of bacteria to adhere to the dental enamel [29]. The pH and buffer capacity in the parotid saliva of individuals with SjS are much lower when compared with those in normal control individuals. The buffer systems responsible for the human saliva-buffering capacity include bicarbonate, phosphate, and protein. Even a minor drop in pH can result in dental caries or damage to the teeth by erosion [30, 31].

36.3   Additional Dental Needs of the SjS Patient

36.3.1   *Background*

At most medical centers and for rheumatologists in practice, communication with dentists and specialists in Oral Medicine is quite limited. However, rheumatologists need to be familiar with the terminology used by Oral Medicine in order to read the relevant literature published on SjS, and to advise patients regarding particular dental procedures that may influence their medical status. Radiation therapists have developed a close working relationship with Oral Medicine to prevent and treat oral complications, but similar interactions for rheumatologists are uncommon. Therefore, we will review basic terminology and approaches as a background to specific discussions listed below.

Table 36.1 Saliva content and stimulation in normal individuals

Saliva functions
- Saliva also breaks down food caught in the teeth, protecting them from bacteria that cause decay. Furthermore, saliva lubricates and protects the teeth, the tongue, and the tender tissues inside the mouth.
- Saliva also plays an important role in tasting food, by trapping thiols produced from odorless food compounds by anaerobic bacteria living in the mouth. Saliva secretes gustin hormone which is thought to play a role in the development of taste buds.

Stimulation of saliva
- The production of saliva is stimulated both by the sympathetic and parasympathetic nervous systems.
- The saliva stimulated by sympathetic innervation is thicker, and saliva stimulated parasympathetically is more watery.
- Parasympathetic stimulation leads to acetylcholine (ACh) release onto the salivary acinar cells. ACh binds to muscarinic receptors and causes an increased intracellular calcium ion concentration (through the IP3/DAG second messenger system). Increased calcium causes vesicles within the cells to fuse with the apical cell membrane, leading to secretion formation.
- ACh also causes the salivary gland to release kallikrein, an enzyme that converts kininogen to lysyl-bradykinin. Lysyl-bradykinin acts upon blood vessels and capillaries of the salivary gland to generate vasodilation and increased capillary permeability respectively. The resulting increased blood flow to the acinar allows production of more saliva.
- Lastly, both parasympathetic and sympathetic nervous stimulations can lead to myoepithelium contraction which causes the expulsion of secretions from the secretory acinus into the ducts and eventually to the oral cavity.

Contents of saliva
Electrolytes:
- 2–21 mmol/L sodium (lower than blood plasma)
- 10–36 mmol/L potassium (higher than plasma)
- 1.2–2.8 mmol/L calcium (similar to plasma)
- 0.08–0.5 mmol/L magnesium
- 5–40 mmol/L chloride (lower than plasma)
- 25 mmol/L bicarbonate (higher than plasma)
- 1.4–39 mmol/L phosphate
- Iodine (mmol/L usually higher than plasma, but dependent variable according to dietary iodine intake)
- Mucus in saliva mainly consists of mucopolysaccharides and glycoproteins
- Antibacterial compounds (thiocyanate, hydrogen peroxide, and secretory immunoglobulin A)
- Epidermal growth factor or EGF
- Various enzymes. There are three major enzymes found in saliva
- α-amylase (EC3.2.1.1). Amylase starts the digestion of starch and lipase fat before the food is even swallowed
- It has a pH optima of 7.4
- Antimicrobial enzymes that kill bacteria
  - Lysozyme
  - Salivary lactoperoxidase
  - Lactoferrin
  - Immunoglobulin A
  - Proline-rich proteins (function in enamel formation, Ca_2+-binding, microbe killing, and lubrication)

Table 36.1 (continued)

- Minor enzymes include:
  - Salivary acid phosphatases A + B, *N*-acetylmuramoyl-*L*-alanine amidase
  - NAD(P)H dehydrogenase (quinone), superoxide dismutase, glutathione transferase, class 3 aldehyde dehydrogenase, glucose-6-phosphate isomerase, and tissue kallikrein (function unknown)
- Cells: Possibly as much as 8 million human and 500 million bacterial cells per mL. The presence of bacterial products (small organic acids, amines, and thiols) causes saliva to sometimes exhibit foul odor
- Opiorphin, a newly researched pain-killing substance found in human saliva

Tables 36.1 and 36.2 present a series of items that the rheumatologist may need to understand in order to communicate effectively with the dentist. These items include:

- The contents of saliva
- Biofilm
- Dental plaque and accelerated caries
- Structure of dental enamel and its dissolution based on low pH
- Role of fluoride in maintaining oral health
- Dental restorations, including veneers
- Whitening or bleaching agents for cosmetic dentistry

Patients may require:

- Additional visits for their oral hygiene, ranging from every 3 to 6 months
- Topical fluoride treatment after their dental cleaning
- Use of a stronger fluoride applied by dental trays used at night
- Use of calcifying agents such as MI paste
- Topical antibiotics to retard gum recession

In individuals with SjS, there is an increase in dental caries (usually root and incisal caries), appearing as destruction around the necks of the teeth and even on the labial and incisal surfaces [32].

Dental plaque, consisting of more than 500 species of bacteria in a mature state, is a complex biofilm of microbes that adheres to the surfaces of teeth and provides a reservoir for oral microbial pathogens [33]. Streptococci account for approximately 20% of the total number of oral bacteria, and they are predominantly the first colonizers of freshly cleaned enamel surface. These bacteria are also the primary causative agents of biofilm formation and dental caries.

The bacteria normally are dislodged and expelled from the tooth surfaces and oral cavity by the mechanical forces of salivary flow and tongue movement [34]. The alteration of bacterial flora occurs with dryness due to causes other than SjS, including anxiety or medications [14].

Table 36.2 Terminology of oral medicine

Oral biofilm

A biofilm is an aggregate of microorganisms in which cells adhere to each other and/or to oral surfaces. They play a key role in dental decay and oral candidiasis.

Biofilms have been found to be involved in a wide variety of microbial infections in the body: by one estimate, 80% of all infections including dental decay and oral candidiasis. Biofilms also are important in other mucus membranes where they influence local vaginal immunity, ocular infections, sinus and upper respiratory tract infections found more frequently in SS patients. In addition to the lubricating and antibacterial properties, these secretions may influence extracellular polymeric substance (EPS) involved in cellular recognition of specific or nonspecific attachment sites on a surface such as dental enamel, or mucosal membranes.

Dental plaque

Dental plaque is the material that adheres to the teeth and consists of bacterial cells (mainly *Streptococcus mutans* and *Streptococcus sanguinis*), salivary polymers, and bacterial extracellular products. Plaque is a biofilm on the surfaces of the teeth. This accumulation of microorganisms subjects the teeth and gingival tissues to high concentrations of bacterial metabolites which results in dental disease.

Tooth enamel

The high mineral content of enamel, which makes this tissue the hardest in the human body, also makes it susceptible to a demineralization process which often occurs as dental caries. In SS patients, the lack of saliva leads to poor mechanical removal of bacteria, alteration of the biofilm, and a lowering of the oral pH due to the decreased volume of alkaline secretion and proteins with buffering capacity.

Sugars from candies, soft drinks, and even fruit juices play a significant role in tooth decay, and consequently in enamel destruction. The mouth contains a great number and variety of bacteria, and when sucrose, the most common of sugars, coats the surface of the mouth, some intraoral bacteria interact with it and form lactic acid, which decreases the pH in the mouth. Then, the hydroxylapatite crystals of enamel demineralize, allowing for greater bacterial invasion deeper into the tooth. The most important bacterium involved with tooth decay is *Streptococcus mutans*, but the number and type of bacteria varies with the progress of tooth destruction.

Oral hygiene and fluoride

Considering the vulnerability of enamel to demineralization and the daily menace of sugar ingestion, prevention of tooth decay is the best way to maintain the health of teeth in SS patients. Naturally occurring calcium fluoride is not the same as sodium fluoride, a byproduct of the fertilizer industry and the fluoride that is added to drinking water. The recommended dosage of fluoride in drinking water depends on air temperature; in the USA, it ranges from 0.7 to 1.2 mg/L. Fluoride catalyzes the diffusion of calcium and phosphate into the tooth surface, which in turn remineralizes the crystalline structures in a dental cavity. The remineralized tooth surfaces contain fluoridated hydroxylapatite and fluorapatite, which resist acid attack much better than the original tooth did. Thus, despite fluoridation's detractors, most dental health care professionals and organizations agree that the inclusion of fluoride in public water has been one of the most effective methods of decreasing the prevalence of tooth decay.

Dental veneer in cosmetic dentistry

Veneers were invented initially for Hollywood actors to alter the appearance of actors' teeth. At the time, they fell off in a very short time as they were held on by denture adhesive. Today, with improved cements and bonding agents, they typically last 10–30 years.

Table 36.2 (continued)

Veneers are an important tool for the cosmetic dentist. A dentist may use one veneer to restore a single tooth that may have been fractured or discolored, or multiple teeth to create a "Hollywood" type of makeover. Many people have small teeth resulting in spaces that may not be easily closed by orthodontics.

A problem with cosmetic dentistry in SS patients is that areas of underlying decay are no longer visible for detection or accessible to dental care and thus may progress more rapidly to tooth loss.

Tooth whitening or dental bleaching

Dental bleaching, also known as *tooth whitening*, is a common procedure in general dentistry but most especially in the field of cosmetic dentistry. A child's deciduous teeth are generally whiter than the adult teeth that follow. As a person ages, the adult teeth often become darker due to changes in the mineral structure of the tooth, as the enamel becomes less porous. Teeth can also become stained by bacterial pigments, foodstuffs, and tobacco.

There are many methods to whiten teeth: bleaching strips, bleaching pen, bleaching gel, laser bleaching, and natural bleaching. Oxidizing agents such as hydrogen peroxide or carbamide peroxide are used to lighten the shade of the tooth. The oxidizing agent penetrates the porosities in the rod-like crystal structure of enamel and oxidizes interprismatic stain deposits; over a period of time, the dentin layer, lying underneath the enamel, is also bleached. Power or light-accelerated bleaching, sometimes colloquially referred to as laser bleaching, uses light energy to accelerate the process of bleaching in a dental office. Different types of energy can be used in this procedure, with the most common being halogen, LED, or plasma arc.

Although tooth bleaching may be safely done in SS patients in a dentist's office, it should not be done by non-dental individuals who increasingly offer their services at shopping center mall kiosks, spas, salons, or other similar places. In these sites, the "amateurs" greatly accelerate the laser bleaching to save time and this may result in damage to the dental surface and gingival damage.

Even in the dentist's office for the SS patient, it may be necessary to use lesser quantities of lightening agents or to perform on alternate days (rather than on a single day). Even when these precautions are taken, side effects of dental bleaching may include chemical burns from gel bleaching (if a high-concentration oxidizing agent contacts unprotected tissues, which may bleach or discolor mucous membranes) and sensitive teeth. It is worth advising patients who ask that nearly half the initial change in color provided by an intensive in-office treatment (i.e., 1-h treatment in a dentist's chair) may be lost in 7 days. Rebound tooth sensitivity is experienced due to a dehydration of the tooth.

Certain tooth whitening "tooth pastes" have an overall low pH, which can put enamel at risk for decay or destruction by demineralization. Consequently, care should be taken and risk evaluated when choosing a product which is very acidic. Also, tooth whiteners in tooth-pastes work through a mechanical action. They have mild abrasives which aid in the removal of stain but also may weaken dental enamel.

SjS, as well as other conditions including xerostomia associated with aging, also increases a person's likelihood of contracting opportunistic infections such as oral candidiasis and the proliferation of cariogenic microorganisms [35].

A study demonstrated that persons with primary SjS were reported to have higher numbers of cariogenic and acidophilic microorganisms in comparison with those found in control individuals [36].

Another comprehensive study, carried out with interviews and clinical oral examinations of 53 persons with primary SjS and 53 age-matched control individuals, found that those with primary SjS had more teeth extracted, more problems with their teeth in their lifetime, and higher dental expenses, compared with the control group.

In a separate study [37], the number of decayed, missing, or filled teeth was higher in both the younger and older groups of persons with primary SjS, compared with the normal control individuals. The young persons had, on average, seven teeth missing, compared with two missing in the control individuals. Those with primary SjS had more frequent dental visits compared with control individuals.

Even with excellent oral hygiene, individuals with SjS have elevated levels of dental caries, along with the loss of many teeth early in the disease. Pedersen et al. [36] reported that persons, who brushed their teeth with toothpaste containing fluoride and visited their dentist more frequently, still had higher numbers of missing, filled, and decayed teeth, along with a higher gingival index.

Fluoride is an extremely important element in the prevention of dental caries [32, 38–42]. However, certain regions do not maintain fluoridation in the water supply; patients living in these areas are at particular risk. In addition, the increasing use of non-fluoridated bottled water in place of fluoridated tap water is having a profound effect in decreasing fluoride exposure for many patients.

Topical fluoride promotes remineralization of teeth by the development of a crystalline protective veneer at the site of demineralization and inhibition of bacterial metabolism and acid production. Fluoride may be applied in various forms, depending on the severity of disease, including mouth rinses, fluoride gels applied at home in custom-fitted trays, and by dental office-based application of fluoride varnish [32, 38–42].

Chemoprophylaxis – Several approaches may be taken in an effort to reduce oral bacterial flora, including the use of chlorhexidine (CHX), a topical antimicrobial agent, and products containing baking soda, bicarbonate, or xylitol (see below) [32, 43–45]. In addition, CHX has an antifungal affect that may also benefit patients with SjS. CHX may also be used to soak dentures overnight. Dentures may be a source of bacterial infection as well as recurrent candida infection, and patients should not wear dentures overnight.

Polyol sweeteners, such as xylitol and sorbitol that are not fermentable by acid-producing bacteria, are of low cariogenic or noncariogenic potential; they may prevent or limit demineralization and promote the remineralization process. Xylitol may be a useful adjunct to other anti-caries treatments, but should not be considered in patients with SjS as a substitute for fluoride or other well-established interventions [46, 47].

Patients with SjS may have more difficulty wearing dentures because of the decreased moisture in the mouth. No adequately controlled clinical trials have addressed this question. In general, dentures cannot replicate the efficiency and comfort of natural teeth.

There are scattered case reports regarding the ability of patients with SjS to handle dental implants, although the often-poor status of oral tissues and bone loss in SjS patients may cause difficulty. The majority of reports for SjS patients appear favorable, but do not provide long-term follow-up [48, 49]. Decisions regarding use of implants in a given patient with SjS should be made on an individual basis, and the limited evidence should be acknowledged.

The safety of home products for whitening or brightening of teeth in patients with dry mouth and salivary gland dysfunction has not been studied. However, the use of such products should be avoided, since there may be increased risk from the acidity of some over-the-counter products designed for use in patients with normal salivary flow and content.

If professionally applied whitening processes are considered, the use of a rematerializing solution containing calcium phosphate and a fluoride treatment may be beneficial in conjunction with a bleaching treatment. Such procedures should only be performed after consultation by the patient with their dry mouth dentist.

36.4 Particular Oral Needs of the SjS Patient to Be Assessed by the Rheumatologist

The particular needs for evaluation and treatment in SjS patients by the rheumatologist are summarized in Table 36.3. These include:

- Recognition of oral candidiasis, particularly under dentures
- Need for secretagogue therapy
- Recognition of "burning mouth syndrome" out of proportion to objective dryness
- Recognition of medications with anticholinergic medications (often from other physicians)

The response to therapy may be evaluated by ongoing assessment for common clinical signs of dry mouth. These include:

- Difficulty with swallowing or speech due to dryness
- Absence of a pool of saliva on the floor of the mouth
- "Lipstick sign" (spreading of the patient's lipstick onto teeth)
- "Sticking" of a gloved finger to the mucosa
- Frequent occurrence of erythematous candida
- Atrophic glossitis (or lack of papilla) on the tongue
- Dental caries at the gingival margin, especially of the mandibular incisors
- Dry, cracked lips

36.5 Use of Secretagogues

In patients who do not respond adequately to the basic measures described above, and those who continue to have signs or symptoms of dry mouth despite the measures noted above, we suggest additional measures, including the use of muscarinic agonists such as sialogogues.

Table 36.3 Specific precautions for the oral hygiene of the Sjögren's patient

(a) Recognition that a dry mouth is not necessarily a painful mouth. There is a poor correlation between painful mouth and saliva flow. The development of a painful mouth should initiate a search for other causes such as oral yeast infection or a local neuropathy (called burning mouth syndrome).

(b) Dry mouth patients are more difficult to maintain without additional home care protocols. Dental flossing after meals and mechanical stimulation, such as using a soft toothbrush to stimulate the tongue and buccal mucosa at frequent intervals, is useful.

(c) The use of a power toothbrush at home significantly improves brushing efficiency, and requires half the pressure of hand brushing to reduce trauma and overall wear and tear. There are a variety of shapes and sizes of interdental brushes that function as floss alternatives. Another option is a WaterPik, now called WaterFlosser.

(d) Tooth sensitivity may be a problem, and a mild desensitizing toothpaste like Biotene for Sensitive teeth or Pronamel utilizes a different detergent than in most other toothpastes.

Toothpastes should be recommended to enhance the patient's plaque management program. The new Biotene BPF formula contains two extra enzymes that break up attached plaque and reduce buildup and inflammation.

Casein derivatives and lactoperoxidase have been shown to be beneficial in radiation xerostomia.

(e) Frequent breaks during the day for use of sugar-free (as opposed to low sugar) mints or lozenges mechanically stimulate saliva. Also, frequent dental hygiene after meals (or between meals) to remove food debris. A variety of lubricating mouth rinses and sprays may be used to facilitate eating and dental hygiene.

(f) Super dry patients will have a more difficult time tolerating any products with a strong mint flavor. Some patients cannot even tolerate the bland flavor of Oral Balance (GSK); so another product like Align Pharma's Numoisyn Liquid or even the mucositis treatment, Xclair, may be necessary.

Xclair is a cream, indicated for the management of radiation-induced dermatitis and stomatitis, including relief and management of the most common signs and symptoms such as pruritus, erythema, burning, and pain. Xclair is presented in an airless tube containing 50-mL cream. Xclair acts by adhering to the injured tissue to moisturize and reduce the sensitivity of inflamed tissue. It is a hydrolipidic wound dressing, and contains the hydrating, barrier-forming, and moisturizing ingredient sodium hyaluronate, which may favor tissue hydration and therefore benefit the healing process. In this manner, it serves to mitigate the mucosal stress reaction to severe dryness and promote healing of mucosal ulceration.

(g) For dental hygiene procedures, the use of a low-power ultrasonic scaler to debride or deep scale can significantly reduce the risks of tissue trauma. Soft polishing cups that Oscillate, rather than spin, create less heat and do not scuff up tender gum tissues.

(h) Bonding, cements, and crown margins are subject to acid attack, which is more prevalent when there is not adequate salivary output to rinse away food particles or dilute acids.

(i) There is no contraindication to tooth whitening for the average Sjögren's patient. Products should be approved by the American Dental Association to confirm that their testing was done in a scientific manner, and should be buffered pH as much as possible. Directions must be followed exactly since each product may have different exposure times or intervals to obtain optimal results with the less side effects.

(j) Implants, while expensive, do provide an alternative when tooth loss has been unavoidable. According to Yale's Dr. Frazio at a recent California Dental Association meeting, the only contraindications would be smoking, or the lack of commitment on the part of the patient to do what it takes to maintain the health of the implants. The medical workup should focus on any condition or medications that would compromise the healing process.

Table 36.3 (continued)

Implants in SS patients remain at the "state of an art" stage since there is no clear standard for the timing of different stages in the implant process (i.e., when the posts are uncovered and the implant inserted), and thus experience with SS patients should be carefully researched by the patient prior to this expensive procedure.

(k) SS patients may be doing everything right but continue to achieve bad results in terms of progressive dental decay and enamel loss.

Several products that have been used in radiation xerostomia and have been used in SS patients in our clinic

(a) MI paste and MI paste plus Recalcitrant.

(b) Xclair for oral mucositis.

MI Paste contains the active ingredient RECALDENT™ (CPP-ACP), a special milk-derived phosphopeptide that binds calcium and phosphate to tooth surfaces, plaque, and surrounding soft tissue. *MI Paste* is a water-based, sugar-free cream that is applied directly to the tooth surface or oral cavity. *Also improves* fluoride uptake as well as soothing sensitive surfaces – making patient compliance easier.

MI Paste Plus is similar to *MI Paste*, but is enhanced with a form of fluoride (900 ppm) to further promote remineralization and protect teeth from caries development. Since the fluoride acts in conjunction with RECALDENT™ (CPP-ACP), it is reported more effective than fluoride alone. Patients are instructed to apply a pea-sized amount to their teeth every 4 h. The minerals not only provide the necessary building blocks for the remineralization that maintains the status quo, but also binds with acids to neutralize the oral pH, reducing the patient's risk of further tooth loss.

Caphasol is an orally available agent suggested to retard calcium loss.

Use of a systemic sialogogue (administered orally) is indicated in patients with more than very mild salivary dysfunction, who do not achieve sufficient salivary excretion with topical stimulants such as those described above. Two muscarinic agonists, pilocarpine and cevimeline, increase salivary flow and improve symptoms of dry mouth [22, 50–57]. Pilocarpine and cevimeline are most effective in SjS patients with early disease and thus greater residual excretory capacity. A double-blind trial has recently been reported for a buccal insert that releases pilocarpine [58] and the early promising results have not yet been confirmed [59].

Their use of cholinergic secretagogues may sometimes be limited by poor tolerance, largely due to cholinergic side effects including undesirable increased/excessive perspiration. Although very uncommon, patients should also be cautioned about driving at night or performing hazardous activities in reduced lighting, because they may experience altered visual acuity or impaired depth perception.

Pilocarpine, a muscarinic agonist that stimulates predominantly muscarinic M3 receptors, can significantly increase aqueous secretions in patients with residual salivary gland function. The usual dose is 5 mg three or four times/day. It is most effective when taken four times/day because of its short duration of action. We thus suggest that patients try to take the medication four times daily if they do not receive adequate symptomatic relief with three times daily dosing. Side effects, including sweating, abdominal pain, flushing, or increased urination, may limit its use. In some patients with unacceptable levels of side effects at the full dose, a reduced dose of 2.5–3.75 mg three times daily, or 5 mg twice daily may still provide benefit.

In addition to effects upon xerostomia, pilocarpine may improve symptoms of ocular dryness, although without any objective change in tear production.

In the largest randomized trial that demonstrated the benefit of pilocarpine, 357 patients were randomly assigned to receive either pilocarpine (5 or 2.5 mg every 6 h) or placebo for 12 weeks. The following findings were observed:

- A significantly greater proportion of patients receiving pilocarpine (5 mg), compared with those who received placebo, experienced improvement in global assessments of symptoms of both dry mouth and dry eye (61% vs. 31%, and 42% vs. 26%, respectively).
- There was no difference in benefit found between pilocarpine 2.5 mg every 6 h and placebo.
- Sweating and increased urinary frequency were both more common with pilocarpine 5 mg compared with placebo (43% vs. 7% and 10% vs. 2%, respectively).
- No serious adverse events occurred, and only 3% of patients taking pilocarpine 5 mg withdrew from the study due to drug-related adverse events.
- The overall withdrawal rate did not differ between the three groups (6–7%).

There are no published studies that have examined the long-term efficacy of pilocarpine in patients with SjS.

Due to the potential for pilocarpine to stimulate the muscarinic M2 receptor, theoretical cardiac or lung (asthmatic complications) might occur, and therefore, patients with these historical features were excluded from clinical trials of pilocarpine or cevimeline [22, 50, 60–64]. However, clinical practice with these agents in patients with radiation xerostomia (who frequently have a long history of smoking and cardiac disease) has not shown this to be a clinically significant problem [55].

Cevimeline is taken three times a day (optimally about half an hour before meals), and can be taken up to four times a day (including an additional tablet at bedtime to help with nocturnal dryness).

- Cevimeline has a longer half-life in serum, and longer occupancy on receptor, which correlates with patient salivation profile [55].
- Pilocarpine is taken four times a day, and the patients typically experience a brief "spurt" of saliva due to its relatively short half-life in the sera.

The two drugs have not been compared directly. Issues that determine choice principally include cost to the patient, convenience, individual clinical response, and tolerance of adverse effects.

The choice between pilocarpine (Salagen®) and cevimeline (Evoxac®) is largely determined by individual factors, since both appear similarly effective. However, it has been the experience of several SjS centers that the longer half-life of cevimeline leads to improved tolerance and lower side effects.

Some patients do not respond sufficiently well to the muscarinic agonists to justify continued use, especially when cholinergic side effects are present. However, in those with an inadequate response, it is important to examine the patient carefully to rule out oral candidiasis, which may be responsible for a lack of symptomatic improvement with use of a secretagogue. The examination should include removal of upper dentures and determining if signs such as angular cheilitis are present.

When initiating therapy with these agents:

- We suggest gradually increasing the dose and taking it about 30 min before meals.
- We increase the dose gradually (starting once/day for a week).
- We add a proton pump inhibitor if needed to avoid gastric bloating and sudden onset of sweating.
- We suggest a trial of at least 3-months duration if the medication is tolerated, since the response is frequently delayed.
- If patients do not tolerate one preparation, they may try the other preparation.

Major side effects of cevimeline include excessive sweating, nausea, rhinitis, diarrhea, and visual disturbances. Use of lower doses in patients with poor tolerance of the full dose has been reported. Efficacy in lower dosing is obtained by dissolving the desired fraction of a 30-mg capsule's contents in water, or to employ a "rinse-and-spit" regimen (also called "cevimeline gargle") to minimize systemic absorption [64].

In randomized placebo-controlled trials, cevimeline significantly increases salivary flow and patient's "oral quality of life" [65]. The efficacy of cevimeline was illustrated in a study that randomly assigned 197 patients with either primary or secondary SjS to cevimeline or placebo [66]. The following outcomes were observed:

- Patients' global assessments of dryness were improved significantly more often by cevimeline 30 mg three times daily than by TID doses of 15 mg or placebo (65%, 32%, and 35%, respectively).
- The most common adverse events seen more often with the drug (30 or 15 mg TID) than placebo were nausea (21% and 12% vs. 7%), increased sweating (18% and 5% vs. 1%), and diarrhea (16% and 14% vs. 7%).
- Withdrawal from the study for adverse events was more common in patients on cevimeline (30 or 15 mg TID) compared with placebo (16.1% and 13.8% vs. 4.3%, respectively).
- Serious adverse events were seen in <3% of patients, and were not more common with cevimeline.

Drugs that inhibit cytochrome CYP2D6 and CYP3A3 also inhibit the metabolism of cevimeline. Individuals who are known to be deficient in these cytochrome isoenzymes should use cevimeline with caution.

36.5.1 Other Cholinergic Agonists

Bethanechol and pyridostigmine are cholinergic agonist agents that are approved in the USA for use in urinary retention and myasthenia gravis, respectively, but not for SjS. They have mixed muscarinic and nicotinic activity, and are used much less often for SjS because of greater adverse effects (compared with pilocarpine and cevimeline). However, they have been shown to provide palliative care of radiation xerostomia in small double-blind studies [67–69].

Amofostine is an agent that may provide protection of the salivary glands during radiation therapy [70], but was not as effective as pilocarpine in patients with xerostomia after radiation or SjS [71].

Bromhexine (a mucolytic agent) also showed palliative response in radiation xerostomia, and had been suggested for symptomatic treatment in SjS [72–74]. However, this agent has now been withdrawn from the market although it exhibited a good safety profile [75]. These agents have theoretical benefit, but they have not been subject to controlled clinical trials to demonstrate efficacy in SjS. Anecdotal trials of these agents in SjS, as well as amofostine, have been disappointing in our clinic particularly in relation to their cost.

36.5.2 Additional Topical Treatments

- Topical interferon alpha [76]. Although oral interferon alpha was promising in early studies, results were far less encouraging in a subsequent larger well-designed study [77–79]. Further studies will be needed before this medication can be recommended in this setting. However, the use of interferon alpha in patients with hepatitis C and sicca symptoms has exacerbated their dryness complaints.
- Acupuncture and herbal teas [80] that may result in qualitative changes in saliva as well as increased flow in some patients [81].
- Anhydrous crystalline maltose to stimulate masticatory and gustatory response [82].
- Anetholetrithione which exhibited modest benefit in an initial small double-blind trial [83], but subsequent larger trials were not reported.

36.5.3 Systemic Therapy

36.5.3.1 TNF-Alpha Blockers

Short-term studies with infliximab, a TNF-blocker, showed significant improvements in SjS symptoms in an initial open trial [84]. However, randomized, double-blind, placebo-controlled studies showed no indication of increased efficiency in persons treated with infliximab [85]. Randomized, double-blind, placebo-controlled studies with etanercept also showed no reduction of sicca symptoms in SjS [86–88].

Rituximab, known for its tolerability, is an anti-CD20 antibody that is effective in persons with various autoimmune diseases. Several small controlled studies have shown a mild increase in saliva flow in a subset of patients with early disease [89–91]. Salivary biopsies from treated patients have also shown decreases in lymphocytic infiltrates [92, 93].

Epratuzumab, directed against the B-cell epitope CD22, appears to function by modulation of B-cells than by depletion of these cells from the circulation [94]. Steinfeld et al. presented preliminary results in the treatment of primary SjS including increased salivary flow in the drug-treated cohort. The study consisted of 16 Caucasian individuals, two of whom discontinued due to complications. However, ten persons reported adverse events, which included acute infusion, dental abscess, transient ischemic attack with secondary seizure, and osteoporotic fracture. Non-serious adverse events included headache, paresthesia, and acute infusion reaction, which resolved quickly [94].

Recently, a monoclonal anti-BAFF antibody (belimumab) has shown promising results in SLE leading to FDA approval. Trials of belimumab are just beginning [95, 96].

36.6   Oral Candidiasis

Oral candidiasis, a common complication of SjS, occurs in more than one-third of patients [97–99]. Symptoms include a painful mouth, sometimes with a burning sensation, and sensitivity to spicy or acidic foods. Oral candidiasis is particularly frequent following antibiotic treatment or the use of glucocorticoids (see "Clinical Manifestations of Oropharyngeal and Esophageal Candidiasis").

Oral candidiasis is one of the most common oral infections. In 1980, an inverse relationship between salivary flow rates and the level of Candida infection was described [100]. Persons with SjS have also been reported to have *Candida albicans* more frequently than the general population at a given salivary flow rate, indicating a role for qualitative anti-candida factors such as lysozyme content in saliva [101, 102].

Findings in SjS patients with oral candidiasis include:

- Diffuse or patchy erythema, and (less often), white patches on the mucosal surfaces.
- The tongue, buccal mucosa, palate, lips, and the corners of the lips may be affected.
- There may be loss of tongue papillae.
- Angular cheilitis and atrophic changes of the buccal mucosa are common manifestations in SjS.

In patients with SjS and oral candidiasis, several particular factors require consideration. Because most antifungal preparations for oral use contain sugar to improve taste, such agents should not be used immediately before bed without following with a thorough tooth brushing.

An alternative oral "off-label" approach preferred by some experts is use of topical Nystatin Vaginal tablets (100,000 units/tablet) sucked on like a lozenge three to four times/day for 7–10 days. These tablets do not contain fermentable carbohydrate in the carrier.

- We initially treat with clotrimazole (200 mg/day) for 5 days, and treat angular cheilitis using topical clotrimazole cream.
- We advise use of a compounded oral mouth rinse of the type recommended by radiation therapists for mucositis.

- The rinse should be used for 2 min (rinse plus gargle) three times/day for 2–3 weeks.
- These rinses are known by various names, such as "Stanford Mouth Rinse" or "Miracle Mouthwash."
- We use a mixture containing:

  Mylanta (aluminum hydroxide/magnesium hydroxide) 240 mL (as a vehicle)
  Diphenhydramine 20 mL
  Nystatin 20 mL
  Doxycycline 20 mL

- The components can be ordered separately and mixed by the patient.
- Variations of this mouth rinse may contain viscous lidocaine, low-dose glucocorticoids, or brompheniramine/pseudoephedrine elixir.
- Several mouth rinses used by radiation therapists may also be helpful, such as:

  A homemade remedy of 12 tsp. salt and 1/2 tsp. baking soda in 8 oz water
  A wound rinse with aloe vera extract
  Carafate suspension as a rinse used twice per day

There is some concern in patients with severe salivary dysfunction that insufficient local (salivary) levels of medication may be reached with use of systemic medications. Thus, in dry mouth patients who do not respond adequately to systemic medications within 7–10 days, switching to a topical oral antifungal is suggested.

In patients with more persistent oral fungal disease, we recommend the use of nystatin vaginal troches (100,000 units) that are sucked on daily with water sweetened with an artificial sweetener (to improve the taste). Treatment twice daily for up to 4–6 weeks may be required.

- Alternatives include:

  - Miconazole oral gel (sugar-free, 24 mg/mL=20 mg/g), 5–10 mL four times/day, held in the mouth before swallowing
  - Amphotericin lozenges (10 mg) four times daily

36.7 Treatment and Management of Cutaneous Manifestations

36.7.1 Treatment of Dry Skin in SjS Is Similar to Managing Xerosis in Other Conditions

1. The patient should moisturize the skin with a fragrance-free cream moisturizer once or twice a day. Moisturizing is performed immediately after bathing or showering, while the skin is still damp, to prevent further evaporation from the skin. Sometimes in cases of extreme dryness, an ointment is suggested, for its barrier and protective properties (such as petrolatum jelly or Aquaphor®).

If ointment is used, then application should be onto damp skin, as the ointment itself does not contain water. Excess greasiness can be blotted with a towel. Sometimes a moisturizing cream with beta- or alpha-hydroxy acid, or urea, can add extra moisture, but in cases of cracks in the skin, these will sting and irritate.

2. Excessive, long, hot showers or baths should be avoided, in addition to heavily fragranced cleansers.

3. Cleansing of the skin: The usual recommendation is to cleanse with a moisturizing soap such as Dove® fragrance-free bar, or a soap-free cleanser such as Cetaphil® gentle cleanser or Aquanil® cleanser.

   If the xerosis leads to pruritis, then safe anti-pruritic topical treatments are recommended.

4. Over-the-counter lotions containing menthol, camphor (Sarna Anti-Itch Lotion®), 2% lidocaine (Neutrogena Norwegian Formula Soothing Relief Anti-Itch Moisturizer®), and pramoxine (Aveeno Anti-Itch Concentrated Lotion®) are readily available.

5. Oral antihistamines should be used with caution because of their anticholinergic effects. Fexofenidine (Allegra) does not cross the blood-brain barrier and may have slightly less dryness as a side effect. Over-the-counter sleeping medications that contain hydroxyzine (Atarax) or diphenhydramine (Benadryl) are very drying, and may contribute to sleep disturbance.

6. Topical corticosteroids: We generally do not like to use topical corticosteroids, especially the ultra-potent ones, but even the mid-potency ones – for more than a couple of weeks at a time. In the case of inflammatory skin findings, local treatment with potent topical steroids can augment systemic treatments.

   Sometimes topical corticosteroids are used for pruritus, but their use should be limited due to long-term side effects such as skin atrophy, tachyphylaxis, and absorption.

7. We always suggest constant daily sun protection for patients with autoimmune conditions. Because the wavelength of light causing sun sensitivity in autoimmune conditions may not be in the UVB spectrum (290–320 nm), patients should use a broad-spectrum sunscreen.
   - SPF factors refer to UVB protection only, so patients cannot count on simply the SPF factor.
   - Most sunscreens available now have added UVA protection (290–320 nm), commonly from chemical UVA-absorbing compounds, such as Parsol 1789 (avobenzone).

8. We prefer physical sun blocks, since wavelengths outside of both UVB and UVA may affect the patient with autoimmune disease.
   - Physical sun blocks contain titanium dioxide or zinc oxide, which reflect rays.
   - One commonly available sun block is Neutrogena Sensitive Skin Sun Block SPF-30®, which uses purely titanium dioxide as its active ingredient.

9. The most effective protection is sun-protective clothing, since it will not wear off as sunscreens do. This includes hats, sun glasses, UV-protective lip balm, long-sleeved shirts (some clothing is sun-repellent).

Obviously, avoiding excess sun contact altogether is prudent, such as trying to stay indoors during the intense sunlight hours of 10 a.m. to 2–4 p.m.

10. Mucous-promoting compounds. Study of the tear film and saliva has shown that SjS symptoms are more than the simple absence of aqueous secretions. In particular, the lubricating film contains a series of mucins and proteins in an emulsified gel. A lipid layer prevents subsequent evaporation. As many of the extraglandular symptoms of SjS may result from decreased lubrication, such as chronic upper airway dryness or vaginal dryness, these agents may part of future treatments.
Agents that are currently in trial (particularly for oral and ocular) include:

(a) Diquafosol, an agonist of the P2Y2 receptor that stimulates net chloride transfer from the serosal to the mucosal side of epithelial membranes [103, 104].

(b) 15-S Hete, an arachidonic acid metabolite, acts as a mucin secretagogue and has been shown to stimulate mucin I production [105].

(c) Rebamide [106], ecabet sodium [107], and gefarnate [108] have been used in Japan as gastroprotective agents because of their mucus secretary action.

36.7.2 Vaginal Dryness

A gynecologic examination is useful to rule out other causes of painful intercourse and other causes of vaginal dryness.

Sexual considerations: When vaginal dryness does occur as part of SjS, the spouse or partner needs to be reassured that this is a "physiological" problem, and not related to a failure of sexual arousal. Psychological fear of discomfort may further exacerbate the problem. Sterile lubricants such as Astroglide®, KY Brand® jelly or Surgilube® are helpful (and should be liberally applied to both partners for maximal comfort) Table 36.4 [109, 110].

• Despite liberal application of lubrication to the female, if the partner's penis is not well lubricated, the female SjS patient will likely experience discomfort during and after intercourse.

Lubricants such as Maxilube® and Astroglide® have slightly different characteristics when compared with KY Brand® jelly or Surgilube®, and yet, share the common characteristics of being water-soluble and non-irritating. This also holds true for the new non-hormonal vaginal moisturizer Replens®, which may be used, unassociated with intercourse. For those patients who do not like the gel-type lubricants, Lubrin® vaginal inserts are now available.

Finding the right preparation for a specific individual is often a matter of trial and error inasmuch as satisfaction with each lubricant is a matter of personal preference. The patient needs to be frank with her physician regarding her satisfaction or dissatisfaction with a particular preparation. The physician also needs to assure the female SjS patient that her male partner should also be sensitive to her needs, and actively participate in preparations to help maximize sexual satisfaction for both partners.

Table 36.4 Vaginal dryness and dyspareunia in the SS patient

• Insertional dyspareunia
– Lubrication difficulties
Lack of knowledge of sexual response
Lack of arousal
Postmenopausal atrophy
– Vulvitis – infectious or irritative
– Vaginitis – infectious or irritative
– Vaginismus
– Psychological concerns
• Pain in a specific area of vulva or vagina
– Hymenal ring difficulty
– Old scars, lesions, abscesses, gland enlargement
– Vulvitis – infectious or irritative
– Vaginitis – infectious or irritative
• Pain with deep penetration
– Masses or uterine enlargement
– Endometriosis
– Adhesions
– Vaginismus
– Condyloma accuminata
– Psychological concerns

The external use of preparations containing petrolatum or oils that "seal in" moisture, such as Vaseline® or cocoa butter, as well as "scented" or "flavored" preparations may lead to maceration and irritation of the sensitive and fragile vaginal mucosal lining, and are to be avoided.

Vaginal dryness in perimenopausal or postmenopausal women is often related to vaginal atrophy because of declining estrogen levels, and therefore may respond to vaginal topical estrogen creams such as Estrace® (if tolerated without irritation). Cortisone creams are not beneficial in this situation.

If vaginal yeast infection occurs, prompt treatment with clotrimazole topical cream, vaginal suppositories (Gynelotrimin®), or p.o. gluconazole 150 mg is safe and effective. Oral gluconazole's benefit is that it can be started earlier in the day, rather than waiting until bedtime to use cream or suppository. With yeast infection, prompt treatment is essential to avoid rapid escalation of the infection during the day, along with higher level of discomfort for the patient.

On the external vulvar surface, dryness may be treated with lubricating creams, as would other skin surfaces (see section on skin dryness). Several patients have reported considerable satisfaction with the use of a thin film of vitamin E oil [111] used on the vulva once or twice a day.

An issue of concern to female SjS patients has been whether or not estrogen/hormone replacement therapy (HRT) at the time of menopause is harmful to their condition [112]. With regard to estrogen replacement in general, the clinical evidence is controversial whether the risks of blocking osteoporosis and reducing cardiovascular mortality adequately offset the small increase in risk in breast cancer.

It is also worth noting that the subset of women who had previous hysterectomy/ ovariectomy was not found to have increased risk of breast cancer on receiving estrogen replacement [113].

Of importance, some women feel that estrogen replacement improves their quality of life, in terms of mood elevation and by reducing hot flashes and hormone-related vaginal dryness [114–116]. Part of this improvement may relate to the interconversion of hormones to include DHEA, which appears to have beneficial effects on local mucosal surfaces [117] as well as improving mucosal secretory function [118].

Earlier investigators were concerned that estrogen might have a negative influence on SjS or SLE based on animal studies. At our clinic, we have not seen any deterioration of SjS related to either estrogen replacement therapy or low estrogen forms of oral contraceptives.

Because of this, we encourage adequate estrogen replacement for the properly screened postmenopausal SjS patient who feels that it improves their quality of life. Although the data has not been formally collected in SjS, there have been extensive trials on the use of oral contraceptives and estrogen replacement in SLE patients [114, 115, 119]. These studies have indicated safety in terms of breast cancer and disease activity. However, caution with regard to blood clot risk remains, particularly in the patient with circulating anti-coagulants or a past history of thromboembolic disease.

Nonetheless, estrogens would not be the agent of choice to deal with either postmenopausal osteoporosis or elevated lipid profiles. Other therapeutic alternatives for osteoporosis (alendronate, Fosamax®, and residronate, Actonel®) and other agents for lowering cholesterol (such as statins) are now available, and estrogens are now not the agents of choice for these medical issues.

36.7.3 Special Precautions at the Time of Surgery

SjS patients have particularly unique needs at the time of surgery. Patients with ocular dryness are at increased risk for corneal abrasions in operating rooms (generally have low-humidity environments), and particularly in the postoperative recovery room, where non-humidified oxygen is blown across their face at a time when they are still too groggy to have adequate blink reflex.

Therefore, we have recommended application of an ocular ointment or gel prior to surgery.

Patients are subject to severe dryness of the mouth as a consequence of their disease but are told to be "NPO" for at least 12 h before surgery (and often longer if they are a later operative case in the day). We have found that patients can safely use their oral mouth sprays for comfort preoperatively, while not having the risk of gastric contents and aspiration during anesthesia. If possible, patients should request from their surgeons that they be placed in an early slot in the OR schedule.

The anesthesiologist will need to take special precautions with oral intubations, as these patients have "fragile" teeth and often have expensive dental reconstructions and restorations including implants.

Therefore, it is important for the patient to make certain that a "heads-up" note is recorded in – or better yet – on the front – of the chart.

Patients with SjS often have very dry upper airways and minimal use of anticholinergic agents to control tracheal secretions. The tenacious mucus secretions may predispose to mucus inspissations and postoperative obstructions. The use of humidified oxygen and mucolytics may help minimize this process.

Although anesthesiologists and surgeons are familiar with precautions regarding NSAIDs and bleeding risk, they are often less familiar with the relatively long duration of agents such as the new biologic agents. Although most of the literature about increased rate of infection after joint replacements deal with TNF inhibitors, it is likely that similar caveats will apply to additional biologic agents as they become available.

Finally, steroid coverage for "stress" levels may be required in patients on chronic steroids. Also, oral candida is quite common in the postoperative patient who has been on steroids and recent antibiotic therapy.

Patients should also be permitted to have their eye and mouth moisturizers and other appropriate remedies at bedside if hospitalized.

Acknowledgments This chapter includes the contributions to patient care provided by the Scripps Oral Health Clinic (headed by Dr. John Weston) and our dedicated Oral Hygienists including Laurie Powell and Joanne Snyder who specialize in Sjögren's syndrome, as well to our Dermatology associates particularly Drs. Alice Liu and Judith Kopersky, and our Gynecology and Urology associates particularly Drs. John Willems and John Naitoh.

References

1. Locker D, Clarke M, Payne B. Self-perceived oral health status, psychological well-being, and life satisfaction in an older adult population. J Dent Res. 2000;79:970.
2. Meijer JM, Meiners PM, Huddleston Slater JJR, Spijkervet FKL, Kallenberg CGM, Vissink A, et al. Health-related quality of life, employment and disability in patients with Sjogren's syndrome. Rheumatology. 2009;48:1077.
3. Landi F, Russo A, Liperoti R, Cesari M, Barillaro C, Pahor M, et al. Anticholinergic drugs and physical function among frail elderly population. Clin Pharmacol Ther. 2006;81:235–41.
4. Fox RI. Sjogren's syndrome. Lancet. 2005;366:321–31.
5. Bookman AAM, Shen H, Cook RJ, Bailey D, McComb RJ, Rutka JA, et al. Whole stimulated salivary flow: correlation with the pathology of inflammation and damage in minor salivary gland biopsy specimens from patients with primary Sjögren's syndrome but not patients with sicca. Arthritis Rheum. 2011;63:2014–20.
6. Stern ME, Beuerman RW, Fox RI, Gao J, Mircheff AK, Pflugfelder SC. A unified theory of the role of the ocular surface in dry eye. Adv Exp Med Biol. 1998;438:643–51.
7. Stern ME, Gao J, Siemasko KF, Beuerman RW, Pflugfelder SC. The role of the lacrimal functional unit in the pathophysiology of dry eye. Exp Eye Res. 2004;78:409–16.
8. Valls Sole J, Graus F, Font J, Pou A, Tolosa ES. Normal proprioceptive trigeminal afferents in patients with Sjogren's syndrome and sensory neuronopathy. Ann Neurol. 1990;28:786–90.

9. Bergdahl M. Salivary flow and oral complaints in adult dental patients. Community Dent Oral Epidemiol. 2000;28:59–66.
10. Bergdahl M, Bergdahl J. Burning mouth syndrome: prevalence and associated factors. J Oral Pathol Med. 1999;28:350–4.
11. Femiano F, Scully C. Burning mouth syndrome (BMS): double blind controlled study of alpha-lipoic acid (thioctic acid) therapy. J Oral Pathol Med. 2002;31:267–9.
12. Grushka M, Ching V, Epstein J. Burning mouth syndrome. Adv Otorhinolaryngol. 2006;63: 278–87.
13. Speciali J, Stuginski-Barbosa J. Burning mouth syndrome. Curr Pain Headache Rep. 2008; 12:279–84.
14. Bergdahl M, Bergdahl J. Low unstimulated salivary flow and subjective oral dryness: association with medication, anxiety, depression, and stress. J Dent Res. 2000;79:1652.
15. Vriezekolk JE, Geenen R, Hartkamp A, Godaert GL, Bootsma H, Kruize AA, et al. Psychological and somatic predictors of perceived and measured ocular dryness of patients with primary Sjogren's syndrome. J Rheumatol. 2005;32:2351–5.
16. Strietzel F, Lafaurie G, Bautista M, Alajbeg I, Pejda S, Vuleti L, et al. Efficacy and safety of an intraoral electrostimulation device for xerostomia relief: a multicenter randomized trial. Arthritis Rheum. 2011;63:180–90. Epub 28 Dec 2010.
17. Strietzel F, Martìn Granizo R, Fedele S, Lo Russo L, Mignogna M, Reichart P, et al. Electrostimulating device in the management of xerostomia. Oral Dis. 2007;13:206–13.
18. Fedele S, Wolff A, Strietzel F, Lopez R. Neuroelectrostimulation in treatment of hyposalivation and xerostomia in Sjogren's syndrome: a salivary pacemaker. J Rheumatol. 2008;35: 1489.
19. Fox RI, Liu AY. Sjogren's syndrome in dermatology. Clin Dermatol. 2006;24:393–413.
20. Schiffman S, Miletic I. Effect of taste and smell on secretion rate of salivary IgA in elderly and young persons. J Nutr Health Aging. 1999;3:158–64.
21. Daniels T. Sjogren's syndrome: clinical spectrum and current diagnostic controversies. Adv Dent Res. 1996;10:3.
22. Al-Hashimi I. The management of Sjogren's syndrome in dental practice. J Am Dent Assoc. 2001;132:1409–17; quiz 60–1.
23. Al-Hashimi I. Sjogren's syndrome: diagnosis and management. Womens Health. 2007;3: 107–22.
24. Nagy K, Urban E, Fazekas O, Thurzo L, Nagy E. Controlled study of lactoperoxidase gel on oral flora and saliva in irradiated patients with oral cancer. J Craniofac Surg. 2007;18: 1157–64.
25. Warde P, Kroll B, O'Sullivan B, Aslanidis J, Tew-George E, Waldron J, et al. A phase II study of Biotene in the treatment of postradiation xerostomia in patients with head and neck cancer. Support Care Cancer. 2000;8:203–8.
26. Temmel A, Quint C, Schickinger-Fischer B, Hummel T. Taste function in xerostomia before and after treatment with a saliva substitute containing carboxymethylcellulose. J Otolaryngol. 2005;34:116.
27. Schubert MM, Peterson DE, Lloid ME. Oral complications. In: Thomas ED, Blume KG, Forman SJ, editors. Hematopoietic cell transplantation. Oxford: Blackwell Science; 1999. p. 751–63.
28. MacFarlane T, Mason D. Changes in the oral flora in Sjogren's syndrome. J Clin Pathol. 1974;27:416.
29. Ayars GH, Altman LC, Fretwell MD. Effect of decreased salivation and pH on the adherence of Klebsiella species to human buccal epithelial cells. Infect Immun. 1982;38:179.
30. Zero DT. Etiology of dental erosion – extrinsic factors. Eur J Oral Sci. 1996;104:162–77.
31. Larsen M, Nyvad B. Enamel erosion by some soft drinks and orange juices relative to their pH, buffering effect and contents of calcium phosphate. Caries Res. 2000;33:81–7.
32. Newbrun E. Current treatment modalities of oral problems of patients with Sjogren's syndrome: caries prevention. Adv Dent Res. 1996;10:29–34.

33. Paster B, Boches S, Galvin J, Ericson R, Lau C, Levanos V, et al. Bacterial diversity in human subgingival plaque. J Bacteriol. 2001;183:3770.
34. Daniels T, Fox P. Salivary and oral components of Sjogren's syndrome. Rheum Dis Clin North Am. 1992;18:571.
35. Astor FC, Hanft KL, Ciocon JO. Xerostomia: a prevalent condition in the elderly. Ear Nose Throat J. 1999;78:476–9.
36. Pedersen A, Bardow A, Nauntofte B. Salivary changes and dental caries as potential oral markers of autoimmune salivary gland dysfunction in primary Sjogren's syndrome. BMC Clin Pathol. 2005;5:4.
37. Christensen L, Petersen P, Thorn J, SchiØdt M. Dental caries and dental health behavior of patients with primary Sjogren's syndrome. Acta Odontol Scand. 2001;59:116–20.
38. Castillo JL, Milgrom P. Fluoride release from varnishes in two in vitro protocols. J Am Dent Assoc. 2004;135:1696–9.
39. Castillo JL, Milgrom P, Kharasch E, Izutsu K, Fey M. Evaluation of fluoride release from commercially available fluoride varnishes. J Am Dent Assoc. 2001;132:1389–92; quiz 459–60.
40. Daniels T, Fox PC. Salivary and oral components of Sjogren's syndrome. Rheum Dis Clin North Am. 1992;18:571–89.
41. Mann J, Karniel C, Triol CW, Sintes JL, Garcia L, Petrone ME, et al. Comparison of the clinical anticaries efficacy of a 1500 NaF silica-based dentifrice containing triclosan and a copolymer to a 1500 NaF silica-based dentifrice without those additional agents: a study on adults in Israel. J Clin Dent. 1996;7:90–5.
42. Pfarrer AM, White DJ, Featherstone JD. Anticaries profile qualification of an improved whitening dentifrice. J Clin Dent. 2001;12:30–3.
43. Banting DW, Papas A, Clark DC, Proskin HM, Schultz M, Perry R. The effectiveness of 10% chlorhexidine varnish treatment on dental caries incidence in adults with dry mouth. Gerodontology. 2000;17:67–76.
44. Epstein JB, Loh R, Stevenson-Moore P, McBride BC, Spinelli J. Chlorhexidine rinse in prevention of dental caries in patients following radiation therapy. Oral Surg Oral Med Oral Pathol. 1989;68:401–5.
45. Johansson G, Andersson G, Edwardsson S, Bjorn AL, Manthorpe R, Attstrom R. Effects of mouthrinses with linseed extract Salinum without/with chlorhexidine on oral conditions in patients with Sjogren's syndrome. A double-blind crossover investigation. Gerodontology. 2001;18:87–94.
46. Ship JA, McCutcheon JA, Spivakovsky S, Kerr AR. Safety and effectiveness of topical dry mouth products containing olive oil, betaine, and xylitol in reducing xerostomia for polypharmacy-induced dry mouth. J Oral Rehabil. 2007;34:724–32.
47. Sintes JL, Escalante C, Stewart B, McCool JJ, Garcia L, Volpe AR, et al. Enhanced anticaries efficacy of a 0.243% sodium fluoride/10% xylitol/silica dentifrice: 3-year clinical results. Am J Dent. 1995;8:231–5.
48. Isidor F, Brondum K, Hansen HJ, Jensen J, Sindet-Pedersen S. Outcome of treatment with implant-retained dental prostheses in patients with Sjogren syndrome. Int J Oral Maxillofac Implants. 1999;14:736–43.
49. Payne AG, Lownie JF, Van Der Linden WJ. Implant-supported prostheses in patients with Sjogren's syndrome: a clinical report on three patients. Int J Oral Maxillofac Implants. 1997;12:679–85.
50. Ramos-Casals M, Brito-Zerón P. New approaches in Sjögren's syndrome therapy. Expert Rev Clin Immunol. 2007;3:195–204.
51. Peluso G, De Santis M, Inzitari R, Fanali C, Cabras T, Messana I, et al. Proteomic study of salivary peptides and proteins in patients with Sjogren's syndrome before and after pilocarpine treatment. Arthritis Rheum. 2007;56:2216–22.
52. Wu CH, Hsieh SC, Lee KL, Li KJ, Lu MC, Yu CL. Pilocarpine hydrochloride for the treatment of xerostomia in patients with Sjögren's syndrome in Taiwan-A double-blind, placebo-controlled trial. J Formos Med Assoc. 2006;105:796–803.

53. Bhamra J, Wong J, Gohill J. Oral pilocarpine for the treatment of keratoconjunctivitis sicca with central corneal irregularity. J Cataract Refract Surg. 2003;29:2236–8.
54. Vivino FB. The treatment of Sjogren's syndrome patients with pilocarpine-tablets. Scand J Rheumatol Suppl. 2001;115:1–9; discussion 9–13.
55. Fox RI, Konttinen Y, Fisher A. Use of muscarinic agonists in the treatment of Sjogren's syndrome. Clin Immunol. 2001;101:249–63.
56. al-Hashimi I, Taylor SE. A new medication for treatment of dry mouth in Sjogren's syndrome. Tex Dent J. 2001;118:262–6.
57. Fox RI, Stern M, Michelson P. Update in Sjogren syndrome. Curr Opin Rheumatol. 2000;12:391–8.
58. Gibson J, Halliday JA, Ewert K, Robertson S. A controlled release pilocarpine buccal insert in the treatment of Sjögren's syndrome. Br Dent J. 2007;202:E17.
59. Yeoman C. A controlled release buccal insert. Br Dent J. 2007;202:404–5.
60. Leung KCM, McMillan AS, Wong MCM, Leung WK, Mok MY, Lau CS. The efficacy of cevimeline hydrochloride in the treatment of xerostomia in Sjögren's syndrome in southern Chinese patients: a randomised double-blind, placebo-controlled crossover study. Clin Rheumatol. 2008;27:429–36.
61. Yamada H, Nakagawa Y, Wakamatsu E, Sumida T, Yamachika S, Nomura Y, et al. Efficacy prediction of cevimeline in patients with Sjögren's syndrome. Clin Rheumatol. 2007;26:1320–7.
62. Yamada H, Nakagawa Y, Wakamatsu E, Sumida T, Yamachika S, Nomura Y, et al. Efficacy prediction of cevimeline in patients with Sjögren's syndrome. Clin Rheumatol. 2007;26: 1320–7.
63. Suzuki K, Matsumoto M, Nakashima M, Takada K, Nakanishi T, Okada M, et al. Effect of cevimeline on salivary components in patients with Sjogren syndrome. Pharmacology. 2005;74:100–5.
64. Takagi Y, Kimura Y, Nakamura T. Cevimeline gargle for the treatment of xerostomia in patients with Sjogren's syndrome. Ann Rheum Dis. 2004;63:749.
65. Mavragani CP, Moutsopoulos HM. Conventional therapy of Sjogren's syndrome. Clin Rev Allergy Immunol. 2007;32:284–91.
66. Petrone D, Condemi JJ, Fife R, Gluck O, Cohen S, Dalgin P. A double-blind, randomized, placebo-controlled study of cevimeline in Sjoegren's syndrome patients with xerostomia and keratoconjunctivitis sicca. Arthritis Rheum. 2002;46:748–54.
67. Epstein JB, Burchell JL, Emerton S, Le ND, Silverman S. A clinical trial of bethanechol in patients with xerostomia after radiation therapy: a pilot study. Oral Surg Oral Med Oral Pathol. 1994;77:610–4.
68. Llorente I, Lizcano F, Alvarez R, Diez N, Sopena M, Gil MJ, et al. Cholinergic modulation of spontaneous hypothalamic-pituitary-adrenal activity and its circadian variation in man. J Clin Endocrinol Metab. 1996;81:2902–7.
69. Bhalla R, Swedler WI, Lazarevic MB, Ajmani HS, Skosey JL. Myasthenia gravis and scleroderma. J Rheumatol. 1993;20:1409–10.
70. Bohuslavizki KH, Brenner W, Klutmann S, Hubner RH, Lassmann S, Feyerabend B, et al. Radioprotection of salivary glands by amifostine in high-dose radioiodine therapy. J Nucl Med. 1998;39:1237.
71. Olver IN. Xerostomia: a common adverse effect of drugs and radiation. Aust Prescriber. 2006;29:97–8.
72. Misawa M, Ohmori S, Yanaura S. Effects of bromhexine on the secretions of saliva and tears. J Pharmacol. 1985;39:241–50.
73. Avisar R, Savir H, Machtey I, Ovaknin L, Shaked P, Menache R, et al. Clinical trial of bromhexine in Sjogren's syndrome. Ann Ophthalmol. 1981;13:971.
74. Frost-Larsen K, Isager H, Manthorpe R. Sjogren's syndrome treated with bromhexine: a randomised clinical study. Br Med J. 1978;1:1579.

75. Jayaram S, Desai A. Efficacy and safety of Ascoril expectorant and other cough formula in the treatment of cough management in paediatric and adult patients – a randomised double-blind comparative trial. J Indian Med Assoc. 2000;98:68.
76. Barnard DL. Interferon-alpha. Amarillo Biosciences. Curr Opin Investig Drugs. 2002;3: 693–7.
77. Khurshudian AV. A pilot study to test the efficacy of oral administration of interferon-alpha lozenges to patients with Sjogren's syndrome. Oral Surg Oral Med Oral Pathol Oral Radiol Endod. 2003;95:38–44.
78. Cummins MJ, Papas A, Kammer GM, Fox PC. Treatment of primary Sjogren's syndrome with low-dose human interferon alfa administered by the oromucosal route: combined phase III results. Arthritis Rheum. 2003;49:585–93.
79. Shiozawa S, Tanaka Y, Shiozawa K. Single-blinded controlled trial of low-dose oral IFN-alpha for the treatment of xerostomia in patients with Sjogren's syndrome. J Interferon Cytokine Res. 1998;18:255–62.
80. Blom M, Dawidson I, Angmar-MÅnsson B. The effect of acupuncture on salivary flow rates in patients with xerostomia* 1. Oral Surg Oral Med Oral Pathol. 1992;73:293–8.
81. Dawidson I, Angmar-Mânsson B, Blom M, Theodorsson E, Lundeberg T. Sensory stimulation (acupuncture) increases the release of calcitonin gene-related peptide in the saliva of xerostomia sufferers* 1. Neuropeptides. 1999;33:244–50.
82. Fox PC, Cummins MJ, Cummins JM. Use of orally administered anhydrous crystalline maltose for relief of dry mouth. J Altern Complement Med. 2001;7:33–43.
83. Epstein J, Decoteau W, Wilkinson A. Effect of sialor in treatment of xerostomia in Sjogren's syndrome. Oral Surg Oral Med Oral Pathol. 1983;56:495–9.
84. Steinfeld SD, Demols P, Salmon I, Kiss R, Appelboom T. Infliximab in patients with primary Sjögren's syndrome: a pilot study. Arthritis Rheum. 2001;44:2371–5.
85. Mariette X, Ravaud P, Steinfeld S, Baron G, Goetz J, Hachulla E, et al. Inefficacy of infliximab in primary Sjögren's syndrome: results of the randomized, controlled Trial of Remicade in Primary Sjögren's Syndrome (TRIPSjS). Arthritis Rheum. 2004;50:1270–6.
86. Moutsopoulos NM, Katsifis GE, Angelov N, Leakan RA, Sankar V, Pillemer S, et al. Lack of efficacy of etanercept in Sjögren's syndrome correlates with failed suppression of TNF alpha and systemic immune activation. Ann Rheum Dis. 2008;67:1437–43.
87. Zandbelt MM, de Wilde P, van Damme P, Hoyng CB, van de Putte L, van den Hoogen F. Etanercept in the treatment of patients with primary Sjögren's syndrome: a pilot study. J Rheumatol. 2004;31:96–101.
88. Sankar V, Brennan MT, Kok MR, Leakan RA, Smith JA, Manny J, et al. Etanercept in Sjogren's syndrome: a twelve-week randomized, double-blind, placebo-controlled pilot clinical trial. Arthritis Rheum. 2004;50:2240–5.
89. Zapata LF, Agudelo LM, Paulo JD, Pineda R. Sjogren keratoconjunctivitis sicca treated with rituximab. Cornea. 2007;26:886–7.
90. Devauchelle-Pensec V, Pennec Y, Morvan J, Pers JO, Daridon C, Jousse-Joulin S, et al. Improvement of Sjögren's syndrome after two infusions of rituximab (anti-CD20). Arthritis Rheum. 2007;57:310–7.
91. Pijpe J, van Imhoff GW, Vissink A, van der Wal JE, Kluin PM, Spijkervet FK, et al. Changes in salivary gland immunohistology and function after rituximab monotherapy in a patient with Sjögren's syndrome and associated MALT lymphoma. Ann Rheum Dis. 2005;64: 958–60.
92. Meijer JM, Pijpe J, Vissink A, Kallenberg C, Bootsma H. Treatment of primary Sjogren's syndrome with rituximab: extended follow-up, safety and efficacy of retreatment. Ann Rheum Dis. 2009;68:284.
93. Meijer JM, Meiners P, Vissink A, Spijkervet F, Abdulahad W, Kamminga N, et al. Effectiveness of rituximab treatment in primary Sjögren's syndrome: a randomized, double blind, placebo controlled trial. Arthritis Rheum. 2010;62:960–8.

94. Steinfeld SD, Tant L, Burmester GR, Teoh NK, Wegener WA, Goldenberg DM, et al. Epratuzumab (humanised anti-CD22 antibody) in primary Sjogren's syndrome: an open-label phase I/II study. Arthritis Res Ther. 2006;8:R129.

95. d'Arbonneau F, Pers JO, Devauchelle V, Pennec Y, Saraux A, Youinou P. BAFF-induced changes in B cell antigen receptor-containing lipid rafts in Sjogren's syndrome. Arthritis Rheum. 2006;54:115–26.

96. Pers JO, d'Arbonneau F, Devauchelle-Pensec V, Saraux A, Pennec YL, Youinou P. Is periodontal disease mediated by salivary baff in Sjogren's syndrome? Arthritis Rheum. 2005;52:2411–4.

97. Rhodus NL, Michalowicz BS. Periodontal status and sulcular *Candida albicans* colonization in patients with primary Sjogren's syndrome. Quintessence Int. 2005;36:228–33.

98. Azuma T, Takei M, Yoshikawa T, Nagasugi Y, Kato M, Otsuka M, et al. Identification of candidate genes for Sjogren's syndrome using MRL/lpr mouse model of Sjogren's syndrome and cDNA microarray analysis. Immunol Lett. 2002;81:171–6.

99. Rhodus NL, Bloomquist C, Liljemark W, Bereuter J. Prevalence, density, and manifestations of oral *Candida albicans* in patients with Sjogren's syndrome. J Otolaryngol. 1997;26:300–5.

100. Tapper-Jones L, Aldred M, Walker D. Prevalence and intraoral distribution of *Candida albicans* in Sjogren's syndrome. J Clin Pathol. 1980;33:282.

101. Samaranayake YH, Samaranayake LP, Wu PC, So M. The antifungal effect of lactoferrin and lysozyme on *Candida krusei* and *Candida albicans*. APMIS. 1997;105:875–83.

102. Samaranayake L, MacFarlane T. Factors affecting the in-vitro adherence of the fungal oral pathogen *Candida albicans* to epithelial cells of human origin. Arch Oral Biol. 1982;27:869–73.

103. Samarkos M, Moutsopoulos HM. Recent advances in the management of ocular complications of Sjogren's syndrome. Curr Allergy Asthma Rep. 2005;5:327–32.

104. Tauber J, Davitt WF, Bokosky JE, Nichols KK, Yerxa BR, Schaberg AE, et al. Double-masked, placebo-controlled safety and efficacy trial of diquafosol tetrasodium (INS365) ophthalmic solution for the treatment of dry eye. Cornea. 2004;23:784–92.

105. Profita M, Sala A, Riccobono L, Pace E, PaternÚ A, Zarini S, et al. 15 (S)-HETE modulates LTB4 production and neutrophil chemotaxis in chronic bronchitis. Am J Physiol Cell Physiol. 2000;279:C1249.

106. Oka H, Nakano H, Kimata T, Matsuda T, Ozaki S. Effect of rebamipide for the treatment of xerostomia in patients with Sjogren's syndrome. Progr Med. 2004;24:205–10.

107. Ichikawa T, Ishihara K, Hayashida H, Hiruma H, Saigenji K, Hotta K. Effects of ecabet sodium, a novel gastroprotective agent, on mucin metabolism in rat gastric mucosa. Dig Dis Sci. 2000;45:606–13.

108. Nakamura M, Endo K, Nakata K, Hamano T. Gefarnate stimulates secretion of mucin-like glycoproteins by corneal epithelium in vitro and protects corneal epithelium from desiccation in vivo. Exp Eye Res. 1997;65:569–74.

109. Carsons S. A review and update of Sjogren's syndrome: manifestations, diagnosis, and treatment. Am J Manag Care. 2001;7:433–43.

110. Graziottin A. Clinical approach to dyspareunia. J Sex Marital Ther. 2001;27:489–501.

111. Fleming Cole N, Toy EC, Baker B. Sjogren's syndrome. Prim Care Update Ob Gyns. 2001;8:48–51.

112. Johnson EO, Skopouli FN, Moutsopoulos HM. Neuroendocrine manifestations in Sjogren's syndrome [In Process Citation]. Rheum Dis Clin North Am. 2000;26:927–49.

113. Colditz GA, Hankinson SE, Hunter DJ, Willett WC, Manson JAE, Stampfer MJ, et al. The use of estrogens and progestins and the risk of breast cancer in postmenopausal women. N Engl J Med. 1995;332:1589–93.

114. Buyon JP, Kalunian KC, Skovron ML, Petri M, Lahita R, Merrill J, et al. Can women with systemic lupus erythematosus safely use exogenous estrogens? JCR: J Clin Rheumatol. 1995;1:205.

115. Buyon JP, Petri MA, Kim MY, Kalunian KC, Grossman J, Hahn BH, et al. The effect of combined estrogen and progesterone hormone replacement therapy on disease activity in systemic lupus erythematosus: a randomized trial. Ann Intern Med. 2005;142:953–62.
116. Petri M. Long-term outcomes in lupus. Am J Manag Care. 2001;7:S480–5.
117. Sullivan DA, Belanger A, Cermak JM, Berube R, Papas AS, Sullivan RM, et al. Are women with Sjögren's syndrome androgen-deficient? J Rheumatol. 2003;30:2413–9.
118. Petri MA, Lahita RG, van Vollenhoven RF, Merrill J, Schiff M, Ginzler EM, et al. Effects of prasterone on corticosteroid requirements of women with systemic lupus erythematosus. Arthritis Rheum. 2002;46:1820–9.
119. Petri M. Exogenous estrogen in systemic lupus erythematosus: oral contraceptives and hormone replacement therapy. Lupus. 2001;10:222–6.

Chapter 37
Treatment of B-Cell Lymphoma

Michael Voulgarelis and Haralampos M. Moutsopoulos

Contents

37.1 Introduction

Sjögren's syndrome (SS) displays the highest incidence of malignant lymphoprolif-erative disorders among all of the autoimmune diseases. This association was high-lighted in studies performed at the National Institutes of Health in the 1970s [1, 2] and verified in a meta-analysis that estimated the risk of Non-Hodgkin's lymphoma (NHL) among the classic autoimmune diseases [3]. This meta-analysis reported that the possibility of an overt malignant lymphoproliferation is higher among SS patients (random effects standardized incidence rate (SIR) of 18.9 [95% confidence interval 9.4, 37.9]). By comparison, the SIRs for lymphoma among patients with systemic lupus erythematosus and rheumatoid arthritis were 7.52 and 3.25, respectively [3].

M. Voulgarelis (✉) • H.M. Moutsopoulos
Department of Pathophysiology, School of Medicine, National University of Athens,
Athens, Greece

M. Ramos-Casals et al. (eds.), *Sjögren's Syndrome*,
DOI 10.1007/978-0-85729-947-5_37, © Springer-Verlag London Limited 2012

Thus, along with *Helicobacter pylori*–positive gastric mucosa–associated lymphoid tissue (MALT) lymphomas, SS is a paradigm of antigen-driven lymphomatous evolution [4].

Clinical studies on SS-related lymphoma have been hampered by their relatively low incidence, the consequent challenges in performing large prospective studies, the lack of a universal approach to treatment, and by the absence of consensus in hematopathology with regard to nomenclature and classification. Despite these limitations, significant progress in the field has been recognized in recent years.

The life-time prevalence of NHL development in SS patients ranges between 5% and 10%, with the median age at lymphoma diagnosis being 58 years (range 33–82 years) and the median time from SS diagnosis to lymphoma evolution 7.5 years [1, 5, 6]. More than 98% of SS-associated lymphomas are of B-cell origin, of which 80% are low-grade lymphomas. These low-grade lymphomas include extranodal marginal zone (MZ) tumors of the MALT type (52.5%) and nodal MZ lymphomas (NMZL) (12.5%). Follicular and lymphoplasmacytic lymphomas occur much less commonly. High-grade, diffuse large B-cell lymphomas (DLBCL) account for 17.5% of lymphoma cases in SS [6].

In this review, we present current treatment approaches in patients with SS-associated B-cell NHLs and emphasize the need for tailored therapy according to the lymphoma subtype and patients' individual clinical characteristics. We highlight recent advances in the natural history of SS-related lymphomas that influence therapeutic strategies, explore existing controversies in the field, and indicate areas that require additional investigation.

37.2 Marginal Zone (MZ) Lymphomas

The three major subtypes of MZ lymphomas are extranodal MZ B-cell lymphomas of the MALT type (MALT lymphoma), primary splenic lymphomas, and NMZL. Each of these MZ lymphoma types represents a clinically and prognostically unique subcategory within the present World Health Organization (WHO) classification [7]. MALT lymphomas represent the vast majority of MZ lymphomas, whereas the other two entities are relatively rare disorders. MALT lymphomas were named after the lymphoid micro-anatomic compartment that nourishes its presumed normal counterpart, the MZ. The MZ is situated around the follicular mantle at the periphery of the splenic white pulp, as well as at the periphery of lymphoid follicles (Fig. 37.1). The MZ fosters B-cell populations of varied maturation stages that, although functionally heterogeneous, share the capacities for plasma cell differentiation and homing to certain tissue compartments (Fig. 37.2).

MZ lymphomas are the most common type of tumors encountered in SS patients [5, 6, 8]. According to one study, patients with SS exhibited a 28-fold higher risk of developing a MZ lymphoma compared with the general population [9]. Two recent, population-based Scandinavian studies reported a somewhat lower risk [9, 10].

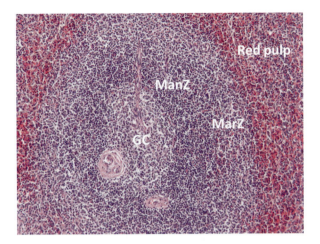

Fig. 37.1 Splenic lymphoid follicle: Structure and elements. The lymphoid follicle has a pale-staining germinal centers (*GC*) in which B-cells are proliferating. Note the presence of a mantle zone (*ManZ*) that contains small lymphocytes and an outer marginal zone (*MarZ*) that contains larger lymphocytes that are less packed than cell in the ManZ. Outside the MarZ is the red pulp. MarZs are more evident in splenic follicles than lymph node follicles (H&E, ×200)

37.2.1   *Extranodal Marginal Zone Lymphomas of MALT Type*

As a rule, MALT lymphomas are indolent. They are located at mucosal and non-mucosal extranodal sites that contain epithelium, usually columnar epithelium [11, 12]. The majority of these sites are normally devoid of any organized lymphoid element, but the neo-formation of an acquired MALT component, elicited by certain external anti-genic challenges, precedes MALT lymphoma development. Although MALT lympho-mas are pathogenetically associated with diverse stimuli such as infection (*Helicobacter pylori*) or autoimmune insults (Hashimoto thyroiditis), all appear to derive from neo-plastic transformation of MZ B lymphocytes [13–15]. The histological features of MALT lymphoma closely simulate the original lymphoepithelial complexes of Peyer's patches. Characteristic features include reactive lymphoid follicles, with or without colonization by neoplastic cells of MZ and/or monocytoid morphology (centrocyte-like cells) that infiltrate the overlying epithelium (lymphoepithelial lesions). These neo-plastic cells are admixed with small B lymphocytes and plasma cells that may or may not be neoplastic [16] (Fig. 37.3).

Lymphoepithelial sialadenitis, the histologic hallmark of SS, is characterized by a lymphoid population that surrounds and infiltrates the salivary ducts. Lymphoepithelial lesions result from the disorganization and proliferation of ductal epithelial cells [17]. These lesions, which appear first as small clusters, progres-sively organize into lymphoid follicle-like structures that contain germinal centers. The phenotype of these immunocompetent cells, mainly primed CD4+ T lympho-cytes, suggests the formation of activated follicular structures in which activated B-cells produce autoantibodies [18–20]. This MALT component, acquired

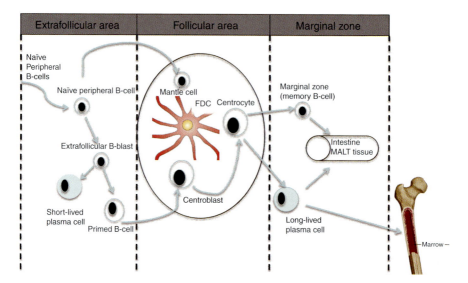

Fig. 37.2 B-cell maturation in the peripheral lymph nodes. After leaving the bone marrow, the naive mature B-cells initially migrate to the outer region of the lymph node in the "primary" follicles to later transfer to the follicle mantles. Subsequently, these IgM+/IgD + cells come into contact with antigen and transform into proliferating extrafollicular B blasts, from which short-lived plasma cells and "primed" B-cells are derived. These "primed" B-cells stimulate and sustain the germinal center reaction, during which they transform into rapidly proliferating centroblasts. During the mitotic proliferation and differentiation of the centroblasts into centrocytes, somatic mutations in the variable region of the immunoglobulin genes emerge in a randomized manner. The centrocytes with mutations that lead to an increase in the affinity of the immunoglobulin receptor differentiate further, enabling them to pass out of the germinal center into the marginal zone to become long-lived plasma cells or "memory" B-cells. The long-lived plasma cells predominantly populate the bone marrow and organs that are directly exposed to foreign antigens (gastrointestinal tract). Memory IgM+CD27+ B-cells are the counterpart of MZ cells and possess preferential homing to mucosa-associated lymphoid tissue sites (Peyer's patches, bronchus, larynx)

Fig. 37.3 Lymphoepithelial lesions in MALT lymphoma of salivary gland. Centrocyte-like cells surround the salivary ducts and infiltrate the epithelium to form lymphoepithelial lesions (*arrow*). Within the lesions, the majority of the intraepithelial lymphocytes have a similar morphology to the neoplastic cells of the surrounding lymphomatous infiltrate. (H&E, × 200). *MALT* mucosa-associated lymphoid tissue

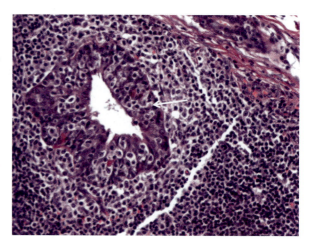

secondarily to the autoimmune process, represents the substrate from which B-cell lymphomatous proliferation develops.

The distinction between lymphoepithelial sialadenitis with features of acquired MALT and MALT lymphoma remains both obscure and controversial, because clonally expanded populations of B-cells have been detected in both conditions. The distinction still relies upon the identification of particular morphological features. The presence of centrocyte-like, monocytoid and plasmacytoid cells that form broad halos around epithelial nests or broad strands and interconnect lymphoepithelial lesions are features consistent with a neoplastic process (Fig. 37.4). Other features indicating MALT lymphoma include the secondary infiltration of the reactive germinal centers by malignant lymphocytes, the presence of atypical plasma cells that contain Dutcher bodies (nuclear inclusions), clusters of histiocytes, and overt fibrosis. All the above, along with monoclonality confirmed by immunophenotyping, establish the MALT lymphoma diagnosis [17].

In SS patients, MZ lymphomas of the MALT type are primarily low-grade and localized (stage I and II) to extranodal areas [5] (Table 37.1). The salivary glands are the most commonly affected site, but other common extranodal sites are the stomach, nasopharynx, ocular adnexa, skin, liver, kidney, and lung. Twenty percent of patients display involvement of more than one extranodal site at diagnosis, illustrating the preferential migration of these cells to multiple mucosal sites. This fact emphasizes the importance of extensive staging procedures in SS patients with MALT lymphomas.

Loco-regional lymph node involvement is common with MALT lymphomas, but generalized peripheral lymphadenopathy is extremely rare. Major salivary gland enlargement, particularly of both parotid glands, is the typical presenting symptom. Most patients display indolent disease with good performance status and the absence of B symptoms, splenomegaly, and bone marrow infiltration. Elevated levels of lactate dehydrogenase (LDH) or beta 2-microglobulin levels are unusual. SS patients with MALT lymphomas frequently also have concurrent vasculitis affecting the peripheral nerves, skin, and kidneys. Anemia, lymphopenia, paraproteinemia, and mixed monoclonal cryoglobulinemia (type II) contribute further to a distinctive clinical syndrome that is not encountered in MALT lymphomas that are unrelated to SS.

Regardless of the affected site at presentation, diagnostic studies should include the standard lymphoma staging procedures and the examination of Waldeyer's ring with complete blood count; basic biochemical studies; serum protein electrophoresis; and assays for lactate dehydrogenase, beta 2-microglobulin, and cryoglobulins. Computed tomographic scans of the chest, abdomen, and pelvis are also appropriate, as is bone marrow biopsy (Table 37.2). The initial staging should include a gastroduodenal endoscopy with multiple biopsies from gastro-esophageal junction, each region of the stomach, and the duodenum. *H. pylori* infection also needs to be either confirmed or excluded. Fresh biopsy and washings material should be available for cytogenetic studies in addition to routine histology and immunohistochemistry.

Sites commonly involved by MALT lymphomas may require special diagnostic procedures. Ultrasonography and magnetic resonance imaging are useful for investigations of the thyroid, soft tissues (hard palate), salivary glands, and orbits. Primary bronchial mucosa–associated lymphoid tissue lymphoma requires histological

Fig. 37.4 Parotid MALT lymphoma in Sjögren's syndrome. (**a**) Neoplastic marginal zone cells infiltrate around salivary duct remnants. The lymphoid cells form broad strands interconnecting lymphoepithelial lesions (H&E, ×200) (*arrow*). (**b**) Atypical lymphoid cells diffusely positive for CD20 (immunostaining with L26 antibody ×100). (**c**) In addition, there were about four times more lambda light-chain-positive plasma cells than kappa light-chain-positive cells

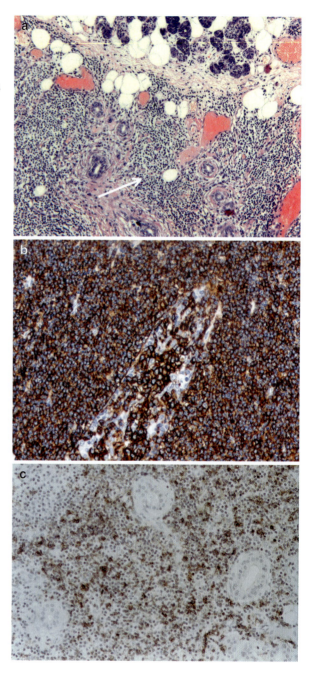

Table 37.1 Clinical characteristics of Sjögren's syndrome patients with MALT lymphomas

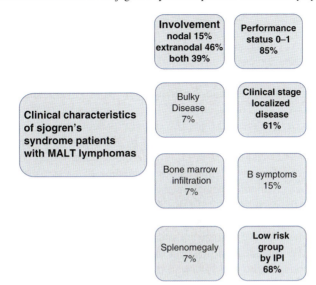

Bulky Disease: Tumor mass size >7 cm

B symptoms: Unexplained weight loss of >10% of body weight in 6 months; unexplained, persistent or recurrent fever >38°C; recurrent drenching night sweats

IPI: International prognostic index. One point is assigned for each of the following parameters: Age greater than 60 years, stage III or IV, elevated serum LDH, ECOG/Zubrod performance status of 2, 3, or 4, and more than 1 extranodal site. The sum of the points allotted correlates with the following risk groups: Low risk (0–1 points), Low-intermediate risk (2 points), High-intermediate risk (3 points), and High risk (4–5 points)

Table 37.2 Staging for MALT lymphoma in Sjögren's syndrome

History

Physical examination

CT scan (neck, thorax, abdomen)

Laboratory tests

• Blood count

• LDH levels

• Immunofixation

• Liver and renal function

• HCV, HIV serology

• Cryoglobulins

• Functional thyroid tests

• C4 levels

• Albumin levels

• Beta-2 microglobulin

Bone marrow biopsy

Gastric endoscopy

Optionally, based on symptoms

• Endoscopic ultrasound

• Bronchoscopy and lavage

• Orbit MRI and ophthalmologic examination

assessment by bronchoscopy. Any pulmonary mass or pleural effusion detected should be examined histopathologically. The difficulty in staging MALT lymphoma lies in the application of traditional staging systems for nodal-type lymphoma in extranodal MALT lymphoma. The Ann Arbor system is based on the extension from contiguous nodes and can be misleading in MALT lymphomas, because the involvement of multiple extranodal sites may not reflect truly disseminated disease.

Several studies demonstrate that non-gastric MALT lymphomas in the general population have a good outcome [21, 22]. Five-year survival rates have ranged from 86 to 100%. Despite the fact that 30% of these patients present with disseminated disease, their outcome remains unaffected by the multi-focal nature of the lymphoma (5-year survival of 90%) [23]. Furthermore, none of the conventional oncologic approaches appear to influence the outcome of these patients. It has been suggested that chemotherapeutic intervention may be ineffective in preventing recurrence in the early stage of the disease [23].

Some patients with persistent disease can be allowed to go untreated for prolonged periods of time yet have normal life spans. A retrospective analysis by Ambrosetti et al. reported no significant differences in outcomes among SS patients with salivary MALT lymphomas who underwent no treatment or received a variety of treatment modalities, including surgery, radiotherapy, and chemotherapy [24]. This is consistent with a study conducted by our department, in which SS patients with salivary MALT lymphomas had a quite uncomplicated clinical course with a median overall survival of 6.4 years. Notably, at a median follow-up of 6 years, treated and untreated patients with MALT lymphomas showed the same overall survival [5]. Conversely, patients with nodal involvement or advanced disease, defined by concomitant nodal and extranodal and/or bone marrow infiltration, exhibit worse prognoses [23, 25].

The international prognostic index defines various risk groups according to clinical and laboratory parameters including age, stage, involvement of more than one extranodal site, lactate dehydrogenase level, and performance status. Patients determined to be at high risk of death by this index also have a poor prognosis [26].

The natural history of MALT lymphomas suggests a two-stage dissemination process. During the initial phase, the tumors spread to other MALT sites. In the second phase, the lymph nodes and bone marrow become affected [23]. Consequently, treatment should be "patient *and* case tailored," taking into account the site and stage of the lymphoma along with the international prognostic index and clinical characteristics of the individual patient. In addition, bulky tumor, serologic markers such as elevated beta 2-microglobulin or reduced albumin levels, and the presence of a large-cell component in tissue histology at diagnosis are also linked to poor outcomes [26, 27].

37.2.2 Therapeutic Approaches of MALT Lymphomas

For SS patients with MALT lymphoma localized to the salivary glands or other regions (stage IE), a "wait and watch" policy is appropriate. Chemotherapy is reserved for patients with disseminated lymphoma that infiltrates multiple (not regional) lymph nodes and/or bone marrow, as well as for those who fall into the high-risk category according to the international prognosis index. This strategy may be especially appropriate for elderly patients who have asymptomatic disease, as well as for those with substantial comorbidities that preclude a vigorous therapeutic approach.

Alkylating agents (cyclophosphamide, chlorambucil), purine analogues (fludarabine, cladribine), and anti-CD20 monoclonal antibody therapy are all suitable options for disseminated disease, but these recommendations have not been substantiated by large patient series and randomized trials [28–30]. In patients with disseminated MALT lymphoma at presentation who do not have SS, single chemotherapeutic agents such as alkylating agents and nucleoside analogues achieve a 75% complete remission rate, with projected 5-year event-free and overall survival rates of 50% and 75%, respectively [28]. However, responses differ dramatically according to whether patients have gastric or non-gastric involvement of their MALT lymphomas; patients without gastric involvement fare substantially worse [30].

In a study conducted by our department, 75% of patients with SS-associated MALT lymphomas achieved complete responses following treatment with 2-chloro-2-deoxyadenosine [31]. OSS features, namely xerostomia, parotid gland enlargement, salivary flows, and hyposthenuria, also showed improvement, and the disappearance of cryoglobulins and monoclonal bands within the urine was also observed. In addition to its direct cytotoxic potential, 2-chloro-2-deoxyadenosine has been associated with a profound T-cell depletion. The potential implication of antigen-specific T-cells in MALT lymphoma pathogenesis explains the favorable effect of this agent in these lymphomas [32]. When considering this type of treatment, it is important to weigh the indolent nature of these malignancies against the potentially severe adverse effects that may accompany purine analogue administration.

Anti-CD20 monoclonal antibody strategies may also have a place in the management of MALT lymphoma. High response rates are particularly observed in untreated patients [29]. Preliminary studies have documented benefits of B-cell depletion with an anti-CD20 monoclonal antibody for the glandular and extraglandular manifestations of SS patients [33–35]. The overall response rate appears to be on the order of 75%. However, anti-CD20 treatments are not universally effective in SS patients with MALT lymphomas [36]. Responses may differ according to the particular tissues involved because this treatment may fail to eliminate distinct B-cell sub-populations, e.g., MZ cells. Anti-CD20 treatments may also be antagonized by microenvironmental factors that promote B-cell survival, as recently has been described in a murine model of SS [37, 38].

Recurrences of MALT lymphoma at the same or different nodal or extranodal sites have been reported in 25–35% of patients, even years after the achievement complete responses. This highlights the need for life-long follow-up [29]. The roles of higher doses of rituximab (or other B-cell depletion strategies), maintenance treatment, and combination therapy with conventional chemotherapeutic agents require further exploration. All of these approaches have proven beneficial in other types of lymphoma [39]. The combination of anti-CD20 monoclonal antibody administration with fludarabine or 2-chloro-2-deoxyadenosine has been reported to achieve a high complete response rate in both gastric and non-gastric MALT lymphomas [40, 41]. The concomitant use of an anti-CD20 monoclonal antibody with

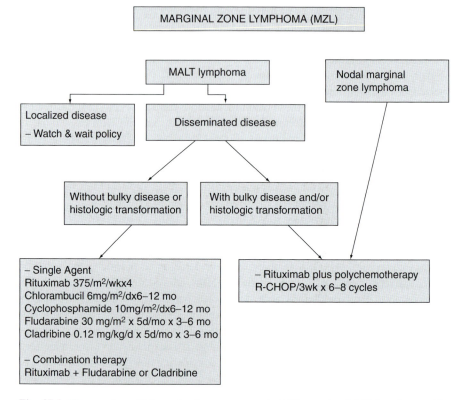

Fig. 37.5 Therapeutic guidelines for the management of SS-associated MZ lymphomas. No established guidelines have been developed for the treatment of extranodal salivary MALT lymphomas in SS patients. Our policy for the management of these lymphomas is presented in this figure. In localized disease, a wait and see policy is adopted with close follow-up. If lymphoma is disseminated with nodal and bone marrow involvement or the patients have several risk factors according to IPI, single agent chemotherapy such as chorambucil, 2cda, or rituximab is administered. Doxorubicin-based combined chemotherapy should be reserved for patients who have a high-grade transformation or high tumor burden as indicated by high LDH levels, a tumor mass greater than 7 cm, and bulky regional nodal involvement. In our experience, the use of R-CHOP regimen as a first-line treatment appears to be effective in SS patients with NMZLs

2-chloro-2-deoxyadenosine increases the response rate and quality of response, significantly prolonging the time to treatment failure. In addition, an increased number of patients treated with this combination proved negative for minimal residual disease, which correlates with a longer time to treatment failure [41]. Figure 37.5 illustrates our algorithm for the management of MZ lymphomas in SS patients.

Prospective, multicenter, large series, randomized, double-blinded studies of SS patients with MALT lymphoma are needed to compare different chemotherapy regimens and determine the optimal approach for patients with disseminated or relapsing disease. Potentially active drugs could also include those that target the inhibition of the $NF\kappa B$ pathway, the downstream molecular product of the translocations involving MALT1 gene, such as bortezomid. The frequency of translocations involving

MALT1 appears to be low in SS patients with non-gastric MALT lymphomas. In contrast, t(11;18)(q21;q21) which involves the MALT1 gene frequently occurs in patients with gastric MALT lymphoma and SS, which may explain, in part, why these patients are largely resistant to *H. pylori* eradication therapy [42]. Interestingly, the t(11;18)(q21;q21), specific to MALT-type lymphoma, is found in 18–24% of patients with gastric MALT lymphoma. In addition to antimicrobial therapy failure, this specific translocation is accompanied by a resistance to alkylating agents but is a marker for sensitivity to an anti-CD20 monoclonal antibody [43–45].

37.2.3 Nodal Marginal Zone B-Cell Lymphomas (NMZL): Histology, Differential Diagnosis, and Outcome

Patients with NMZL have worse outcomes compared to those with MALT lymphomas. The 5-year survival rates in NMZL range between 50% and 70% [46]. The survival curves for NMZL do not display any plateau, suggesting that disease is not with current treatments. The 5-year event-free survival is approximately 30%. The estimated median time to progression ranges between 1 and 2 years [47]. At diagnosis, 20% of patients have lymph node histology that reveals an increased percentage of large cells (>20%) and a high mitotic rate, indicating a transformation to diffuse large B-cell lymphoma [47].

More than two-thirds of SS patients with NMZL present with an advanced stage, displaying peripheral, abdominal nodal involvement and splenomegaly [6]. The nodal spread of MALT lymphoma in a patient with SS could resemble a NMZL, because the lymph node histologies in these conditions share several morphological features. However, isolated or disseminated lymphadenopathy in the absence of extranodal lesions should alert the clinician to the possibility of NMZL. NMZL may show different patterns of lymph node infiltration such as "marginal zone"-like/ perifollicular, nodular, diffuse, or a combination of patterns [48] (Fig. 37.6). As a consequence, it is impossible to distinguish NMZL from MALT lymphoma by morphology or immunohistochemistry. Only thorough clinical staging can confirm a NMZL in the absence of concurrent extranodal involvement (Table 37.3).

37.2.4 Managing NMZL

NMZLs resemble other primary nodal B-cell lymphomas such as follicular with respect to B symptoms, elevated serum concentrations of lactate dehydrogenase, performance status, and international prognosis index. NMZL represents a therapeutic dilemma because precise therapeutic guidelines do not exist, owing largely to the absence of data from studies with substantial numbers of cases. The current therapies for NMZL are heterogeneous and determined by the age of the patient and the clinical stage aggressiveness of the tumor. NMZL typically has a short time to progression. Feasible treatment options include polychemotherapy with anthracycline-based chemotherapy combined with an anti-CD20 monoclonal antibody. In our experience,

Fig. 37.6 SS-associated nodal marginal zone B-cell lymphoma (NMZL). (**a**) Lymph node infiltration by NMZL is characterized by a predominant population of small- to medium-sized centrocyte-like, monocytoid B-cells and scattered transformed B-cells (H&E, ×400). (**b**) Staining (anti-CD21 ×200) for follicular dendritic cells (DDCs) reveals overrun follicles by showing residual meshwork of FDCs indicative of follicular colonization. The tumor cells surround reactive follicles and expand into the interfollicular areas. These results, together with the histological findings, confirmed that the lesion represented a B-cell marginal zone lymphoma. The clinical staging confirms the diagnosis of NMZL in the absence of extranodal involvement

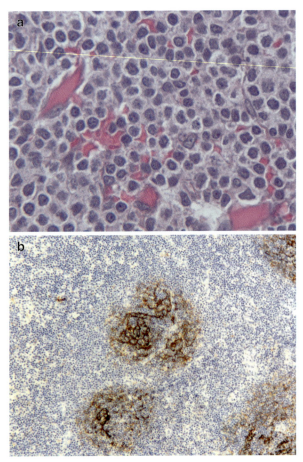

the use of R-CHOP (a regimen comprising an anti-CD20 monoclonal antibody plus cyclophosphamide/doxorubicin/vincristine/prednisone) as a first-line treatment appears to be effective in SS patients with NMZL, although long-term results are still needed [49–51]. In young patients who experience disease relapses, autologous bone marrow transplantation should be considered [52].

37.3   Diffuse Large B-Cell Lymphomas

37.3.1   Histology and General Considerations

In some patients with SS, lymphomas tend to evolve toward less differentiated (higher grade) cell types [5]. The transition from benign chronic lymphoepithelial sialadenitis to indolent MALT lymphomas and possibly to high-grade lymphoma,

Table 37.3 Clinical and histological features of 26 SS patients who developed marginal zone B-cell lymphoma

	MALT (%) lymphoma	Nodal marginal zone lymphoma (%)
Cases	21/26 (80.8)	5/26 (19.2)
Sex		
Male	1(4.8%)	0 (0)
Female	20 (95.2%)	5 (100)
Age		
Mean ± SD	50.71 ± 11.6	48 ± 9.4
Range	30–74	37–61
Ann Arbor stage		
I–II	16 (76.2)	1 (20)
III–IV	5 (23.8)	4 (80)
Nodal involvement	3 (14.3)	5 (100)
Extranodal involvement[a]	21(100)	1 (20)
Both nodal and extranodal	3 (14.3)	1 (20)
Bulky disease[b]	1 (4.8)	1 (20)
B-symptoms[c]	2 (9.5)	1 (20)
Splenomegaly	2 (9.5)	4 (80)
Bone marrow involvement	4 (19)	3 (60)

[a]Parotid gland, submandibular salivary gland, lacrimal gland, lung
[b]Tumor mass size >7 cm
[c]Unexplained weight loss of >10% of body weight in 6 months; unexplained, persistent or recurrent fever >38°C; recurrent, drenching night sweats

e.g., DLBCL, represents a multi-step process caused by genetic alterations such as p53 allelic loss and mutations, hypermethylation of p15 and p16 genes, and p16 gene deletions [53, 54]. The histological transformation of MALT lymphoma to DLBCL is heralded by the emergence of an increased number of transformed blasts that form sheets or clusters, which eventually effaces the preceding MALT lymphoma (Fig. 37.7). It is unclear how many DLBCLs arise from preexisting MALT, nodal or follicular lymphomas. Immunohistochemical, karyotypic, and genotypic studies have provided convincing proof that the supervening large-cell lymphomas arise from the same clone as the low-grade lymphomas [53]. Thus, the majority of high-grade lymphomas in SS patients may represent blastic-variance of either MZ B-cell or follicular center cell lymphomas.

SS patients with DLBCLs tend to be older than those with MALT lymphomas, with a median age at diagnosis of 58.4 versus 50.7 years respectively [6]. During transformation, the clinical picture is characterized by further nodal and extranodal dissemination [5]. The histologic transformation to high-grade lymphoma always denotes a poor prognosis. Consequently, it is crucial to identify de novo and secondary DLBCLs in SS patients since median overall survival is estimated at less than 2 years [5].

Fig. 37.7 Diffuse large
B-cell lymphoma in Sjögren's
syndrome. Lymph node
biopsy demonstrates a diffuse
proliferation of large
lymphoid cells that have
totally effaced the
architecture

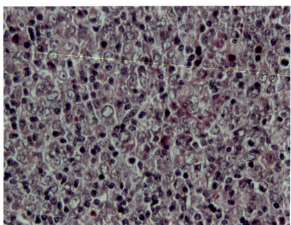

37.3.2 Treatment of DLBCL

Combined chemotherapy is recommended for patients with de novo or transformed DLBCL [50, 51]. A number of aggressive induction regimens have been used and evaluated in clinical studies, but large randomized trials have reported that the less aggressive classical CHOP chemotherapy (cyclophosphamide/doxorubicin/vincristine/prednisone) has comparable CR and overall survival rates. However, the median survival of SS patients with DLBCL treated with CHOP is estimated to be only 1.8 years [5]. The presence of B symptoms and a large tumor diameter (>7 cm) are independent death risk factors. In addition, CHOP therapy combined with an anti-CD20 monoclonal antibody (R-CHOP) has been shown to have a significant clinical effect in DLBCL among the general population, increasing both response rate and survival. These observations prompted us to use this regimen for the treatment of six SS patients with aggressive NHL [50, 51]. A major finding of our study was that R-CHOP induced sustained CR in all SS patients for a follow-up period of 2 years. Moreover, the extranodal manifestations of these patients, such as peripheral neuropathy and skin vasculitis, resolved after 8 cycles of R-CHOP. The remission of these symptoms and signs was accompanied by a decrease in the circulating mixed cryoglobulins as well as an increase in C4 complement component levels, indicating that this regimen effectively controls both the autoimmune and neoplastic process.

SS patients with unfavorable IPI score and involvement of more than one extranodal site are at a much higher risk of CNS disease, and should therefore be given CNS prophylaxis with intrathecal methotrexate injections [55]. Specific extranodal sites appear to be more frequently associated with CNS involvement, namely the testes, paranasal sinuses, hard palate, orbit, paravertebral masses, and bone marrow. Our observations warrant larger controlled trials to assess the effectiveness of this regimen.

37.4 Conclusions

SS-associated lymphomas are a heterogeneous group of malignancies. The most common subtype, accounting for up to 60% of lymphomas, is MZ lymphoma of MALT type. Recently, significant advances in our understanding of the morphology, phenotype, etiology, pathogenesis, and natural history, as well as the use of WHO classification of lymphoid neoplasms, have begun to elucidate the differences between MALT lymphoma and other lymphoproliferative disorders, enabling the identification of prognostic tissue markers. Beyond chemotherapy, a variety of new treatment options have emerged in the management of patients with SS MALT lymphoma, with B-cell depletion with monoclonal antibody therapy being the most significant. Nevertheless, the lack of large multicenter studies and the rarity of the disease prevent the proposal of a definite treatment approach.

Patients with low-grade lymphoma types, especially MALT lymphomas, including those with disseminated extranodal disease, should be managed conservatively with an anti-CD20 monoclonal antibody or other mild chemotherapeutic agents. In contrast, disease features that indicate high-grade disease are markers for poor prognosis. In patients who are otherwise young and fit, aggressive, multi-agent approaches to treatment may be indicated.

References

1. Kassan SS, Thomas TL, Moutsopoulos HM, et al. Increased risk of lymphoma in sicca syndrome. *Ann Intern Med.* 1978;89:888-92.
2. Bunim JJ, Talal N. Development of malignant lymphoma in the course of Sjogren's syndrome. *Trans Assoc Am Physicians.* 1963;76:45-56.
3. Zintzaras E, Voulgarelis M, Moutsopoulos HM. The risk of lymphoma development in autoimmune diseases: a meta-analysis. *Arch Intern Med.* 2005;165:2337-44.
4. Suarez F, Lortholary O, Hermine O, et al. Infection-associated lymphomas derived from marginal zone B cells: a model of antigen-driven lymphoproliferation. *Blood.* 2006;107:3034-44.
5. Voulgarelis M, Dafni UG, Isenberg DA, et al. Malignant lymphoma in primary Sjogren's syndrome: a multicenter, retrospective, clinical study by the European Concerted Action on Sjogren's Syndrome. *Arthritis Rheum.* 1999;42:1765-72.
6. Baimpa E, Dahabreh IJ, Voulgarelis M, et al. Hematologic manifestations and predictors of lymphoma development in primary Sjögren syndrome: clinical and pathophysiologic aspects. *Medicine (Baltimore).* 2009;88:284-93.
7. Harris NL, Jaffe ES, Diebold J, et al. The World Health Organization classification of hematological malignancies report of the Clinical Advisory Committee Meeting, Airlie House, Virginia, November 1997. *Mod Pathol.* 2000;13:193-207.
8. Royer B, Cazals-Hatem D, Sibilia J, et al. Lymphomas in patients with Sjogren's syndrome are marginal zone B-cell neoplasms, arise in diverse extranodal and nodal sites and are not associated with viruses. *Blood.* 1997;90:766-75.
9. Smedby KE, Hjalgrim H, Askling J, et al. Autoimmune and chronic inflammatory disorders and risk of non-Hodgkin lymphoma by subtype. *J Natl Cancer Inst.* 2006;98:51-60.
10. Theander E, Henriksson G, Ljungberg O, et al. Lymphoma and other malignancies in primary Sjogren's syndrome: a cohort study on cancer incidence and lymphoma predictors. *Ann Rheum Dis.* 2006;65:796-803.

11. Pelstring RJ, Essell JH, Kurtin PJ, Cohen AR, Banks PM. Diversity of organ site involvement among malignant lymphomas of mucosa-associated tissues. *Am J Clin Pathol.* 1991;96:738-45.
12. Dogan A, Du M, Koulis A, et al. Expression of lymphocyte homing receptors and vascular addressins in low-grade gastric B-cell lymphomas of mucosa-associated lymphoid tissue. *Am J Pathol.* 1997;151:1361-9.
13. Bahler DW, Swerdlow SH. Clonal salivary gland infiltrates associated with myoepithelial sialadenitis (Sjogren's syndrome) begin as nonmalignant antigen-selected expansions. *Blood.* 1998;91:1864-72.
14. Martin T, Weber JC, Levallois H, et al. Salivary gland lymphomas in patients with Sjogren's syndrome may frequently develop from rheumatoid factors B cells. *Arthritis Rheum.* 2000;43:908-16.
15. D'Elios MM, Manghetti M, Almerigogna F, et al. Different cytokine profile and antigen-specificity repertoire in Helicobacter pylori-specific T cell clones from the antrum of chronic gastritis patients with or without peptic ulcer. *Eur J Immunol.* 1997;27:1751-5.
16. Isaacson PG, Spencer J. Malignant lymphoma of mucosa-associated lymphoid tissue. *Histopathology.* 1987;11:445-62.
17. DiGiuseppe JA, Corio RL, Westa WH. Lymphoid infiltrates of the salivary glands: pathology, biology and clinical significance. *Curr Opin Oncol.* 1996;8:232-7.
18. Stott DI, Hiepe F, Hummel M, et al. Antigen-driven clonal proliferation of B cells within target tissue of an autoimmune disease. The salivary glands of patients with Sjogren's syndrome. *J Clin Invest.* 1998;102:938-46.
19. Adamson TC, Fox RI, Frisman DM, et al. Immunohistologic analysis of lymphoid infiltrates in primary Sjogren's syndrome using monoclonal antibodies. *J Immunol.* 1983;130:203-8.
20. Boumba D, Skopouli FN, Moutsopoulos HM. Cytokine mRNA expression in the labial salivary gland tissues from patients with primary Sjogren's syndrome. *Br J Rheumatol.* 1995;34:326-33.
21. Zinzani PL, Magagnoli M, Galieni P, et al. Nongastrointestinal low-grade mucosa-associated lymphoid tissue lymphoma: analysis of 75 patients. *J Clin Oncol.* 1999;17:1254-8.
22. Zucca E, Conconi A, Pedrinis E, et al. Nongastric marginal zone B-cell lymphoma of mucosa-associated lymphoid tissue. *Blood.* 2003;101:2489-95.
23. Thieblemont C, Berger F, Dumontet C, et al. Mucosa-associated lymphoid tissue lymphoma is a disseminated disease in one third of 158 patients analyzed. *Blood.* 2000;95:802-6.
24. Ambrosetti A, Zanotti R, Pattaro C, et al. Most cases of primary salivary mucosa-associated lymphoid tissue lymphoma are associated either with Sjoegren syndrome or hepatitis C virus infection. *Br J Haematol.* 2004;126:43-9.
25. Montalbán C, Castrillo JM, Abraira V, et al. Gastric B-cell mucosa-associated lymphoid tissue (MALT) lymphoma. Clinicopathological study and evaluation of the prognostic factors in 143 patients. *Ann Oncol.* 1995;6:355-62.
26. Thieblemont C, Bastion Y, Berger F, et al. Mucosa-associated lymphoid tissue gastrointestinal and nongastrointestinal lymphoma behavior: analysis of 108 patients. *J Clin Oncol.* 1997;15:1624-30.
27. Radaszkiewicz T, Dragosics B, Bauer P. Gastrointestinal malignant lymphomas of the mucosa-associated lymphoid tissue: factors relevant to prognosis. *Gastroenterology.* 1992;102:1628-38.
28. Hammel P, Haioun C, Chaumette MT, et al. Efficacy of single-agent chemotherapy in low-grade B-cell mucosa-associated lymphoid tissue lymphoma with prominent gastric expression. *J Clin Oncol.* 1995;13:2524-9.
29. Conconi A, Martinelli G, Thiéblemont C, et al. Clinical activity of rituximab in extranodal marginal zone B-cell lymphoma of MALT type. *Blood.* 2003;102:2741-5.
30. Jäger G, Neumeister P, Brezinschek R, et al. Treatment of extranodal marginal zone B-cell lymphoma of mucosa-associated lymphoid tissue type with cladribine: a phase II study. *J Clin Oncol.* 2002;20:3872-7.
31. Voulgarelis M, Petroutsos G, Moutsopoulos HM, et al. 2-chloro-2-deoxyadenosine in the treatment of Sjogren's syndrome-associated B cell lymphoproliferation. *Arthritis Rheum.* 2002;46:2248-9.
32. Hussell T, Isaacson PG, Crabtree JE, et al. Helicobacter pylori-specific tumour-infiltrating T cells provide contact dependent help for the growth of malignant B cells in low-grade gastric lymphoma of mucosa-associated lymphoid tissue. *J Pathol.* 1996;178:122-7.
33. Pijpe J, van Imhoff GW, Vissink A, et al. Changes in salivary gland immunohistology and function after rituximab monotherapy in a patient with Sjogren's syndrome and associated MALT lymphoma. *Ann Rheum Dis.* 2005;64:958-60.

34. Pijpe J, van Imhoff GW, Spijkervet FK, et al. Rituximab treatment in patients with primary Sjogren's syndrome: an open-label phase II study. *Arthritis Rheum.* 2005;52:2740-50.
35. Seror R, Sordet C, Guillevin L, et al. Tolerance and efficacy of rituximab and changes in serum B cell biomarkers in patients with systemic complications of primary Sjögren's syndrome. *Ann Rheum Dis.* 2007;66:351-7.
36. Quartuccio L, Fabris M, Moretti M, et al. Resistance to rituximab therapy and local BAFF overexpression in Sjögren's syndrome-related myoepithelial sialadenitis and low-grade parotid B-cell lymphoma. *Open Rheumatol J.* 2008;2:38-43.
37. De Vita S, Dolcetti R, Ferraccioli G, et al. Local cytokine expression in the progression toward B cell malignancy in Sjögren's syndrome. *J Rheumatol.* 1995;22:1674-80.
38. Gong Q, Ou Q, Ye S, et al. Importance of cellular microenvironment and circulatory dynamics in B cell immunotherapy. *J Immunol.* 2005;174:817-26.
39. Hainsworth JD, Litchy S, Burris HA 3rd, et al. Rituximab as first-line and maintenance therapy for patients with indolent non-Hodgkin's lymphoma. *J Clin Oncol.* 2002;20:4261-7.
40. Salar A, Domingo-Domenech E, Estany C, et al. Combination therapy with rituximab and intravenous or oral fludarabine in the first-line, systemic treatment of patients with extranodal marginal zone B-cell lymphoma of the mucosa-associated lymphoid tissue type. *Cancer.* 2009;115:5210-7.
41. Orciuolo E, Buda G, Sordi E, et al. 2CdA chemotherapy and rituximab in the treatment of marginal zone lymphoma. *Leuk Res.* 2010;34:184-9.
42. Streubel B, Huber D, Wohrer S, et al. Frequency of chromosomal aberrations involving MALT1 in mucosa-associated lymphoid tissue lymphoma in patients with Sjogren's syndrome. *Clin Cancer Res.* 2004;10:476-80.
43. Lévy M, Copie-Bergman C, Gameiro C, et al. Prognostic value of translocation t(11;18) in tumoral response of low-grade gastric lymphoma of mucosa-associated lymphoid tissue type to oral chemotherapy. *J Clin Oncol.* 2005;23:5061-6.
44. Liu H, Ruskon-Fourmestraux A, Lavergne-Slove A, et al. Resistance of t(11;18) positive gastric mucosa-associated lymphoid tissue lymphoma to Helicobacter pylori eradication therapy. *Lancet.* 2001;357(9249):39-40.
45. Martinelli G, Laszlo D, Ferreri AJ, et al. Clinical activity of rituximab in gastric marginal zone non-Hodgkin's lymphoma resistant to or not eligible for anti-Helicobacter pylori therapy. *J Clin Oncol.* 2005;23:1979-83.
46. Berger F, Felman P, Thieblemont C, et al. Non-MALT marginal zone B-cell lymphomas: a description of clinical presentation and outcome in 124 patients. *Blood.* 2000;95:1950-6.
47. Nathwani BN, Anderson JR, Armitage JO, et al. Marginal zone B-cell lymphoma: a clinical comparison of nodal and mucosa-associated lymphoid tissue types Non-Hodgkin's Lymphoma Classification Project. *J Clin Oncol.* 1999;17:2486-92.
48. Shin SS, Sheibani K. Monocytoid B-cell lymphoma. *Am J Clin Pathol.* 1993;99:421-5.
49. Koh LP, Lim LC, Thng CH. Retreatment with chimeric CD 20 monoclonal antibody in a patient with nodal marginal zone B-cell lymphoma. *Med Oncol.* 2000;17:225-8.
50. Voulgarelis M, Giannouli S, Anagnostou D, et al. Combined therapy with rituximab plus cyclophosphamide/doxorubicin/vincristine/prednisone (CHOP) for Sjogren's syndrome-associated B-cell aggressive non-Hodgkin's lymphomas. *Rheumatology (Oxford).* 2004;43:1050-3.
51. Voulgarelis M, Giannouli S, Tzioufas AG, et al. Long-term remission of Sjögren's syndrome-associated aggressive B-cell non-Hodgkin's lymphomas following administration of combined B-cell depletion therapy and CHOP (cyclophosphamide, doxorubicin, vincristine, prednisone). *Ann Rheum Dis.* 2006;65:1033-7.
52. Brown JR, Gaudet G, Friedberg JW, et al. Autologous bone marrow transplantation for marginal zone non-Hodgkin's lymphoma. *Leuk Lymphoma.* 2004;45:315-20.
53. Rossi D, Gaidano G. Molecular heterogeneity of diffuse large B-cell lymphoma: implications for disease management and prognosis. *Hematology.* 2002;7:239-52.
54. Neumeister P, Hoefler G, Beham-Schmid C, et al. Deletion analysis of the p16 tumor suppressor gene in gastrointestinal mucosa-associated lymphoid tissue lymphomas. *Gastroenterology.* 1997;112:1871-5.
55. Pui CH, Thiel E. Central nervous system disease in hematologic malignancies: historical perspective and practical applications. *Semin Oncol.* 2009;36(4 Suppl 2):S2-16.

Chapter 38
Classic Immunosuppressive and Immunomodulatory Drugs

Clio P. Mavragani and Stuart S. Kassan

Contents

38.1 Introduction

Symptoms of Sjögren's syndrome (SS) are chronic and can sometimes be devastating, compromising patients' quality of life to a major degree. Despite the advances in our understanding of the pathogenesis of SS, its therapy remains largely empiric, symptomatic, and focused on alleviating sicca symptoms. Eye lubricants, saliva substitutes, and stimulators of the glandular secretion are the cornerstones of therapy in SS. Despite the autoimmune nature of the disorder, evidence for the use of immunosuppressive agents, the mainstay of therapy of diseases of autoimmune origin, is scarce. In an attempt to alleviate the symptoms of SS by altering the natural disease process, a number of immunosuppressive agents have been tested in clinical studies, mostly with unsatisfactory or questionable results (Table 38.1).

C.P. Mavragani (✉)
Department of Experimental Physiology, School of Medicine, University of Athens,
Athens, Greece

S.S. Kassan
University of Colorado Health Sciences Center, Denver, CO, USA

M. Ramos-Casals et al. (eds.), *Sjögren's Syndrome*,
DOI 10.1007/978-0-85729-947-5_38, © Springer-Verlag London Limited 2012

Table 38.1 Effect of immunomodulating or immunosuppressive medications in the treatment of primary Sjögren's syndrome

Immunomodulatory agent	Formulation and dose	Effect
Hydroxychloroquine	200 mg daily	No improvement in sicca symptoms. Inhibition of glandular cholinesterase activity, increased salivary soluble interleukin-2 receptor in primary Sjögren's syndrome
		Improvement of subjective/objective measures of eye dryness
NSAIDs		Improvement of musculoskeletal complaints
Corticosteroids	Systemic (0.5–1 mg/kg body weight daily)	Limited evidence of improvement
	Local	Induction of corneal lesions
Azathriopine	0.5–1 mg/kg body weight daily	Autoimmune liver disease, interstitial lung involvement, renal disease
Cyclophosphamide	0.5–1 g/m^2 of body surface/month for 6 months	Refractory to steroids; glomerulonephritis, necrotic vasculitis, severe neurological involvement
Methotrexate	0.2 mg/kg body weight weekly	Improvement in subjective measures/polyarthritis
		No improvement of objective indices of dry mouth
Cyclosporine	5 mg/kg body weight daily	Improvement of subjective measures of xerostomia
		Retardation of evolution of histopathological lesions

38.2 Antimalarials

Early studies failed to suggest a substantial role of hydroxychloroquine (HCQ) in alleviating sicca symptoms despite this medication's ability to reduce inflammatory markers within saliva and serum markers of B-cell hyperreactivity, e.g., hypergammaglobulinemia and autoantibody levels [1, 2]. However, recent data from an open-label, 48-week prospective study of 32 pSS patients suggested that HCQ use led to improvement of subjective symptoms of eye dryness and delayed disease progression. The latter was evidenced by the worsened objective dryness scores (Shirmer's test, lissamine green, tear break-up time) in the control group 3 months after treatment cessation. Levels of B-cell-activating factor (BAFF) [3, 4] within the tears of patients in the HCQ group were significantly reduced [5]. Another study suggested a potential role of HCQ in improving salivary hypofunction through inhibition of cholinesterase activity within salivary glands [6].

Although its utility in treating sicca symptoms is debatable, HCQ seems to be beneficial for musculoskeletal complaints such as arthralgias, myalgias, fibromyalgia-like features, and the non-erosive polyarthropathy that is sometimes associated with pSS [1, 2, 7]. Vasculitis has been reported after HCQ cessation in one case [8].

38.3 Nonsteroidal Anti-inflammatory Drugs (NSAIDs)

Data on the use of NSAIDs in the management of pSS are scarce. These medications can be used with appropriate caution in patients with musculoskeletal complaints.

38.4 Glucocorticoids

Although evidence for a beneficial role of glucocorticoids in the alleviation of local symptoms is limited to non-existent [9, 10], these agents play an important role in the management of extraglandular disease manifestations such as interstitial lung disease, glomerulonephritis, autoimmune liver disease, nervous system involvement, and vasculitis. The starting dose of glucocorticoids varies according to clinical judgment and the specific pSS manifestation, but for serious complications generally equates to a daily prednisone dose on the order of 0.5–1 mg/kg of body weight [7, 11, 12]. For CNS involvement, intravenous pulses of methylprednisolone (1 g/day for 3 consecutive days) have been employed but there are no controlled data and no consensus about the appropriate approach to that challenging subset of patients in general. Topical glucocorticoid use in the eyes has been associated with corneal lesions in patients with pSS, and therefore should be employed cautiously [13].

38.5 Azathioprine

Given the promising therapeutic results of azathioprine in terms of reduction of the extent of lymphocytic infiltration in NZB/NZW F1 hybrid mice [14], the role of low-dose azathioprine (1 mg/kg body weight/day) was examined in a 6-month, double-blind, placebo-controlled trial in 25 pSS patients. The authors observed no therapeutic benefit in terms of symptoms, signs, or serologic or histologic markers, but did report a considerable number of reported adverse effects [15]. The authors concluded that azathioprine was unsuitable for the treatment of SS. There may be some patient subsets with particular disease manifestations, however, in which azathioprine use is appropriate. The medication is occasionally used in pSS in patients with interstitial lung disease, glomerulonephritis, and nervous system involvement [7].

38.6 Cyclophosphamide

Cyclophosphamide is reserved for serious or life-threatening conditions such as glomerulonephritis refractory to prednisolone, systemic necrotizing vasculitis, or severe neurological involvement. Because of extrapolations from studies of cyclophosphamide in systemic lupus erythematosus, the medication is usually administered intravenously (0.5–1 g/m^2 of body surface/month) for a total of 6 months.

Cyclophosphamide use is associated with a high risk of bone marrow suppression, infertility, and cancer development. This latter complication is particularly relevant to pSS patients who already have an elevated risk of lymphomagenesis. One study estimated that the risk of lymphoma among pSS patients treated with cyclophosphamide is increased 100-fold over the baseline population risk [16]. As noted elsewhere in this book, pSS patients with purpura, mixed monoclonal cryoglobulinemia, and low complement C4 levels comprise an especially high-risk group in terms of lymphoma [17].

38.7 Methotrexate

Methotrexate is a well-established immunoregulatory and anti-inflammatory agent that modulates many of the pro-inflammatory cytokines found within the histopathological SS lesions [18]. Methotrexate (0.2 mg/kg of body weight/week) administered with or without prednisone (<10 mg/day) appears to be an effective approach to managing the polyarthritis sometimes associated with pSS [7]. An open-label trial of 0.3 mg/kg administered weekly alleviated the subjective symptoms of dry mouth and eyes and decreased the frequency of parotid gland enlargement, dry cough, and purpura. However, no effect on the flow rates of the lacrimal or salivary glands was observed [19]. Thus, the use of methotrexate is reserved optimally for mild-to-moderate extraglandular features of the disease.

38.8 Cyclosporine

Cyclosporine acts by inhibiting interleukin-2 production by activated helper T cells. Because the lymphocytic infiltration of the labial minor salivary glands in SS consists mainly of activated memory helper T cells [20], there was strong rationale for a trial cyclosporine, administered at a dose of 5 mg/kg body weight/day [21]. Although subjective improvements were observed in xerostomia and there was some indication of stabilization of the histopathological lesions of SS, no changes in the objective indices of lacrimal and parotid flows were observed.

In contrast, cyclosporine eyedrops have had a substantial impact on the ocular sicca component of SS. The topical application of cyclosporine eyedrops (0.05% or 0.1% twice daily) has been shown to be effective in two parallel multicenter trials, leading to significant improvement in two objective measures (corneal staining, Schirmer's values) and three subjective outcomes of dry eye disease (blurred vision, need for concomitant artificial tears, physician's evaluation of a global response).

38.9 Conclusion

Despite the progress, management of SS remains largely empirical. Until the etiology of the condition is understood more fully, treatment of SS will remain mostly symptomatic. Classic categories of immunosuppressive regimens do not appear to modify the natural history of this disorder in most patients, although restricted use for these medications has been advocated, in certain circumstances.

References

1. Tishler M, Yaron I, Shirazi I, et al. Hydroxychloroquine treatment for primary Sjogren's syndrome: its effect on salivary and serum inflammatory markers. Ann Rheum Dis. 1999;58:253–6.
2. Manoussakis MN, Moutsopoulos HM. Antimalarials in Sjogren's syndrome – the Greek experience. Lupus. 1996;5 Suppl 1:S28–30.
3. Groom J, Kalled SL, Cutler AH, et al. Association of BAFF/BLyS overexpression and altered B cell differentiation with Sjogren's syndrome. J Clin Invest. 2002;109:59–68.
4. Mariette X, Roux S, Zhang J, et al. The level of BLyS (BAFF) correlates with the titre of autoantibodies in human Sjogren's syndrome. Ann Rheum Dis. 2003;62:168–71.
5. Yavuz S, Asfuroglu E, Bicakcigil M, et al. Hydroxychloroquine improves dry eye symptoms of patients with primary Sjogren's syndrome. Rheumatol Int. 2011;31:1045–9. Epub Mar 23, 2010.
6. Dawson LJ, Caulfield VL, Stanbury JB, et al. Hydroxychloroquine therapy in patients with primary Sjogren's syndrome may improve salivary gland hypofunction by inhibition of glandular cholinesterase. Rheumatology (Oxford). 2005;44:449–55.
7. Mavragani CP, Moutsopoulos NM, Moutsopoulos HM. The management of Sjogren's syndrome. Nat Clin Pract Rheumatol. 2006;2:252–61.
8. Okan G, Karaaslan M, Büyükbabani N. Systemic vasculitis developing after hydroxychloroquine interruption in a patient with Sjögren's syndrome. Clin Exp Dermatol. 2010;35:442–3. Epub Nov 3, 2009.
9. Zandbelt MM, van den Hoogen FH, de Wilde PC, et al. Reversibility of histological and immunohistological abnormalities in sublabial salivary gland biopsy specimens following treatment with corticosteroids in Sjogren's syndrome. Ann Rheum Dis. 2001;60:511–3.
10. Fox PC, Datiles M, Atkinson JC, et al. Prednisone and piroxicam for treatment of primary Sjogren's syndrome. Clin Exp Rheumatol. 1993;11:149–56.
11. Kaufman I, Schwartz D, Caspi D, et al. Sjogren's syndrome – not just Sicca: renal involvement in Sjogren's syndrome. Scand J Rheumatol. 2008;37:213–8.
12. Hawley RJ, Hendricks WT. Treatment of Sjogren syndrome myelopathy with azathioprine and steroids. Arch Neurol. 2002;59:875; author reply 876.
13. Linardaki G, Moutsopoulos HM. The uncertain role of immunosuppressive agents in Sjogren's syndrome. Cleve Clin J Med. 1997;64:523–6.
14. Yeoman CM, Franklin CD. The treatment of Sjogren's disease in NZB/NZW F1 hybrid mice with azathioprine: a two-stage study. Clin Exp Rheumatol. 1994;12:49–53.
15. Price EJ, Rigby SP, Clancy U, et al. A double blind placebo controlled trial of azathioprine in the treatment of primary Sjogren's syndrome. J Rheumatol. 1998;25:896–9.
16. Moutsopoulos HM, Balow JE, Lawley TJ, et al. Immune complex glomerulonephritis in sicca syndrome. Am J Med. 1978;64:955–60.
17. Skopouli FN, Dafni U, Ioannidis JP, et al. Clinical evolution, and morbidity and mortality of primary Sjogren's syndrome. Semin Arthritis Rheum. 2000;29:296–304.
18. Boumba D, Skopouli FN, Moutsopoulos HM. Cytokine mRNA expression in the labial salivary gland tissues from patients with primary Sjogren's syndrome. Br J Rheumatol. 1995;34:326–33.
19. Skopouli FN, Jagiello P, Tsifetaki N, et al. Methotrexate in primary Sjogren's syndrome. Clin Exp Rheumatol. 1996;14:555–8.
20. Skopouli FN, Fox PC, Galanopoulou V, et al. T cell subpopulations in the labial minor salivary gland histopathologic lesion of Sjogren's syndrome. J Rheumatol. 1991;18:210–4.
21. Drosos AA, Skopouli FN, Costopoulos JS, et al. Cyclosporin A (CyA) in primary Sjogren's syndrome: a double blind study. Ann Rheum Dis. 1986;45:732–5.

Chapter 39
New Immunosuppressive Agents for the Treatment of Sjögren's Syndrome

Steven Carsons

Contents

Despite the significant success in many immune-mediated disorders of disease-modifying antirheumatic drugs (DMARDs) such as methotrexate and azathioprine, the demonstration of DMARD efficacy for the control of sicca and extraglandular symptoms of Sjögren's syndrome (SS) has been elusive. This chapter will discuss potential applications of newer DMARDs for the management of primary SS (pSS) (Table 39.1).

39.1 Leflunomide

Leflunomide (LEF) is an oral immunosuppressive agent approved by the US FDA and the European Commission for use in rheumatoid arthritis (RA). Recently, the European Medicines Agency approved LEF for the treatment of psoriatic arthritis

S. Carsons
Division of Rheumatology, Allergy and Immunology, Winthrop-University Hospital, Mineola, NY, USA

Department of Medicine, Stony Brook University School of Medicine, Stony Brook, NY, USA

M. Ramos-Casals et al. (eds.), *Sjögren's Syndrome*,
DOI 10.1007/978-0-85729-947-5_39, © Springer-Verlag London Limited 2012

Table 39.1 Oral agents with potential disease-modifying activity for Sjögren's syndrome

DMARD	Possible mechanism of action	Other known and proposed uses
Leflunomide	Orotic acid dehydrogenase inhibitor	RA
Mycophenolic acid	Inosine monophosphate dehydrogenase inhibitor	Prophylaxis of organ transplant rejection, SLE
Interferon-α	Anti-viral; inhibition of B cell proliferation	HBV, HCV, HCL, CML
Mizoribine	Inosine monophosphate dehydrogenase inhibition	Prophylaxis of renal transplant rejection; immune-mediated GN
Rebamipide	Cytoprotection via enhancement of local PG synthesis; growth factor production	Peptic ulcer disease, IBD, Behcet's disease
Diquafosol	Enhanced epithelial secretion via purine receptor agonism	Dry eye syndromes
Cladribine	Purine nucleoside analogue	HCL, MS
Fingolimod	Sphingosine-1 phosphate receptor modulation	MS

SLE systemic lupus erythematosus, *RA* rheumatoid arthritis, *HBV* hepatitis B virus infection, *HCV* hepatitis C virus infection, *HCL* hairy cell leukemia, *CML* chronic myelogenous leukemia, *GN* glomerulonephritis, *IBD* inflammatory bowel disease, *MS* multiple sclerosis

(PsA). LEF, a derivative of isoxazole, rapidly converts to its active form known as A77-1726 in the intestinal mucosa [1]. LEF is a potent inhibitor of orotic acid dehydrogenase which, in turn, results in pyrimidine synthesis inhibition. This preferentially prevents expansion of the lymphocyte ribonucleotide pool and thus, proliferation of activated T lymphocytes. LEF may exert similar action on other immune cells including monocyte/macrophages and B lymphocytes and may inhibit additional enzymes involved in lymphocyte activation and signaling such as tyrosine kinase [2]. Of note, LEF has an exceedingly long half-life (14–18 da.) and is excreted via renal and fecal routes. Blocking enterohepatic recirculation with cholestyramine or charcoal reduces half-life approximately 15-fold and is clinically useful when the drug needs to be rapidly eliminated. LEF is not dialyzable.

Approximately 5% of subjects in RA clinical trials receiving LEF developed liver function test abnormalities. These usually occur during the first 6 months of therapy and resolve in follow-up [3]. Serious LEF-induced hepatotoxicity is thought to be rare [4]. Nevertheless, in 2010, the FDA issued a warning regarding LEF use and the risk of liver injury. Diarrhea occurred in 17% of patients in LEF clinical trials [5], usually within the first 3 months of therapy, and may be associated with the administration of a loading dose. Diarrhea may resolve with continued LEF therapy. A post-marketing survey of greater than 2000 RA LEF-treated patients in Japan identified 29 individuals with interstitial lung disease. Sixty-nine percent had baseline interstitial lung disease prior to initiation of therapy. A review panel determined that the relationship of LEF therapy to the development of interstitial lung disease was probable in 3 and possible in 11 [6]. LEF is teratogenic in rabbits and rats and is contraindicated in pregnancy.

Women and men on LEF who are contemplating conceiving a child should stop LEF and purge existing drug with cholestyramine. Elimination of drug should be documented by serum levels <0.02 mg/L 2 weeks apart. This course should be followed in cases of accidental pregnancy while on LEF.

A pilot study has been published examining the use of LEF for pSS. van Woerkom et al. [7] performed a 24-week, open-label pilot study of LEF (20 mg weekly) on 15 women with pSS. All patients fulfilled the European-American Consensus Criteria and had positive labial salivary gland biopsy (focus score ≥ 1). Fourteen of the fifteen patients reached the 24 week endpoint. Twelve attained the 20% overall response endpoint while seven attained the 50% overall response endpoint. Significant improvements from baseline were seen in fatigue scores, serum immunoglobulin concentrations, and rheumatoid factor levels. The Schirmer test improved by 33%. Two patients developed liver function test abnormalities and two became leucopenic. Two patients also developed lupus-like cutaneous lesions de novo and three additional patients had exacerbations of existing lupus-like skin lesions. Antibodies to ds-DNA were not measured as part of this study.

Two additional studies published in abstract form have suggested a role for LEF in pSS. An open-label study in 17 patients who failed glucocorticoid therapy demonstrated an improvement in symptoms and laboratory studies on LEF [8]. A study of laboratory parameters in 18 patients treated with LEF suggested efficacy for SS [9]. Thus, it appears that LEF may be useful in a subset of patients with SS. Additional study is needed to determine the safety in patients with features of cutaneous lupus erythematosus.

39.2   Interferon-α

Although the precise etiology of SS is unknown, it is presumed that an environmental trigger stimulates the innate immune system which results in the enhanced elaboration of interferon-α by plasmacytoid dendritic cells. Viral infections are good candidates for this trigger. Despite this, levels of IFN-α have been reported to be depressed in Sjögren's syndrome. It is hypothesized that therapy with oral IFN may restore salivary gland function. Shiozawa et al. performed a 6-month single-blinded controlled trial involving 56 SS patients who received either 150 IU of IFN or 250 mg of sucralfate orally [10]. This study demonstrated a significant increase in salivary flow by the Saxon test for the IFN group, although only 50% of the IFN-treated individuals responded. Seven of the nine IFN responders who underwent re-biopsy of minor salivary glands showed improvement in the degree of lymphocytic infiltration.

Ship et al. [11] examined the effect of multiple dosages of oral IFN lozenges in a phase II placebo-controlled trial over a 12-week period in 111 patients. Complete response was defined as a 25% improvement in the VAS for oral dryness and a 0.05 g/min increase in unstimulated salivary flow. The percentages of patients who achieved complete remission were numerically but not statistically higher in the groups receiving higher IFN doses (150 IU t.i.d., 450 IU o.d., and 450 IU t.i.d.) compared to the low-dose (150 IU o.d.) or placebo groups. Increases in stimulated salivary flow did reach significance for the 150 IU t.i.d. group by week 12.

A phase III trial examined the efficacy of the 150 IU t.i.d.dose of IFN in 497 patients with pSS [12]. Treated patients had a significant increase in unstimulated whole salivary flow. Improvement in unstimulated whole salivary flow correlated with improvement in symptom scores for ocular and oral dryness. The primary endpoint of this study (increases in salivary flow and VAS for oral dryness) was not met. To date, oral low-dose IFN has not received approval for the treatment of SS. Yamada et al. [13] treated three patients with pSS and progressive, relapsing demyelinating polyneuropathy with interferon-α three million units three times weekly. The patients had previously failed therapy with glucocorticoids, multiple immunosuppressive agents, and IVIg. All three patients experienced significant improvement in their neurological symptoms and electrophysiologic parameters. In addition, improvement was noted in mononuclear infiltration upon repeat minor salivary gland biopsy and in SS-A and SS-B titers. Because the development of SS and SLE was described in an HCV patient treated with interferon-α 2b [14], a degree of caution should be used in considering IFN-α for therapy of SS.

39.3   Mycophenolic Acid

Mycophenolic acid (MPA) is an oral immunosuppressive agent established for suppression of transplant rejection. More recently, MPA has been shown to be efficacious in the treatment of lupus nephritis. MPA selectively inhibits inosine monophosphate (IMP) dehydrogenase. Inosinic acid is the ribonucleotide of hypoxanthine and is the initial nucleotide formed in purine synthesis. Since proliferation of activated T and B lymphocytes is dependent on de novo purine synthesis, IMP dehydrogenase inhibition by MPA has proven useful for the treatment of autoimmune disease.

Willeke et al. [15] conducted a prospective open-label pilot study of MPA in 11 patients fulfilling American-European Consensus Criteria for pSS. MPA was administered in the form of mycophenolate sodium (MPS) starting with 360 mg daily and increasing to a maximum of 1,440 mg daily; a dose equivalent to 2 g of mycophenolate mofetil (MMF). Eight patients completed the study. Two patients withdrew due to adverse affects (GI intolerance and vertigo). One patient was withdrawn following hospitalization for pneumonia. Significant improvement was noted in VAS for sicca complaints and requirement for artificial tears. Although there was some improvement in the Schirmer test, this was not significant. It was noted, however, that a major improvement in glandular function was noted in two patients with relatively short disease duration. Significant reduction was seen in levels of gamma globulins, total IgM, and rheumatoid factor. Further study of mycophenolate in early SS patients appears warranted.

39.4 Mizoribine

Another IMP dehydrogenase inhibitor, mizoribine, was originally developed as an antifungal agent in Japan. Initially approved in that country for the suppression of renal transplant rejection, mizoribine has subsequently been used to treat RA, SLE nephritis, and idiopathic nephrotic syndrome [16]. Nakayamada et al. conducted a multicenter open-label clinical trial in 59 patients who fulfilled the Japanese Ministry of Health and Welfare's diagnostic criteria for SS. The patients were treated with mizoribine 50 mg t.i.d. for 16 weeks [17]. The authors noted a significant improvement in salivary secretion volume (measured at 2 min), patients' assessments of dry mouth and dry eye symptoms, and physician global assessment. Differences in immunological parameters, including total immunoglobulins and levels of Ro and La antibodies, were not noted. Approximately 30% of patients experienced adverse events, the most common of which were liver function test abnormalities, cytopenias, and gastrointestinal symptoms. These authors also examined response to mizoribine in relation to the degree of histologic change on minor salivary gland biopsy [18]. Patients with moderate degrees of lymphocytic infiltration, fibrosis, and acinar atrophy demonstrated superior responses to mizoribine as compared to those with mild or severe degrees of these histologic categories. As shown for the other IMPDH inhibitor, mycophenolate (above) in preliminary studies, patients with earlier stages of disease may be responsive to these agents.

39.5 Rebamipide

Rebamipide is a cytoprotective agent used in Japan primarily to treat peptic ulcer disease [19]. Rebamipide inhibits NSAID-induced gastric mucosal damage in animals. Its major mechanism of action was believed initially to be enhancement of local prostaglandin synthesis accomplished by induction of COX-2 and upregulation of EP4 receptor gene expression, ultimately resulting in the stimulation of mucus secretion. More recently, rebamipide has been shown to enhance the local production of growth factors such as epidermal growth factor (EGF), hepatocyte growth factor (HSF), and vascular endothelial growth factor (VEGF). Rebamipide also induces heat shock proteins and anti-oxidant mechanisms, such as the inhibition of lipid peroxidation.

Because rebamipide is believed to exert its positive effects on ulcer healing via the promotion of tissue healing, its potential efficacy in chronic inflammatory disorders has been studied. Rebamipide administered per rectum has demonstrated efficacy in inflammatory bowel disease. Studies have shown positive results in stomatitis secondary to Behcet's disease. Because of its protective effect on mucosa, rebamipide has been studied for xerostomia in SS. In a double-blind placebo-controlled trial, Sugai et al. [20] administered rebamipide at a dose of 100 mg t.i.d. to 104 subjects with SS. Patients with pSS but not secondary SS treated with rebamipide demonstrated a significant increase in salivary secretion at weeks 2, 4, and 8. For all SS subjects, there was a trend toward improvement in overall dry mouth symptoms and objective dry mouth findings, but these differences were not statistically significant. Approximately two-thirds of patients in the active and placebo groups experienced adverse effects. The majority of these were gastrointestinal symptoms that did not lead to withdrawal from the study. There were no significant differences between the rebamipide and control groups in the incidence or type of adverse events experienced.

39.6   Diquafosol

Diquafosol is a water-soluble dinucleotide (diuridine tetraphosphate) in development as a topical ocular surface disease-modifying agent for dry eye including that caused by SS [21]. Diquafosol is a selective purine receptor agonist targeted toward the stimulation of $P2Y_2$ receptors. Topical diquafosol stimulates these receptors at the ocular surface, resulting in stimulation of secretion from multiple components of the ocular surface. $P2Y_2$ receptor stimulation stimulates fluid and ion secretion at the conjunctival surface via non-glandular mechanisms. In addition, diquafosol enhances goblet cell mucin production. $P2Y_2$ receptors have been shown to be present on the Meibomian gland and are thought to stimulate ocular lipid production. Thus, diquafosol appears to be capable of increasing tear production and restoring tear composition to a more normal state. Several phase III trials have been conducted comparing diquafosol to placebo. All trials demonstrated an improvement in corneal staining, although not all endpoints were met for all trials [22]. Diquafosol remains a potentially important treatment for dry eye in SS.

39.7   Cladribine

Cladribine (2-chloro-2-deoxy adenosine; 2-Cda) is a purine nucleoside analogue with selective activity toward lymphocytes and monocytes. 2-Cda may also function by epigenetic mechanisms including inhibition of DNA methylation and is especially active in CD4+, CD8+ T lymphocytes and CD19+ B cells [23]. Initially approved for hairy cell leukemia, 2-Cda has been used to inhibit progression in CLL, both B cell neoplasms. Accordingly, 2-Cda has also been studied in autoimmune disorders including lupus nephritis. Most recently, oral 2-Cda has demonstrated efficacy in relapsing multiple sclerosis [24].

Voulgarelis et al. [25] reported on four patients who had pSS as well as some aspect of lymphoproliferative disorder including lymphoma or cryoglobulinemia with an IgM kappa monoclonal component. Three of four patients had long-term remission of the B cell–associated lymphoproliferative process. Some SS symptoms improved, including parotid swelling and oral dryness. A randomized study of oral cladribine in SS, particularly for those with lymphoproliferative features, would be required to demonstrate clinical utility for the exocrine and lymphoproliferative features of SS.

39.8 Fingolimod

Fingolimod (FTY 720) is a modulator of sphingosine-1-phosphate receptor (SIP_1) signaling. Effects of fingolimod on lymphocytes are mediated in part by SIP_1 antagonism and include inhibition of egress from secondary lymphoid tissue and suppression of IFN-gamma secretion from CD4+ lymphocytes. Recently, clinical trials have demonstrated efficacy of fingolimod for relapsing multiple sclerosis [26], and thus, may be useful in other autoimmune disorders including SS. An SIP_1 modulator capable of inhibiting lymph node egress of activated T cells that subsequently target lacrimal and salivary glands would be a particularly useful property for a therapeutic agent in SS. While to date, there are no clinical trials of fingolimod in pSS, Sekiguchi and colleagues demonstrated the presence of SIP_1 in inflammatory cells, vascular endothelium, and salivary gland epithelium in biopsies of minor salivary glands. SIP_1 expression was enhanced in biopsies from patients with advanced disease. SIP_1 enhanced gamma-interferon production from CD4+ cells. SIP_1-mediated enhancement was greater in CD4+ cells obtained from SS patients [27]. Further investigation of the therapeutic potential of fingolimod in animal models of SS may provide data leading to performance of clinical trials.

References

1. Kaltwasser JP, Behrens F. Leflunomide: long-term clinical experience and new uses. Expert Opin Pharmacother. 2005;6:787–801.
2. Fox RI, Herrmann ML, Frangou CG, et al. How does leflunomide modulate the immune response in rheumatoid arthritis? BioDrugs. 1999;12:301–15.
3. van Roon EN, Tim L, Jansen TL, et al. Leflunomide for the treatment of rheumatoid arthritis in clinical practice. Drug Saf. 2004;27:345–52.
4. Available from: www.rheumatology.org/publications/hotline/0303TNFL.asp. (accessed october 11, 2011)
5. van Riel PL, Smolen JS, Emery P, et al. Leflunomide: a manageable safety profile. J Rheumatol Suppl. 2004;71:21–4.
6. Cannon GW, Strand V, Simon LS, et al. Interstitial lung disease in rheumatoid arthritis patients receiving leflunomide. Arthritis Rheum (Abstr). 2004;50:209.
7. van Woerkom JM, Kruize AA, Geenen R, et al. Safety and efficacy of leflunomide in primary Sjögren's syndrome: a phase II pilot study. Ann Rheum Dis. 2007;66:1026–32.
8. Scagliusi P, D'Amore M, Scagliusi A, et al. Le nuove terapie nella syndromedi Sjögren: efficacia della Leflunomide. Reumatismo. 2004;56(3 Suppl 3):271 (Abstract P04).
9. Benucci M, LI Gobbi F, Pierfederici P. Modificazioni dei parametric della scintigrafia delle ghiandole salivary in corso di terapia con leflunomide in pazienti con syndrome di Sjögren. Reumatismo. 2004;56(3 Suppl 3):324 (Abstract P112).

10. Shiozawa S, Tanaka Y, Shiozawa K. Single-blinded controlled trial of low-dose oral IFN-alpha for the treatment of xerostomia in patients with Sjögen's syndrome. J Interferon Cytokine Res. 1998;18:255–62.

11. Ship JA, Fox PC, Michalek JE, et al. Treatment of primary Sjögren's syndrome with low-dose natural human interferon-alpha administered by the oral mucosal route: a phase II clinical trial. IFN Protocol Study Group. J Interferon Cytokine Res. 1999;19(8):943–51.

12. Cummings MJ, Papas A, Kramer GM, Fox PC. Treatment of primary Sjögren's syndrome with low-dose human interferon ala administered by the oromucosal route: combined phase III results. Arthritis Rheum. 2003;49(4):585–93.

13. Yamada S, Nishimiya J, Nakajima T, Taketazu F. Interferon alfa treatment for Sjögren's syndrome associated neuropathy. J Neurol Neurosurg Psychiatry. 2005;76:576–8.

14. Onishi S, Nagashima T, Kimura H, et al. Systemic lupus erythematosus and Sjögren's syndrome induced in a case by interferon-alpha used for the treatment of hepatitis C. Lupus. 2010;19:753–5.

15. Willeke P, Schlüter B, Becker H, et al. Mycophenolate sodium treatment in patients with primary Sjögren syndrome: a pilot trial. Arthritis Res Ther. 2007;9:R115.

16. Moutsopoulos HM, Fragoulis GE. Is mizoribine a new therapeutic agent for Sjögren's syndrome? Nat Rev Rheumatol. 2008;4:350–1.

17. Nakayamada S, Saito K, Umehara H, et al. Efficacy and safety of Mizoribine for the treatment of Sjögren's syndrome: a multicenter open-label clinical trial. Mod Rheumatol. 2007;17:464–9.

18. Nakayamada S, Fujimoto T, Nonomura A, et al. Usefulness of initial histological features for stratifying Sjögren's syndrome responders to mizoribine therapy. Rheumatology. 2009;48:1279–82.

19. Arakawa T, Higuchi K, Fujiwara AY, et al. 15th anniversary of rebamipide: looking ahead to the new mechanisms and new applications. Dig Dis Sci. 2005;50 Suppl 1:S3–11.

20. Sugai S, Takahashi H, Ohta S, et al. Efficacy and safety of rebamipide for the treatment of dry mouth symptoms in patients with Sjögren's syndrome: a double-blind placebo-controlled multicenter trial. Mod Rheumatol. 2009;19:114–24.

21. Samarkos M, Moutsopoulos HM. Recent advances in the management of ocular complications of Sjögren's syndrome. Curr Allergy Asthma Rep. 2005;5:327–32.

22. Fischbarg J. Diquafosol tetrasodium. Inspire/Allegan/Santen. Curr Opin Investig Drugs. 2003;4:1377–83.

23. Spurgeon S, Yu M, Phillips JD, Epner EM. Cladribine: not just another purine analogue? Expert Opin Investig Drugs. 2009;18:1169–81.

24. Giovannoni G, Comi G, Cook S, et al. A placebo-controlled trial of oral cladribine for relapsing multiple sclerosis. N Engl J Med. 2010;362:416–26.

25. Voulgarelis M, Petroutsos G, Moutsopoulos HM, Skopouli FN. 2-cholo-2'-deoxiadenosine in the treatment of Sjögren's syndrome-associated B cell lymphoproliferation. Arthritis Rheum. 2002;46:2248–9.

26. Cohen JA, Barkhof F, Comi G, et al. Oral fingolimod or intramuscular interferon for relapsing multiple sclerosis. N Engl J Med. 2010;362:402–15.

27. Sekiguchi M, Iwasaki T, Kitano M, et al. Role of sphingosine 1-phosphate in the pathogenesis of Sjögren's syndrome. J Immunol. 2008;180:1921–8.

Chapter 40
B-Cell-Targeted Therapies in Sjögren's Syndrome

Xavier Mariette

Contents

X. Mariette
Hôpital Bicêtre, Assistance Publique-Hôpitaux de Paris (AP-HP),
Université Paris-Sud 11, Le Kremlin Bicêtre, France

Institut Pour la Santé et la Recherche Médicale (INSERM), Paris, France

M. Ramos-Casals et al. (eds.), *Sjögren's Syndrome*,
DOI 10.1007/978-0-85729-947-5_40, © Springer-Verlag London Limited 2012

40.1 B-Cell Hyperactivity in Sjögren's Syndrome

40.1.1 Evidence of B-Cell Hyperactivity

B-cell hyperactivity has been recognized for a long time in Sjögren's syndrome (SS). More than 30 years ago, Talal et al. demonstrated an increased level of beta-2-microglobulin in the serum of patients with SS [1]. More than 20 years ago, Moutsopoulos et al. detected increased levels of immunoglobulin light chains within the sera of patients with SS [2].

B-cell activation in SS is initially polyclonal but can progress to monoclonal B-cell lymphoproliferation [3]. A relative risk of lymphoma of 44 was reported by Kassan et al. in 1978 [4]. A recent study in Sweden and a meta-analysis found a somewhat lower (but still substantially elevated) relative risk, on the order of 16–18 [5, 6]. Lymphomas in SS are prone to develop at sites of inflammation (salivary glands) mediated by infiltrating B-lymphocytes [7, 8]. B-cell hyperactivity in primary SS is evidenced by a polyclonal hypergammaglobulinemia, the presence of autoantibodies such as anti-SSA/Ro and anti-SSB/La, high levels of rheumatoid factor [9], elevated concentrations of beta-2-microglobulin, and free immunoglobulin light chains in the serum. Gottenberg et al. recently demonstrated that serum beta-2-microglobulin and free light chain levels correlated with systemic involvement of the disease [10, 11].

40.1.2 An Increase in BAFF Could Explain B-Cell Hyperactivity in SS

A cytokine known as B-cell-activating factor of the tumor necrosis factor family (BAFF), also called B-lymphocyte stimulator (BLyS), TALL-1, THANK, zTNF4, TNFSF13b, or TNFSF20, plays a crucial role in the differentiation and survival of B-cells. Three distinct receptors are essential to normal BAFF physiology: (1) B-cell maturation antigen (BCMA); (2) transmembrane activator, calcium-modulator and cyclophilin ligand interactor (TACI); and (3) BAFF receptor (BAFFR or BR3) [12, 13]. BAFF is produced principally by monocytes, dendritic cells, and macrophages [14].

BAFF transgenic mice first develop a disease that mimics systemic lupus erythematosus (SLE) before evolving a sialadenitis that resembles SS. These mice also have a two-fold elevated risk of lymphoma [15].

40.1.2.1 Serum BAFF in SS

One year after the first link between BAFF in SLE in humans, Groom et al. demonstrated elevated serum levels of BAFF in SS patients [16]. Correlations between serum BAFF concentrations, IgG, and rheumatoid factor levels were reported in 2003 [17]. Moreover, patients with anti-SSA/Ro and/or anti-SSB/La antibodies were shown to have higher serum concentrations of BAFF compared to those without those antibodies. These findings have been confirmed in other studies [18–20].

40.1.3   BAFF Is Secreted by Resident Cells of Target Organs of Autoimmunity

The first report by Groom et al. in 2002 showed the presence of BAFF within the lymphocytic salivary infiltrate that is characteristic of primary SS. Lavie et al. subsequently demonstrated that both the T-cells of the infiltrate and the epithelial cells could express BAFF [21]. Deridon et al. suggested that the B-cells of the infiltrate that are the target of BAFF and express the different receptors could also express the ligand, leading to an autocrine pathway way for BAFF secretion and activation of B-cells [22].

Several groups have demonstrated that salivary epithelial cells express and secrete BAFF, both in patients with SS and in healthy subjects [22, 23]. This expression is increased by stimulation with type 1 or type 2 interferon (IFN) [23]. Salivary epithelial cells from patients with SS seem to be more susceptible to the effects of type 1 INF.

SLE and SS share many characteristics, including the presence of an IFN signature in both peripheral blood mononuclear cells and target organs of the respective diseases (e.g., the salivary glands in SS and the kidneys in SLE) [24–26]. It has been shown that stimulation of salivary epithelial cells by poly(I:C) or infection of the cells by reovirus, a double-stranded RNA virus, induces BAFF secretion by salivary epithelial cells [27]. Thus, BAFF is a possible bridge between innate and adaptive immunity in SS.

40.1.4   Increase of BAFF Could Explain the Lack of Efficacy of TNF Inhibition in SS

Two randomized controlled trials, one with infliximab [28] and one with etanercept [29], demonstrated the lack of efficacy of TNF inhibition in SS. Primary SS patients in the etanercept group but not in the placebo group experienced an increase in type 1 IFN levels and BAFF secretion following etanercept administration, possibly explaining the failure of the anti-TNF strategy [30].

40.2   Rituximab in SS

40.2.1   The Different Studies Assessing Rituximab in SS

Rituximab, a monoclonal anti-CD20 antibody, is approved for the treatment of rheumatoid arthritis that is refractory to TNF inhibition. Targeting B-cells also appears to be a promising treatment strategy in SS. The use of rituximab to treat lymphomas complicating SS has been the subject of case reports [31–38] as well as three case series [39–41] (Table 40.1). In two of these case series [39, 41], the

Table 40.1 Open and controlled studies of rituximab in primary Sjögren's syndrome

Reference	Type of study	Number of patients	Indications of RTX	Efficacy for systemic features	Efficacy for fatigue	Efficacy for objective dryness	Efficacy for subjective dryness	Decrease in RF and of IgG	Infusion reactions
Pijpe 2005 [39]	Open	15	Lymphoma (7/15) Early SS (2.3 years) (8/15)	Yes[a]: 3/7 (43%) / NM	No / Yes	No / Yes if residual salivary flow	No / Yes if residual salivary flow	Yes (RF) / No (IgG)	3 SSR, 2 IRR
Seror 2007 [40]	Open	16	Lymphoma (5/16) Systemic features (9.5 years) (11/16)	Yes[a]: 4/5 (80%) Yes: 9/11 (82%)	NM	No: 2/16 (18%)	No: 5/16 (36%)	Yes (both)	2 SSR, 2 IRR
Devauchelle 2007 [41]	Open	16	SS (13.3 years)	1/2 (interstitial pneumonitis)	Yes	No	Yes	No (except IgA RF)	2 IRR
Dass 2008 [42]	RCT	17 (8 on RTX)	SS (7.7 years) Anti-SSA +	NR	Yes in the RTX group P<0.001	No	No	Yes (RF) No (IgG)	1 SSR, 2 IRR
Meijer 2010 [43]	RCT	30 (20 on RTX)	Early SS (5.5 years) RF + Anti-SSA + residual salivary flow	Yes P=0.03 (RTX vs placebo)	Yes P=0.023 (RTX vs placebo)	Yes P=0.038 (RTX vs placebo)	Yes P<0.05 (RTX vs placebo)	Yes (both) P<0.05 (RTX vs placebo)	1 SSR

IRR infusion-related reaction, *NR* not relevant, *NM* not mentioned, *RCT* randomized controlled trial, *SSR* serum sickness-like reaction

[a]Efficacy on lymphoma

efficacy of rituximab appeared to be restricted to patients with early disease. The third open study focused on patients with extraglandular complications of SS, because B-cell hyperactivity is more pronounced in this category of patients [40]. Rituximab appeared to have a strong impact on the systemic features of SS in that study, e.g., the parotidomegaly, synovitis, and cryoglobulinemic vasculitis. However, patients experienced no improvement in either subjective assessments or objective measurements of their sicca symptoms.

The first randomized, controlled trial of rituximab in SS included only 17 patients without any systemic complications [42]. Fatigue, assessed by a visual analogic scale (VAS), was the primary end-point. Fatigue improved significantly in the rituximab group and not in the placebo group (50% improvement versus 20%, respectively).

Another randomized, controlled trial demonstrated efficacy of RTX on stimulated salivary flow, the primary end-point, as well as on systemic complications, symptoms of oral and ocular dryness, and fatigue [43]. A significant decrease in rheumatoid factor level was also observed. Two larger randomized trials are now under way, one in France and one in the UK.

40.2.2 Safety of Rituximab

Serum sickness appears to be a common complication of rituximab in SS. Up to 15% of SS patients treated with rituximab present with a serum sickness-like disease 3–7 days after rituximab infusion (fever, arthralgia, and purpura). Cases of serum sickness have also been described in open studies of rituximab in lupus. The higher frequency of serum sickness disease in SS may be due to hypergammaglobulinemia, which is much more common in SS and SLE than in RA. This complication is benign in most cases but serves as a contraindication to further treatment with rituximab.

The risk of severe infections is a potential issue with rituximab, as with other biologic agents. In RA, the rate of severe infections has been reported to be approximately 2.3/100 patients-years in clinical trials [44] and approximately 5.0/100 patient-years in patients followed in registries [45]. In RA, low serum IgG level, which is rare in SS, is a risk factor of severe infections [45]. Some cases of progressive multifocal leukoencephalopathy (PML) have been described in patients with autoimmune diseases treated with rituximab, but not in any SS patient to date [46]. Assessments of the role of rituximab in causing PML is challenging because most patients reported to date have received intensive immunosuppression with other medications before receiving rituximab.

40.2.3 Increase of BAFF After Rituximab Therapy

Serum BAFF levels increase after rituximab. This has been demonstrated in RA [47, 48], SLE, and SS [49, 50]. The increase has been attributed in part to the disappearance of B-cells in the peripheral blood and the consequent failure of BAFF to bind to its receptor. Two independent studies have also shown that a true homeostatic feedback mechanism exists, characterized by increased BAFF mRNA expression in monocytes following the administration of rituximab [48, 49]. In theory, the increase in BAFF after rituximab could favor the stimulation of new autoimmune B-cells. Another potential biologic target in SS, therefore, is BAFF itself, with inhibition of BAFF via a targeted monoclonal antibody or another strategy. The implications of depleting B-cells and inhibiting BAFF simultaneously remain unclear at the present time. However, targeted BAFF inhibition strategies are in advanced stages of testing in SLE (see below).

40.3   Other B-Cell-Targeted Therapies

40.3.1   Epratuzumab

Epratuzumab, an anti-CD22 monoclonal antibody, has been studied in an open-label trial of 15 patients [51]. This anti-B-cell antibody leads to only partial B-cell depletion (50% in blood). In this open study, improvements of dryness, fatigue, and pain VAS were observed. Moreover, salivary flow appeared to improve in patients with early disease. A controlled trial is now necessary to confirm these data.

40.3.2   BAFF-Targeted Therapy

BAFF is clearly implicated in pathogenesis of SLE and SS. The role of APRIL is less clear, but APRIL could play an important role in the local stimulation of B-cells within the synovium of RA patients. Thus, neutralizing BAFF or APRIL is an appealing approach to the treatment of human autoimmune disease. Two different drugs are currently under development (Fig. 40.1):

- Belimumab is a monoclonal anti-BAFF antibody which targets only BAFF.
- Atacicept is a TACI-Fc molecule that targets both BAFF and APRIL.

Two large phase 2 studies (400–500 patients each) of belimumab have been reported. In RA, the results are rather disappointing with around 30% ACR 20 response in all belimumab groups versus 15% in the placebo group [52]. This may be explained by the fact that, as indicated above, B-cell activation in RA may not be driven only by BAFF. In SLE, the results are more encouraging. Although the primary end-point (decrease of SLEDAI of more than three points) was not achieved in the whole study including 449 patients, the analysis restricted to the 70% of patients with antinuclear antibodies or anti ds-DNA antibodies showed a significant effect of belimumab for decreasing activity of the disease measured by SLEDAI and anti ds-DNA antibody level [53]. Thus, two phase 3 studies including each more

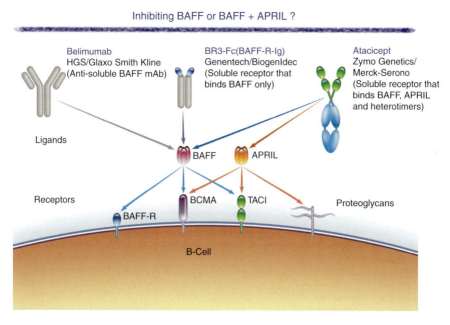

Fig. 40.1 Three treatment strategies for the inhibition of BAFF or BAFF+APRIL. Note: The BR3-Fc development program has been suspended

than 800 patients each have been conducted in SLE and have achieved their primary efficacy end-point [54, 55]. The tolerance of belimumab in these different studies was good. Preliminary phase 2 studies in SS have just begun. Phase 2 studies with atacicept did not demonstrate any efficay in RA but are still in progress in SLE.

40.4 Conclusion

B-cell modulation is clearly a promising therapy in SS, but its utility will likely be limited to certain patient subsets. The design details of future studies in SS will therefore be critical. Initial studies should focus on patients with systemic complications, early disease, and unequivocal evidence of B-cell hyperactivity. The validation of a consensus activity score of the disease recently developed [56] will be helpful in conducting future trials.

References

1. Talal N, Grey HM, Zvaifler N, et al. Elevated salivary and synovial fluid beta2-microglobulin in Sjögren's syndrome and rheumatoid arthritis. Science. 1975;187:1196–8.
2. Moutsopoulos HM, Steinberg AD, Fauci AS, et al. High incidence of free monoclonal lambda light chains in the sera of patients with Sjogren's syndrome. J Immunol. 1983;130(6):2663–5.

3. Ioannidis JP, Vassiliou VA, Moutsopoulos HM. Long-term risk of mortality and lymphoproliferative disease and predictive classification of primary Sjogren's syndrome. Arthritis Rheum. 2002;46:741–7.
4. Kassan SS, Thomas TL, Moutsopoulos H, et al. Increased risk of lymphoma in sicca syndrome. Ann Intern Med. 1978;89:888–92.
5. Theander E, Henriksson G, Ljungberg O, et al. Lymphoma and other malignancies in primary Sjogren's syndrome: a cohort study on cancer incidence and lymphoma predictors. Ann Rheum Dis. 2006;65:796–803.
6. Zinteras E, Voulgarelis M, Moutsopoulos HM. The risk of lymphoma development in autoimmune diseases: a meta-analysis. Arch Intern Med. 2005;165:2337–44.
7. Royer B, Cazals-Hatem D, Sibilia J, et al. Lymphomas in patients with Sjogren's syndrome are marginal zone B-cell neoplasms, arise in diverse extranodal and nodal sites and are not associated with viruses. Blood. 1997;90:766–75.
8. Voulgarelis M, Dafni UG, Isenberg DA, et al. Malignant lymphoma in primary Sjogren's syndrome: a multicenter, retrospective, clinical study by the European Concerted Action on Sjogren's Syndrome. Arthritis Rheum. 1999;42:1765–72.
9. Bende RJ, Aarts WM, Riedl RG, et al. Among B cell non-Hodgkin's lymphomas, MALT lymphomas express a unique antibody repertoire with frequent rheumatoid factor reactivity. J Exp Med. 2005;201:1229–41.
10. Gottenberg JE, Busson M, Cohen-Solal J, et al. Correlation of serum B lymphocyte stimulator and beta2 microglobulin with autoantibody secretion and systemic involvement in primary Sjogren's syndrome. Ann Rheum Dis. 2005;64(7):1050–5.
11. Gottenberg JE, Aucouturier F, Goetz J, et al. Serum immunoglobulin free light chain assessment in rheumatoid arthritis and primary Sjögren's syndrome. Ann Rheum Dis. 2007;66(1): 23–7.
12. Schneider P, MacKay F, Steiner V, et al. BAFF, a novel ligand of the tumor necrosis factor family, stimulates B cell growth. J Exp Med. 1999;189:1747–56.
13. Moore PA, Belvedere O, Orr A, et al. BLyS: member of the tumor necrosis factor family and B lymphocyte stimulator. Science. 1999;285:260–3.
14. Nardelli B, Belvedere O, Roschke V, et al. Synthesis and release of B-lymphocyte stimulator from myeloid cells. Blood. 2001;97:198–204.
15. Mackay F, Woodcock SA, Lawton P, et al. Mice transgenic for BAFF develop lymphocytic disorders along with autoimmune manifestations. J Exp Med. 1999;190:1697–710.
16. Groom J, Kalled SL, Cutler AH, et al. Association of BAFF/BLyS overexpression and altered B cell differentiation with Sjogren's syndrome. J Clin Invest. 2002;109:59–68.
17. Mariette X, Roux S, Zhang J, et al. The level of BLyS (BAFF) correlates with the titre of autoantibodies in human Sjogren's syndrome. Ann Rheum Dis. 2003;62:168–71.
18. Jonsson M, Szodoray P, Jellestad S, et al. Association between circulating levels of the novel TNF family members APRIL and BAFF and lymphoid organization in primary Sjögren's syndrome. J Clin Immunol. 2005;25(3):189–201.
19. Pers JO, Daridon C, Devauchelle V, et al. BAFF overexpression is associated with autoantibody production in autoimmune diseases. Ann N Y Acad Sci. 2005;1050:34–9.
20. Pers JO, d'Arbonneau F, Devauchelle-Pensec V, et al. Is periodontal disease mediated by salivary BAFF in Sjögren's syndrome? Arthritis Rheum. 2005;52:2411–4.
21. Lavie F, Miceli-Richard C, Quillard J, et al. Overexpression of BAFF in T cells infiltrating labial salivary glands from patients with Sjögren's syndrome. J Pathol. 2004;202:496–502.
22. Daridon C, Devauchelle V, Hutin P, et al. Aberrant expression of BAFF by B lymphocytes infiltrating the salivary glands of patients with primary Sjögren's syndrome. Arthritis Rheum. 2007;56:1134–44.
23. Ittah M, Miceli-Richard C, Gottenberg JE, et al. B-cell activating factor of the TNF family (BAFF) is expressed under stimulation by interferon in salivary gland epithelial cells in primary Sjögren's syndrome. Arthritis Res Ther. 2006;8:R51.

24. Bave U, Nordmark G, Lofgren T, et al. Activation of the type-I interferon system in primary SS. Arthritis Rheum. 2005;52:1185–95.
25. Hjelmervik TO, Petersen K, Jonassen I, et al. Gene expression profiling of minor salivary glands clearly distinguishes primary Sjogren's syndrome patients from healthy control subjects. Arthritis Rheum. 2005;52:1534–44.
26. Gottenberg J, Cagnard N, Lucchesi C, et al. Activation of interferon pathways and plasmacytoid dendritic cell recruitment in target organs of primary Sjögren's syndrome. Proc Natl Acad Sci USA. 2006;103:2770–5.
27. Ittah M, Miceli-Richard C, Gottenberg JE, et al. Viruses induce high expression of B cell-activating factor by salivary gland epithelial cells through Toll-like receptor- and type-I interferon-dependent and -independent pathways. Eur J Immunol. 2008;38(4):1058–64.
28. Mariette X, Ravaud P, Steinfeld S, et al. Inefficacy of infliximab in primary Sjögren's syndrome. Results of the randomized controlled trial of Remicade in primary Sjögren's syndrome (TRIPSS). Arthritis Rheum. 2004;50:1270–6.
29. Sankar V, Brennan MT, Kok MR, et al. Etanercept in Sjogren's syndrome: a twelve-week randomized, double-blind, placebo-controlled pilot clinical trial. Arthritis Rheum. 2004;50:2240–5.
30. Mavragani CP, Niewold TB, Moutsopoulos NM, et al. Augmented interferon-alpha pathway activation in patients with Sjögren's syndrome treated with etanercept. Arthritis Rheum. 2007;56:3995–4004.
31. Somer BG, Tsai DE, Downs L, et al. Improvement in Sjogren's syndrome following therapy with rituximab for marginal zone lymphoma. Arthritis Rheum. 2003;49(3):394–8.
32. Voulgarelis M, Giannouli S, Anagnostou D, et al. Combined therapy with rituximab plus cyclophosphamide/doxorubicin/vincristine/prednisone (CHOP) for Sjogren's syndrome-associated B-cell aggressive non-Hodgkin's lymphomas. Rheumatology (Oxford). 2004;43(8):1050–3.
33. Harner KC, Jackson LW, Drabick JJ. Normalization of anticardiolipin antibodies following rituximab therapy for marginal zone lymphoma in a patient with Sjogren's syndrome. Rheumatology (Oxford). 2004;43(10):1309–10.
34. Ramos-Casals M, Lopez-Guillermo A, Brito-Zeron P, et al. Treatment of B-cell lymphoma with rituximab in two patients with Sjögren's syndrome associated with hepatitis C virus infection. Lupus. 2004;13(12):969–71.
35. Pijpe J, van Imhoff GW, Vissink A, et al. Changes in salivary gland immunohistology and function after rituximab monotherapy in a patient with Sjögren's syndrome and associated MALT lymphoma. Ann Rheum Dis. 2005;64(6):958–60.
36. Ahmadi-Simab K, Lamprecht P, Nolle B, et al. Successful treatment of refractory anterior scleritis in primary Sjögren's syndrome with rituximab. Ann Rheum Dis. 2005;64(7):1087–8.
37. Ring T, Kallenbach M, Praetorius J, et al. Successful treatment of a patient with primary Sjögren's syndrome with rituximab. Clin Rheumatol. 2006;25(6):891–4.
38. Voulgarelis M, Giannouli S, Tzioufas AG, et al. Long term remission of Sjögren's syndrome associated aggressive B cell non-Hodgkin's lymphomas following combined B cell depletion therapy and CHOP (cyclophosphamide, doxorubicin, vincristine, prednisone). Ann Rheum Dis. 2006;65(8):1033–7.
39. Pijpe J, van Imhoff GW, Spijkervet FK, et al. Rituximab treatment in patients with primary Sjögren's syndrome: an open-label phase II study. Arthritis Rheum. 2005;52:2740–50.
40. Seror R, Sordet C, Guillevin L, et al. Tolerance and efficacy of rituximab and changes in serum B cell biomarkers in patients with systemic complications of primary Sjögren's syndrome. Ann Rheum Dis. 2007;66:351–7.
41. Devauchelle-Pensec V, Pennec Y, Morvan J, et al. Improvement of Sjögren's syndrome after two infusions of rituximab (anti-CD20). Arthritis Rheum. 2007;57:310–7.
42. Dass S, Bowman SJ, Vital EM, et al. Reduction of fatigue in Sjogren's syndrome with rituximab: results of a randomised, double-blind, placebo controlled pilot study. Ann Rheum Dis. 2008;67:1541–4.

43. Meijer JM, Meiners PM, Vissink A, et al. Effectiveness of rituximab treatment in primary Sjögren's syndrome: a randomized, double-blind, placebo-controlled trial. Arthritis Rheum. 2010;62:960–8.
44. Salliot C, Dougados M, Gossec L. Risk of serious infections during rituximab, abatacept and anakinra treatments for rheumatoid arthritis: meta-analyses of randomised placebo-controlled trials. Ann Rheum Dis. 2009;68:25–32.
45. Gottenberg JE, Ravaud P, Bardin T, et al. Risk factors for severe infections in patients with rheumatoid arthritis treated with rituximab in the autoimmunity and rituximab registry. Arthritis Rheum. 2010 Sep;62(9):2625–32.
46. Carson KR, Evens AM, Richey EA, et al. Progressive multifocal leukoencephalopathy after rituximab therapy in HIV-negative patients: a report of 57 cases from the Research on Adverse Drug Events and Reports project. Blood. 2009;113:4834–40.
47. Cambridge G, Stohl W, Leandro MJ, et al. Circulating levels of B lymphocyte stimulator in patients with rheumatoid arthritis following rituximab treatment: relationships with B cell depletion, circulating antibodies, and clinical relapse. Arthritis Rheum. 2006;54:723–32.
48. Toubi E, Kessel A, Slobodin G, et al. Macrophage function changes following rituximab treatment in patients with rheumatoid arthritis. Ann Rheum Dis. 2007;66(6):818–20.
49. Lavie F, Miceli-Richard C, Ittah M, et al. Increase of B-cell activating factor of the TNF family (BAFF) after rituximab: insights into a new regulating system of BAFF production. Ann Rheum Dis. 2007;66(5):700–3.
50. Pers JO, Devauchelle V, Daridon C, et al. BAFF-modulated repopulation of B lymphocytes in the blood and salivary glands of rituximab-treated patients with Sjögren's syndrome. Arthritis Rheum. 2007;56:1464–77.
51. Steinfeld SD, Tant L, Burmester GR, et al. Epratuzumab (humanised anti-CD22 antibody) in primary Sjögren's syndrome: an open-label phase I/II study. Arthritis Res Ther. 2006; 8(4):R129.
52. Stohl W, Chatham W, Weisman M, et al. Belimumab (BmAb), a novel fully human monoclonal antibody to B-lymphocyte stimulator (BLyS), selectively modulates B-cell sub-populations and immunoglobulins in a heterogeneous rheumatoid arthritis subject population. Arthritis Rheum. 2005;52:S444.
53. Wallace DJ, Stohl W, Furie RA, et al. A phase II, randomized, double-blind, placebo-controlled, dose-ranging study of belimumab in patients with active systemic lupus erythematosus. Arthritis Rheum. 2009;61(9):1168–78.
54. Navarra S, Ilianova E, Bae SC, et al. Belimumab, a blys-specific inhibitor, reduced disease activity, flares, and steroid use in patients with seropositive systemic lupus erythematosus (SLE): BLISS-52 study. EULAR 2010 meeting, poster SAT0204, Rome, 2010.
55. van Vollenhoven RF, Zamani O, Wallace DJ, et al. Belimumab, a blys-specific inhibitor, reduces disease activity and severe flares in seropositive sle patients: BLISS-76 study. EULAR 2010 meeting, oral presentation, Rome, 2010.
56. Seror R, Ravaud P, Bowman S, et al. EULAR Sjogren's Syndrome Disease Activity Index (ESSDAI): development of a consensus systemic disease activity index in primary Sjogren's syndrome. Ann Rheum Dis. 2010;69(6):1103–9.

Chapter 41
Other Biological Therapies in Primary Sjögren's Syndrome

Pilar Brito-Zerón, Cándido Diaz-Lagares, M. Jose Soto-Cárdenas, Manuel Ramos-Casals, and Munther A. Khamashta

Contents

P. Brito-Zerón • C. Diaz-Lagares
Sjögren Syndrome Research Group (AGAUR), Laboratory of Autoimmune Diseases Josep Font, Institut d'Investigacions Biomèdiques August Pi i Sunyer (IDIBAPS), Barcelona, Spain

M.J. Soto-Cárdenas
Department of Medicine, University of Cadiz, Department of Internal Medicine, Hospital Puerta del Mar, Cadiz, Spain

M. Ramos-Casals (⊠)
Spanish Group of Autoimmune Diseases (GEAS), Spanish Society of Internal Medicine (SEMI), Sjögren Syndrome Research Group (AGAUR), Laboratory of Autoimmune Diseases Josep Font, Institut d'Investigacions Biomèdiques August Pi i Sunyer (IDIBAPS), Department of Autoimmune Diseases, ICMD Hospital Clínic, Barcelona, Spain

M.A. Khamashta
Lupus Research Unit, The Rayne Institute, King's College London School of Medicine at Guy's, King's and St Thomas' Hospitals, St Thomas' Hospital, London, UK

M. Ramos-Casals et al. (eds.), *Sjögren's Syndrome*,
DOI 10.1007/978-0-85729-947-5_41, © Springer-Verlag London Limited 2012

41.1   Introduction

Sjögren's syndrome (SS) is a systemic autoimmune disease that mainly affects the exocrine glands and usually presents as persistent dryness of the mouth and eyes. SS typically affects white perimenopausal women, with an incidence of 4–5 cases per 100,000. At present, there is no treatment capable of modifying the evolution of SS and the therapeutic approach is based on symptomatic replacement or stimulation of glandular secretions, using substitutive and oral muscarinic agents. Extraglandular involvement requires organ-specific therapy generally based upon some combination of glucocorticoids and immunosuppressive agents, similar to that applied in patients with systemic lupus erythematosus (SLE) [1]. The use of biological agents targeting molecules and receptors involved in the etiopathogenesis of primary SS, most of which have been evaluated in SLE, opens a new era in the therapeutic management of patients with primary SS. B cell targeted therapies, especially rituximab, are the most promising agents in primary SS currently. Other promising B cell targeted therapies include epratuzumab and belimumab. T cell targeted agents (efalizumab, abatacept, alefacept) should currently be considered possible future options [2]. In this chapter, we review the potential use of biological agents targeting cytokines and T cell adhesion molecules involved in the etiopathogenesis of primary SS.

41.2   Cytokine Targeted Therapies

A possible role of cytokines in the etiopathogenesis of primary SS has been suggested by several studies [3]. Unfortunately, the recent excellent results obtained in rheumatic diseases using agents blocking some cytokines (such as anti-TNF agents for RA and spondyloarthropathies) have not been confirmed in systemic autoimmune diseases such as SLE or primary SS.

41.2.1   Infliximab

Recent studies have analyzed the role of infliximab for the treatment of primary SS (Table 41.1). In a single-center, open-label pilot study, Steinfeld et al. [4] found an improvement in clinical and functional parameters in 16 patients with primary SS treated with 3 infusions of infliximab (3 mg/kg) at 0, 2, and 6 weeks. The same authors [5] evaluated the safety and efficacy of a maintenance regimen of infliximab in 10 of the 16 patients with primary SS who received additional infusions of infliximab for 1 year. A statistically significant decrease in global and local disease manifestations was observed in all ten patients, although the main improvement was only observed in subjective symptomatology, with no changes in the erythrocyte

Table 41.1 New and possible therapeutic approaches in primary SS using biological agents

B cell targeted therapies
- Rituximab (anti-CD20)
- Ocrelizumab (humanized anti-CD20)
- Epratuzumab (anti-CD22)
- Belimumab (anti-BAFF)

T cell targeted therapies
- Efalizumab (anti-CD11a)
- Alefacept (anti-CD2)
- Abatacept (anti-CD80/86)

Cytokine targeted therapies
- Infliximab (anti-TNF)
- Etanercept (anti-TNF)
- Tocilizumab (anti-IL6r)
- Anakinra (anti-IL1)
- Ustekinumab, briakinumab (anti-IL12/23)
- Rontalizumab, sifalimumab (anti-IFNα)
- Anti-IL10
- Anti-IL17

Complement targeted therapies
- Eculizumab (anti-C5a/C5b-9)

sedimentation rate or IgG levels. Treatment was generally well tolerated, and the main side effect was a mild, self-limiting infusion reaction in 4 (40%) patients (one of them presenting with generalized rash, fever and arthralgia), while 2 (20%) developed infectious processes (enteritis and tonsillitis).

Other authors have reported successful responses in some patients with extraglandular features. Caroyer et al. [6] reported the successful treatment of a severe sensory neuropathy with infliximab, while Pessler et al. [7] reported a successful response to infliximab in an 11-year-old girl with polyarthritis, suggesting that TNF-alpha blockers have a role in the treatment of arthritis in pediatric SS.

However, the key study for evaluating the therapeutic effect of infliximab in primary SS was published by Mariette et al. in 2004 [8]. These authors conducted a multicenter, randomized, double-blind, placebo-controlled trial including a total of 103 patients with primary SS. The patients were assigned randomly to receive infliximab infusions (5 mg/kg) or placebo at weeks 0, 2, and 6 and were followed for 22 weeks. At week 10, 26.5% of patients receiving placebo and 27.8% of patients treated with infliximab had a favorable overall response ($p=0.89$). At week 22, 20.4% of the placebo group and 16.7% of the infliximab group had a favorable response. In addition, the two groups did not differ in any of the secondary end points over the 22 weeks of the trial. Thus, although infliximab might play a role in the treatment of specific severe refractory extraglandular features, the results of this controlled trial indicate clearly that anti-TNF agents should not be considered as a first-line option for the treatment of primary SS.

Table 41.2 Therapeutic role of biological agents targeting cytokines and T cell adhesion molecules in primary SS: reported studies

Biological agent	Authors (reference)	Patients	Study design	Efficacy
Infliximab	Steinfeld et al. [4]	16	Open label	Response
	Mariette et al. [8]	103	Randomized, double-blind, placebo-controlled	No response
Etanercept	Sankar et al. [9]	28	Randomized, double-blind, placebo-controlled	No response
	Zandbelt et al. [10]	15	Open label	No response
Anakinra	University of Oslo	–	Phase II	Study completed, no publications provided
Efalizumab	NIDCR	–	Phase II	Study completed, no publications provided

NIDCR National Institute of Dental and Craniofacial Research (US)

41.2.2   Etanercept

Two studies performed in small series of patients have demonstrated a limited beneficial effect of etanercept in primary SS (Table 41.2). Sankar et al. [9] conducted a 12-week randomized, double-blind, placebo-controlled trial of etanercept. Twenty-eight patients received 25 mg of etanercept or placebo (vehicle) by twice-weekly subcutaneous injection. Of the 14 patients taking etanercept, 11 had primary SS and 3 had SS associated with rheumatoid arthritis. Baseline measures did not differ between the two groups. Three etanercept-treated patients and one placebo-treated patient did not complete the trial. Five etanercept-treated patients and three placebo-treated patients showed improvement from baseline in the primary outcome variable at 12 weeks, but the difference was not statistically significant. There were no significant differences between the groups for changes in subjective measures of oral or ocular symptoms (by visual analog scale), the IgG level, Schirmer I test result, van Bijsterveld score, or salivary flow. However, the ESR had decreased in the etanercept group compared with baseline [9].

Zandbelt et al. [10] evaluated the effect of etanercept on sicca, systemic, and histological signs of 15 patients with primary SS who were treated with 25-mg etanercept subcutaneously twice per week during 12 weeks, with follow-up visits at weeks 18 and 24. No increase of salivary or lacrimal gland function was observed in any patient. In four patients, a decrease of fatigue complaints was noted, which was also reflected by decreased scores in the MFI [*MFI questionnaire? What does MFI stand for?*] questionnaire. A repeated treatment up to 26 weeks showed the same results. The authors concluded that etanercept 25 mg twice weekly did not appear to reduce sicca symptoms and signs in SS and did not affect minor salivary gland biopsy results.

These two studies showed no evidence to suggest that treatment with etanercept at a dosage of 25 mg twice weekly was clinically efficacious in SS. Recent studies have investigated the underlying pathogenic mechanisms that may explain this lack of efficacy. Moutsopoulos et al. [11] linked the inefficacy of etanercept with the absence of suppression of TNF-alpha and other markers of immune activation observed in SS patients treated with etanercept. Those results suggested that TNF-alpha is a pivotal cytokine in the pathogenesis of primary SS.

Another study [12] found that interferon (IFN)-alpha activity and BAFF levels are elevated in the plasma of patients with SS treated with etanercept in comparison with controls, suggesting that etanercept exacerbated the overexpression of IFN-alpha and BAFF [12]. These findings may also explain the apparent lack of efficacy observed for etanercept in SS.

41.2.3 Interferon Alpha

Recent studies have suggested a pivotal of the INF pathway in the pathogenesis of primary SS [13], with some IFN-related genes such as STAT4 and IRPF5 being overexpressed [14, 15]. Three controlled studies evaluated the use of oral IFN-α (150 IU daily). A small, controlled trial (12 patients) suggested a beneficial effect on the unstimulated salivary flow rate and ocular/oral dryness [16], while a single-blinded, sucralfate-controlled trial [17] found a significant, time-dependent increase in the production of whole saliva at 3 months but not at 6 months. In contrast, a large placebo-controlled trial including 497 patients [18] found significant improvement in only one of 28 outcomes evaluated (unstimulated whole saliva, $p = 0.01$) and a higher percentage of adverse events (40% vs 25% in the placebo group, $p < 0.001$). The limited benefits observed in these studies allow considering that the blockade of this cytokine may be a better potential therapeutic intervention [19]. Anti-IFN monoclonal antibodies are under development in SLE [19].

41.2.4 Emerging Anticytokine Therapies

Recent studies have analyzed the blockade of other cytokines as a possible therapeutic option in patients with RA, SLE, psoriasis, and Crohn's disease, including monoclonal antibodies against IL-6, IL-10, IL-12, IL-17, IL-18, or IL-23 [20–25]. The IL-6R antagonist tocilizumab has been recently approved for treatment of rheumatoid arthritis (RA) in Europe, Japan, and the USA [26], while monoclonal antibodies against IL-12 and IL-23 (ustekinumab and ABT-874) are currently evaluated for the treatment of moderate-to-severe psoriasis [27, 28]. Other studies are testing an IL-18-binding protein in RA and psoriasis [19]. Recent studies have reported an increased expression of these cytokines (IL12, IL17, IL18, IL23) in primary SS [29–31], and it seems reasonable that some of these anti-cytokine therapies might also be tested in primary SS in the future.

41.3   T Cell Targeted Therapies

Adhesion molecules participate in many stages of the immune response, regulating leukocyte circulation, lymphoid cell homing to tissues and inflammatory sites, migration across endothelial cells, and T cell stimulation. During the T cell immune response, adhesion molecules form a specialized junction between the T cell and the antigen-presenting cell. For this reason, in the search for new therapeutic agents, many researchers have focused their attention on targeting adhesion molecules. Most of these efforts are intended to develop drugs for autoimmune diseases. Therapeutic agents such as efalizumab and alefacept have been approved by the FDA for the treatment of some inflammatory autoimmune diseases such as psoriasis [32].

After the initiation of the autoimmune process in primary SS, autoantigens are expressed on the surface of epithelial cells, with T lymphocytes migrating to exocrine tissue and being activated in situ and B cells producing autoantibodies locally [33]. Several studies have recently analyzed the role of T cell dysfunction in the pathogenesis of primary SS.

41.3.1   Efalizumab

Efalizumab (Raptiva®) is a humanized monoclonal antibody that targets the CD11a component of leukocyte function–associated antigen-1 (LFA-1), preventing its binding to intercellular adhesion molecules. Blocking this interaction results in interference with T cell activation and reactivation, inhibition of leukocyte extravasation, and adherence to keratinocytes in psoriatic epidermis. Some studies have suggested a potential role for LFA-1 in controlling the migration of lymphocytes to exocrine glands in SS [34, 35], with the implication that efalizumab might be a treatment strategy worth testing.

Efalizumab was approved by the FDA and EMEA for the treatment of psoriasis [36]. Unfortunately, it has recently been withdrawn after 5 years of use because of three cases of progressive multifocal leukoencephalopathy [37]. An ongoing phase II study sponsored by the National Institute of Dental and Craniofacial Research, which had been recruiting patients since 2006, had to be suspended.

41.3.2   Alefacept

Alefacept (Amevive®) is a selective immunomodulating drug that blocks the LFA–3/ CD2 interaction necessary for the activation and proliferation of memory effector T cells by binding to the CD2 expressed on the T cell surface. Among biological agents, alefacept has demonstrated the longest remission in psoriasis [38], and appears to be well tolerated, even with long-term use. Alefacept was approved by the FDA in January 2003 for the treatment of chronic plaque psoriasis [39]. However, the primary concern with alefacept is T lymphocyte depletion. Because the CD4+ count is reduced by alefacept, it should be monitored on a regular basis to ensure it does not drop below 250 cells/µL. The reported side effects are minor and include: headache, nasopharyngitis, rhinitis, influenza, upper respiratory tract infections, pruritus, arthralgia, fatigue, nausea, and elevated liver enzymes. Severe infections and malignancies have not been linked to the use of alefacept, and few patients develop anti-alefacept antibodies. Alefacept seems to be a safe biological therapy for moderate-to-severe chronic plaque psoriasis with few side effects reported and will probably be tested in coming years in patients with systemic autoimmune diseases such as SLE, RA, and SS.

41.3.3 Abatacept

Abatacept (Orencia®) is a soluble fusion protein that consists of the extracellular domain of human cytotoxic T lymphocyte–associated antigen 4 (CTLA-4) linked to the modified Fc portion of human IgG1. Specifically, abatacept blocks the CD80 and CD86 ligands on the surface of antigen-presenting cells that interface with the T cell's CD28 receptor to activate T cells.

Abatacept has recently been approved for the treatment of rheumatoid arthritis refractory to other agents and seems to be more immunosuppressive than TNF-alpha blockers. The combination of abatacept and a TNF-alpha-blocking agent does not seem to be more effective than either agent alone. Because abatacept has the ability to suppress T cell function, it is a potential treatment for psoriasis and other autoimmune conditions involving T cell driven pathologic processes. However, a recent controlled trial in patients with RA showed an increased rate of serious adverse events in patients receiving abatacept in combination with other biologic therapies [40], including a trend to a higher incidence of neoplasms (7% vs 2%). Therefore, abatacept should not be used in combination with other biologics to treat RA. Further long-term studies and postmarketing surveillance are required to assess for longer-term harms and sustained efficacy [41].

Recent evidence suggests that CTLA-4, an immune attenuator, contributes significantly to homeostatic control of T helper cell proliferation, and has a critical immunoregulatory role in the downregulation of T cell activation. Only two studies have been carried out in patients with primary SS. The first found no significant differences in the CTLA-4 polymorphisms of Tunisian patients with SS compared with the control group [42], while a recent study by Downie-Doyle et al. [43] described insignificant differences in haplotype frequencies of Australian SS patients compared with controls. A controlled trial of abatacept is under way in the Netherlands.

41.4 Conclusion

New therapeutic approaches in primary SS using biological agents are centered on correcting lymphocytic dysfunction, with agents directed at modifying T cell dysfunction or diminishing B cell hyperactivity. B cell targeted therapies seem to be the most promising agents in primary SS, especially rituximab (anti-CD20). Rituximab has demonstrated therapeutic efficacy in the treatment of associated extraglandular and lymphoproliferative processes, although data from large randomized, double-blind, placebo-controlled studies are not yet available. Other promising B cell targeted therapies include agents against CD22+ cells (epratuzumab) and therapies antagonizing Blys/BAFF (belimumab). It seems logical that these agents may play a role in modifying the etiopathogenic events of patients with primary SS, a disease characterized by B cell hyperactivity.

The excellent results of TNF targeted therapies in RA led to these agents being tested in patients with primary SS. However, controlled studies showed a lack of efficacy of infliximab and etanercept in primary SS. Strategies based on T cell targeted therapies (efalizumab, abatacept, alefacept) should be considered as possible future therapeutic options, although the poor response obtained with anti-TNF agents (which may be considered as partially directed against T cells) might suggest a similar limited response.

In the near future, biological agents will play key roles in the treatment of severe SS, broadening the therapeutic options for patients with this disease. However, the possible risks and benefits of using these agents should be balanced carefully. Assessments of the risk of serious adverse events versus the potential benefits of treatment must be made on a patient-by-patient basis.

References

1. Ramos-Casals M, Tzioufas AG, Stone JH, Sisó A, Bosch X. Treatment of primary Sjögren syndrome: a systematic review. JAMA. 2010;304:452–60.
2. Ramos-Casals M, Brito-Zerón P. Emerging biological therapies in primary Sjögren's syndrome. Rheumatology (Oxford). 2007;46:1389–96.
3. Ramos-Casals M, Font J. Primary Sjögren's syndrome: current and emergent aetiopathogenic concepts. Rheumatology (Oxford). 2005;44:1354–67.
4. Steinfeld SD, Demols P, Salmon I, Kiss R, Appelboom T. Infliximab in patients with primary Sjögren's syndrome: a pilot study. Arthritis Rheum. 2001;44:2371–5.
5. Steinfeld SD, Demols P, Appelboom T. Infliximab in primary Sjögren's syndrome: one-year followup. Arthritis Rheum. 2002;46:3301–3.
6. Caroyer JM, Manto MU, Steinfeld SD. Severe sensory neuronopathy responsive to infliximab in primary Sjögren's syndrome. Neurology. 2002;59:1113–4.
7. Pessler F, Monash B, Rettig P, Forbes B, Kreiger PA, Cron RQ. Sjogren syndrome in a child: favorable response of the arthritis to TNFalpha blockade. Clin Rheumatol. 2006;25:746–8.
8. Mariette X, Ravaud P, Steinfeld S, et al. Inefficacy of infliximab in primary Sjögren's syndrome: results of the randomized, controlled Trial of Remicade in Primary Sjogren's Syndrome (TRIPSS). Arthritis Rheum. 2004;50:1270–6.
9. Sankar V, Brennan MT, Kok MR, et al. Etanercept in Sjögren's syndrome: a twelve-week randomized, double-blind, placebo-controlled pilot clinical trial. Arthritis Rheum. 2004;50:2240–5.
10. Zandbelt MM, de Wilde P, van Damme P, Hoyng CB, van de Putte L, van den Hoogen F. Etanercept in the treatment of patients with primary Sjögren's syndrome: a pilot study. J Rheumatol. 2004;31:96–101.
11. Moutsopoulos NM, Katsifis GE, Angelov N, Leakan RA, Sankar V, Pillemer S, et al. Lack of efficacy of etanercept in Sjögren syndrome correlates with failed suppression of tumour necrosis factor alpha and systemic immune activation. Ann Rheum Dis. 2008;67:1437–43.

12. Mavragani CP, Niewold TB, Moutsopoulos NM, Pillemer SR, Wahl SM, Crow MK. Augmented interferon-alpha pathway activation in patients with Sjögren's syndrome treated with etanercept. Arthritis Rheum. 2007;56:3995–4004.
13. Mavragani CP, Crow MK. Activation of the type I interferon pathway in primary Sjögren's syndrome. J Autoimmun. 2010;35(2):225–31. PubMed PMID:20674271.
14. Mariette X, Gottenberg JE. Pathogenesis of Sjögren's syndrome and therapeutic consequences. Curr Opin Rheumatol. 2010;22:471–7.
15. Miceli-Richard C, Gestermann N, Ittah M, et al. The CGGGG insertion/deletion polymorphism of the IRF5 promoter is a strong risk factor for primary Sjögren's syndrome. Arthritis Rheum. 2009;60:1991–7.
16. Cummins MJ, Papas A, Kammer GM, Fox PC. Treatment of primary Sjögren's syndrome with low-dose human interferon alfa administered by the oromucosal route: combined phase III results. Arthritis Rheum. 2003;49:585–93.
17. Ship JA, Fox PC, Michalek JE, Cummins MJ, Richards AB. Treatment of primary Sjögren's syndrome with low-dose natural human interferon-alpha administered by the oral mucosal route: a phase II clinical trial. IFN Protocol Study Group. J Interferon Cytokine Res. 1999;19:943–51.
18. Shiozawa S, Tanaka Y, Shiozawa K. Single-blinded controlled trial of low-dose oral IFN-alpha for the treatment of xerostomia in patients with Sjögren's syndrome. J Interferon Cytokine Res. 1998;18:255–62.
19. Roescher N, Tak PP, Illei GG. Cytokines in Sjögren's syndrome: potential therapeutic targets. Ann Rheum Dis. 2010;69:945–8.
20. Smolen JS, Maini RN. Interleukin-6: a new therapeutic target. Arthritis Res Ther. 2006;8:407.
21. Llorente L, Richaud-Patin Y, Garcia-Padilla C, et al. Clinical and biologic effects of anti-interleukin-10 monoclonal antibody administration in systemic lupus erythematosus. Arthritis Rheum. 2000;43:1790–800.
22. Koenders MI, Joosten LA, van den Berg WB. Potential new targets in arthritis therapy: interleukin (IL)-17 and its relation to tumour necrosis factor and IL-1 in experimental arthritis. Ann Rheum Dis. 2006;65 Suppl 3:iii29–33.
23. Isenberg D, Rahman A. Systemic lupus erythematosus – 2005 annus mirabilis? Nat Clin Pract Rheumatol. 2006;2:145–52.
24. Strand V, Singh JA. Newer biological agents in rheumatoid arthritis: impact on health-related quality of life and productivity. Drugs. 2010;70:121–45.
25. Singh JA, Beg S, Lopez-Olivo MA. Tocilizumab for rheumatoid arthritis. Cochrane Database Syst Rev. 2010;7:CD008331.
26. Nam JL, Winthrop KL, van Vollenhoven RF, et al. Current evidence for the management of rheumatoid arthritis with biological disease-modifying antirheumatic drugs: a systematic literature review informing the EULAR recommendations for the management of RA. Ann Rheum Dis. 2010;69:976–86.
27. Menter A. The status of biologic therapies in the treatment of moderate to severe psoriasis. Cutis. 2009;84(4 Suppl):14–24.
28. Kuhn A, Luger TA. Psoriasis: is ustekinumab superior to etanercept for psoriasis? Nat Rev Rheumatol. 2010;6:500–1.
29. Vosters JL, Landek-Salgado MA, Yin H, et al. Interleukin-12 induces salivary gland dysfunction in transgenic mice, providing a new model of Sjögren's syndrome. Arthritis Rheum. 2009;60:3633–41.
30. Katsifis GE, Rekka S, Moutsopoulos NM, Pillemer S, Wahl SM. Systemic and local interleukin-17 and linked cytokines associated with Sjögren's syndrome immunopathogenesis. Am J Pathol. 2009;175:1167–77.
31. Sakai A, Sugawara Y, Kuroishi T, Sasano T, Sugawara S. Identification of IL-18 and Th17 cells in salivary glands of patients with Sjögren's syndrome, and amplification of IL-17-mediated secretion of inflammatory cytokines from salivary gland cells by IL-18. J Immunol. 2008;181:2898–906.

32. Jois SD, Jining L, Nagarajarao LM. Targeting T cell adhesion molecules for drug design. Curr Pharm Des. 2006;12:2797–812.
33. Konttinen YT, Kasna-Ronkainen L. Sjögren's syndrome: viewpoint on pathogenesis. One of the reasons I was never asked to write a textbook chapter on it. Scand J Rheumatol Suppl. 2002;116:15–22.
34. Mikulowska-Mennis A, Xu B, Berberian JM, Michie SA. Lymphocyte migration to inflamed lacrimal glands is mediated by vascular cell adhesion molecule-1/alpha(4)beta(1) integrin, peripheral node addressin/l-selectin, and lymphocyte function-associated antigen-1 adhesion pathways. Am J Pathol. 2001;159:671–81.
35. Bolstad AI, Eiken HG, Rosenlund B, Alarcon-Riquelme ME, Jonsson R. Increased salivary gland tissue expression of Fas, Fas ligand, cytotoxic T lymphocyte-associated antigen 4, and programmed cell death 1 in primary Sjögren's syndrome. Arthritis Rheum. 2003;48:174–85.
36. Papp KA, Henninger E. Evaluation of efalizumab using safe psoriasis control. BMC Dermatol. 2006;6:8.
37. Gadzia J, Turner J. Progressive multifocal leukoencephalopathy in two psoriasis patients treated with efalizumab. J Drugs Dermatol. 2010;9(8):1005–9.
38. Papp KA. The long-term efficacy and safety of new biological therapies for psoriasis. Arch Dermatol Res. 2006;298:7–15.
39. Dunn LK, Feldman SR. Alefacept treatment for chronic plaque psoriasis. Skin Therapy Lett. 2010;15:1–3.
40. Weinblatt M, Combe B, Covucci A, Aranda R, Becker JC, Keystone E. Safety of the selective costimulation modulator abatacept in rheumatoid arthritis patients receiving background biologic and nonbiologic disease-modifying antirheumatic drugs: a one-year randomized, placebo-controlled study. Arthritis Rheum. 2006;54:2807–16.
41. Maxwell LJ, Singh JA. Abatacept for rheumatoid arthritis: a Cochrane systematic review. J Rheumatol. 2010;37:234–45.
42. Hadj Kacem H, Kaddour N, Adyel FZ, Bahloul Z, Ayadi H. HLA-DQB1 CAR1/CAR2, TNFa IR2/IR4 and CTLA-4 polymorphisms in Tunisian patients with rheumatoid arthritis and Sjögren's syndrome. Rheumatology (Oxford). 2001;40:1370–4.
43. Downie-Doyle S, Bayat N, Rischmueller M, Lester S. Influence of CTLA4 haplotypes on susceptibility and some extraglandular manifestations in primary Sjögren's syndrome. Arthritis Rheum. 2006;54:2434–40.

Chapter 42
Experimental Therapies in Sjögren's Syndrome

Arjan Vissink, Hendrika Bootsma, Fred K.L. Spijkervet,
and Cees G.M. Kallenberg

Contents

42.1 Introduction

Sjögren's syndrome (SjS) is an autoimmune inflammatory disorder of exocrine glands that has a particular predilection for the lacrimal and salivary glands. Dry mouth and dry eyes are frequently proffered as presenting symptoms [1, 2]. These are in many cases accompanied by several nonspecific symptoms, such as malaise

A. Vissink • F.K.L. Spijkervet
Department of Oral and Maxillofacial Surgery, University Medical Center Groningen, University of Groningen, Groningen, The Netherlands

H. Bootsma • C.G.M. Kallenberg (✉)
Department of Rheumatology and Clinical Immunology, University Medical Center Groningen, University of Groningen, Groningen, The Netherlands

M. Ramos-Casals et al. (eds.), *Sjögren's Syndrome*,
DOI 10.1007/978-0-85729-947-5_42, © Springer-Verlag London Limited 2012

and fatigue [3]. In addition, extraglandular manifestations such as purpura, polyneuropathy, and arthritis can be present even as presenting signs of the disease [2]. The occurrence of lymphomas is another important issue in SjS that requires timely diagnosis and treatment [4]. This enlarges the possibilities for therapies aimed to slow down, stop, or even reverse the further development of SjS. This chapter describes experimental therapies that are aimed at reducing disease activity or reversing the progression of SjS [5].

42.2 Progression and Disease Activity in SjS

To rate the true value of a particular treatment aimed to slow down, stop or reverse the further development of SjS and its related health problems, it is of utmost importance to have access to tools that permit reliable rating of disease activity and progression. When applying such tools, one can reliably show whether a particular treatment has a verifiable effect on the various problems SjS patients encounter. Assessments based on these tools might also provide clues for understanding the mechanism underlying the observed treatment effect. A number of such tools are in development or in clinical use in SjS.

42.2.1 Saliva

Within the wide spectrum of clinical manifestations of SjS, salivary gland dysfunction is one of the key manifestations [6–10]. Thus, sialometry has both diagnostic and prognostic importance (Fig. 42.1). Since the amount and composition of saliva reflect the effects of the autoimmune process in the salivary glands, sialochemistry may also be valuable in diagnosis, assessment of prognosis, and evaluation of treatment [7]. For example, the salivary concentration of protein-conjugated acrolein, a marker of cell and tissue damage, correlates highly with disease severity in SjS [8].

In contrast to whole saliva, analysis of gland-specific saliva can reveal sequential involvement of particular glands, reflecting the ongoing autoimmune process in individual major salivary glands. By using glandular saliva, patients with SjS may frequently be diagnosed at an earlier stage, and progression and/or effects of therapeutic intervention can be measured in a noninvasive way (Fig. 42.1) [10]. This concept is consistent with studies showing progressive destruction of salivary gland tissue in patients with longer disease duration [11].

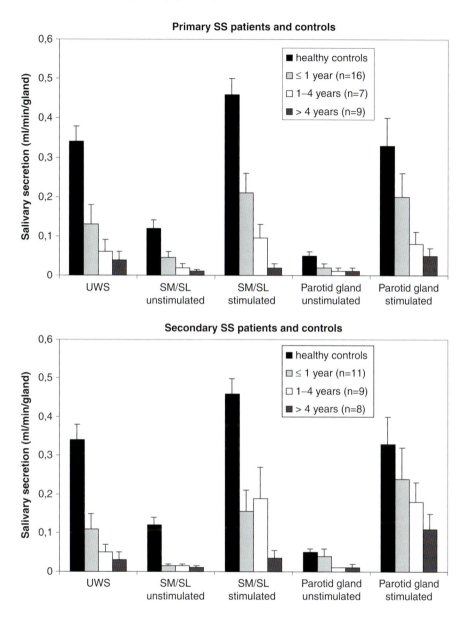

Fig. 42.1 Relation between disease duration, i.e., the time from first complaints induced by or related to oral dryness until referral, and mean salivary flow rates (mean ± SEM). *UWS* unstimulated whole saliva, *SM/SL* submandibular/sublingual glands [15]

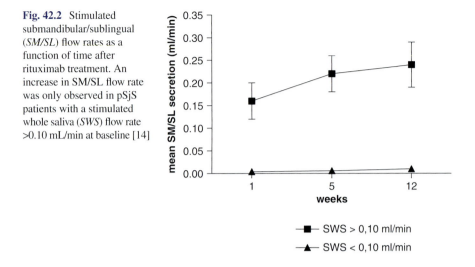

Fig. 42.2 Stimulated submandibular/sublingual (*SM/SL*) flow rates as a function of time after rituximab treatment. An increase in SM/SL flow rate was only observed in pSjS patients with a stimulated whole saliva (*SWS*) flow rate >0.10 mL/min at baseline [14]

It has been proposed that determination of glandular flow rates is not only important in the diagnostic workup of SjS, but might also serve as a parameter for assessing the potential for intervention [10, 12]. Patients with early disease benefit most from stimulatory agents such as pilocarpine, potentially because these patients have sufficient residual secretory tissue. In contrast, such agents are of little to no value in patients bereft of secretory function. Furthermore, early SjS patients have the highest concentrations of salivary sodium, which is related to more severe disease manifestations [13, 14]. This argues for early diagnosis and immediate treatment of patients with early onset pSjS, who often have residual salivary gland function and report the highest levels of fatigue.

A recent intervention study with B cell depletion in patients with SjS showed that only patients with sufficient residual gland function (i.e., those with early disease) responded well to treatment designed to improve sicca symptoms (Fig. 42.2) [15]. It seems that some residual salivary gland tissue is necessary for either recovery or regeneration of secretory gland tissue after intervention therapy [15, 16]. Thus, gland-specific sialometry is not only of paramount importance for diagnosing patients with early onset SjS, but also crucial in identifying patients who may benefit from intervention therapy.

42.2.2 Serum

Serum may contain a variety of markers that can be used to diagnose SjS, to characterize disease activity and progression, to recognize patients who may develop extraglandular manifestations, to identify patients with an increased risk of developing lymphoma, and to evaluate the effect of a biologic intervention. As an example, a decrease in the level of rheumatoid factor following B cell depletion therapy with rituximab in primary SjS patients might be a useful serum parameter to assess the treatment effect [17, 18]. In addition, analysis of changes in immune activation markers, such as cytokines involved in lymphocyte activation and inflammation, might serve as a biomarker for responses to therapy or recurrence of disease.

42.2.3   Labial or Parotid Tissue

Although both labial and parotid biopsies are valid to diagnose SjS [19], detailed immunohistopathologic analyses of parotid biopsies are particularly useful to correlate with clinical findings such as salivary flow rate and the composition of saliva. The parotid gland can be sampled repeatedly through incisional biopsy procedures [16]. This approach is very useful when looking in detail into the assumed achievements of intervention therapies [15, 17, 20] and in getting insight into the mechanisms underlying the return of salivary secretion.

42.3   Molecular Targets for Potential Therapeutic Interventions

Biological agents targeting specific molecules have been introduced in various systemic autoimmune diseases, in particular in rheumatoid arthritis (RA). Biological agents most frequently applied in autoimmune diseases are monoclonal antibodies, soluble receptors, and molecular imitators functioning as false ligands [21]. These biological agents enhance or replace conventional immunosuppressive therapy. In contrast to the situation with RA, no biological agent has yet been approved for the treatment of SjS, but several phase II and III studies have been or are currently being conducted (Tables 42.1 and 42.2) [22–25]. The biological agents used in SjS trials are interferon-alpha (IFN-α), agents that inhibit tumor necrosis factor-alpha (TNF-α), and agents that interfere with B cell function through either depleting or non-depleting mechanisms (anti-CD20, anti-CD22). Although no trials have yet been published with B cell activating factor (BAFF) antagonists and agents blocking co-stimulation, these pathways also offer promising therapeutic approaches [26]. A number of monoclonal antibodies against interleukins (IL) or IL receptors (IL-R) are currently under consideration for use in SjS. The same is true for monoclonal antibodies against IL-6, IL-6R, IL-7, IL-12/IL-13, and IL-17.

42.3.1   Interferons

Interferons are proteins with antiviral activity and potent immunomodulating properties. SjS patients have an activated type I IFN system (Fig. 42.3) [27]. Such a role for IFN-α appears to contradict the reports described below purporting to indicate

Table 42.1 Cytokines as therapeutic targets for the treatment of SjS based on the availability and/
or development of cytokine-directed drugs [24]

Target	Main effect	Rationale for blocking in SjS	Stage of drug development
IFNα	Antiviral, pro- and anti-inflammatory, important for NK cell activity	Decreasing inflammation, reverse Th1 type immune response. Administration of IFNα: enhancing NK cell activity?	Anti-IFNα monoclonal antibody: single dose suppressed IFN signature in SLE, multiple dose phase I study completed Administration of IFNα: multiple parenteral formulations approved, oral lozenge in clinical studies. In SjS, only an effect on salivary secretion was observed, not on the other SjS parameters assessed.
BAFF	B cell development, maturation, survival	Decreasing B cell activation, prevention of GC formation and lymphomagenesis, reduction of autoantibodies	Phase III studies have shown efficacy in SLE. A study in SjS is currently undertaken.
IL-6	B cell proliferation and plasma cell formation, acute phase response, T cell stimulation and recruitment	Decreasing systemic and local inflammation, decreasing B cell activation, decreasing plasma cell formation, reduction of autoantibodies	Phase III studies in RA successfully completed, pilot study in SLE showed normalization of B cell repertoire
IL-7	Growth factor in early T cell development. Stimulation of growth, proliferation, survival and differentiation of mature, naïve, and memory T cells	Decreasing proinflammatory and tissue-destructive responses	Not yet available for administration in humans
IL-12/ IL-23	Differentiation into Th1 type immune response	Decreasing inflammation, reduction of GC formation, and lymphomagenesis	Phase III clinical trial in psoriasis successfully completed, phase II for Crohn's disease currently undertaken
IL-17	Proinflammatory, clearing of extracellular pathogens, major role in autoimmunity	Reverse autoimmunity, reducing inflammation	Phase II clinical trial for RA, Crohn's disease and psoriasis currently undertaken

BAFF B cell–activating factor, *GC* germinal center, *NK* natural killer, *RA* rheumatoid arthritis, *SLE* systemic lupus erythematosus, *SjS* Sjögren's syndrome, *Th1* T-helper type 1

Table 42.2 Potential B cell and T cell targets, monoclonal antibodies, and other treatments used for B cell depletion or modifying T cell stimulation in patients with SjS [25]

Direct targeting of B cells

CD-20 antigen

    Rituximab (chimeric monoclonal antibody)

    Ocrelizumab (humanized monoclonal antibody)

    Ofatumumab (humanized monoclonal antibody)

    Veltuzumab (humanized monoclonal antibody)

    TRU-015 (engineered protein)

CD-22 antigen

    Epratuzumab (humanized monoclonal antibody)

Indirect targeting of B cells

B cell activator belonging to the extracellular TACI receptor domain (BAFF)

    Belimumab (LymphoStat B: fully human monoclonal antibody against BAFF)

BAFF receptors

    Anti-BR3

    Atacicept (IgG Fc fused to the extracellular TACI receptor domain)

    Briobacept/B3-Fc (IgG Fc fused to the extracellular BAFF receptor, BR3 domain)

T cell–dependent activation of B cells

    Abatacept (fully human soluble co-stimulation modulator)

Direct targeting of T cells

IL-2Rα receptor

    Basiliximab (chimeric monoclonal antibody)

    Daclizumab (humanized monoclonal antibody)

CD3

    Muromonab (chimeric antibody)

CD52 (present on all lymphocytes)

    Alemtuzumab (humanized monoclonal antibody)

TACI transmembrane activator and calcium modulator and cyclophylin ligand interactor

that low doses of IFN-α administered via the oromucosal route increase the unstimulated salivary output. It is hypothesized that oral IFN-α treatment acts by increasing saliva secretion via upregulation of aquaporin 5 transcription without significantly influencing the underlying autoimmune process [27, 28].

In a number of phase II studies, treatment of primary SjS patients with IFN-α administered via the oromucosal route (by dissolving lozenges) was demonstrated to be effective and safe [29–32]. Manifestations of treatment efficacy included improvement in salivary output and reduced complaints of xerostomia. Based on these promising results, a randomized, parallel group, double-blind, placebo-controlled clinical trial of 497 patients with primary SjS was conducted. This trial failed to demonstrate a significant effect on the primary endpoints (visual analogue scale (VAS) for oral dryness and stimulated whole salivary flow) in the IFN-α group relative to the placebo group, but there was a significant increase in unstimulated whole saliva in the patients treated with IFN-α. This increase correlated positively with improvement in 7 of 8 symptoms associated with oral and ocular dryness. No adverse events were observed [28]. In conclusion, no clinical evidence for the efficacy of IFN-α treatment in pSjS patients has been shown yet, but improvement of unstimulated whole saliva secretion was observed. Further research is needed to objectify the effect of IFN-α on salivary gland tissue.

IFN-γ is the major cytokine involved in the Th1 response that is instrumental to clear intracellular pathogens (Fig. 42.3). INF-γ is increased in peripheral blood mononuclear cells in primary SjS patients with Raynaud's phenomenon compared to both primary SjS patients without Raynaud's phenomenon and healthy controls [33]. Moreover, IFN-γ is overexpressed by infiltrating cells in the salivary glands of patients with primary SjS, but reaches normal systemic levels in the same patients [23, 34]. Furthermore, IFN-γ reduces the growth of human salivary glands in a concentration-dependent way [35, 36], suggesting that IFN-γ impedes damage repair in the salivary gland [23]. No trials of IFN-γ treatment in pSjS have been reported in the literature yet.

42.3.2 Cytokines

42.3.2.1 TNF-α

TNF-α is a proinflammatory cytokine produced by monocytes, macrophages, mast cells, CD4+ T cells, endothelial cells, and epithelial cells (Fig. 42.3) [23, 25]. TNF-α upregulates apoptosis inducing the death receptor Fas. In combination with INF-γ, TNF-α sensitizes cells, e.g., human salivary gland cells, to apoptosis. There are three main biological agents targeting TNF-α: the chimeric monoclonal IgG1 antibody infliximab, the receptor fusion protein etanercept, and the fully humanized monoclonal antibody adalimumab. In primary SjS, TNF-α targeting treatment could not be proven to be of benefit in reducing the complaints of patients with primary SjS (see chapter on other biological therapies).

42.3.2.2 IL-6

IL-6, a potent proinflammatory cytokine, is involved in acute phase reactions and both B cell and T cell responses (Fig. 42.3). IL-6 was found to be consistently high in the saliva and serum of patients with primary SjS but not healthy controls. Moreover, this cytokine is expressed highly in the salivary glands of SjS patients but not in subjects with sicca complaints only. Tocilizumab, a monoclonal antibody directed against the IL-6 receptor, exhibits efficacy and a good safety profile in RA and is approved for the treatment of that condition [37]. The same antibody led to normalization of the peripheral B lymphocyte repertoire in a pilot study in patients with SLE [38]. B cell abnormalities, comparable between SjS and SLE,

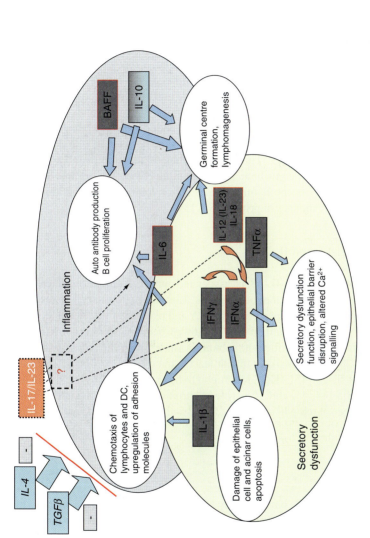

Fig. 42.3 The effect of key cytokines on the different aspects of SjS. An imbalance in the local expression of pro- and anti-inflammatory cytokines leads to chronic inflammation and salivary gland dysfunction. Proinflammatory cytokines are shown in *dark gray*, anti-inflammatory in *green boxes*. IL-10 is a bipolar cytokine with known pro- and anti-inflammatory characteristics, shown in *green and gray*. The effects of cytokines on the most important pathological processes (*white ovals*) are shown by *blue arrows*. The effect of some cytokines on each other is shown in *orange arrows*. IL-4 and transforming growth factor (TGF) β are expressed at low levels or not detectable in SjS (*dotted lines*) but data on this are not yet available. Cytokines in the *red framed boxes* depict cytokines that may provide a good target for therapy. *BAFF* B cell–activating factor, *DC* dendritic cell, *TNF-α* tumor necrosis factor-alpha [42]

are characterized by a shift to increased plasma cell and memory B cell populations. Thus, blocking IL-6 or its receptor may have a beneficial effect on both the local inflammatory process and systemic autoimmunity in SjS (see chapter on other biological therapies).

42.3.2.3 IL-7

IL-7 is an immunoregulatory cytokine that, in particular, is recognized for its role in T cell homeostasis. IL-7 serves as a growth factor in early T cell development and can stimulate the growth, proliferation, survival, and differentiation of mature, naïve, and memory T cells. Expression of IL-7 in human salivary glands was shown to be higher in patients with primary SjS compared with patients who have non-SjS sicca syndrome. Moreover, levels of IL-7 expression correlated with local and peripheral disease activity in SjS. Thus, IL-7-mediated induction of inflammatory cytokines in SjS probably contribute to the immunopathology of this disease. Blockade of IL-7 or IL-7 receptors might be an option to prevent proinflammatory and tissue-destructive responses in primary SjS [39].

42.3.2.4 IL-12, IL-18, and IL-23

Overexpression of IL-12 and IL-18 is associated with inflammation, decreased salivary gland function, and lymphomagenesis. Limited preliminary studies with an IL-18-binding protein were performed in RA and psoriasis [40]. A monoclonal antibody against the p40 subunit of IL-12 showed beneficial effects in Crohn's disease and psoriasis [41]. As the p40 subunit is shared with the recently discovered cytokine IL-23 [42], it is likely that at least some of the beneficial effects are due to blockade of IL-23 [43]. IL-23 was found to be expressed at high levels in the salivary gland in SjS [44, 45] and, if its role in chronic inflammation could be confirmed, blocking the shared p40 subunit of IL-12 and IL-23 would be an appealing treatment strategy.

42.3.2.5 IL-17

IL-17-secreting CD4+ T cells have recently been identified as a specific subset with an important role in inflammation and autoimmunity. SjS patients have increased expression of IL-17 in the salivary glands [44–46] and higher levels in the serum as compared to healthy controls [44]. Further studies are needed to establish the role of IL-17 in humans, but this cytokine is another potential therapeutic target.

42.3.2.6 Anti-cytokine Therapies: Prerequisites and Potential Drawbacks

Successful cytokine-based therapies must have a reasonable safety profile, should reduce inflammation systemically and locally, and should restore the secretory function. Because of redundancy in the cytokine network, targeting a single candidate may not achieve all criteria. Therefore, for an effective therapeutic response, it may be necessary to use a combination of cytokine targets concomitantly or sequentially or target downstream effector molecules shared by several cytokines. A major limitation of these approaches is the increased risk of potentially severe side effects. Local delivery of cytokines or their inhibitors, e.g., by gene therapy, is an appealing alternative to systemic treatment that would greatly improve the risk:benefit ratio of cytokine-based therapy. This approach has been applied successfully in animal models [47, 48]. The increasing availability of biological agents and the potential of gene therapy are exciting, but identifying the right target remains a challenge that can only be overcome by a better understanding of the pathogenesis of SjS.

42.3.3 B Cell Activating Factors

BAFF, also known as BLyS (for *B lymphocyte stimulator*), is a B cell activating factor that acts as a positive regulator of B cell function and expansion (Fig. 42.3). BAFF is a cytokine that prevents apoptosis of autoreactive cells [26]. Different forms of BAFF are present in serum due to translational modifications, principally glycosylation [49]. BAFF levels are elevated in serum and saliva in SjS patients, but no correlation could be shown between serum and saliva levels [50]. However, circulating levels of BAFF in pSjS patients are a marker for disease activity [51].

Two human BAFF antagonists have been developed. One is a human antibody (anti-BLyS, belimumab) that binds to soluble BAFF. The other is a fusion protein of one of the BAFF receptors [52, 53]. SjS patients with elevated BAFF concentrations, hypergammaglobulinemia, elevated levels of autoantibodies, and B cell lymphoma associated with SjS would be candidates for anti-BAFF treatment [54].

Belimumab has recently been shown to be modestly effective in SLE, particularly in those who are serologically active, and to have consistent effects on disease activity, serological parameters, and glucocorticoid sparing [55–57]. A belimumab trial in primary SjS is currently being performed in France.

42.3.4 B and T Cell Receptors

42.3.4.1 Rituximab

Anti-CD20 (rituximab) is a chimeric humanized monoclonal antibody specific for the B cell surface molecule CD20. CD20 is expressed on the surface of normal and malignant pre-B and mature B lymphocytes, but not on plasma cells. CD20 mediates B cell proliferation and differentiation. In retrospective [58, 59], prospective open-label [15, 20, 60, 61], and double-blind, randomized, placebo-controlled trials [18, 21], rituximab was shown to be effective for at least 6–9 months in patients with primary SjS who have active disease. The intervention appeared to improve both subjective and objective complaints, and regeneration of salivary gland tissue was observed in responders [16].

Retreatment with rituximab resulted in a similar good clinical response [58]. In addition, it was shown that timing of B cell repopulation was modulated by BAFF [60]. Baseline serum levels of BAFF were negatively correlated with time to reconstitution. Inefficacy of rituximab occurred when BAFF was produced by either the secretory component of salivary gland cells or by infiltrating B cells [62, 63].

42.3.4.2 Epratuzumab

Epratuzumab is a fully humanized monoclonal antibody specific for the B cell surface molecule CD22. CD22, expressed on the surface of normal mature and malignant B lymphocytes, appears to be involved in the regulation of B cell activation through B cell receptor signaling and cell adhesion [64]. In an open-label phase I/II study that involved 16 primary SjS patients, improvements were observed in the Schirmer test, unstimulated whole salivary flow rate, and the VAS score for fatigue. Remarkably, the number of responders was higher 6 months after the administration of epratuzumab than at an earlier time point [65]. Thus, epratuzumab seems promising as a treatment agent in SjS, but controlled studies are awaited.

42.3.4.3 Abatacept

Abatacept, a biological agent not yet tested in SjS, is a construct of the CTLA4 molecule and the Fc-portion of human IgG that selectively targets the CD80/CD86:CD28 co-stimulatory signal required for full T cell activation and T cell dependent activation of B cells (Table 42.2). Abatacept, currently used for the treatment of RA and juvenile idiopathic arthritis, is safe and effective in patients with moderately or severely active RA who have not responded to TNF-α therapy [66, 67]. Given the novel mechanism of action of abatacept and the recognized role of activated T cells and B cells in the immunopathogenesis of primary SjS, selective modulation of co-stimulation represents a rational therapeutic approach in this disorder. Abatacept is a good potential alternative to B cell depletion therapy in patients who tolerate B cell depletion poorly or in whom depletion is not well tolerated or ineffective. Furthermore, abatacept is a fusion protein, and may therefore have a more favorable side effect profile than rituximab, which is a chimeric monoclonal antibody. A trial with abatacept in the treatment of pSjS is currently being performed in the Netherlands.

42.4 Gene Therapy

Gene transfer refers to a technology that delivers a segment of DNA into target cells or tissues. Gene transfer can involve the direct introduction of a gene or cDNA into diseased cells to restore normal function. Alternatively, the target cells can be normal, but are used to produce a functional, secreted protein to correct malfunctions in other cells and tissues [47]. Currently, gene transfer has been studied in a variety of animal models, but no clinical gene transfer studies have been conducted on patients with SjS to date. Currently, a phase I study is underway in individuals with radiation-induced salivary hypofunction to see whether human aquaporin 1 gene transfer is safe and effective in humans (http://www.clinicaltrials.gov/ct/show/ NCT00372320). The initial results are promising.

Potential target genes in gene therapy for SjS-damaged hyposalivation include inflammatory mediators, cytokine inhibitors, apoptotic molecules, cell–cell interaction, and intracellular molecules [68]. Administration of a recombinant adeno-associated virus encoding the human IL10 transgene (rAAVhIL10) vector to a SjS mouse model resulted in an increased salivary flow and a reduction of the inflammatory response in submandibular glands [69]. A recombinant serotype 2 adeno-associated virus encoding the human vasoactive intestinal peptide (VIP) transgene (rAAV2hVIP), administered to the submandibular gland of female mice, resulted in an increase of salivary flow rate [70]. Thus, local (gene) therapy of the exocrine component of SjS seems to be clinically most appropriate.

Local delivery of an immunomodulatory and anti-apoptotic transgene could reduce gland inflammation by affecting multiple downstream targets. Moreover, a combination of transgenes, e.g., an NFκB inhibitor combined with an anti-CD4 antibody, FasL or VIP, may be particularly useful [48, 70]. However, it recently was shown that transfection of a mouse submandibular gland with serotype 2 adeno-associated virus encoding the TNF receptor type 1 resulted in a negative effect on salivary gland function in SjS, suggesting that local TNF blockade does not have a beneficial effect in SjS. In contrast, TNF blockade even might worsen salivary gland function in SjS [71].

No gene transfer studies have yet been initiated in humans.

42.5 Stem Cell Therapy

Stem cell research has begun to explore the unique qualities of adult salivary gland stem cells as well as their vast clinical potential. Although many questions remain to be answered, significant progress has been made during the last few years. Adult (somatic or tissue-derived) stem cells are generally organ restricted and only form cell lineages of the organ from which they originate (unipotent) and therefore do not form teratomas. Like any other adult stem cell population, salivary gland adult stem cells are undifferentiated but reside between differentiated cells (stem cell niche). Adult stem cells are able to self-renew and can differentiate to yield all specialized cell types. Formation, maintenance, and repair of the tissue in which they reside are the primary roles of the adult stem cell [72].

In a mouse model, Lombaert et al. [73] recently discovered a population of c-Kit+cells within salivary gland tissue with the capability to restore radiation-induced damage to salivary glands in rodents. C-Kit+cells are cells expressing CD117, also called KIT or C-kit receptor, a cytokine receptor that binds to stem cell factor and causes these cells to grow. Stem cell-containing salispheres were cultured from rodent submandibular glands. Cells from these spheres expressed many stem cell markers (e.g., Sca-1, c-Kit, Musashi-1) in vitro and were able to differentiate into all salivary gland lineages. Following stem cell enrichment, c-Kit+cells were able to regenerate and completely restore submandibular gland function in irradiated secondary recipients three months after transplantation, indicative of two essential characteristics of stem cells, the capability to self-renew and to differentiate into all lineages of an organ. Salispheres grown from human parotid and submandibular salivary glands also contained c-Kit+cells and showed self-renewal and differentiation capacities in vitro, bringing human clinical application of such therapy within reach.

In the future, cell-based therapies may restore not only the function of salivary glands damaged by irradiation, but also the functioning of glands damaged by other disorders, e.g., SjS. In order for this approach to be successful, the antibodies responsible for SjS should first be blocked or the stem cells should be modified in such a way that they do not express antigens that are targeted by these antibodies [72].

42.6   Conclusion

SjS has a substantial impact on patients' quality of life and their daily activities [3]. There is a great need to develop effective therapies aimed to slow down, stop, or reverse the further development of SjS. Many agents that might exert such an effect are in development or are currently studied in phase I and II trials. Moreover, it has been shown that a particular agent is not as effective in the one SjS patient compared to another SjS patient. Better characterization of SjS patients by well-defined response criteria, e.g., by means of disease activity and progression scores, by assessing saliva composition and secretion, and/or by selective serum parameters, might help in selecting those SjS patients in whom it is worthwhile to use a particular type of biological [5]. Finally, the data collected by applying these assessment tools might also point to mechanisms underlying the pathogenesis, disease activity, and disease progression in (subsets of) SjS patients.

References

1. Kalk WW, Mansour K, Vissink A, et al. Oral and ocular manifestations in Sjögren's syndrome. J Rheumatol. 2002;29:924–30.
2. Fox RI. Sjögren's syndrome. Lancet. 2005;366(9482):321–31.
3. Meijer JM, Meiners PM, Huddleston Slater JJ, et al. Health-related quality of life, employment and disability in patients with Sjögren's syndrome. Rheumatology (Oxford). 2009;48: 1077–82.
4. Zintzaras E, Voulgarelis M, Moutsopoulos HM. The risk of lymphoma development in autoimmune diseases: a meta-analysis. Arch Intern Med. 2005;165:2337–44.

5. Vissink A, Bootsma H, Spijkervet FKL, Hu S, Wong DT, Kallenberg CGM. Current and future challenges in primary Sjögren's syndrome. Curr Pharm Biotechnol Rev. 2010; (in press).
6. Mignogna MD, Fedele S, Lo RL, Lo ML, Wolff A. Sjögren's syndrome: the diagnostic potential of early oral manifestations preceding hyposalivation/xerostomia. J Oral Pathol Med. 2005;34:1–6.
7. Kalk WW, Vissink A, Spijkervet FK, Bootsma H, Kallenberg CG, Nieuw-Amerongen AV. Sialometry and sialochemistry: diagnostic tools for Sjögren's syndrome. Ann Rheum Dis. 2001;60:1110–6.
8. Higashi K, Yoshida M, Igarashi A, et al. Intense correlation between protein-conjugated acrolein and primary Sjögren's syndrome. Clin Chim Acta. 2010;411(5–6):359–63.
9. Vitali C, Bombardieri S, Jonsson R, et al. Classification criteria for Sjögren's syndrome: a revised version of the European criteria proposed by the American-European Consensus Group. Ann Rheum Dis. 2002;61:554–8.
10. Kalk WW, Vissink A, Stegenga B, Bootsma H, Nieuw Amerongen AV, Kallenberg CG. Sialometry and sialochemistry: a non-invasive approach for diagnosing Sjögren's syndrome. Ann Rheum Dis. 2002;61:137–44.
11. Kalk WW, Vissink A, Spijkervet FK, Möller JM, Roodenburg JL. Morbidity from parotid sialography. Oral Surg Oral Med Oral Pathol Oral Radiol Endod. 2001;92:572–5.
12. Pijpe J, Kalk WW, Bootsma H, Spijkervet FK, Kallenberg CG, Vissink A. Progression of salivary gland dysfunction in patients with Sjögren's syndrome. Ann Rheum Dis. 2007;66:107–12.
13. Pedersen AM, Bardow A, Nauntofte B. Salivary changes and dental caries as potential oral markers of autoimmune salivary gland dysfunction in primary Sjögren's syndrome. BMC Clin Pathol. 2005;5:4.
14. Pedersen AM, Reibel J, Nordgarden H, Bergem HO, Jensen JL, Nauntofte B. Primary Sjögren's syndrome: salivary gland function and clinical oral findings. Oral Dis. 1999;5:128–38.
15. Pijpe J, van Imhoff GW, Spijkervet FK, et al. Rituximab treatment in patients with primary Sjögren's syndrome: an open-label phase II study. Arthritis Rheum. 2005;52:2740–50.
16. Pijpe J, Meijer JM, Bootsma H, et al. Clinical and histologic evidence of salivary gland restoration supports the efficacy of rituximab treatment in Sjögren's syndrome. Arthritis Rheum. 2009;60:3251–6.
17. Meijer JM, Meiners PM, Vissink A, et al. Effective rituximab treatment in primary Sjögren's syndrome: a randomised, double-blind, placebo-controlled trial. Arthritis Rheum. 2010;62:960–8.
18. Meiners PM, Vissink A, Kallenberg CG, Kroese FG, Bootsma H. Treatment of primary Sjögren's syndrome with anti-CD20 therapy (rituximab). A feasible approach or just a starting point? Expert Opin Biol Ther. 2011 Aug 7. [Epub ahead of print].
19. Pijpe J, Kalk WW, van der Wal JE, et al. Parotid gland biopsy compared with labial biopsy in the diagnosis of patients with primary Sjögren's syndrome. Rheumatology (Oxford). 2007;46:335–41.
20. Meijer JM, Pijpe J, Vissink A, Kallenberg CG, Bootsma H. Treatment of primary Sjögren syndrome with rituximab: extended follow-up, safety and efficacy of retreatment. Ann Rheum Dis. 2009;68:284–5.
21. Kourbeti IS, Boumpas DT. Biological therapies of autoimmune diseases. Curr Drug Targets Inflamm Allergy. 2005;4:41–6.
22. Meijer JM, Pijpe J, Bootsma H, Vissink A, Kallenberg CG. The future of biologic agents in the treatment of Sjögren's syndrome. Clin Rev Allergy Immunol. 2007;32:292–7.
23. Roescher N, Tak PP, Illei GG. Cytokines in Sjögren's syndrome. Oral Dis. 2009;15:519–26.
24. Roescher N, Tak PP, Illei GG. Cytokines in Sjögren's syndrome: potential therapeutic targets. Ann Rheum Dis. 2010;69(6):945–8.
25. Tobón GJ, Saraux A, Pers JO, Youinou P. Emerging biotherapies for Sjögren's syndrome. Expert Opin Emerg Drugs. 2010;5:269–82.

26. d'Arbonneau F, Pers JO, Devauchelle V, Pennec Y, Saraux A, Youinou P. BAFF-induced changes in B cell antigen receptor-containing lipid rafts in Sjögren's syndrome. Arthritis Rheum. 2006;54:115–26.

27. Båve U, Nordmark G, Lövgren T, et al. Activation of the type I interferon system in primary Sjögren's syndrome: a possible etiopathogenic mechanism. Arthritis Rheum. 2005;52: 1185–95.

28. Cummins MJ, Papas A, Kammer GM, Fox PC. Treatment of primary Sjögren's syndrome with low-dose human interferon alfa administered by the oromucosal route: combined phase III results. Arthritis Rheum. 2003;49:585–93.

29. Shiozawa S, Tanaka Y, Shiozawa K. Single-blinded controlled trial of low-dose oral IFN-alpha for the treatment of xerostomia in patients with Sjögren's syndrome. J Interferon Cytokine Res. 1998;18:255–62.

30. Ferraccioli GF, Salaffi F, De Vita S, et al. Interferon alpha-2 (IFN alpha 2) increases lacrimal and salivary function in Sjögren's syndrome patients. Preliminary results of an open pilot trial versus OH-chloroquine. Clin Exp Rheumatol. 1996;14:367–71.

31. Ship JA, Fox PC, Michalek JE, Cummins MJ, Richards AB. Treatment of primary Sjögren's syndrome with low-dose natural human interferon-alpha administered by the oral mucosal route: a phase II clinical trial. J Interferon Cytokine Res. 1999;19:943–51.

32. Khurshudian AVA. A pilot study to test the efficacy of oral administration of interferon-alpha lozenges to patients with Sjögren's syndrome. Oral Surg Oral Med Oral Pathol Oral Radiol Endod. 2003;95:38–44.

33. Willeke P, Schlüter B, Schotte H, Domschke W, Gaubitz M, Becker H. Interferon-gamma is increased in patients with primary Sjögren's syndrome and Raynaud's phenomenon. Semin Arthritis Rheum. 2009;39:197–202.

34. Oxholm P, Daniels TE, Bendtzen K. Cytokine expression in labial salivary glands from patients with primary Sjögren's syndrome. Autoimmunity. 1992;12:185–91.

35. Wu AJ, Kurrasch RH, Katz J, Fox PC, Baum BJ, Atkinson JC. Effect of tumor necrosis factor-alpha and interferon-gamma on the growth of a human salivary gland cell line. J Cell Physiol. 1994;161:217–26.

36. Daniels PJ, Gustafson SA, French D, Wang Y, DePond W, McArthur CP. Interferon-mediated block in cell cycle and altered integrin expression in a differentiated salivary gland cell line (HSG) cultured on Matrigel. J Interferon Cytokine Res. 2000;20:1101–9.

37. Smolen JS, Beaulieu A, Rubbert-Roth A, OPTION Investigators, et al. Effect of interleukin-6 receptor inhibition with tocilizumab in patients with rheumatoid arthritis (OPTION study): a double-blind, placebo-controlled, randomised trial. Lancet. 2008;371(9617): 987–97.

38. Illei GG, Shirota Y, Yarboro CH, et al. Tocilizumab in systemic lupus erythematosus: data on safety, preliminary efficacy, and impact on circulating plasma cells from an open-label phase I dosage-escalation study. Arthritis Rheum. 2010;62:542–52.

39. Bikker A, van Woerkom JM, Kruize AA, et al. Increased expression of interleukin-7 in labial salivary glands of patients with primary Sjögren's syndrome correlates with increased inflammation. Arthritis Rheum. 2010;62:969–77.

40. Tak PP, Bacchi M, Bertolino M. Pharmacokinetics of IL-18 binding protein in healthy volunteers and subjects with rheumatoid arthritis or plaque psoriasis. Eur J Drug Metab Pharmacokinet. 2006;31:109–16.

41. Ding C, Xu J, Li J. ABT-874, a fully human monoclonal anti-IL-12/IL-23 antibody for the potential treatment of autoimmune diseases. Curr Opin Investig Drugs. 2008;9: 515–22.

42. Oppmann B, Lesley R, Blom B, et al. Novel p19 protein engages IL-12p40 to form a cytokine, IL-23, with biological activities similar as well as distinct from IL-12. Immunity. 2000;13:715–25.

43. Kikly K, Liu L, Na S, Sedgwick JD. The IL-23/Th(17) axis: therapeutic targets for autoimmune inflammation. Curr Opin Immunol. 2006;8:670–5.

44. Katsifis GE, Rekka S, Moutsopoulos NM, Pillemer S, Wahl SM. Systemic and local interleukin-17 and linked cytokines associated with Sjögren's syndrome immunopathogenesis. Am J Pathol. 2009;175:1167–77.
45. Nguyen CQ, Hu MH, Li Y, Stewart C, Peck AB. Salivary gland tissue expression of interleukin-23 and interleukin-17 in Sjögren's syndrome: findings in humans and mice. Arthritis Rheum. 2008;58:734–43.
46. Sakai A, Sugawara Y, Kuroishi T, Sasano T, Sugawara S. Identification of IL-18 and Th17 cells in salivary glands of patients with Sjögren's syndrome, and amplification of IL-17-mediated secretion of inflammatory cytokines from salivary gland cells by IL-18. J Immunol. 2008;181:2898–906.
47. Kok MR, Baum BJ, Tak PP, Pillemer SR. Use of localised gene transfer to develop new treatment strategies for the salivary component of Sjögren's syndrome. Ann Rheum Dis. 2003;62:1038–46.
48. Lodde BM, Baum BJ, Tak PP, Illei G. Experience with experimental biological treatment and local gene therapy in Sjögren's syndrome: implications for exocrine pathogenesis and treatment. Ann Rheum Dis. 2006;65:1406–13.
49. Le Pottier L, Bendaoud B, Renaudineau Y, Youinou P, Pers JO, Daridon C. New ELISA for B cell-activating factor. Clin Chem. 2009;55:1843–51.
50. Pers JO, d'Arbonneau F, Devauchelle-Pensec V, Saraux A, Pennec YL, Youinou P. Is periodontal disease mediated by salivary BAFF in Sjögren's syndrome? Arthritis Rheum. 2005;52:2411–4.
51. Szodoray P, Jellestad S, Alex P, et al. Programmed cell death of peripheral blood B cells determined by laser scanning cytometry in Sjögren's syndrome with a special emphasis on BAFF. J Clin Immunol. 2004;24:600–11.
52. Baker KP, Edwards BM, Main SH, et al. Generation and characterization of LymphoStat-B, a human monoclonal antibody that antagonizes the bioactivities of B lymphocyte stimulator. Arthritis Rheum. 2003;48:3253–65.
53. Ramanujam M, Davidson A. The current status of targeting BAFF/BLyS for autoimmune diseases. Arthritis Res Ther. 2004;6:197–202.
54. Szodoray P, Jonsson R. The BAFF/APRIL system in systemic autoimmune diseases with a special emphasis on Sjögren's syndrome. Scand J Immunol. 2005;62:421–8.
55. Jacobi AM, Huang W, Wang T, et al. Effect of long-term belimumab treatment on B cells in systemic lupus erythematosus: extension of a phase II, double-blind, placebo-controlled, dose-ranging study. Arthritis Rheum. 2010;62(1):201–10.
56. Navarra SV, Guzman RM, Gallacher AE, BLISS-52 Study Group. Efficacy and safety of belimumab in patients with active systemic lupus erythematosus: a randomised, placebo-controlled, phase 3 trial. Lancet. 2011;377(9767):721–31. doi:10.1016/S0140-6736(10)61354-62. Published online Feb 7.
57. Stone JH. BLISS! Lupus learns its lessons. Lancet. 2011;377(9767):693–4. Published online Feb 7.
58. Seror R, Sordet C, Guillevin L, et al. Tolerance and efficacy of rituximab and changes in serum B cell biomarkers in patients with systemic complications of primary Sjögren's syndrome. Ann Rheum Dis. 2007;66:351–7.
59. Gottenberg JE, Guillevin L, Lambotte O, et al. Tolerance and short term efficacy of rituximab in 43 patients with systemic autoimmune diseases. Ann Rheum Dis. 2005;64(6):913–20.
60. Devauchelle-Pensec V, Pennec Y, Morvan J, et al. Improvement of Sjögren's syndrome after two infusions of rituximab (anti-CD20). Arthritis Rheum. 2007;57:310–7.
61. Dass S, Bowman SJ, Vital EM, Ikeda K, Pease CT, Hamburger J, et al. Reduction of fatigue in Sjögren syndrome with rituximab: results of a randomised, double-blind, placebo-controlled pilot study. Ann Rheum Dis. 2008;67(11):1541–4.
62. Pers JO, Devauchelle V, Daridon C, et al. BAFF-modulated repopulation of B lymphocytes in the blood and salivary glands of rituximab-treated patients with Sjögren's syndrome. Arthritis Rheum. 2007;56:1464–77.

63. Daridon C, Devauchelle V, Hutin P, et al. Aberrant expression of BAFF by B lymphocytes infiltrating the salivary glands of patients with primary Sjögren's syndrome. Arthritis Rheum. 2007;56:1134–44.

64. Carnahan J, Wang P, Kendall R, et al. Epratuzumab, a humanized monoclonal antibody targeting CD22: characterization of in vitro properties. Clin Cancer Res. 2003;9(10 Pt 2): 3982S–90S.

65. Steinfeld SD, Tant L, Burmester GR, et al. Epratuzumab (humanized anti-CD22 antibody) in primary Sjögren's syndrome: an open-label Phase I/II study. Arthritis Res Ther. 2006;8:R129.

66. Genovese MC, Schiff M, Luggen M, et al. Efficacy and safety of the selective co-stimulation modulator abatacept following 2 years of treatment in patients with rheumatoid arthritis and an inadequate response to anti-tumour necrosis factor therapy. Ann Rheum Dis. 2008;67: 547–54.

67. Choy EH. Selective modulation of T cell co-stimulation: a novel mode of action for the treatment of rheumatoid arthritis. Clin Exp Rheumatol. 2009;27(3):510–8.

68. Kagami H, Wang S, Hai B. Restoring the function of salivary glands. Oral Dis. 2008;14: 15–24.

69. Kok MR, Yamano S, Lodde BM, et al. Local adeno-associated virus-mediated interleukin 10 gene transfer has disease-modifying effects in a murine model of Sjögren's syndrome. Hum Gene Ther. 2003;14:1605–18.

70. Lodde BM, Mineshiba F, Wang J, et al. Effect of human vasoactive intestinal peptide gene transfer in a murine model of Sjögren's syndrome. Ann Rheum Dis. 2006;65:195–200.

71. Vosters JL, Yin H, Roescher N, Kok MR, Tak PP, Chiorini JA. Local expression of tumor necrosis factor-receptor 1: immunoglobulin G can induce salivary gland dysfunction in a murine model of Sjögren's syndrome. Arthritis Res Ther. 2009;11:R189.

72. Coppes RP, Stokman MA. Stem cells and the repair of radiation-induced salivary gland damage. Oral Dis. 2010;17(2):143–53.

73. Lombaert IM, Brunsting JF, Wierenga PK, et al. Rescue of salivary gland function after stem cell transplantation in irradiated glands. PLoS One. 2008;3:e2063.

Index

M. Ramos-Casals et al. (eds.), *Sjögren's Syndrome*,
DOI 10.1007/978-0-85729-947-5, © Springer-Verlag London Limited 2012